Chamberlain's Symptoms and Signs in Clinical Medicine

Chamberlain's Symptoms and Signs in Clinical Medicine

An Introduction to Medical Diagnosis

12TH EDITION

Colin Ogilvie, MD, FRCP

*Consultant Physician to the Royal Liverpool Hospital,
the Liverpool Regional Cardiothoracic Centre and the
King Edward VII Hospital, Midhurst*

Christopher C. Evans, MD, FRCP, FRCPI

*Consultant Physician to the Royal Liverpool
Hospital and the Liverpool Regional
Cardiothoracic Centre*

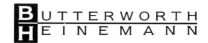

BUTTERWORTH
HEINEMANN

Butterworth–Heinemann
Linacre House, Jordan Hill, Oxford OX2 8DP
A division of Reed Educational and Professional Publishing Ltd

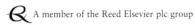 A member of the Reed Elsevier plc group

OXFORD BOSTON JOHANNESBURG
MELBOURNE NEW DELHI SINGAPORE

First published 1936
Reprinted 1936
Second edition 1938
Reprinted 1940, 1941
Third edition 1943
Reprinted 1944, 1945
Fourth edition 947
Reprinted 1948, 1950
Fifth edition 1952
Sixth edition 1957
Seventh edition 1961
Reprinted 1964
Eighth edition 1967
Ninth edition 1974
Reprinted 1978, 1979
Tenth edition 1980
Reprinted 1983
Eleventh edition 1987
Twelfth edition 1997

British Library Cataloguing in Publication Data
Chamberlain's symptoms and signs in clinical medicine: an
  introduction to medical diagnosis – 12th ed
  1. Diagnosis
  I. Title II. Ogilvie, Colin III. Evans, Christopher C.
  616'.075

Library of Congress Cataloguing in Publication Data
Chamberlain's symptoms and signs in clinical medicine: an
  introduction to medical diagnosis – 12th ed/Colin Ogilvie,
  Christopher C. Evans
  p. cm.
  Includes index
  1. Diagnosis. 2. Symptomatology. I. Chamberlain, E. Noble
  (Ernest Noble), 1899–1974. II. Evans, Christopher C. III. Title
  RC71.C53 1997
  616.07'5–dc21
  DNLM/DLC for Library of Congress 97–5699 CP

ISBN 0 7506 2030 7
      0 7506 3683 1 Butterworth–Heinemann International Edition

Text Management: John Ormiston

Design and Illustration:

Printed and bound in Great Britain

Contents

Contributors

Michael D.W. Lye, MD, FRCP
Professor of Geriatric Medicine, University of
Liverpool

Robin M. Philpott, MB, FRC Psych
Consultant Psychiatrist in Old Age, North Mersey
Community NHS Trust

Simon W. Ryan, MD, FRCP, DCH
Reader in Child Health, University of Liverpool

George B. Wyatt, MB, FRCP, FFPHM, FFCM, DTM
and H, DCH
Senior Lecturer in Tropical Medicine, Liverpool
School of Tropical Medicine

Preface to the Twelfth Edition

It is 60 years since the first edition of *Chamberlain's Symptoms and Signs* was published. There have been more significant changes in medical diseases, methods of investigations and treatment and in medical education techniques in the decade since the previous edition than in any other.

The need to hear and record the patient's history, and to elicit and interpret physical signs remains paramount in medical practice. In an era of increasing medical litigation, accurate records of history and examination in hospital and general practice serve to strengthen the defence of the doctor. Recent changes in medical education are directed to problem-solving techniques, which rely on evidence-based medicine that require access to a computer. However, we still believe that comprehensive texts, illustrated with contemporary and common disease states, will remain a valuable source of clinical instruction for students and qualified medical staff.

In this edition we take into account that, in the past decade, AIDS and age-related illnesses have assumed considerable importance, iatrogenic and self-inflicted disorders have increased, and keyhole surgical techniques have removed tell-tale diagnostic scars. We illustrate signs where appropriate with modern diagnostic imaging, such as MRI and CT scans, ultrasonography and echocardiography.

There are three new chapters. Dr Robin Philpott has produced separate chapters on psychiatry and neurology (previously one chapter), Professor Michael Lye highlights the additional skills required to deal with elderly patients, and there is a new and final chapter on the diagnosis of death. Dr Steven Ryan and Dr George Wyatt have rewritten the examination of children and tropical diseases chapters, respectively, and the nervous system has been extensively revised by Dr Chris Earl. We are grateful to them all.

Of the remaining chapters, revision has been shared with colleagues to whom we are indebted, including Dr Ian Gilmore (digestive system), Dr Ralph Perry (cardiovascular system), Dr Richard Clark (haemopoietic system), Professor Gareth Williams (endocrine system), and Dr Ronald Finn and Dr Gordon Bell (renal, urinary and genital systems).

More tables have been introduced for ease of learning and understanding, and a comprehensive revision of the illustrations has resulted in nearly 150 new photographs, the majority in colour. We are grateful to all the patients illustrated who have consented to their photographs being published in this edition.

A separate list of acknowledgements for illustrations is given elsewhere, but we are also grateful to Mr David Adkins and Staff of the Medical Illustration Department of the Royal Liverpool University Hospital. Our secretaries, Mrs Ruth White, Mrs Barbara Mann and Miss Lisa Gurrell, have willingly undertaken tedious typing duties and both authors are grateful to Dr Geoff Smaldon and his colleagues at the publishers for their encouragement and forbearance during the long gestation of this edition.

Acknowledgements

We gratefully acknowledge the generosity of colleagues who have permitted us to reproduce single or multiple pictures:

Dr M.M. Arnold
Dr R.C. Bucknall
Dr A.T. Carty
Dr R.G. Charles
Mr R.J. Donnelly
Dr A. Ellis
Dr S. Evans
Miss J.V. Evans
Dr C.J. Garvey
Dr R.D. Griffiths
Dr J. Harper
Mr M.J. Hershman

Mr K. Jones
Mr S.B. Kaye
Dr G.H.R. Lamb
Mr J.N. McGalliard
Mr G.A. McLoughlin
Mr R.D. Page
Dr A. Robbers
Professor I. Siegel
Dr J.P. Vora
Dr M.J. Walshaw
Dr R.G. Wilks

The history and general principles of examination

INTRODUCTION: THE STUDENT'S APPROACH TO THE PATIENT

It is natural for the student to be apprehensive when first approaching a patient. He fears that sick people will not welcome a nervous and clumsy beginner and that he can be of no help to them. This is the time for him to remember that many patients find comfort in the knowledge that their own suffering may serve, through the observations of students, to ease the burden of those who follow, perhaps even their own children. But the student has more than this to offer the patient. He can be a 'friend at court', a messenger between the fearful patient and the awesome doctor. Time and again, students have discovered facts vital to diagnosis or management that had previously been withheld because of the patient's fear, the doctor's haste or the forbidding retinue that accompanies the physician on his round. The student should approach his patient with humility and gratitude, but also with quiet confidence and pride in the responsibility which will be his for the remainder of his life.

Clinical medicine is above all a matter of communication between people, and the quality of the student's relationship with patients and colleagues could decide his success or failure as a physician. It is no exaggeration to say that even facial expression, tone of voice and manner of movement can affect the ability to elicit the patient's story and to lead him back to health. For it is in such outward signs that we display those attitudes of mind – impatience, boredom, embarrassment, disbelief and reproach – which act as a barrier to communication with others. In the presence of his patient the student must master his emotions, clear his mind of distracting thoughts and avoid all appearances of haste. His manner should be alert and attentive, yet gentle and sympathetic. Without these qualities, he will neither obtain the facts needed for diagnosis nor effectively convey the advice essential to management.

Before confronting the patient, the student must not only have composed his own attitude but he should also have anticipated, so far as possible, the likely attitude of the particular patient he has come to see. He must be ready for the resigned and sometimes resentful manner of the patient with chronic incurable disease, the frightened questioning from those with recent alarming symptoms, the desperate pleading of the patient in acute pain, the inattention and unresponsiveness of the seriously ill. He must also adapt himself to the patient's ethnic, social, educational and intellectual background and use forms of speech which he can understand.

Whether in a hospital ward or the patient's home, it is wise to speak first to those who are looking after the patient. The nurse or relative in charge will indicate whether the patient is available for examination. So far as possible, patients should not be disturbed during meal times, when they have visitors or while they are undergoing diagnostic or therapeutic procedures. The attendant will also be able to say whether, because of the patient's present mental or physical state, any special precautions are needed. The student can thus be forewarned of language difficulty, emotional traits or any defects of memory, concentration, hearing or speech which might call for some modification of his approach.

Before attempting to obtain a formal clinical history, the student should introduce himself and ask if he may put some questions about the illness which took the patient to his doctor. He should then make sure that the patient is as free as possible of any immediate physical or mental discomfort. Except in urgent cases, it is preferable to postpone the interview rather than try to elicit the history of a patient who is drowsy from drugs, or feeling sick, or wanting to visit the toilet. In general, it is best to interview the patient alone and to call later upon a relative for information which is not obtainable from the patient. When it comes to the physical examination, an attendant should be present to help the patient undress or change position or, where appropriate, to act as chaperone.

GUIDE TO HISTORY RECORDING

THE PRESENTING PROBLEM

Some patients come out at once with their story; others remain silent. The former must not be interrupted except to steer them away from irrelevancy. The latter should be gently encouraged rather than questioned. In other words, the patient's history should whenever possible be received, not taken.

Most patients expect the doctor to make the first move. After a few words to put the patient at his ease, he must find out why the patient has come. The conventional opening question 'What do you complain of?' is not always suitable. Some patients have no real symptoms but feel obliged to mention a minor discomfort in answer to this question when in fact they have come with a problem rather than a pain. The more sympathetic question 'What can I do to help you?' sometimes brings a more revealing answer. However, more than one approach may have to be made before the appropriate response is obtained; a list of suggested alternatives is given below.

Whether the patient is presenting with a symptom or a problem, this should be recorded *in the patient's own words*, along with a note of its duration. If the patient's own words consist of a diagnosis (e.g. bronchitis, angina) rather than a symptom (e.g. cough, chest pain), he must be asked to indicate how this condition affects him. The symptoms and not the 'diagnosis' are then recorded, thus: Cough: 3 months. Chest pain: 1 week.

Questionnaire
- *What do you feel wrong with yourself?*
- *In what way do you feel ill?*
- *What can I do to help you?*
- *Tell me why you've come to see me.*
- *What took you to the doctor? (for patients who have already seen another doctor)*

THE ANTECEDENT HISTORY

The aim of this part of the history is to sketch in the patient's personal and family background. Although it is chronologically appropriate to record this antecedent history before the history of the present condition, it may be best to take the main history first, especially from patients who have come with their story well prepared; if the flow is interrupted, they could easily forget what they had intended to say. On the other hand, reticent or frightened patients may be put at ease by answering a few simple questions about home and family before attempting to describe the illness for which they are seeking help.

The facts elicited in this part of the history may have bearing on management as well as diagnosis. For example, the physical fitness of a relative or the presence of stairs in the patient's house may determine whether he can be nursed at home while a previous illness can sometimes contraindicate the use of a drug for the present illness.

The antecedent history includes *past health, family history* and *social or personal history*.

Past health

Patients often omit trauma (accidents and operations) or mishaps in pregnancy (miscarriages, 'toxaemia') when asked about previous illnesses. Specific inquiry should therefore be made about these. Patients may also forget transient minor illness which, though unimportant to them at the time, may have a significant relationship to their present problem. Typical examples of this are a minor dental procedure prior to the onset of subacute bacterial endocarditis or an episode of diplopia in a patient presenting years later with paraplegia due to multiple sclerosis. Where a direct link between past and present illness is clear, it is better to record the earlier illness as part of the history of the present condition than to relegate it to past health.

Questionnaire
- *Have you had any serious illness in the past?*
- *How did it affect you?*
- *Any operations or bad injuries?*
- *Any stillbirths, miscarriages or problems in pregnancy?*
- *Have you ever been to hospital?*
- *Have you missed time from work because of illness?*
- *Have you ever visited your doctor before?*
- *Have you ever had (here list illnesses possibly relevant to present complaint)*

Family history

The main purpose here is to find out whether there are in the family any diseases relevant to the patient's own illness. The possible causes for a disease affecting more than one member of a family are:

1 Environmental: transmission of infection, poverty, common dietary or smoking habits, poor hygiene, etc.
2 Coincidental, as in the case of common diseases, such as cancer.
3 Heredity: many diseases 'run' in families but most of those transmitted by known modes of inheritance are relatively rare.

Fear of acquiring or transmitting a family disease is a common cause for seeking medical advice and these patients may have anxiety symptoms simulating the illness which they dread.

The past and present health and, where applicable, the age and cause of death of all first-degree relatives are recorded and the patient should also be asked whether any relative has had symptoms similar to his own.

Inquiry about consanguinity may be relevant in certain rare inherited diseases.

Questionnaire
- *Are you married?*
- *Is your wife/husband well?*
- *Do you have children? (record age and sex)*
- *Have they ever been seriously ill?(record details)*
- *Have you lost any children? (record age and cause of death)*
- *Do you have brothers and sisters? (record age and sex)*
- *Have they ever been seriously ill? (record details)*
- *Have you lost any brothers or sisters? (record age and cause of death)*
- *Are both your parents living? (if not, give age and cause of death)*
- *Have they ever been seriously ill? (record details)*
- *Do you know of anyone in the family with symptoms like yours?*
- *Do you know of any disease affecting more than one member of your family?*

Social history
The questions asked under this heading are designed to uncover anything in the patient's personal life relevant to either the cause or management of his illness. We need, therefore, to know about his work, hobbies, habits, environment at home, visits abroad, domestic and marital life and any potential source of mental stress.

Questionnaire
- *Are you working?*
- *What exactly do you do? (record hours, physical activity, potential hazards, travelling)*
- *How long have you done this job?*
- *What jobs have you done before, starting when you left school? (record as above)*
- *What do you do in your spare time? (hobbies, sport, etc.)*
- *Are your meal-times regular?*
- *When is your main meal?*
- *Do you or did you smoke? (record duration, number of cigarettes/cigars/pipes per day)*
- *Do you or did you take alcohol? (record type and amount)*
- *Do you or did you take drugs of any kind? (record type and amount)*
- *Have you been abroad? (record where and when)*

- *Tell me about your home (rooms, stairs, toilet facilities, state of repair)*
- *Who is living in the same house?*
- *Have any been ill recently?*
- *Do you keep animals at home?*
- *Is all well at home and at your work?*
- *Have you had any recent worries or stresses?*

History of present condition
The patient is now encouraged to tell his story in his own words. Questions should be confined to those needed to establish the date and mode of onset of each symptom, its chronological development to the present day (see Figure 1.1) and its precise nature along with any associated phenomena. Leading questions must not be asked, although alternatives can be offered. For example: 'Did your pain come suddenly or gradually?' is permitted; 'Did your pain come suddenly?' is not.

When the patient has finished his story and answered 'No' to the question: 'Have you any other symptoms at all?', he may then be asked leading questions to ensure that no symptom has been forgotten. A list of symptoms that may be elucidated is given in Table 1.1.

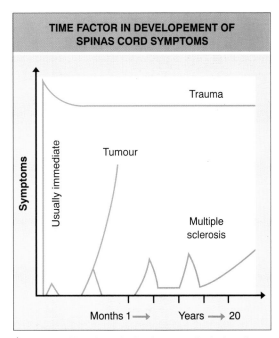

▲ Figure 1.1 Time factor in development of spinal cord symptoms

◀ Table 1.1

SYMPTOM REVIEW			
Gastrointestinal	**Cardio-respiratory**	**Neurological**	**Others**
Appetite	Cough	Blackouts	Urinary symptoms
Indigestion	Sputum	Vertigo	Menstrual symptoms
Nausea	Haemoptysis	Headaches	Skin rashes
Vomiting	Dyspnoea	Visual changes	Joint pains
Dysphagia	Palpitations	Hearing changes	Swellings
Constipation	Leg swelling	Pareses	Weight change
Diarrhoea	Chest pain	Paraesthesiae	Sweats
Abdominal pain	Wheeze	Tremors	
Bleeding			

Questionnaire
Onset (record for each symptom in chronological order)
- *When did your (symptom) first start?*
- *Were you perfectly well before then?*
- *Have you ever had anything like this before?*
- *Did your (symptom) come suddenly one day or gradually?*
- *What were you doing when it came on? (if onset sudden)*
Development (record for each symptom in chronological order)
- *What has happened to your (symptom) since then?*
- *Coming and going? (record frequency, duration and relationship if any to physiological or environmental factors)*
  Getting worse or better? (record whether the change has been gradual; if not, then when it occurred and whether related to physiological or environmental factors)
Description (pain given here as an example)
- *Show me where you feel your pain.*
- *Does it move anywhere?*
- *What kind of pain is it? Aching, stabbing, throbbing, gripping?*
- *How bad is it? Does it make you stop what you're doing?*
- *How often do you get it? (record whether continuous or number of times per day, week month or year)*
- *How long does it last?*

- *Does it come at any special times?*
- *Does anything bring it on or make it worse?*
- *Does anything relieve it? What do you do when it comes on?*
- *Do you feel anything else wrong at the same time?*

THE PHYSICAL EXAMINATION

The physical examination begins during the taking of the history because certain abnormalities – of mood, speech, posture and movement, for example – are then more evident than when the patient is asked to lie still and silent on a couch. The history usually points to the system or part of the body to be examined first and in greatest detail. Systematic examination follows (Figure 1.2) and should comprise the following:

1 General inspection of the whole body for external evidence of disease: wasting, dehydration, obesity, jaundice, pallor, cyanosis, rashes, swellings, abnormal stature or development, abnormal facial characteristics and pathological changes in the skin, hair or nails.
2 The digestive system: mouth, oesophagus, stomach and intestines, liver, gallbladder, hernial orifices, rectum, faeces and vomitus.
3 The genito-urinary system: kidneys, bladder, genitalia, breasts and urine.
4 The respiratory system: nose, paranasal sinuses, throat, airways, lungs and sputum.
5 The cardiovascular system: heart, peripheral veins and arteries and blood pressure.

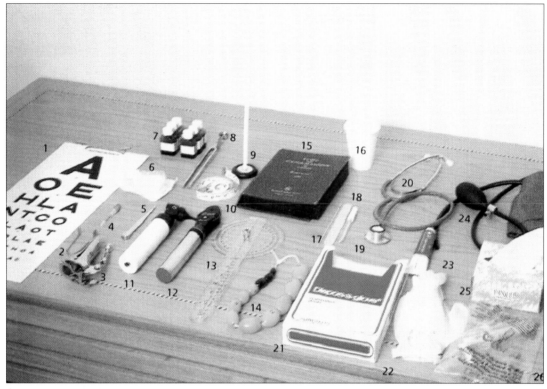

▲ **Figure 1.2 Instruments used for clinical examination** (reproduced from *Clinical Examination of the Patient* by John Lumley and Pierre-Marc G. Bouloux, Butterworth–Heinemann, 1994)

1	Snellen chart
2	Nasal speculum
3	Vaginal speculum
4	Sterile pin
5	Two point retractor
6	Cotton wool
7	Bottles of odorants
8	Tuning fork
9	Patellar hammer
10	Tape measure
11	Auroscope
12	Ophthalmoscope
13	Goniometer
14	Beads for testicular sizing
15	Test charts for colour vision
16	Cup
17	Wooden stick
18	Wooden spatula
19	Thermometer
20	Stethoscope
21	Box of disposable gloves
22	Disposable gloves
23	Lubricant
24	Cuff of sphygmomanometer
25	Tissues
26	Disposable proctoscope

6 The haemopoietic system: lymph nodes, spleen, liver and blood.

7 The skeletal system: gait, posture, joints, muscles and bones.

8 The nervous system: cerebration, speech, cranial nerves and motor and sensory systems.

9 The psychological state.

10 The endocrine system: thyroid gland, hair distribution, physical and sexual development.

11 The special sense organs: eyes, ears, nose.

Although the physical findings are recorded in systems, the examination should be adapted for the patient's convenience. For example, the neck, spine and loins can be examined as well as the lungs when the patient sits up.

SOME IMPORTANT AND COMMON SYMPTOMS

There follows a brief account of some important and common symptoms which may arise in more than one system of the body: pain, headache, loss of consciousness and weight loss.

PAIN
Pathways and causation

Pain is transmitted from pain receptors (nociceptors) in skin, muscles, skeleton, blood vessels, viscera and membranes through a system of fine afferent nerve fibres. It is then conveyed via the posterior nerve roots and the spinothalamic tracts to the thalamus and ascending bulbar reticular system, and there is evidence to suggest that recognition of pain and the associated emotional disturbances lies in the thalamus, though the localization of pain may be a function of the cerebral cortex. The nerve fibres which transmit pain are of two kinds: large myelinated A fibres and small unmyelinated C fibres. It has been suggested that the former exert an inhibitory effect upon the perception of pain.

The stimuli productive of pain are several, and an understanding of them contributes to the interpretation of pain as a system of disease. It is unnecessary here to deal with physiological responses to painful stimuli, e.g. a pin-prick or burn, but sensory nerve endings in the skin and mucous membranes are so rich that pain is easily evoked and easily localized, whereas in some viscera, e.g. the gastrointestinal tract and heart, the nerve endings are more scattered and this may account partly for the less precise distribution of the pain and its deep character. Further, some tissues, e.g. the lung and visceral pleura and the alimentary tract, are normally insensitive to stimuli that affect the skin (cutting and burning), though a diseased organ, as in appendicitis or gastric ulceration, may be painful to the touch or squeezing especially if the peritoneum is inflamed. On the other hand, colicky pain in the bowel may be caused by distension or obstruction which may act through the sensory nerve endings or by pulling on mesenteric vessels, for it is well established that pain may be caused by traction or distension of arteries. Such visceral sensations are probably carried out by the sympathetic nervous system while peritoneal and parietal pleural pains are conveyed by somatic afferents. A spontaneous burning pain in the face or limbs may rarely result from a localized thalamic lesion.

Whether physical causes act by producing chemical changes is difficult to prove in short-acting stimuli such as a cut, but they may do so when the pain persists after the physical agent has been removed, e.g. after a blow or irradiation. However, delayed pain of this kind may be conveyed by nerve fibres which conduct at a slower rate. More certainly, some types of pain are essentially due to chemical agents, noxious or rendered so by the condition of the tissue upon which they act.

Thus substances such as histamine, acetylcholine and 5-hydroxytryptamine are responsible for pain in allergic processes, and HCl, when introduced experimentally into the stomach, can be shown to aggravate the pain of an active peptic ulcer. The pain of ischaemic origin, as in angina or intermittent claudication, is presumed to be due to metabolites resulting from oxygen insufficiency, though the nature of the metabolites is not yet known. Conversely, neurones concerned with pain perception

have been found to possess opiate receptors and the brain produces its own endogenous analgesic, endorphin, to which these receptors are sensitive.

In interpreting the origin of pain it must be realized that while the skin is very sensitive and pain is easily localized to the affected segments of the spinal cord this is not so in visceral and deep somatic pains (muscles and periosteum) in which the painful stimuli may be received by many segments of the cord and even affect neighbouring segments. This is seen in conditions such as perforation of an ulcer, angina or even intestinal colic in which the pain may be widespread.

Pain may also be 'referred' to other areas of the body which are innervated from the same segments as the viscus involved. Pleural pain may radiate to the abdominal wall, biliary colic pain may spread to the scapular area, and central diaphragmatic lesions may cause pain in the shoulder-tip (4th cervical segment).

It may be noticed that the position of the pain does not always decide the organ from which it is arising, but factors that modify the pain may do so. Thus a central chest pain is not always anginal and if it is constantly provoked by swallowing suggests an oesophageal lesion. Similarly, a hypogastric pain may suggest a vesical origin if it is associated with dysuria, a uterine origin if it is related to menstruation, or an intestinal pain if it is modified by bowel action.

Clinical aspects

One of the commonest of complaints, pain can vary in significance from diagnostic certainty to misleading confusion.

The patient who describes a band-like sensation across the chest which occurs on walking and which is quickly relieved by rest leaves little doubt that he is suffering from angina pectoris. On the contrary, the individual who changes the description from pain in the chest to a throbbing or bumping sensation and cannot even place his hand with accuracy over the area of discomfort does little to help in the diagnosis. None the less, there are few of us who have not experienced pain and have realized that it is not always easy to find suitable adjectives to describe it or even to locate it precisely.

Tolerance must be shown (as in all questioning) and questions framed in differing ways to make sure whether the answers are the same.

The duration of the pain and whether it is continuous or wavelike may also be significant.

Then the severity should be ascertained. It may vary from degrees expressed by such words as 'terrible', 'agonizing' or 'excruciating' to 'slight' or 'annoying'. Wrong usage of words by patients is common. Thus 'acute' is often used to mean severe rather than of short duration, and 'chronic' may imply very bad instead of prolonged.

Allowance must also be made for the variation in the emotional response to pain. The same painful stimulus whether in health or disease may be regarded merely as an annoyance by one, but as intolerable by another even though pain threshold varies little between individuals. This may also be bound up with anxiety connected with the cause and seriousness of the pain, and often if the patient can be reassured that the underlying pathology is trivial he will cease to complain so much. In these days of widespread (though sometimes inaccurate) familiarity with coronary artery disease, any pain in the chest is regarded with more alarm than, say, a pain in the lumbar region, though the former may be no more serious and even less severe. It is very important not to regard unexplained pain as non-existent. Continued review with an open mind may sometimes eventually reveal an unexpected cause.

If this proves not to be the case, it must equally be recognized that pain can be psychogenic in origin or due to such trivial causes that the state of mind is responsible for its apparent severity.

This is particularly so in nervous apprehensive subjects and in those suffering from emotional strain, especially anxieties in the home or at work.

Psychogenic pain is rarely of constant pattern, and if the patient is seen often there will usually be considerable contradiction in the story, and the patient will often have consulted many doctors but is reluctant to believe those who blame the condition on 'nerves'.

Unlike the malingerer, a rare individual concerned solely with making profit out of his alleged pain, the psychoneurotic deserves and requires sympathetic but firm handling if he is to improve. He may have genuine pain but tends to magnify it if apprehensive or wishing to gain sympathy.

Examination

This may be negative, as so often in peptic ulcer or angina, but it must be directed in the first place to the area of the pain. Here, exploration of structures such as the skin and muscles and superficial blood vessels and nerves may supply the answer. Examples are seen in pain associated with herpes zoster; tenderness of muscles in 'rheumatism'; and poor arterial pulsation in intermittent claudication.

Often the pain originates in deeper structures – notably the viscera – and care is necessary to identify the source of such pain by those methods of clinical examination and special investigations appropriate to the structure suspected, as described in subsequent chapters.

Shock is a feature of many forms of severe pain, especially the deep pain of grave visceral lesions.

Muscle spasm or 'guarding' in muscle supplied from the same segments of the cord is particularly common in abdominal lesions and of great diagnostic importance. It may also, as a protective measure, restrain breathing, as in pleurisy or limit the movement of an injured joint.

Hyperaesthesia is also closely bound up with certain types of pain. It implies that an area of the body responds to a non-noxious stimulus with pain, or that undue pain is caused by a noxious stimulus.

The phenomenon may be observed commonly in the sensitivity of a burn to light touch, but it may also be associated with deeper lesions, e.g. superficial tenderness over the abdominal wall in inflammatory processes such as appendicitis with peritonitis.

The objectives of the questions about pain may be summarized as follows:

1 To ascertain the site and distribution of the pain and whether these are constant. This enables the observer to decide whether the pain falls into an anatomical pattern consistent with an organic origin or whether the pattern is so bizarre as to suggest a psychogenic source in a patient who is unfamiliar with anatomy and physiology.
  Allowance must be made for unusual distribution of pain which is not uncommon and quite genuine and for true physical pain with a psychogenic overlay.
2 To determine the character and severity of the pain. This is often most difficult and depends on the intelligence, emotional stability and descriptive ability of the patient. With a reliable historian many pains can give important leads to diagnosis, as witness the pain of peripheral arterial disease, renal colic and duodenal ulcer.
3 To find out what makes the pain better or worse. Familiar examples are the ease given by food and antacids in peptic ulceration, the precipitation of angina by physical effort and its relief by rest, the aggravation of pleural pain by deep breathing and its cessation if breathing is momentarily stopped.
4 To determine specific time relationships of pain, e.g. nocturnal pain in peptic ulcer, monthly pain in dysmenorrhoea, and morning headaches of cerebral tumour.
5 To assess the individual's personality and response to other discomforts of life so as to decide whether the pain might be wholly or partly psychogenic. Inquiry should be made about specific emotional disturbances and whether they are likely to be temporary or prolonged.

6 To elicit symptoms constantly associated with the pain, e.g. haematuria in renal colic or jaundice in biliary colic.

HEADACHE

Headache is the term used by patients to describe a variety of head pains and discomforts and is one of the commonest of all symptoms (Figure 1.3).

The brain itself, the inner meninges and the ependyma are insensitive to pain. Headache must therefore arise from the blood vessels, nerves or dura or it may be referred from extracranial structures. Headache is mediated by the branches of the trigeminal nerve and/or the upper 3 cervical nerves.

Cause

Intracranial

Space-occupying lesions such as tumour, haematoma or abscess increase intracranial pressure and cause headache by stretching or distortion of the dura and blood vessels. Raised intracranial pressure and meningeal irritation are responsible for the headache of intracranial haemorrhage and meningitis. Contrary to popular belief, hypertension is rarely a cause of headache except when it is complicated by cerebral haemorrhage or encephalopathy. The headache of migraine is associated with abnormal dilation of both intra- and extracranial vessels.

Extracranial

Head pains may be referred posteriorly from the neck or anteriorly from facial structures. Compression of upper cervical nerve roots in patients with spondylosis is a common cause of occipital headache. 'Tension' headaches of psychogenic origin have been attributed to spasm of the nuchal and scalp muscles. Head pains referred from the face include ocular causes such as glaucoma and refractory errors, nasal sinusitis, dental caries and temporo-mandibular arthritis. Headache of extracranial origin may also arise in blood vessels (migraine; temporal arteritis), nerves (trigeminal and post herpetic neuralgia) or bone (trauma; metastases; Paget's disease).

Systemic

Headache is often the symptom of a systemic condition such as fever, metabolic disorders (e.g. uraemia) or toxic states (e.g. alcohol excess, drugs). Vasodilatation of both intra- and extracerebral vessels may be the mechanism of headache in some of these cases.

When these organic causes of headache have been excluded, there remains a large group of patients in

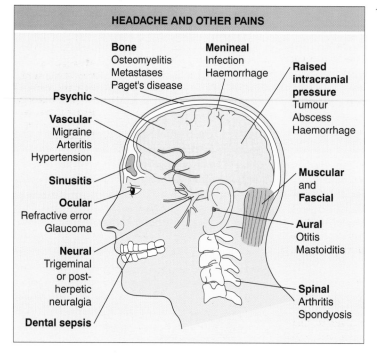

◀ Figure 1.3 Headache and other pains

HEADACHE AND OTHER PAINS

Bone
Osteomyelitis
Metastases
Paget's disease

Menineal
Infection
Haemorrhage

Raised intracranial pressure
Tumour
Abscess
Haemorrhage

Psychic

Vascular
Migraine
Arteritis
Hypertension

Sinusitis

Ocular
Refractive error
Glaucoma

Neural
Trigeminal
or post-
herpetic
neuralgia

Dental sepsis

Muscular and Fascial

Aural
Otitis
Mastoiditis

Spinal
Arthritis
Spondyosis

whom headache is either of pyschogenic origin or due to a transient and trivial cause, such as prolonged study, exhausting exercise, dietary indiscretion or sleep deprivation.

DIAGNOSIS
Symptoms
Character
The character of headache is of limited value in diagnosis. Migraine and intracranial causes of headache tend to be throbbing in nature and neuralgic pains shooting while psychogenic tension headaches may be described in a variety of terms such as a feeling of pressure, tightness, burning or pricking.

Site
In general, headache arising from facial structures (eyes, teeth, sinuses, etc.) is referred to the frontal or temporal regions and headache of cervical or meningeal origin to the occiput. Neuralgic pain occurs in the distribution of the affected nerve and arteritic pain at the site of the affected artery (commonly the temporal). The headache of migraine is characteristically unilateral but often becomes generalized later in the attack. A complaint of pressure on the top of the head suggests a tension headache. The site of the headache is a poor guide to the location of an intracranial lesion; in particular, space-occupying lesions in the posterior fossa may, by causing internal hydrocephalus with distension of the lateral ventricles, give rise to frontal headache.

Age of onset
Psychogenic and tension headaches and – at the other extreme – headaches due to cerebral tumour may occur at all ages. Migraine is the commonest cause for recurrent headaches starting in childhood or youth. Characteristic through not necessarily common causes of headache first presenting in the elderly are giant cell (temporal) arteritis, post herpetic neuralgia, cervical spondylosis, glaucoma and Paget's disease.

Periodicity
Migraine tends to recur at varying intervals over many years with periods of complete freedom. Psychogenic headaches are often daily in occurrence and increase towards the end of the day. The headache of raised intracranial pressure is usually worse on waking in the morning while the frontal headache of sinusitis more often develops after rising in the morning.

Factors influencing headache
Stooping aggravates the headache of raised intracranial pressure. Migrainous headaches are made worse by noise, light and exertion and relieved by a vasoconstrictor drug. Chewing may precipitate bouts of trigeminal neuralgia and the head pains referred from the teeth or temporo-mandibular joints. The occipital headache of cervical spondylosis may be affected by the movements or posture of the neck.

Associated symptoms
Migraine is commonly preceded by a transient neurological aura which passes off as the headache develops. This most often takes the form of a 'fortification' (zigzag) spectrum in one half of the visual field. Photophobia is a common accompaniment of both migraine and meningitis. Vomiting is also a feature of migraine and of headache due to raised intracranial pressure.

Signs
Of an intracranial cause
Papilloedema, neck rigidity and focal neurological signs must be excluded in all patients with persistent headache.

Of an extracranial cause
The eyes, ears, nose and teeth must be examined especially to exclude glaucoma, aural or nasal discharge, sinus tenderness and dental caries or abscess. The skin of forehead and scalp are inspected for herpetic vesicles or scars and the cranium palpated for any abnormal swellings. In giant cell arteritis, the temporal or occipital artery may be inflamed, tender and pulseless (see Figure 1.4). Painful restriction of cervical spine move-

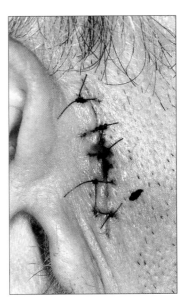

◀ **Figure 1.4 Recent biopsy of right superficial temporal artery in a case of temporal arteritis causing headache**

ments will be found in patients with headache due to cervical spondylosis. Systemic causes of headache – fever especially – must also be excluded.

In the great majority of patients with headache, no abnormal signs will be found and in most of these there will be no organic lesion. However, in cases of severe or persistent headache without obvious cause, further investigation will be needed. Tests which may help in the elucidation of headache include radiographs of skull, sinuses, cervical spine and chest, a CAT scan of the head and, in cases of suspected meningitis, CSF examination.

LOSS OF CONSCIOUSNESS
This may be transient (blackout) or lasting (coma).

Blackouts
The commonest cause for a sudden transient loss of consciousness is a simple postural syncope or 'faint'. This diagnosis should only be made if consciousness is lost when the patient is upright and returns within seconds of lying flat and also if predisposing causes can be identified. These include sudden or prolonged standing especially in a hot atmosphere and conditions inducing vasovagal reflexes such as pain, fear, emotional shock, micturition, defaecation, cough and pressure over the carotid sinus. Postural faints may also result from hypotensive drugs and from an autonomic neuropathy as in diabetes. The common factor is a transient reduction of cerebral blood flow due to loss of vasomotor tone in dependent parts such as the legs and splanchnic bed; bradycardia may also occur. In the case of syncope associated with defaecation, micturition and cough, an additional cause is raised intrathoracic pressure diminishing venous return and cardiac output. When a single cough is followed by a blackout, the possibility of cough induced epilepsy should be considered.

The symptoms and signs of a simple syncope are a feeling of faintness, nausea and sometimes blurred vision preceding the attack, weakness, sweats, pallor, a feeble slow pulse and hypotension. Rapid and complete recovery when the patient lies flat supports the diagnosis. Momentary convulsive movements or even incontinence may occur in profound syncope but, in these cases, epilepsy should always be excluded.

Syncope caused by loss of blood may be mistaken for a simple faint when internal bleeding (e.g. gastro-intestinal or retro-peritoneal) is unaccompanied by pain, distension or visible haemorrhage. Consciousness may quickly return when the patient lies flat but nausea, pallor, sweats and hypotension tend to persist, dyspnoea is common and there is usually tachycardia rather than bradycardia.

A similar situation may result from a vascular catastrophe such as myocardial infarction or pulmonary embolism when these occur without chest pain. Unconsciousness may be sudden and transient and the pulse may be either fast or slow but circulatory failure with hypotension persist after the patient lies down and other cardiac or respiratory features appear: dyspnoea, cyanosis, cardiac dysrhythmia, jugular venous engorgement, gallop rhythm, basal lung crackles, etc.

In the conditions discussed so far, sudden transient loss of consciousness is likely to occur only in the upright posture: standing or sitting. When such attacks happen in bed or recur after the patient has fallen to the ground, three possibilities must be considered: cardiac dysrhythmia, a cerebrovascular lesion and epilepsy. In older subjects, particularly, sudden transient blackouts may result from a cardiac dysrhythmia or cardiac asystole due to heart block (Stokes–Adams attacks). There may be no warning except for momentary palpitations and faintness. Because abnormalities of rhythm can be so short-lived, palpation of a peripheral pulse should be the first step in the examination of a patient who has just had a blackout.

A second important cause of sudden transient blackout especially in the elderly is narrowing or occlusion of arteries supplying the brain. There are three possible mechanisms for the transience of such a lesion: 'spasm', occlusion by a small friable clot which disintegrates after impaction or pre-existing stenosis of major vessels supplying the cerebral circulation. Spasm is a doubtful entity, except perhaps during a hypertensive crisis or an attack of migraine. Transient loss of consciousness associated with vertebral or carotid arterial stenosis may result from small emboli arising from the site of the stenosis or from anything which lowers systemic blood pressure and thereby further diminishes flow through the stenosed vessel. Blackouts from this cause may be distinguished from a simple postural faint if there are focal cerebral symptoms or sequelae. In the carotid circulation, these usually consist of ipsilateral visual loss ('amaurosis fugax') or contralateral hemiparesis. In the vertebro-basilar circulation, vertigo, loss of balance, hemianopia and diplopia are characteristic symptoms.

There are two other syndromes in which blackouts result from vertebro-basilar insufficiency: the 'Sistine Chapel syndrome' and 'subclavian steal'. In the first of these, the blackout is brought on by extreme movements of the neck diminishing blood flow through a vertebral artery already narrowed by atheroma. In its classical form, it afflicts elderly tourists craning to admire Michaelangelo's paintings on the roof of the Sistine Chapel in Rome. Stenosis of the subclavian artery proximal to the origin of the vertebral artery may result in the arm deriving its blood supply from the vertebral circulation in which the flow of blood is thereby reversed (subclavian steal). This syndrome is characterized by sudden transient blackouts, sometimes associated with other features of vertebrobasilar insufficiency and often provoked by vigorous use of the arm on the affected side. A final example of narrowing of an artery supplying the brain leading to momentary loss of consciousness is aortic stenosis. The blackout typically occurs on effort and may be preceded by anginal pain.

Minor epilepsy

Minor epilepsy should always be thought of as a cause of blackouts especially in children. Features which help distinguish minor forms of epilepsy from other causes of sudden transient loss of consciousness are the lack of any relationship to posture and the momentary duration of the attacks. Indeed, the attack may be so brief that the patient remains upright and is sometimes not even aware that anything untoward has happened although they tend to drop any object they may be holding at the time. Some patients experience sensory hallucinations or a feeling of déja vu, especially in temporal lobe epilepsy, and observers may notice transient movements of the face, eyes or limbs which can either be convulsive or purposive.

Major epilepsy

In major epilepsy, loss of consciousness is usually more prolonged and may have to be differentiated from other causes of coma as well as of transient blackouts. Table 1.2 shows the main differences between epileptic fits and syncopal faints.

◄ Table 1.2

DIFFERENCES BETWEEN FITS AND FAINTS		
	Fits	**Faints**
Precipitating cause	Usually none	Sudden or prolonged standing, pain, haemorrhage, fear, unpleasant sights and smells
Warning	Brief aura – sensory, psychic, or motor	Sense of expected loss of consciousness
Mode of onset	Instantaneous unconsciousness	Develops over minutes
Cry	Guttural on falling	None
Colour	Cyanosis/pallor	Intense pallor
Sweating	Rare	Common
Rigidity	Present (grand mal)	Absent
Convulsions	Present often (grand mal)	Rare
Incontinence	Common	Rare
Injury	Common	Occasional
Tongue biting	Common	None
After-effects	Sleep, altered behaviour, headache	Limpness and exhaustion
Pulse	Normal or rapid	Poor volume; slow
BP	Normal	Low
Local neurological signs	In focal epilepsy, Babinski when unconscious	None
EEG	Abnormal	Normal

For hysterical fits (now rare), see page 281.

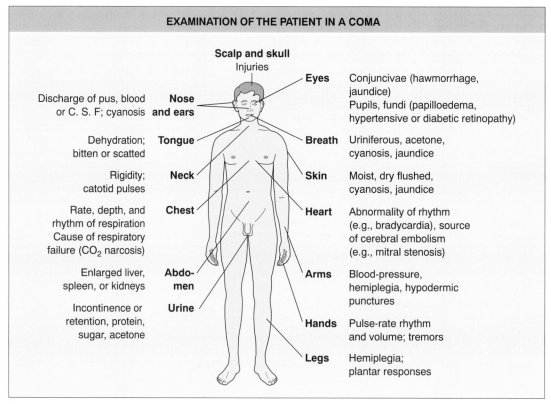

EXAMINATION OF THE PATIENT IN A COMA

Scalp and skull
Injuries

Eyes — Conjuncivae (hawmorrhage, jaundice)
Pupils, fundi (papilloedema, hypertensive or diabetic retinopathy)

Discharge of pus, blood or C. S. F; cyanosis — **Nose and ears**

Dehydration; bitten or scatted — **Tongue**

Breath — Uriniferous, acetone, cyanosis, jaundice

Rigidity; catotid pulses — **Neck**

Skin — Moist, dry flushed, cyanosis, jaundice

Rate, depth, and rhythm of respiration Cause of respiratory failure (CO_2 narcosis) — **Chest**

Heart — Abnormality of rhythm (e.g., bradycardia), source of cerebral embolism (e.g., mitral stenosis)

Enlarged liver, spleen, or kidneys — **Abdomen**

Arms — Blood-pressure, hemiplegia, hypodermic punctures

Incontinence or retention, protein, sugar, acetone — **Urine**

Hands — Pulse-rate rhythm and volume; tremors

Legs — Hemiplegia; plantar responses

▲ Figure 1.5 Examination of the patient in a coma

SUDDEN BLACKOUTS: EYE WITNESS CHART	
Time of day	
Place of attack	
Precipitating causes:	hot atmosphere, emotion, pain, postural change, exertion, etc.
Posture at onset:	standing, sitting, lying
Cry	
Colour:	pallor, flushed, cyanosed
Pulse:	rate, rhythm, volume
Movements:	convulsive or purposive; focal or general
Injury or incontinence	
Duration	
Symptoms on recovery:	headache, confusion, dysphasia, paresis, etc.

▲ Table 1.3

Table 1.3 lists the observations to be recorded by the witness of a sudden blackout.

Coma

This is defined as a state of unconsciousness from which the patient cannot be roused. It may gradually supervene in the last stages of many chronic diseases, but the present comments concern those forms which develop rapidly or unexpectedly and thus offer a problem for diagnosis in the casualty department or in the home (see Figure 1.5 and Table 1.4).

History should always be sought from relatives concerning the previous health of the patient with special reference to hypertension, previous strokes or coronary disease, renal disease, epilepsy, diabetes and the taking of drugs such as insulin or sedatives. If a witness of the onset is available, he should be questioned about the possibility of trauma or alcoholism, the occurrence of headaches or convulsions, and also whether the onset was sudden or gradual. In the absence of relatives, a search of the patient's personal effects may reveal clues in the form of a diabetic or epileptic card, or narcotic drugs.

◀ Table 1.4

COMA: COMMON CAUSES AND DIAGNOSTIC SIGNS	
The cause	**Diagnostic signs**
Trauma	Skull or scalp injury Blood or CSF from nose or ears
Vascular	Hemiplegia; hypertension; neck rigidity (if subarachnoid haemorrhage)
Neoplasm	Focal CNS signs. Papilloedema
Infections	Pus from nose or ears. Neck rigidity. Fever
Epilepsy	History or signs of convulsions Tongue scarred or bleeding
2 Metabolic	
Uraemia	Uriniferous breach. Dehydration. Twitching Retinopathy. Proteinuria
Diabetes	Acetone on breath. Dehydration. Retinopathy (micro-aneurysms). Sugar and ketones in urine
Hypoglycaemia	Sweats. Twitching. Babinski's sign may be present
CO_2 narcosis	Sweats. Central cyanosis. Signs of lung disease Papilloedema
Hepatic	Jaundice. Splenomegaly. Haematemesis Flapping tremor
Myxoedema	Puffy face. Dry skin. Bradycardia. Low temperature
3 Toxic	
Alcohol	Smell of breath. Flushed face (Look carefully for head injury)
Narcotic drugs	Pinpoint pupils (opiates) Shallow breathing. Cyanosis. Skin puncture marks

Physical examination of the unconscious patient (Figure 1.5) is obviously limited by the patient's inability to co-operate. This applies particularly to the discovery of paralysis which may be an important sign of a localized cerebral cause for the coma. However, a hemiplegia (see also page 254) can usually be revealed by raising both arms or both legs and then letting them fall. The paralysed limb falls limply and heavily to the bed, the opposite side retaining sufficient normal tone to allow it to sink more gently. In lighter degrees of coma, paralysis can be detected by applying a painful stimulus to the part and observing whether there is any movement of withdrawal, e.g. flexion of the knee or screwing up of the face. It is essential that the examination should be systematic so that no important signs are overlooked. One system is to start at the top of the head looking for signs of trauma and finish at the soles of the feet by eliciting the plantar responses. This system is illustrated in Figure 1.5. Certain signs, such as abolition of the tendon reflexes and incontinence or retention of urine, are common to many forms of coma, but those signs which are of value in differential diagnosis are listed in Table 1.4.

Loss of Weight
Presentation
Some patients become aware of weight loss because they weigh themselves regularly, others because they or their relatives have noticed thinning of the face or ill-fitting clothes. In the case of children, inadequate gain rather than loss of weight may be the presenting complaint (see Chapter 14).

History
The amount and duration of weight loss (if known) must be recorded, as must whether this loss has occurred against a background of steady or fluctuating weight.

Recent changes in diet, habit or circumstances are noted. Examples include a change from maternal to matrimonial cooking, the irregularity of meals arising from a change in occupation and loss of interest in food among those compelled to live alone by separation or bereavement.

An assessment of appetite and the quantity of food consumed should be made in relation to the build and physical activity of the patient.

Certain psychogenic disorders may lead to the deliberate avoidance of food due in some cases to fear of obesity. These include anorexia nervosa and bulimia (self-induced vomiting). Severe anorexia is also a characteristic symptom of depression but in anxiety states the appetite can be either impaired or increased.

Symptoms that point to a possible organic cause for weight loss must now be elicited if they have not already been volunteered. To establish the state of appetite and whether any reduction is due to anorexia or to fear of eating is of considerable value in differential diagnosis (see Table 1.5). Other symptoms of potential relevance to organic causes of weight loss are difficulties in chewing, dysphagia, nausea and vomiting, indigestion, abdominal pains or distension, changes in bowel action or faecal appearances, thirst, polyuria, excessive sweating and persistent cough.

Examination

The first step in examination is to weigh the patient stripped to underwear on an accurate scale. If no previous record of weight is available and there is no clinical suspicion of organic disease, the patient should be weighed again a few weeks later before being submitted to extensive investigation.

Evidence of recent weight loss should be sought in the shape of ill-fitting clothing or skin. A fold of skin is drawn out between finger and thumb and then released. A large area of fold and a slow return on release will be found in those who have recently lost weight but this sign also occurs in cases of dehydration and in the elderly.

A full physical examination is now carried out with particular reference to common and important causes of weight loss (see Table 1.5).

1 Inspect the mucosae for anaemia or jaundice.
2 Record temperature.
3 Inspect the mouth for inadequate dentitian, painful mucosal lesions and ability to swallow fluids and solids without coughing.
4 Examine the abdomen for tenderness, distension, free fluid, hepatomegaly and malignant masses.
5 Look for evidence of thyrotoxicosis: sweating, tremors, enlarged thyroid, tachycardia (see Chapter 7).
6 Test the urine for glycosuria.
7 Inspect the faeces for melaena or steatorrhoea.
8 Exclude pulmonary tuberculosis by clinical and radiographic examination of the lungs.

WEIGHT LOSS AND APPETITE	
Cause of weight loss	**Appetite**
Oro-pharyngeal lesions	Normal. May be afraid to eat (due to pain or cough)
Oesophageal obstruction	Normal or reduced. May be afraid to eat (pain or vomiting)
Gastric carcinoma	Reduced
Gastric ulcer	Reduced or afraid to eat (pain)
Widespread (especially intra-abdominal) cancer	Reduced
Malabsorption syndromes	Normal
Fevers (especially tuberculosis)	Normal or reduced
Thyrotoxicosis	Normal or increased
Diabetes mellitus	Normal or increased
Depression	Reduced
Anxiety states	Increased or reduced (e.g. by fear of obesity)

▲ Table 1.5

TABLE OF SYMPTOMS

This table must not be regarded as complete, but it will serve as a skeleton outline to which the student can add after further reading and experience in the wards. Fuller details of the symptoms of disease are given in each chapter and will suggest the type of question to be asked and will explain the reason why the questions are set out here. Those symptoms which have just been dealt with more fully are not included here.

Symptom	Questions	Examination
Blood in faeces *Blood in urine* *(haematuria)*	See Examination of faeces, page 70 1 Amount. Colour of urine (bright red: smoky) 2 Relation to micturition (before, during, after) 3 Pain (renal or bladder) 4 Other urinary symptoms	1 Urinary system 2 Microscopy of urine 3 Haemopoietic system 4 Cardiovascular system
Collapse	1 Patient's description of what happened 2 Did he fall? Was he unconscious? 3 Associated symptoms (dizziness, sweating , pallor, pain, diarrhoea, fever, haemorrhage) 4 Food or drugs taken 5 Previous health. Any similar collapse before? 6 Onlooker's observations	1 For evidence of poisoning, infections, intestinal derangement and internal haemorrhage 2 Cardiovascular system 3 Central nervous system
Constipation	1 Recent or longstanding 2 Normal habits 3 Partial or absolute 4 If partial, is it increasing? 5 Associated symptoms (pain, vomiting) 6 Any alternation with diarrhoea	1 Intestinal tract (abdominal and rectal examination) 2 Examine for general state of health, especially loss of weight 3 Character of stools
Coughing of blood *(Haemoptysis)*	1 Evidence that the blood was coughed (blood bright red, frothy, etc.) 2 Amount of blood. Was the sputum subsequently stained? 3 Previous symptoms of respiratory or heart disease	1 Respiratory system 2 Cardiovascular system 3 Haemopoietic system
Decreased quantity of urine (oliguria, anuria)	I Amount passed and frequency 2 Fluid intake 3 Duration of symptom 4 Appearance of urine 5 Other symptoms of renal or heart disease 6 Drugs taken	1 Cardiovascular system 2 Urinary system 3 Distinguish from retention
Diarrhoea	1 Recent or of long duration. Intermittent or persistent 2 Frequency of motions and their character 3 Any fever or loss of weight 4 Food eaten. Other persons affected 5 Recent overseas travel	1 Intestinal tract (abdominal and rectal examination) 2 Examination of faeces

Symptom	Questions	Examination
Difficulty in breathing (dyspnoea)	1 Personal or family history of asthma 2 Relation to effort – degree? 3 Relation to posture – on lying down? 4 Associated symptoms: wheeze, cough, haemoptysis, chest pain	1 Respiratory system 2 Cardiovascular system 3 Anaemia
Difficulty in micturition (dysuria)	1 Exact nature (e.g. in starting, in force of stream, in inhibition) 2 If accompanied by pain	1 Urinary system 2 Nervous system
Difficulty in swallowing (dysphagia)	1 Site – high or low 2 Whether for fluids or only solids 3 Whether increasing 4 History of possible trauma to oesophagus (hot liquids; corrosive poisons) 5 Loss of weight 6 Pain 7 Cough on swallowing	1 Neck and chest – clinically 2 Oesophagus – radiologically 3 Heart and great vessels – clinically and radiologically 4 Mouth, pharynx and larynx 5 Central nervous system 6 For anaemia
Dizziness (vertigo)	1 Continuous or paroxysmal 2 Does patient tend to fall in a particular direction? 3 Severity (does he fall?) 4 Variation with posture 5 Associated phenomena, e.g. vomiting, deafness, tinnitus	1 Ears, including labyrinthine function 2 Nervous system 3 Cardiovascular system 4 Eyes 5 Evidence of toxaemia
Double vision (diplopia)	1 Is the object seen double with one eye (monocular) or with both eyes (binocular)? (Test objectively) 2 Does the diplopia increase on looking to the right, left, upwards or downwards?	1 Close each eye in turn to see if diplopia is monocular or binocular 2 In monocular diplopia examine for local disease of the eye 3 In binocular diplopia test integrity of cranial nerves, especially external muscles of orbit 4 Examine central nervous system
Flatulence	1 Relation to meals 2 Whether wind belched or passed per anus 3 Is the flatus offensive?	1 Observe for air-swallowing 2 Examine gastrointestinal tract and associated viscera
Frequency of micturition	1 Number of times urine is passed in 24 hours 2 Whether at night or in daytime or both 3 Amount of urine passed each time 4 If accompanied by pain	1 Urinary system 2 Nervous system

Symptom	Questions	Examination
Inability to pass urine (retention) (Exclude decreased quantity of urine)	1 Sudden onset or increasing difficulty 2 Any psychical trauma 3 Symptoms of urological or neurological disease	1 Abdomen for distension of bladder 2 If distension, examine for surgical causes of retention (especially and prostatic enlargement), and also nervous system. Catheterize if necessary 3 Do not overlook retention in any severe illness, especially with clouding of consciousness
Incontinence of faeces	1 Is the symptom occasional or persistent? 2 Is there a call to stool? 3 Is the patient conscious of defaecation?	1 Anus, rectum and colon 2 Nervous system 3 General condition with special reference to mental state and consciousness
Incontinence of urine	1 Does it occur only at night (in which case the term 'enuresis' is used)? 2 Does the urine dribble away all the time or only periodically?	1 Urinary system 2 Nervous system 3 Vaginal causes 4 Mental state
Increased quantity of urine (polyuria)	1 Approx. amount passed and frequency 2 Appearance of urine 3 Whether continually or only occasionally present. Mainly day or night 4 Is there undue thirst?	1 Urinary system, including urinanalysis and specific gravity 2 Endocrine organs (especially for diabetes mellitus and insipidus)
Indigestion	1 Exact definition, e.g. pain, flatulence, anorexia 2 Relation to food and bowel movement 3 General health; diet 4 Relief from antacids	1 Digestive system 2 Other systems for signs of ill health 3 Irritative pain arising from other systems e.g. root irritation
Involuntary movements (tremors, choreiform movements, spasms, etc.)	1 Parts of body affected 2 Effect of voluntary muscular action and sleep upon 3 Continuous or occasional	1 Nervous system 2 Evidence of toxaemia, e.g. in fevers, thyrotoxicosis, renal, respiratory or hepatic failure
Loss of power (paresis, paralysis)	1 Sudden or gradual 2 Portion of body involved and extent 3 Whether maximum at onset or increasing 4 Previous attacks 5 Other symptoms of nervous disease	1 Nervous system 2 Other systems which may give indications of the cause, e.g. sites of embolus formation, malignant disease, etc.

Loss of speech (aphasia and dysarthria)	1 Mode of onset, sudden or gradual
	2 Does patient understand speech (e.g. execute a simple command given without signs)?
	3 Does he understand written words, e.g. will he execute a command given in writing?
	4 Does the patient speak? If so, is the speech intelligible?
	5 Can he write?
		1 Nervous system, especially:
		  (a) Intellectual function
		  (b) For evidence of paralysis of limbs
		  (c) For evidence of paralysis of muscles of articulation (larynx, tongue, etc.)

Nausea	1 Whether related to food 2 Whether accompanied by vomiting 3 Is the patient taking any medicines?	1 Gastrointestinal tract and associated viscera 2 Nervous system

Symptom	Questions	Examination
Noises in the ears or head	1 Types of noise, e.g. singing, buzzing, voices, etc. 2 Are the noises persistently or occasionally present?	1 Ears (deafness, vertigo, aural pain or discharge) 2 Cardiovascular system, especially arteries and blood pressure 3 Nervous system 4 Evidence of mental instability
Numbness, tingling pins and needles (paraesthesiae: dysaesthesiae)	1 Extent and distribution 2 Sudden or gradual onset 3 Periodic or continuous	1 Nervous system, especially for involvement of peripheral nerves or sensory tracts 2 Cardiovascular system, especially peripheral vessels
Obesity	1 Family history 2 Sudden or gradual onset	1 Distribution of fat 2 Endocrine organs 3 Generalized or localized 4 Habits of diet and exercise 5 If associated with pain
Pallor (anaemia)	1 The patient's usual colour 2 Whether of sudden or gradual appearance 3 Has there been any haemorrhage? 4 Any symptoms of anaemia? (See page 187)	1 Haemopoietic system. Blood count in all cases 2 Other systems or tissues, affections of which are known to produce anaemia
Palpitation	1 Whether in attacks. If so, mode of onset and offset, with particular reference to suddenness 2 Is the heart rate known? Does it vary? 3 Consciousness of irregularity 4 Whether the patient has been taking drugs 5 Association with emotion and exercise	1 Cardiovascular system 2 Nervous system
Rashes	1 Duration and associated symptoms 2 Distribution 3 Is there: (a) pain, (b) itching? 4 Is the patient taking drugs? 5 Contact with infectious diseases or known irritants	1 Distribution and character of rash 2 Presence of fever and signs of toxaemia 3 If the rash has disappeared the same questions should be asked even though objective confirmation may be impossible
Sore tongue and mouth	1 Duration 2 Patchy (e.g. ulcers) or diffuse 3 Whether taking any medicines 4 Diet 5 Any dysphagia	1 Digestive system, especially tongue, teeth and buccal mucosa 2 Haemopoietic system
Swelling of abdomen	1 Sudden or gradual onset 2 Total duration 3 Whether the swelling varies in size 4 Whether body-weight is changing 5 Menstrual cycle 6 Alimentary symptoms	For general obesity, tympanites, ascites, enlarged viscera, pregnancy or abdominal tumours

Symptom	Questions	Examination
Swelling of feet (oedema)	1 Whether persistent or only after standing, unilateral or bilateral 2 Degree and duration 3 Other symptoms of cardiac and renal disease, anaemia, etc. 4 Is it limited to the legs or is the face affected?	Confirm the presence of oedema by pressure (pitting) or note 'solid' oedema which does not pit. Then examine: 1 Cardiovascular system, including veins 2 Urine 3 Blood 4 Liver 5 Evidence of malnutrition
Thirst	1 Quantity of fluid taken 2 Is there polyuria? 3 Duration	1 Examine urine (sugar and albumin and specific gravity) 2 Look for causes and evidence of dehydration
Unsteadiness in standing or walking	1 Is it worse in the dark? 2 Is it paroxysmal or persistent? 3 Are there associated symptoms (e.g. motor or sensory disturbances, vertigo, tinnitus or deafness)? 4 Does the patient tend to fall to one particular side? 5 If of short duration, inquire as to possible poisoning, including alcohol and hypnotic drugs	1 Nervous system 2 Ears (labyrinthine function)
Vomiting	1 Frequency and forcibility 2 Relation to meals; time of day 3 Whether preceded by nausea or pain 4 Quantity and nature of vomitus 5 Drugs causing emesis 6 Other associated symptoms, e.g. headache, tinnitus or diarrhoea	1 Digestive system 2 Nervous system 3 Other systems if symptoms suggest involvement, e.g. renal disease
Vomiting of blood (haematemesis)	1 Amount and character of haemorrhage 2 Signs supporting its origin (e.g. other haemorrhages, dyspeptic history) 3 Appearance of stools (melaena) 4 Is patient taking drugs, e.g. aspirin, steroids?	1 Digestive system 2 Haemopoietic system 3 Evidence of bleeding which might have led to swallowing of blood
Yellow skin (jaundice)	1 Is the skin yellow or only sallow? 2 Are the conjunctivae yellow? 3 Is the symptom associated with: (a) pain, (b) gastro-intestinal disturbance, (c) rigors? 4 What is the colour of the urine and stools? 5 Has the patient been taking drugs or having any injections (e.g. chlorpromazine)?	1 Skin and mucosae for signs of present jaundice and anaemia. Distinguish from other types of pigmentation (see page 36) 2 Abdomen (espcially liver, gallbladder and spleen) 3 Urine and stools

The case records

Accurate case records are not only essential for the continuing care of individual patients but may also be required for legal purposes, for research or for the prediction of medical service needs within a particular area. The advent of computers for the storage, retrieval and analysis of medical records has increased rather than lessened the need for precision in the recording of the case history.

The system of case recording to be followed in this chapter is set out on pages 23–7 and consists of five 'Ds': a *description* of the patient, the clinical *data*, the *diagnosis*, the *decisions* made and the *developments* that ensue.

DESCRIPTION OF PATIENT

To avoid any possibility of confusion, the patient's full name (and, where applicable, hospital number) should appear on every page of the case record and on all documents included in the file. Most hospitals and clinics will have a printed sheet for the recording of information needed to identify the patient, but it is the student's duty to ensure that certain basic facts are available in his own records. As a minimum, these should include full name and address, date of birth, sex, race, marital status, next of kin, occupation and the time, date and mode of presentation. This last entry should indicate whether the patient was first seen in his own home, in the surgery or in hospital and, if the latter, whether he attended a clinic or presented as an emergency.

DATA

A list should first be made of the sources from which data are available, and these sources must be stated when the case history is written up. Evidence may be obtained from relatives and from members of the hospital staff or other witnesses to the various stages of the patient's illness. Vital information about the present and previous history, including the results of investigations and surgical procedures, is often available in the family doctor's referral note or in earlier hospital records and in urgent cases should be obtained by telephone. The sifting of this documentary evidence is an important part of the student's task but should not be done until after the patient has been interviewed. These data must be incorporated in the original case sheet even if they do not come to light until long afterwards. For example, it would be wrong to leave unchanged, under the heading 'past history', a patient's statement that her hysterectomy was performed for fibroids, when later it transpires from hospital records that the operation was for carcinoma. This change must be made also in the problem list (see Problems below) although it may be decided not to correct the patient's own original impression of her illness (see Explanation to patient).

The history and physical signs (see Chapter 3), along with any previous case documents, and the results of laboratory and other investigations constitute the basic data from which the diagnosis is made, problems identified and management planned. The history should be recorded under the traditional headings and the physical signs under the appropriate system. The date and hour at which the record is made must be clearly stated.

Although this rigid system of recording is necessary to permit a clear view of the patient's problems, it is equally important that the methods used for eliciting symptoms and signs should remain flexible. The patient's story must be allowed to flow freely with the minimum of interruption or interrogation. The student may find it helpful to write down, in the form of rough notes, what the patient has to say and later reassemble these in chronological order, excluding irrelevant matter and making clear which statements are answers to leading questions rather than volunteered. On writing out his case notes the student may find omissions which send him back to the patient's bedside for further information. He may also recognize that items recorded under past history are in fact an essential part of current illness and should therefore be transferred to the history of the present condition.

Similar principles apply to the recording of the physical examination. It may be more convenient for both patient and examiner, for example, to start with the head and finish at the feet, but the final record, compiled from rough notes made at the bedside, should present the findings according to the system affected; and again, as in the case of the history, the student must return to the patient if any gaps appear in this final systematic record. Whenever possible, diagrams should be used to illustrate abnormal findings. This applies especially to signs in the chest and abdomen, superficial sensory changes, abnormalities in the reflexes and the distribution of rashes or joint lesions. A suitable basic diagram is shown in Figure 2.1.

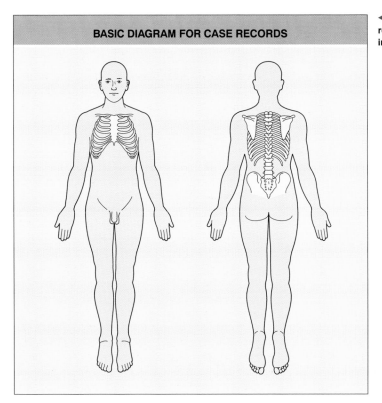

BASIC DIAGRAM FOR CASE RECORDS

◀ **Figure 2.1 Basic diagram for case records to illustrate abnormal findings in physical examination**

It is of the utmost importance to record facts and observations rather than theories and inferences. This applies to the history and physical findings alike. For example, a case history may record as fact a patient's statement that he had pneumonia several years earlier. This could be an erroneous deduction on the part of the patient or his doctor from the symptoms noted at the time. If these consisted of cough, haemoptysis and pleuritic pain, which could equally well have been due to pulmonary infarction, it is these symptoms and not a 'diagnosis' which should appear under past history.

The student must also be particularly careful to record in detail the physical signs which he actually observes rather than the inferences that he draws from them. In the authors' experience, a not uncommon error relates to long-standing facial palsy in which the palpebral fissure may be widened by retraction of the lower eyelid. This may be misinterpreted as narrowing of the opposite palpebral fissure, which is then wrongly attributed to ptosis. Mistakes of this kind would not occur if accurate descriptions were carefully assembled before any attempt was made to interpret them.

DIAGNOSIS

When the student is satisfied that the data are as complete and accurate as possible, he should then briefly summarize the main features in the present history, in chronological order, and those items in the ancillary history which seem potentially relevant either to the chief complaints or to the abnormal signs. This should be followed by a simple list of the abnormal physical findings in each system. To facilitate this, an asterisk can be placed against all positive or relevant items in the ancillary history, the systematic questioning and the physical examination (see Sample case record, page 23).

An attempt is then made to find a single diagnosis which will account for most or all the facts of the case. If some facts do not fit the pattern appropriate to this diagnosis, their accuracy must be checked and the original diagnosis reviewed before two or more separate diagnoses are postulated.

A complete diagnosis would describe the patient's illness in terms of the site (anatomy: where?), nature (pathophysiology: what?) and cause (aetiology: why?)

of the disease process. In most instances, however, the physician has to be satisfied with a differential diagnosis which admits to more than a single possible answer to one or more of these three questions. The alternative diagnoses should be listed in order of probability and reasons given in support of the one which is preferred.

When considering the differential diagnosis, priority must always be given to the problems for which the patient sought medical advice. It is fair to say that in the past more emphasis has sometimes been placed upon diagnostic precision than on defining the actual problems confronting the patient and his physician. In recent years, there has been a move to construct case sheets in terms of such problems and to use the so-called 'problem-orientation' of records as the basis for management decisions.

DECISIONS

PROBLEMS

The first decision to make is which of the patient's problems require attention (investigation, treatment or surveillance) and which, for the time being at least, can be set aside. Two lists of problems are thus compiled: 'active' and 'inactive'. These lists should appear as the front page of the case sheet as well as in the main text (see Plans below), with a number or some other symbol assigned to each problem.

As time passes and more information comes to hand, 'active' problems may be redesignated as 'inactive' (or vice versa) and new problems added to the list. Moreover, old problems are removed if erroneous, or amalgamated if two or more prove to be parts of the same entity. Each change to the problem list is carefully dated.

A 'problem' will only rarely be a complete diagnosis as defined in the previous section. It may consist of a symptom or sign which is not yet fully explained, a clinical syndrome of uncertain cause, a risky habit or occupation, adverse domestic or social circumstances, a predisposition to certain diseases evident in the past or family history, known allergies especially to drugs, an abnormal laboratory finding, a previous operation or a potentially dangerous form of treatment.

PLANS

A plan is devised for each 'active' problem and recorded, under the number and heading of that problem, in the section of the case sheet which follows 'Diagnosis'. The plan is set out in three parts:

1 *Investigations:* These could include ward or laboratory tests, radiographs, consultations, requests for further information about previous health or a social worker's report on the patient's home and working conditions.

2 *Treatment:* This may consist of medicinal therapy, special diets, or physical measures such as irradiation, physiotherapy or surgery. (It should be noted that the precise dosage of drugs and their route of administration are recorded also on a separate chart.) Some indication should be given of the aims and the order of priority of the tests and treatment prescribed, the hazards that may be encountered and the action to be taken if they arise.

3 *Explanation to patient:* What is said to the patient, or even within his hearing, can determine the success or failure of management. 'They don't tell you anything' or 'They all said something different' are only too often the complaints of a patient leaving hospital. Nothing should be done to a patient or said in his presence that has not first been explained, albeit in the simplest terms. Answers to patients' questions given by different members of the staff, whether physician, nurse or student, must be consistent.

It follows that the case records should clearly state what the patient (or, where applicable, the next of kin) is to be told or has been told about the nature, treatment and prognosis of his condition. The form of explanation will vary from one patient to another according to his intelligence, education and temperament. It may be decided, for example, not to reveal to a patient with an inoperable bronchial carcinoma the malignant nature of the lesion. The term used to describe his condition must be written in the case record so that he is not told by successive members of staff that he has 'an ulcer in the tubes', an 'abscess in the lung' and 'an enlarged gland in the chest' – to mention three of the commonly used euphemisms for carcinoma.

DEVELOPMENTS

After the case record has been completed and the initial plans carried out, all subsequent developments should be recorded. These may consist of new symptoms and signs, results of investigations or response to treatment. The results of investigations will usually be filed on sheets separate from the main case record but should also be included in progress notes when they either confirm or refute the original assessment of the case.

Each 'development' should be recorded under the title and number of the problem to which it is relevant and, where appropriate, changes or additions are made to the original problem list on the front sheet (see Problems above, paragraph 2). The initial plans are also reviewed and further plans drawn up in the light of any new developments.

The progress or development of a case can sometimes be best displayed in the form of a graph or chart.

This is done as a nursing routine in the case of pulse rate and temperature, but other examples include the haemoglobin in patients with anaemia, the blood pressure in those on hypotensive drugs, the weight as a measure of fluid balance and the serum bilirubin in patients with jaundice.

THE SYSTEM OF CASE RECORDING

Description	1 Name and address 2 Date of birth 3 Sex 4 Race 5 Marital status 6 Next of kin 7 Occupation 8 Time, date and mode of presentation	Diagnosis	1 Summary of relevant data 2 Differential diagnosis
		Decisions	1 Problems: active or inactive 2 Plans: investigations, treatment, explanation to patient
Data	1 Sources 2 Initial complaint 3 History of present condition 4 Past history 5 Social history 6 Family history 7 Physical signs	Development	1 New symptoms or signs 2 Results of investigations 3 Response to treatment 4 Changes in problems or plans

SAMPLE CASE RECORD

DESCRIPTION OF PATIENT

John Smith, 15 Castle Road, Chester
Born: 21.9.47
Male, Caucasian
Married. Next of kin: Mrs Catherine Smith (wife): same address
Occupation: Builder's labourer
Arrived in Emergency Department, by ambulance at 15.00 hours on 10 January 1994

DATA

Sources

Family doctor's letter, Emergency Department records, previous hospital case sheet, patient's wife.

Initial complaint 10.1.94 15.50 hours

Headaches and confusion: 1 hour (from patient and his wife).

Past history
- Rheumatic fever: 1957.
- Appendicectomy: 1958.
- Gastric ulcer diagnosed by barium meal: 1976 (check previous hospital records). No symptoms in last 8 years.
- Jaundice: anorexia, nausea, dark urine; cleared in 3 weeks; treated at home; no records available: 1979.
- Bronchitis: cough, sputum and wheezing dyspnoea; off work for 4 weeks: February, 1993.

Family history
- Wife has rheumatoid arthritis – cannot manage stairs unaided.
- 2 sons well, aged 10 and 6 years.
- Mother well, aged 78 years. Father died aged 62 years: stroke.
- 1 brother died aged 49 years: heart attack.
- 2 sisters well, aged 36 and 42 years.

Social history

- Home: lives with wife and two sons in 3-bedroom, 2-storey flat.
- Work: builder's labourer.
- Meals: regular and adequate.
- Habits: smokes 30 cigarettes per day. No alcohol or drugs.
- Hobbies: gardening.
- Abroad: to France in 1985. Never in tropics.
- Worries: About his ability to continue work and pay mortgage on flat; also about wife's illness preventing her from looking after the children.

History of present condition

- *4 months ago.* Tires easily. Short of breath, first noticed when digging in the garden and subsequently when playing with the children.
- *6 weeks ago.* Sudden palpitations when gardening. Have recurred at irregular intervals since then, sometimes at rest.
- *Today (history from wife).* Came home for lunch. Slumped over the table. Called out but could not say what was wrong. Wife noticed that his face was twisted and his speech strange. Tried to get up but fell to the floor. Doctor sent for.
- *Doctor's letter.* Found patient stuporose on floor, stertorous breathing, fast irregular pulse, right facial weakness, resisted attempts to undress him. Last seen with bronchitis in 1993. Ambulance sent for.
- *Emergency Department records.* Patient conscious but apparently aphasic. Had a predominantly right-sided convulsive attack with urinary incontinence shortly after arrival. Admitted direct to ward.
  Patient. Since admission, has complained of frontal headache and a confused feeling. Knows where he is and understands what is said but has difficulty in finding the right words.

Systematic questioning

- Appetite good
- No indigestion or vomiting
- Bowels and micturition: normal
- Cough: in mornings; no sputum
- Dyspnoea: as above; no orthopnoea
- No chest or abdominal pain
- No ankle swelling
- Vision and hearing: good
- No dysphagia
- Paraesthesiae: numb feeling in right hand
- No previous fits or faints
- Weight: steady

Physical examination

- Well-nourished man of thin build. Seems apprehensive. Colour, skin, hair, lymph nodes, nails: normal.

RS

- Equal expansion
- Trachea central
- Percussion note, breath sounds, voice sounds: normal
- Basal inspiratory crackles; no wheeze

CVS

- No jugular venous engorgement or oedema
- Pulse: normal volume and rhythm. Rate: 80/min
- BP: 130/85
- Apex: 5th interspace; 9 cm from midline
- Apical lst sound: increased
- No opening snap or 3rd heart sound
- Apical pan-systolic murmur – axilla (gr.2)
- Apical mid-diastolic murmur (gr.3)
- No aortic murmurs.

DS

- Mouth: healthy
- Abdo: no abnormal masses
- Genitalia and rectum: normal

CNS

- Cerebral function: co-operative
- Orientated in time and place
- Understands and obeys the spoken and written word
- Slight delay in finding the right word e.g. in identifying objects
- Cranial nerves: R homonymous hemianopia; slight drooping of R mouth angle
- Trunk: R abdominal reflexes absent
- Limbs: normal power and tone
- Reflexes: see diagram below
- Normal sensation and co-ordination
- Gait: uncertain on legs but can walk unaided and without a limp

Reflexes	R	L
Abdos, upper	–	+
Abdos, lower	–	+
Bic.	++	+
Tric.	++	+
Sup.	+	+
KJ	++	+
AJ	++	+
PLS	↕	↓

DIAGNOSIS

SUMMARY

A 46-year-old man presenting with sudden right-sided weakness and difficulty in speech accompanied by a fast irregular pulse and followed by right-sided convulsions. He had complained of effort dyspnoea for 4 months and bouts of palpitation for 6 weeks. Past illnesses include rheumatic fever, gastric ulcer, jaundice and bronchitis. He smokes cigarettes and has a morning cough. There is a family history of premature vascular disease. On examination, there are mitral systolic and diastolic murmurs, basal lung crackles, a right homonymous hemianopia with right corticospinal tract signs and motor dysphasia.

DIFFERENTIAL DIAGNOSIS

The physical signs in the heart indicate mitral stenosis and regurgitation, probably rheumatic in origin. Paroxysmal atrial fibrillation could account for the palpitations and the irregular pulse noted by the family doctor. The neurological features point to a lesion in the left cerebral hemisphere, probably vascular in view of the sudden onset. Embolism from the left atrium is the most likely cause, but in this heavy smoker with a family history of vascular disease atheroma is an alternative possibility. The effort dyspnoea and bronchitis could result from heavy smoking, from pulmonary congestion due to mitral disease or from a combination of the two.

DECISIONS

These are to go on front page of records.

DECISIONS LIST: PLANS FOR ACTIVE PROBLEMS		
Problems	**Plans**	
	Investigations	*Treatment*
1 Mitral stenosis and regurgiation	ECG. Chest radiograph. Blood count. Electrolytes. Echocardiogram. Cardiologist's opinion – ? catheter or echocardiogram *Explanation* (to patient and wife). Scarred mitral valve in the heart. Probably caused a small clot to break off and lodge in a brain blood vessel. Treatment being given to prevent future clots and tests to decide whether a valve operation is needed and also whether the old gastric ulcer is still active	Continuous heparin infusion: 20,000 units 12 hourly
2 Cardiac dysrhythmia	ECG monitor	
3 R hemiparesis with dysphasia and convulsions	Fasting serum lipids EEG INR – ? anti-coagulants	Physiotherapy Speech therapy Phenytoin sodium 400 mg at night
4 Cigarette smoking		Stop smoking

Problems	Plans	
	Investigations	*Treatment*
1 Mitral stenosis and regurgiation	ECG. Chest radiograph. Blood count. Electrolytes. Echocardiogram. Cardiologist's opinion – ? catheter or echocardiogram	Continuous heparin infusion: 20,000 units 12 hourly
	Explanation (to patient and wife). Scarred mitral valve in the heart. Probably caused a small clot to break off and lodge in a brain blood vessel. Treatment being given to prevent future clots and tests to decide whether a valve operation is needed and also whether the old gastric ulcer is still active	
2 Cardiac dysrhythmia	ECG monitor	
3 R hemiparesis with dysphasia and convulsions	Fasting serum lipids EEG INR – ? anti-coagulants	Physiotherapy Speech therapy Phenytoin sodium 400 mg at night
4 Cigarette smoking		Stop smoking
5 History of bronchitis	Lung function tests	
6 History of jaundice	Liver function tests SH antigen	Warn laboratory
8 Gastric ulcer	Hourly pulse (? bleeding from heparin) Faeces for occult blood. Urgent gastroscopy and Ba. meal (? anti-coagulants). Obtain 1976 hospital records	Proton pump Inhibitor
9 Disabled wife – ? care of children	Social worker	

DECISIONS LIST: PLANS FOR ACTIVE PROBLEMS

DEVELOPMENTS

11.1.94	*10.15 hours*
1	No signs of cardiac failure
	ECG: bifid P waves. Otherwise normal
	Sinus rhythm
	Blood count and electrolytes normal
3	No further convulsions
4	Still smoking – riot act read!
8	No gastric symptoms or signs of bleeding
12.1.94	*11.30 hours*
1 & 2	Complains of palpitations and dyspnoea; basal crackles +. Atrial fibrillation confirmed in ECG.
	Heart rate 130/min.
	Start Digoxin 250 mcg 6-hourly
	Frusemide 40 mg each morning
	Slow-K 1200 mg b.d.
3	INR 13 s (normal)
8	Gastroscopy and Ba meal: no evidence of gastric ulcer
	Faeces negative for occult blood
	Start Warfarin (details)
	Stop Heparin soon (details)

13.1.94	*11.00 hours*
1 & 5	Lung function tests: no evidence of airways obstruction; mild restrictive pattern only.
	Cardiologist opinion: Mitral stenosis and regurgitation with fixed calcified valve. Respiratory symptoms probably due to mitral disease not bronchitis. Will arrange catheter studies with view to mitral valve replacement.
	Patient and wife notified of arrangements.
14.1.94	*10.20 hours*
2	Atrial fibrillation controlled. Heart rate: 84/min.
	Lung bases clear
3	Neurological signs unchanged. Serum lipids: normal
4	Has stopped smoking
6	SH antigen negative: laboratory notified
8	No gastric symptoms or signs of bleeding
9	Social worker: home help obtained for wife. Wife's sister coming to look after children.

External manifestations of disease

INSPECTION OF EXTERIOR OF BODY

While talking to a patient and taking the history outlined in the last chapter, the student should be noting any special characteristics which suggest disease. Such preliminary inspection of the patient as a whole may give clues to diagnosis which could be missed during a detailed examination of the systems. For example, a general slowing of the body's physical or mental activity may be unaccompanied by any focal signs in the early stages of Parkinsonism and hypothyroidism. An impression may also be formed about the general health of the patient and whether he is suffering from any physical discomfort such as pain or dyspnoea. The patient's emotional state and attitude to his illness should also be noted at this stage.

The following observations should then be made:
1 Facial characteristics.
2 Abnormalities in the head and neck.
3 Examination of the mouth (see Chapter 4).
4 Character and distribution of hair.
5 Height and weight.
6 Posture and gait.
7 Skin.
8 Genitalia.
9 Extremities.

FACIAL CHARACTERISTICS

Abnormalities of colour may be most evident in the face but can be reliably detected only in natural light. Screens should, therefore, not be drawn around the bed until colour changes have been excluded. The yellow tint of jaundice is confirmed by inspection of the sclera, and the pallor of anaemia by examining the conjunctival lining of the lower eyelid. Cyanosis, the blue colour imparted by hypoxic blood, is usually best seen in the lips, nose and ears; blueness of the tongue (see page 106) indicates that the cyanosis has a central origin. A deep dusky red colour suggests polycythaemia. The brown pigmentation of Addison's disease may show in the face, especially over areas of friction (e.g. the nasal bridge in those who wear glasses) but, unlike sunburn, it may also occur in the buccal mucosa.

Thickening of the subcutaneous tissues may be seen in acromegaly and myxoedema, and the puffiness of the eyelids in the latter condition may simulate the true subcutaneous oedema of renal disease (Figure 3.1) or superior vena caval obstruction (see Figure 6.9). A puffy swollen face with closure of the eyelids may also occur as an allergic reaction to certain drugs, foods or insect bites. In old age and dehydration (e.g. in diabetes and severe diarrhoea) the skin may be parched and wrinkled.

The condition of the blood vessels should be recorded. Dilated vessels are often seen in mitral disease and in alcoholics: in the former especially on the cheeks, in the latter on the nose but similar changes occur in those who work out of doors. The butterfly rash occurs in rosacea and lupus erythematosus (see page 31 and Figure 3.11). Spider naevi are common in cirrhosis of the liver. All changes in the skin of the face must be compared with those of other parts of the body.

The individual's personality and mood may affect the facial characteristics. This is partly due to the alteration in facial lines and wrinkles which may become modified by pain, fear, anxiety and apathy. Grosser changes may occur in *mental disease* when there may be a stupid expression or a fatuous grin. Changes in character due to alcohol, heroin, morphine, cocaine and other forms of drug addiction may be suspected from the facies. The expression of the drug taker is often shifty, though when deprived he may show agitation and terror. The alcoholic often looks self-satisfied and is plausible in manner.

It is none the less important not to jump to conclusions about alterations in expression because they may

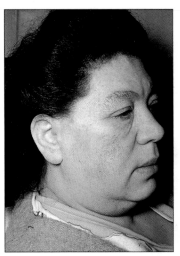

◀ **Figure 3.1
Hypothyroidism**

merely indicate nervousness, shyness, or be evidence of some other psychological imbalance.

Wasting and plumpness may be noticed first in the face, though they should be looked for elsewhere. A notable rounding of the facial contours is not uncommon in patients on corticosteroid therapy ('moon face'). Many nervous diseases such as Parkinsonism and myopathies, which will be described later, have typical facies.

THE EYES

Local diseases of the eyes are beyond the scope of this book and will be considered only in so far as they have a bearing on general medical diagnosis.

Ptosis, squint, irregularity in the pupils and other evidence of oculomotor pareses are of particular importance in the diagnosis of nervous diseases and are considered more fully in Chapter 10, page 226 (see also page 222 for examination of the optic nerve).

Exophthalmos or proptosis (Figure 3.2, see also pages 305–6) is a notable feature of primary hyperthyroidism and may also result, though more rarely, from tumours affecting the orbit or from thrombosis of the cavernous sinus (generally unilateral) (Figure 3.3).

Enophthalmos (recession of the eyes) may occur in serious wasting diseases and dehydration; in the latter, gentle pressure over the closed eye will reveal an abnormal softness and inelasticity of the eyeball. Abnormal hardness on palpation of the closed eye indicates raised intraocular tension (glaucoma) which is an important cause of ocular pain and visual impairment in the elderly.

Inspection of the eyeball itself should take into account abnormalities of the conjunctiva, sclera, cornea, iris and lens.

Conjunctival changes of general medical import include the pallor of anaemia; oedema ('chemosis') due to hypoproteinaemia or impaired venous drainage (Figure 3.4; see also Figure 12.10, page 306); abnormal dryness ('conjunctivitis sicca') in lacrimal gland disease, e.g. Sjögren's syndrome; inflammation in certain infective and allergic disorders such as measles, hay fever or the Stevens–Johnson syndrome (Figure 3.5); increased vascularity imparting a glistening appearance to the eyes in respiratory failure and polycythaemia; haemorrhage

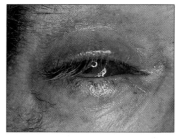

◀ **Figure 3.3 Cavernous sinus thrombosis.** Shows redness and oedema of eyelid, obscuring proptosis. Requires differential diagnosis from erysipelas and insect bites

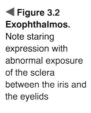

◀ **Figure 3.4 Chemosis and oedema of eyelid due to metastasis in orbit from bronchial carcinoma**

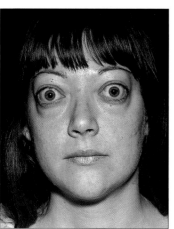

◀ **Figure 3.2 Exophthalmos.** Note staring expression with abnormal exposure of the sclera between the iris and the eyelids

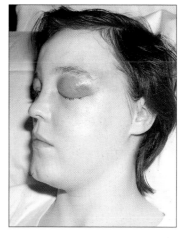

◀ **Figure 3.5 Acute conjunctivitis in Stevens–Johnson syndrome** (see also Figure 3.21)

resulting from blood diseases, fractured skull or violent cough (e.g. whooping-cough).

The sclera is yellow in jaundice and may show inflammatory changes ('episcleritis') in rheumatoid arthritis (see Figure 9.15). Rarely, the blue sclerotics of fragilitas ossium are seen (Figure 3.6).

The commonest abnormality of the *cornea* is arcus senilis which appears as an opalescent ring of lipoid material obscuring the periphery of the iris in elderly subjects. A premature arcus senilis sometimes results from hyperlipidaemia, which may be associated with arterial atheroma.

The cornea may be rendered opaque by the interstitial keratitis of congenital or acquired syphilis. In hepato-lenticular degeneration, a golden-brown deposition of copper (Kayser–Fleischer ring) can sometimes be seen at the periphery of the cornea with the aid of a slit lamp.

The iris

Iritis occurs in rheumatoid arthritis, ulcerative colitis and sarcoidosis, and may be recognized by the discoloration and distortion of the iris and irregularity of the pupil. A rim of iris atrophy also surrounds the Argyll Robertson pupil of neurosyphilis. In albinism, there is lack of pigmentation of the iris, and also of the skin and hair, associated with impaired vision and nystagmus. The eye thus has a pink appearance and the eyelashes are white.

The lens

Diabetes and prolonged hypocalcaemia both predispose to cataract which can sometimes be seen with the naked eye as a grey opacity behind the pupil. A rare abnormality is the curious shimmering movement of the iris caused by the ectopic lens in Marfan's syndrome.

THE LIPS

Indications of ill health may be given by the lips. They are dry and cracked in most illnesses, even of a trivial nature, but *sordes,* a collection of epithelial debris, food and bacteria, are present in the more serious diseases such as uraemia and prolonged fevers. Angular stomatitis, especially with a sore magenta-coloured tongue, may indicate ariboflavinosis (Figure 3.7) but can occur in other deficiency states. Angular stomatitis may also result from ill-fitting dentures and from fungal infections such as candidiasis (thrush).

Herpes simplex, a virus infection of the skin, is recognized as an eruption of vesicles which soon burst and form scabs. It appears not only on the lips but occasionally on other parts of the face (Figure 3.8). The lesions are often described by the patient as 'cold sores'

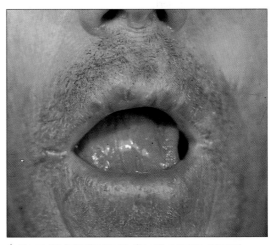

▲ **Figure 3.7 Ariboflavinosis.** Smooth magenta-coloured tongue and angular stomatitis

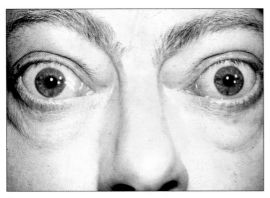

▲ **Figure 3.6 Fragilitas ossium.** The patient, aged 40, had suffered numerous fractures since childhood – spontaneously or from minor injuries

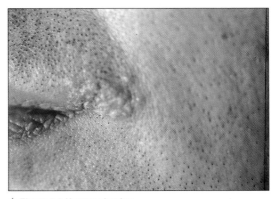

▲ **Figure 3.8 Herpes simplex**

and are a common accompaniment of both upper and lower respiratory tract infections. Herpes simplex is therefore a useful physical sign in the differential diagnosis of pulmonary infection, in which it is commonly present, from pulmonary infarction.

Anaemia and cyanosis are particularly well seen in the lips, but are considered elsewhere. The lips are thick in myxoedema and acromegaly. In the myopathic facies the lower lip is pendulous, exhibiting part of the mucous membrane (see Figure 10.73, page 260). In scleroderma the lips are puckered (see Figure 3.30, page 40) while in Addison's disease they may be pigmented.

THE NOSE

The nose is large in acromegaly, due partly to thickening of the subcutaneous tissues, and partly to bony overgrowth. In hypothyroidism it tends to broaden.

The skin and underlying tissues of the nose may be damaged and destroyed by tuberculous infection *(lupus vulgaris)* or by the granulomatous lesion of sarcoid *(lupus pernio)* or Wegener's granuloma (Figure 3.9). The resulting exposure of the nostrils gives rise to a wolf-like appearance (*L. lupus,* a wolf).

In congenital syphilis the bridge of the nose is depressed, giving a saddle-back appearance (Figure 3.10).

Rosacea is characterized by a reddening of the nose and cheeks, giving the 'butterfly-wings' appearance. It is seen in alcoholics and, in exaggerated form, occurs as the 'strawberry nose'. An appearance similar to rosacea

occurs in lupus erythematosus which may have manifestations in other organs (Figure 3.11).

Perhaps the commonest abnormality of the nose is obstruction to the airway leading to mouth-breathing and a 'nasal' voice; this may be accompanied by discharge (rhinorrhoea) or signs of inflammation over the paranasal sinuses. These changes may reflect allergic or infective conditions of the respiratory tract as a whole and, in particular, can be associated with asthma or bronchiectasis.

Examination of the interior of the nose with a speculum may reveal mucosal changes relevant to systemic disease, e.g. the source of epistaxes in patients with vascular or haematological disorders and nasal polyps in asthmatic subjects.

THE EARS

The ears may be deformed. The usual malformation is an absence of well-defined lobes and a fusion of the ear to the face where the lobe should normally be freely dependant. Ears of this type are common in the mentally compromised and in epileptics. In Down's syndrome (mongolism) the ears are usually large.

Note should be taken of any cyanosis of the periphery of the ear, which may occur in all conditions causing cyanosis. A herpetic eruption may be seen on the ear in the Ramsay–Hunt syndrome (Figure 10.33, page 230). Any discharge from the meatus should be recorded, as it may indicate middle-ear infection and

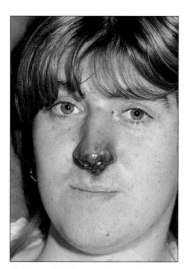

▲ **Figure 3.9 Wegener's granuloma of the nose**

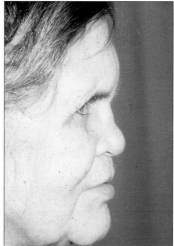

▲ **Figure 3.10 Saddle nose**

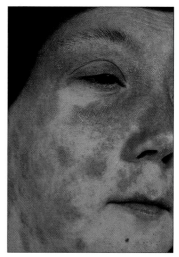

▲ **Figure 3.11 Systemic lupus erythematosus:** typical distribution of rash, including the butterfly-wing appearance on the face

have an important bearing in suspected intracranial abscess. In such cases, the mastoid area should be examined for tenderness and other signs of inflammation. The external auditory meatus and eardrum can be inspected by means of an auroscope (Figure 3.12).

Tophi ('chalk-stones') are collections of uric acid salts which occur in gout. They appear as whitish masses stretching the skin of the ears and sometimes protruding through it (Figure 3.13). They may be seen in other parts of the body.

Abnormalities of hearing
See page 230 *et seq.*

THE SALIVARY AND LACRIMAL GLANDS
The salivary glands may be enlarged. Parotid swellings are situated chiefly in front of the ear. The most important from the physician's point of view is the bilateral painful swelling of these glands caused by *mumps*. In this disease there is pyrexia and it is sometimes complicated by orchitis or a meningo-encephalopathy. Unilateral parotitis is more often due to sepsis, usually associated with a salivary calculus, but may be a feature of typhoid. Swellings beneath the chin may be due to enlargement of the submaxillary or sublingual

glands, but their diagnosis falls more within the scope of surgical practice. Rarely, involvement of salivary and lacrimal glands may be seen in leukaemias, sarcoidosis and Sjögren's syndrome (Figure 3.14).

FACIAL MOVEMENTS
These are considered under the nervous system. They give indications of lesions of the facial nerve, of hypertonicity or hypotonicity of the facial muscles, choreiform movements and other signs of neurological importance.

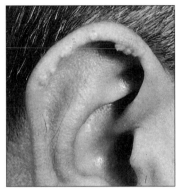

◀ Figure 3.13
Gouty tophi in the ear

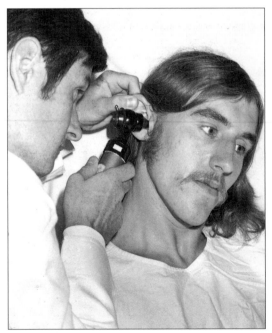

▲ **Figure 3.12 Auroscopy:** to obtain good vision of the eardrum, the auricle is drawn upwards and backwards while the speculum is directed slightly forwards

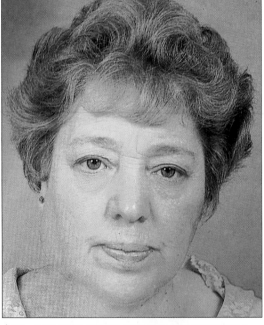

▲ **Figure 3.14 Enlargement of the right parotid gland in a patient with Sjögren's syndrome**

ABNORMALITIES IN THE HEAD AND NECK

The shape and size of the head is sometimes of diagnostic importance. In *hydrocephalus* it is often immense in proportion to the rest of the body, and the forehead appears to overhang the orbits, giving a sunken effect to the eyes, which are directed downwards. In such cases the sutures are unduly separated and the fontanelles enlarged and bulging. See also the Examination of children, Chapter 14.

Frontal bossing occurs in rickets and in congenital syphilis, both rare now.

Generalized gradual enlargement of the head in adults, noticeable to the patient by the increase in the size of his hats, is almost a pathognomonic sign of osteitis deformans (Paget's disease; see Figure 9.1).

The great thickening and prominence of the superciliary arches with the receding forehead above contribute much to the simian appearance of the acromegalic (Figure 3.15).

Lastly, *nodular irregularities* should suggest the possibility of secondary growths or primary tumours of bone or underlying structures such as myeloma or meningioma.

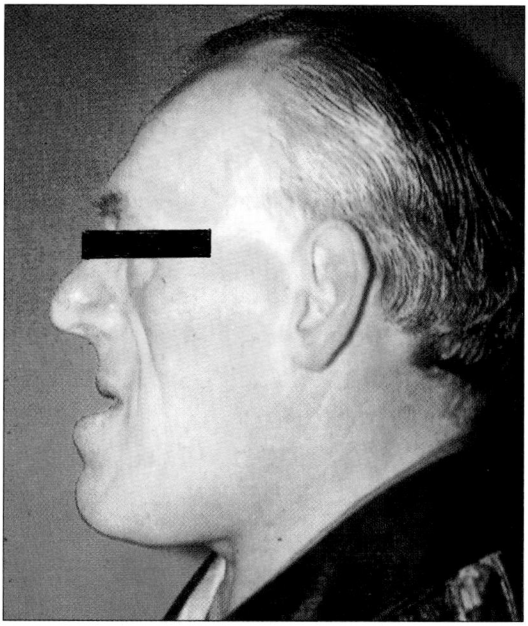

Enlargement of the thyroid gland is known as a *goitre* (Figure 3.16). Note should be taken of the size, regularity or irregularity, consistency and movements of the gland on swallowing. Free movement distinguishes the goitre from enlargement of lymph nodes. When the latter are present, their extent and physical character (page 188) should be observed. In particular, local malignant disease, e.g. of the bronchus, lips or tongue, may produce hard irregular lumps in the neck which contrast with the soft, tender, breaking down masses of septic nodes. Soft or 'rubbery' enlargement of lymph nodes without tenderness suggests a granulomatous lesion such as tuberculosis or sarcoid, a lymphoma (e.g. Hodgkin's disease) or a haematogenous disorder as in leukaemia and glandular fever. (See also The haemopoietic system, Chapter 8.)

The position of the trachea (page 114) and the activity of the accessory muscles of respiration are of importance in respiratory diseases.

Arterial pulsation or lack of it and prominence of the jugular veins may be observed. Their significance is dealt with under the cardiovascular system (pages 142–4).

Examination of the musculoskeletal structures in the neck includes the noting of any abnormal posture such as torticollis, the compensatory hyperextension of ankylosing spondylitis (see Figure 9.18, page 209), and the short 'webbed neck' of Turner's syndrome (see Figure 12.24, page 311). The range of movement of the cervical and temporomandibular joints should be measured (see also Skeletal system, page 202) and the function of the 11th (accessory) cranial nerve examined by testing the power of the sternomastoid muscles (see also Central nervous system, page 232).

▲ Figure 3.15 Acromegaly: prognathism; enlarged nose and ears; prominent superciliary arches

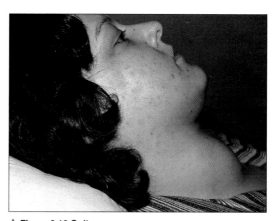

▲ Figure 3.16 Goitre

EXAMINATION OF THE MOUTH

See page 46.

CHARACTER AND DISTRIBUTION OF HAIR

Serious illness can result in dryness and temporary hair fall. In hypothyroidism these characters are especially noticeable, and the hair is thick, coarse and scanty, falling out particularly over the frontal region. The outer third of the eyebrows is also sometimes lost in hypothyroidism. A more complete loss of hair, axillary, pubic and facial, is a feature of anterior hypopituitarism (page 306), Addison's disease in women and chronic hepatic failure (page 78). Total loss of hair (alopecia) may result from cytotoxic drug therapy. In Down's syndrome the hair is silky. Patchy loss of hair occurs in alopecia areata, a condition of unknown cause (but sometimes related to psychogenic illness) and also in secondary syphilis. Loss of hair from the legs in men may be a sign of arterial insufficiency. Excessive hairiness (hirsutism) (Figure 3.17) in the female, especially over the moustache area and limbs, is not necessarily pathological and is common after the

menopause. Grosser distribution over the trunk and limbs with moustache and beard formation requiring shaving call attention to the various types of virilism, especially adrenal.

HEIGHT AND WEIGHT

HEIGHT

The height should be taken into consideration with the age and build of the patient (see also Examination of children, Chapter 14), but although tables of height and weight give a rough indication of the correct proportion between these, they must be interpreted with considerable latitude. Height may be determined by ethnic or genetic factors, and the average height of other members of the patient's race and family must therefore be taken into account.

Excessive height, *gigantism,* suggests overactivity of the anterior lobe of the pituitary gland (excess of growth hormone) occurring before puberty, i.e. before the long bones have attained their full length. Other features of pituitary hyperfunction may also be present (see pages 307–8). A tall, thin build with relatively long limbs is characteristic of *eunuchoidism* (Figure 12.4, page 303) and of Marfan's syndrome.

Small stature, *dwarfism,* may be due to:
1 inherited skeletal anomalies such as achondroplasia or
2 certain diseases acquired in early life before growth is complete. The acquired causes include:
(a) Impaired nutrition from faulty diet or malabsorption (e.g. coeliac disease; cystic fibrosis of pancreas).
(b) Conditions associated with chronic hypoxia such as asthma and congenital heart disease.
(c) In tropical and developing countries especially, chronic infections and infestations.
(d) Endocrine disorders which include hypopituitarism (deficient growth hormone), untreated hypothyroidism (cretinism) and prolonged corticosteroid therapy for asthma or other childhood ailments.
(e) Chronic renal disease with calcium depletion ('renal rickets').

WEIGHT

The weight may be permanently below or above the average, but more significance attaches to a rapid change in weight.

Great *increase in weight* may be a familial characteristic, often occurring at the same age in different members. Although common in middle age, it may even occur in youth. This familial obesity may be aggravated

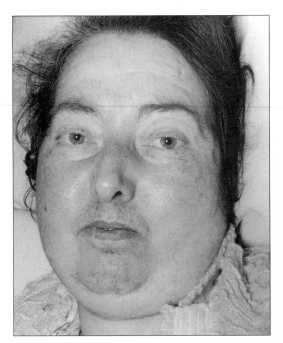

▲ **Figure 3.17 Cushing's syndrome.** Hirsutism and moonface

by over-eating and lack of exercise. Obesity of this kind is of great importance in favouring the development of many diseases, especially those associated with disordered lipid metabolism (diabetes, atheroma, gallstones) and those due to muscular deficiency or gravitational stresses (inguinal and hiatal hernia, diverticulitis, uterine prolapse, varicose veins, osteoarthrosis). Obesity also increases the work and impedes the action of the heart and lungs and will thus aggravate dyspnoea, whatever its cause.

Obesity is seen in childhood as a temporary phenomenon which rectifies itself soon after puberty. More rarely in children or adults it is due to endocrine disturbance as in pituitary-hypothalamic syndromes, certain adrenal diseases, and sometimes in eunuchoidism. Weight increase in hypothyroidism is not due to fat.

Irregular distribution of fat occurs in the rarer lipodystrophies, in some of which the lower part of the body is obese and the upper part emaciated (descending lipodystrophy). In Dercum's disease, adiposis dolorosa, the masses of fat are painful to touch. A special form of localized accumulation of fatty tissue is the *lipoma*, which is often multiple. This is a very common but harmless condition which can be distinguished from other subcutaneous tumours by its soft consistency, lobulated surface and free movement in relation to deeper structures (Figure 3.18).

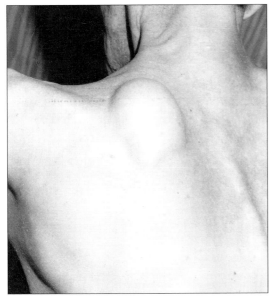

▲ **Figure 3.18 Lipoma**

Decrease of weight is described on pages 13–14.

The term *cachexia* usually implies serious wasting, a greyish or 'earthy' pallor and, frequently, an altered texture of the skin (dry and wrinkled). It is commonly reserved for cases of malignant disease, of which wasting is an essential symptom. Anorexia nervosa gives a similar appearance. Occasionally, the word is applied to the general condition in grave diseases such as leukaemia, chronic renal disease, chronic tuberculosis and so forth.

POSTURE AND GAIT

The posture of a patient sitting in a chair or lying in bed, or the gait as he walks into the consulting room, may provide the first clue to the nature of his disease. Abnormalities are due most often to skeletal or neuromuscular disorders and these are dealt with in Chapters 9 and 10 (see especially pages 241–3).

POSTURE

Skeletal and neurological lesions usually give rise to chronic and persistent disorders of posture such as kyphoscoliosis, ulnar deviation of the fingers, wrist drop and the rigidity of Parkinsonism. Abnormalities of posture arising in other systems are often more acute and transient and result from discomfort, pain or impairment of consciousness rather than from deformity. Patients in respiratory distress, especially of cardiac origin, tend to sit upright clasping their knees or hanging their legs over the edge of the bed. During a severe febrile illness with clouding of consciousness, the patient will lie flat and log-like. In anxiety states and hyperthyroidism, the patient will often sit bolt upright or perched on the edge of the chair, while in cases of depression or thyroid deficiency, a slumped slouching attitude is adopted. Pain may give rise to characteristic postures, as when the patient clutches or supports the affected part or avoids lying on tender areas of the body. In severe abdominal pain, the knees are often drawn up and the body as a whole is 'doubled up'. When the posterior parietal peritoneum is involved, as in carcinoma of the pancreas, relief may be obtained by leaning forwards over the edge of the bed or chair.

GAIT

As in the case of posture, abnormalities of gait due to causes other than skeletal or neuromuscular (see page 243) usually result from discomfort or pain. For example, a limp may be due to painful infective, ulcerative or ischaemic lesions of the skin and subcutaneous tissues of the leg or, more rarely, inflammatory processes involving the psoas muscle in the abdomen. Severe varicose veins, thrombophlebitis and gross oedema of the legs can also cause discomfort on walking, with disturbance of gait. When walking causes dyspnoea, angina or ischaemic pain in the legs, the gait may be slow and cautious with frequent pauses.

SKIN

Some of the points to be observed have been mentioned in describing the skin of the face, but it is necessary to inspect the skin of the whole body.

Undue *sweating* is common in certain infections, and is also usual during the subsidence of any pyrexia. The sweating of pulmonary tuberculosis occurs characteristically during sleep. Sweating is also common in hyperthyroidism and psychoneuroses and in many illnesses which cause exhaustion or severe pain. In most forms of shock there is a cold clammy skin. This may also occur in hypoglycaemia.

Dryness of the skin is also common in fevers in their earlier phases. It is a characteristic of hypothyroidism (see page 304) and of some skin diseases (e.g. ichthyosis), and also results from dehydration.

The degree of pigmentation of the skin should next be noted. Increased pigmentation varying from light to dark shades of brown is a classic sign of Addison's disease (see pages 308–9) (adrenal insufficiency), but should be sought also in the mucous membrane of the mouth. Similar pigmentation may be caused by arsenical poisoning, chronic liver disease, intestinal malabsorption, malignant cachexia and pellagra, but the mucous membranes are rarely affected. The appearance of dirty patients may imitate some of these conditions. *Café au lait* spots may be seen in von Recklinghausen's disease. Pigmentation may also result from chronic venous congestion and is commonly seen in the lower parts of the legs in patients with varicose veins (see Figure 3.47, page 44). Therapeutic irradiation is another cause of localized pigmentation. The possibility that pigmentation is due to sunburn or to racial origin should be ruled out before it is attributed to disease. Patchy loss of pigment ('vitiligo') may occur as a congenital anomaly in healthy people or in association with hyperpigmentation and it is an occasional feature of auto-immune disorders (Figure 3.19(a)). Pallor, cyanosis and jaundice are dealt with elsewhere, but note should be made of the rare yellow of carotinaemia (Figure 3.19(b)), the grey of haemochromatosis and the yellowish raised patches of xanthomatosis. (See xanthelasma, Figure 7.4.)

Blackness of the skin may occur in gangrene, commonly the result of arterial obstruction (see Figure 3.39, page 42).

Excoriation due to scratching may result from irritation of the skin ('pruritus'). This accompanies certain rashes (see below) but can also provide important evidence of systemic disease, such as obstructive jaundice, lymphoma (e.g. Hodgkin's disease) and polycythaemia vera. Pruritus around the vulva is a common early manifestation of diabetes.

Flushing of the skin from transient capillary dilatation most often affects the head and neck, when it is usually due to emotional causes ('blushing') or to hormonal imbalance at the menopause ('hot flushes'). Generalized flushing occurs in fever, hyperthyroidism and hypercarbia. Rarer causes include Hodgkin's disease (in which flushing may be provoked by alcohol) and a carcinoid

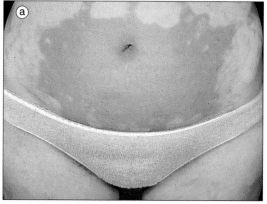

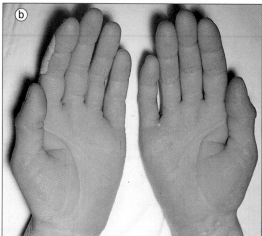

▲ **Figure 3.19 (a) Vitiligo.** (b) Yellowish coloration of hands (also affecting the feet) in a patient consuming large quantities of raw carrots. This may also occur in hypothyroidism

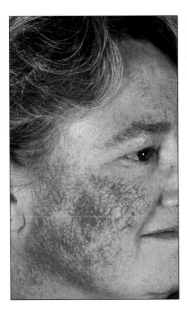

◀ **Figure 3.20 Facial telangiectases as a result of long-term steroid therapy for severe bronchial asthma**

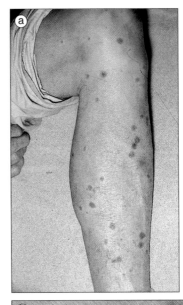

◀ **Figure 3.21 (a) Multiple skin lesions in a man who also had ocular and oral involvement** (same patient as in (b)). (b) Target lesions in Stevens–Johnson syndrome (see also Figure 3.5)

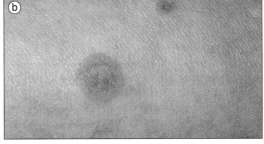

tumour secreting a vasodilatory substance (5-hydrox-ytryptamine) from hepatic metastases. Polycythaemia and chronic vasodilatation due to corticosteroid therapy or alcoholism may give rise to a more persistent cutaneous flush often with telangiectases (Figure 3.20).

The texture of the skin may change. Apart from skin diseases, reference has already been made, in describing facial characteristics, to the increased thickness and coarse texture in myxoedema. This may affect the skin of other parts of the body.

RASHES

Rashes are of great clinical importance. Sometimes the rash is the principal physical sign, as in the exanthemata – for example, measles and chicken-pox; sometimes it is only subsidiary – for example, the purpura of haemorrhagic fevers and certain blood diseases. Drug reaction, whether due to overdose or undue susceptibility, is today among the commonest causes of an unusual rash; barbiturates, antibiotics (e.g. penicillin) and diuretics are specially liable to upset the skin. Drugs may also induce the Stevens–Johnson syndrome in which characteristic 'target' lesions in the skin (Figure 3.21(a) and (b)) are accompanied by conjunctivitis (see Figure 3.5) and mucosal ulceration. A rash is a prominent feature of some vitamin-deficiency diseases, e.g. scurvy and pellagra. The extent and distribution of the rash and how it spreads (centrifugally or centripetally) should be noted; also the site of onset and whether or not there is irritation.

The commoner types of skin eruption are:

1 *Macular,* consisting of coloured spots, not raised above the surrounding skin. Examples are the rashes of measles and glandular fever and less commonly of syphilis and typhoid fever, and the more diffuse and densely distributed spots of scarlet fever. Haemorrhagic rashes, *purpura,* also fall into this category (see Figure 8.1, page 188).

2 *Papular,* or rashes in which the elements are raised into tiny nodes. This type of rash occurs in certain stages of the exanthemas, e.g. chicken pox and in essential diseases of the skin such as lichen planus, eczema and psoriasis (Figure 3.22) in each of which scaling is also present.

3 *Vesicular,* comprised of small blisters or papules, the tops of which are filled with a clear fluid. Good examples are seen in herpes simplex (see The lips, page 30 and Figure 3.8), and herpes zoster, a vesicular rash due to an infection of the posterior root ganglia, and usually distributed in a girdle-like manner around

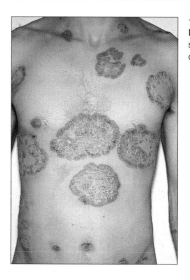

◀ **Figure 3.22 Psoriasis.** Silvery scaling on plaques of chronic psoriasis

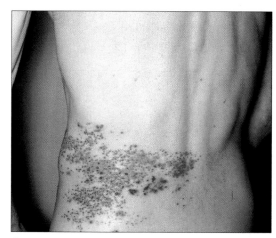

▲ **Figure 3.23 Herpes zoster** ('shingles'). The vesicles in this case are haemorrhagic

one-half of the trunk (to which the disease owes its popular name of 'shingles' (Lat. *cingulum*, a girdle). (Figure 3.23.) Chickenpox is a related disease, and the rash presents somewhat similar characteristics.

4 *Bullous,* consisting of larger blisters generally containing clear fluid. They are well seen in burns and scalds and occasionally in erysipelas. Sometimes they occur in severe nervous lesions and drug intoxication (Figure 3.24). The various forms of pemphigus, of which bullae are the essential features, cannot be considered here.

5 *Pustular,* in many ways resembling a vesicular rash, but in which the little nodules are filled with turbid or purulent instead of clear fluid. Pustules are familiarly seen in acne vulgaris, in which they are non-infective in origin, and to a lesser extent in chickenpox. The malignant pustule of anthrax shows a black centre with surrounding redness.

6 *Nodular* rashes consist of swellings in the skin generally of greater size than the average vesicle or pustule. They are also firmer to touch. An important example of a nodular rash is found in *erythema nodosum* (Figure 3.25). This occurs on the legs, especially the shins, as painful reddish-blue nodules varying in size from a millimetre to several centimetres in diameter. This is commonly due to sarcoidosis, but it may be a response to various infections, especially streptococcal and tuberculous, and also to drugs and other allergens; it may also accompany inflammatory bowel disease. Other examples of a nodular rash are the secondary deposits in the skin of carcinoma or leukaemia, and the deposition of syphilitic, tuberculous and leprous granulation tissue in the form of gummas, tuberculomas and lepromas. Except in the developing countries, these infective forms of granulomas are now relatively less common

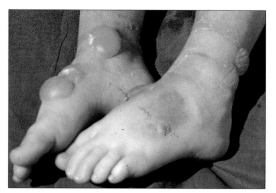

▲ **Figure 3.24 Bullous eruption on the feet due to a reaction to nalidixic acid (Negram) used to treat a urinary infection**

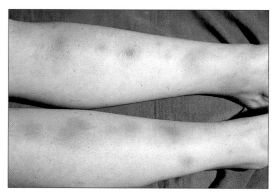

▲ **Figure 3.25 Erythema nodosum**

as a cause of skin nodules than vasculitic granulomas resulting from immune reactions and the purple lesions of Kaposi sarcoma in patients with AIDS. A gross form of nodular change in the skin is neurofibromatosis (Figure 3.26) in which the lesions may be pedunculated (on stalks). Patches of pigmentation (*café au lait* spots) are also found in this condition.

7 *Weals* These are raised areas, sometimes pale, sometimes red, which are often seen in sensitive skins even after slight trauma or exposure to irritants (e.g. nettle stings, insect bites). They may appear as 'writing' on the skin (dermographia, Figure 3.27). They also occur spontaneously in various forms of urticaria and are often an expression of hypersensitivity to foreign proteins either ingested (e.g. shell-fish) or injected (e.g. antitetanic serum). Thus they may have a connection with allergic diseases such as asthma, hay fever and angioneurotic oedema. Other features of a weal are its transient nature and irritable characteristics (itching, burning).

These essential elements of a rash may be accompanied by secondary changes. The area around pustules is usually reddened and swollen from inflammatory reaction. When the pustules burst, *crusts* may form, e.g. in impetigo (see Figure 3.28). *Desquamation* is the name given to shedding of the superficial layers of the epidermis which occurs after many fevers, but is particularly characteristic of scarlet fever and of some drug eruptions. More localized scaling or desquamative rashes include flexural eczema, which, with asthma and hay fever, is a common manifestation of an 'atopic' or allergic state, and also psoriasis which may be associated with a rheumatoid form of arthritis (Figure 3.29). Erosion of the deeper layers of the skin and loss of tissue result in *ulcers;* these may follow infections or injuries, especially when the circulation is abnormal due to varicose veins or arterial atheroma, or when the nerve supply is interrupted. In these cases, the distal parts of the limbs are most often affected. Skin ulcers more rarely result from the breakdown of malignant or granulomatous nodules. *Scars* may be significant of old skin lesions, especially of acne, smallpox, herpes zoster and healed varicose ulcers (see Figure 3.47, page 44). The scars of operations and injuries must not be overlooked, as they may bear upon the present illness.

In many rashes several elements are combined. Thus in smallpox, macules, papules, vesicles and pustules are seen on the skin successively. In allergic purpura, the

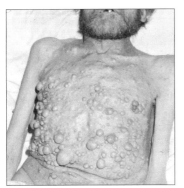

◀ **Figure 3.26 Neurofibromatosis** (von Recklinghausen's disease)

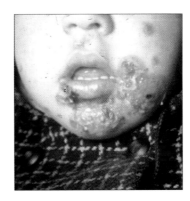

◀ **Figure 3.28 Impetigo**

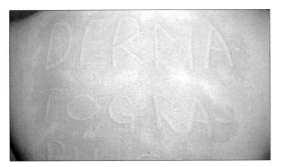

▲ **Figure 3.27 Dermographia**

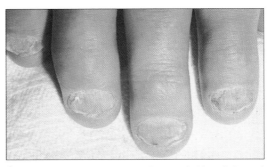

▲ **Figure 3.29 Psoriasis:** arthritis of the terminal interphalangeal joints with deformity and discoloration of the nails

essential haemorrhagic rash is frequently combined with the weals of urticaria.

Pathological changes in the skin, such as *telangiectases,* may be associated with similar lesions in other organs. For example, hereditary haemorrhagic telangiectasia, in which there is multiple localized dilatation of the venules and capillaries in the skin and mucosae, may explain haemorrhages from the nose, lungs, gastrointestinal tract and kidneys. Telangiectasia may also accompany systemic sclerosis (scleroderma) (Figure 3.30) and hepatic disease (spider naevi) and may be seen after irradiation of the skin (Figure 3.31).

In recent years, many cutaneous 'markers' of internal malignant disease have been recognized, especially certain persistent erythematous rashes (see Figure 3.32).

AIDS AND THE SKIN

Florid seborrhoeic dermatitis, widespread herpetic infection and moniliasis of nails, skin and mucus membranes many be found in such immunosuppressed patients. The typical purple nodular lesions of Kaposi's sarcoma are found on the head (Figure 3.33), trunk and limbs and consist of dilated and hypertrophied angiomatous blood vessels (Figure 3.34).

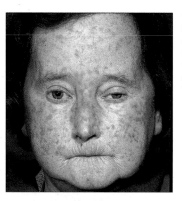

◀ Figure 3.30 Systemic sclerosis, showing puckering of the mouth due to scleroderma, and telangiectasia

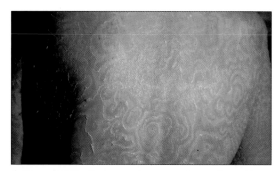

▲ Figure 3.32 Erythema gyratum repens in a patient with bronchial carcinoma

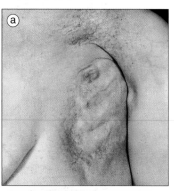

◀ Figure 3.31 Post-radiation telangiectasia. Note also skin scarring.

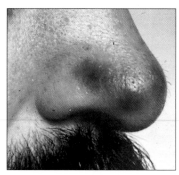

◀ Figure 3.33 Kaposi's sarcoma

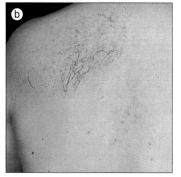

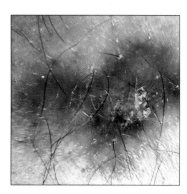

◀ Figure 3.34 Purple angiomatous blood vessels of Kaposi's sarcoma

GENITALIA

The size and form of the genitalia are of especial importance in endocrine disorders (see Chapter 12).

The penis and testes fail to reach adult proportions in several types of infantilism: hypopituitarism, hypothyroidism and eunuchoidism are notable causes. In these cases the normal sexual functions are also in abeyance, and the secondary sex characters (in boys, deepening of the voice, growth of hair on the pubes and in masculine sites) do not develop at puberty. In females the main sign of genital infantilism is the failure to menstruate; the pubic hair may be delayed in appearance, and the general bodily configuration remains sexless without breast development.

By contrast, sexual precocity may be found in adrenal cortical hyperplasia or tumours and in certain rare diseases of the endocrines or brain. Male children may develop a penis of adult proportions at an early age (erection and ejaculation of spermatozoa may occur). Precocious puberty in females may develop along masculine or feminine lines; if the former (premature heterosexual maturation), the clitoris may enlarge and hirsutism appear as in the adrenogenital syndrome; if the latter, the normal sex characteristics, e.g. breast formation and menstruation, are unduly early (Figure 3.35).

The external genital organs may also exhibit evidence of local disease, particularly venereal manifestations such as syphilitic chancre on the penis or vulva, the presence of secondary manifestations of the disease, e.g. condylomas, or the presence of urethral or vaginal discharge in gonorrhoea and other local infections and in non-specific urethritis (see Reiter's syndrome, page 209). Herpes simplex may also affect the genitalia as a sexually transmitted disease.

EXTREMITIES

In certain diseases the shape of the hands may be modified. In myxoedema they are broad and the fingers appear short and stubby from thickening of the subcutaneous tissues. In acromegaly they are large, broad and paw-like (Figure 3.36), but in hypogonadism they are often slender and feminine. Long spidery fingers – arachnodactyly – occur in Marfan's syndrome and are sometimes associated with atrial septal defect or other congenital cardiac anomalies (Figure 3.37).

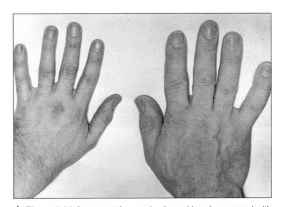

▲ **Figure 3.36 Acromegaly:** spade-shaped hand compared with the normal hand on the left

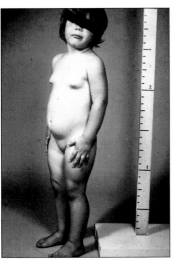

◀ **Figure 3.35 Precocious puberty in a four-year-old**

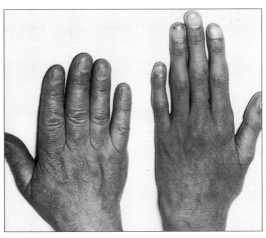

▲ **Figure 3.37 Arachnodactyly.** The spidery fingers are compared with those of a normal hand on the left

The joint affections of the hands are described in Chapter 9. It remains to add that many types of deformity may result from arthritis. Two are worthy of mention here: first, *ulnar deviation* in rheumatoid arthritis, in which the whole hand, but especially the fingers from the metacarpophalangeal joints, is deflected to the ulnar side; secondly, *Heberden's nodes* (Figure 9.21, page 210), bony prominences at the distal interphalangeal joints which occur in osteoarthrosis. Another common deformity of the hand results from fibrous thickening of palmar tissues with flexion of the fingers: Dupuytren's contracture (Figure 3.38). This is usually inherited but may accompany alcoholic cirrhosis of the liver.

Gangrene, causing blackness of the skin, is usually the result of serious and permanent arterial obstruction due to thrombosis complicating atheroma or vasculitis, or to embolism (see also page 182). The toes are most often affected in atheroma (e.g. diabetic gangrene, Figure 3.39) and the fingers in inflammatory vascular conditions associated with a Raynaud phenomenon (e.g. systemic sclerosis, see Figure 7.81, page 181). In this latter condition, the skin of the fingers is taut and shiny, sometimes with telangiectases, and the ends of the fingers may be tapered due to ischaemic resorption of bone. Gangrene may also affect the fingers, forearm or whole leg in drug addicts who have injected their veins or arteries with narcotics through dirty syringes or shared infected needles (Figure 3.40). A special form of gangrene follows the injection of intra-arterial temazepam which may necessitate amputation (see Figure 3.41).

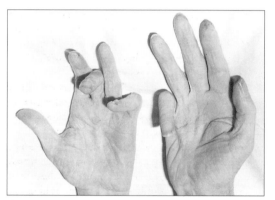

▲ Figure 3.38 Bilateral Dupuytren contractures in a patient with alcoholic cirrhosis of the liver

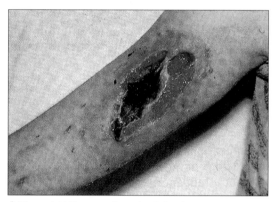

▲ Figure 3.40 Forearm ulceration following repeated IV drug injections

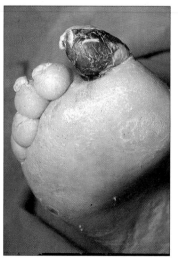

◀ Figure 3.39 Diabetic gangrene

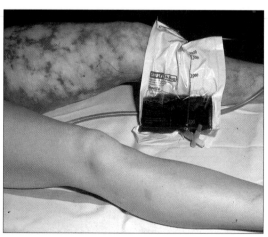

▲ Figure 3.41 Intra-arterial temazepam injection leading to gangrene, muscle necrosis and myoglobinuria

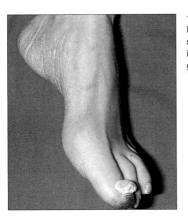

◀ Figure 3.42
Lymphangitis
spreading from an
infected
gangrenous toe

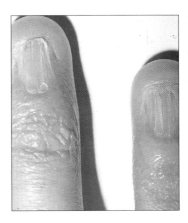

◀ Figure 3.43
Ribbing of the
nails associated
with the
malabsorption
syndrome

In respiratory and cardiac disease, clubbing of the fingers and toes should be sought, but this and the abnormalities of the hands due to nervous diseases will be considered in later chapters.

Traumatic and infective lesions of the hands and feet are common and the latter may be complicated by lymphangitis (Figure 3.42).

Finally, the *nails* should be inspected. Pitting, ribbing and brittleness are often seen after severe illness and in malabsorption syndromes (Figure 3.43). The short irregular nails of the nail-biter may suggest some instability of personality. Koilonychia (spoon-shaped nails) is seen in iron-deficiency anaemias (Figure 3.44, and Figure 8.10, page 195). In psoriasis, the nails may be deformed, pitted and yellow in colour (see Figure 3.29). A rare cause of yellow nails is lymphatic obstruction, usually accompanied by pleural effusion (see Figure 6.42). Leukonychia, abnormal whiteness at the base of the nails, sometimes occurs in chronic liver failure (see

Figure 8.10, page 195) and other conditions associated with hypoalbuminaemia. Splinter haemorrhages may appear beneath the nails in blood diseases and as the result of emboli in bacterial endocarditis (see Figure 3.45). A similar appearance in the nailbed may be caused by small digital infarcts in patients with a vasculitis, e.g. systemic lupus erythematosus.

Tremors are generally seen best in the hands. Apart from neurological causes dealt with on page 238 they may be present in senility, thyrotoxicosis, alcoholism, carbon dioxide retention and in renal and hepatic failure.

The *legs* should be specially inspected for evidence of circulatory disorders, both venous and arterial. Examination of the legs for evidence of deep vein thrombosis is especially important when pulmonary embolism is suspected. This evidence may include tenderness in the thigh or calf, pain in the calf on dorsiflexion of the foot (Homans' sign), pitting oedema or an increase in the girth of one leg when compared with

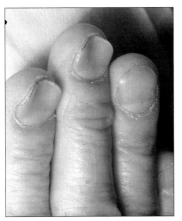

◀ Figure 3.44
Koilonychia

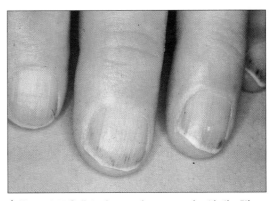

▲ Figure 3.45 Splinter haemorrhages seen best in the 5th
finger. There are also fading lesions in the middle finger

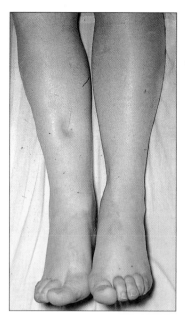

◀ **Figure 3.46
Pitting pretibial
oedema due to
deep vein
thrombosis**

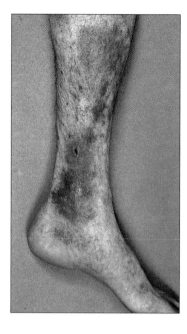

◀ **Figure 3.47
Eczema,
pigmentation and
ulcer scars
associated with
varicose veins**

the other. Venous congestion or obstruction causes pitting oedema which may best be elicited over the tibiae and ankles (see Figure 3.46). Chronic impairment of venous return may lead to varicose veins associated with eczema, pigmentation and ulceration over the lower part of the legs (Figure 3.47). Evidence of arterial ischaemia includes pallor, cyanosis, coldness, loss of hair, anaesthesia and trophic changes such as gangrene (see Figure 3.39).

Because of gravity, haemorrhagic rashes associated with increased capillary fragility as in scurvy and other forms of purpura may be seen best in the lower limbs (see Figure 3.48). Erythema nodosum (see Figure 3.25, page 38) also favours the legs.

Bone deformities such as bow-legs (Figure 3.49), knock-knees and sabre tibiae must also be noted, although these are now relatively uncommon. Deformity of the feet, especially pes cavus, may occur with con-

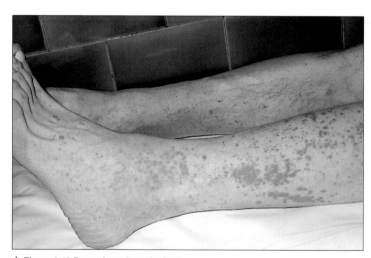

▲ **Figure 3.48 Purpuric rash on the legs**

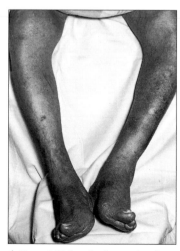

▲ **Figure 3.49 Paget's disease: bow-legs**

genital neurological disorders including syringomyelia and the hereditary ataxias.

The toe nails may be clubbed and may also show evidence of neglect (Figure 3.50).

The *joints* of the lower limb are particularly prone to disease. Osteoarthrosis affects the weight-bearing joints of the hip, knee and ankle; rheumatoid arthritis commonly involves the small joints of the feet, and gout favours the metatarsophalangeal joint of the big toe (see also Chapter 9).

Neurological abnormalities of the legs are described in Chapter 10.

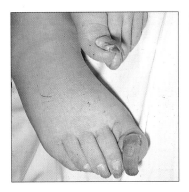

◀ **Figure 3.50**
Onychogryphosis

The digestive system

The digestive system comprises the alimentary tract and the accessory organs and tissues concerned in the digestion of food. It will be convenient to describe the symptoms and objective examination of each part separately, though certain general descriptions of symptoms common to all parts and the method of examining the abdomen as a whole will be necessary.

THE MOUTH

See also the Respiratory system, Chapter 6 and Haemopoietic system, Chapter 8.

SYMPTOMS
Symptoms arising in the mouth include thirst and dryness, increased salivation, loss or disorder of taste, difficulty in speech, chewing or swallowing, soreness and pain.

THIRST AND DRYNESS
Thirst usually reflects the degree of cellular dehydration and can thus result from diminished intake or excessive loss of water, or from increased consumption of salt. Severe diarrhoea, polyuria in diabetes mellitus and renal failure and profuse sweating, especially in fevers, are notable causes, aggravated sometimes because the patient is too weak to drink. Dryness of the mouth from decreased salivation is a familiar transient feature in fear, but it may be more persistent in mouth breathers from nasal obstruction. It may also result from diseases of the salivary glands, e.g. mumps, Sjögren's disease and salivary calculi, and is usual in the states of dehydration causing thirst. In acute illness such dryness may be a useful indication of the necessity for fluids. Drugs such as anticholinergics and antidepressants may produce a dry mouth as may depression even without medication.

INCREASED SALIVATION
This occurs in irritant lesions of the buccal mucosa (e.g. stomatitis, teething in infants), in Parkinsonism (see page 261) and as an accompaniment of nausea (water brash). Salivation is often a distressing symptom of oesophageal obstruction because the normal secretions cannot be swallowed. Anxiety states may produce an increase in saliva, which patients find difficult to swallow.

LOSS OR DISORDER OF TASTE
The sensory nerve endings in the tongue can only distinguish the primary sensations of taste: sweet, bitter, sour, salt. Loss of these sensations usually indicates a lesion of the 7th or 9th or more rarely the mandibular division of the 5th cranial nerves. More often, a patient complaining of loss of 'taste' cannot distinguish those more subtle flavours of food which depend upon the sense of smell. This symptom, which commonly results in anorexia, is rarely due to lesions of the olfactory nerves and more commonly to disease of the nasal mucosa or obstruction of the nasal airway; it may also be caused by drugs such as captopril. The presence of an unpleasant taste in the mouth or a distortion in the flavour of food sometimes occurs in cerebral lesions or as an aura in epilepsy (see page 279), but is also a frequent psychogenic symptom associated with the fear that the breath is offensive to others. An unpleasant taste is in fact only rarely associated with an offensive breath (see page 48). See also Central nervous system, Chapter 10.

DIFFICULTY IN SPEECH, CHEWING OR SWALLOWING
These symptoms can result from diminished salivary secretion, inadequate teeth or an ill-fitting denture and painful conditions of the mouth or throat. The neuromuscular causes are dealt with in Chapter 10.

SORENESS AND PAIN
Soreness of the mucous membrane covering the mouth or tongue is found in the various forms of stomatitis, and inflammation of the buccal mucosa due to local or systemic causes (see below). The soreness is felt especially when very hot or acid foods are taken and during speech, chewing or swallowing. The commonest form of pain arising in the mouth is toothache due to dental caries or periodontal abscess. The pain is constant, aching in character, aggravated by chewing or by cold foods, and it may radiate to the ear, the temple or the orbit.

PHYSICAL SIGNS: EXAMINATION OF THE MOUTH

The examination of the mouth requires a good light, and preferably the use of an electric torch if bright daylight is not available.

THE TEETH

The teeth should be inspected and their number and condition noted. Deficient or carious teeth and ill-fitting false teeth which prevent adequate chewing, or discourage the patient from wearing the denture at meal times, may be contributory causes of dyspepsia. Abnormal formation of the teeth is important in the diagnosis of congenital syphilis in which the incisors may be notched (Hutchinsonian teeth). Discoloration may be due to poor dental hygiene, but is sometimes seen when the fluorine content of water is unduly high. The teeth then show a mottled brownish appearance. This may also be produced by tetracyclines (Figure 4.1). A rare phenomenon is the pink fluorescence of the teeth in congenital porphyria.

THE GUMS

The state of the gums should next be noted. A deep-red congestion with easy bleeding is present when the gums are inflamed (gingivitis), and in pyorrhoea pus can be squeezed from the gum margins. Both in gingivitis and pyorrhoea the teeth are generally affected and are often loose and covered with a greenish-yellow exudate. The gum margins retract. Oral sepsis of this kind may in certain circumstances give rise to bacterial endocarditis or to lung abscess; it can also be an aggravating factor in gastric disorders. The gums are pale in anaemia, and in lead poisoning a blue line may be seen at the gum margin. The blue line is due to a deposit of lead sulphide in the gum tissues; thus it cannot be cleaned away with a pledget of cotton-wool, and it is seen even better if the gum margins between the teeth are transilluminated from behind by a small electric torch. This does not occur in edentulous patients and has become rare. A yellow line may similarly be caused by cadmium sulphide. (See also Haemopoietic system, page 190.) In scurvy the gums are soft and spongy and bleed easily (see also Figure 8.17, page 197). Vincent's angina may cause ulceration and sloughing of the gingiva as well as faucial manifestations. Hypertrophy of the gums may occur in epileptics taking phenytoin over a long period of time (see Figure 10.97, page 280) and also in certain leukaemias (see Figure 8.6, page 190).

THE TONGUE AND BUCCAL MUCOUS MEMBRANE

The normal papillae of the tongue give rise to a furred appearance best seen in the posterior part. Dryness of the tongue is an important sign of dehydration (see page 46) and may be accompanied by thickening, discoloration and 'caking' of the fur.

Anaemia, cyanosis and jaundice may be evident in the tongue. In certain anaemias (pernicious anaemia and iron-deficiency anaemias particularly) the tongue is depapillated, i.e. smooth and shiny and sometimes sore (see page 190). Cyanosis of the tongue is always central in origin (see page 106). The ventral aspect of the tongue must be inspected as haemorrhages, neoplastic ulcer and leucoplakia (Figure 4.2) may only be seen from below.

The tongue is large in acromegaly and in Down's syndrome, and in the latter often fissured. Macroglossia for which no other obvious cause is found may be due to amyloidosis (Figure 4.3).

Paralysis, atrophy, tremors and abnormalities of movement of the tongue and soft palate will be noted incidentally but are referred to under the nervous system.

Small ulcers indicate the presence of stomatitis (see page 49). The more serious ulcers of syphilis and malignant disease should not be overlooked; the former tend to be central and the latter marginal. Leucoplakia may be syphilitic, AIDS related and sometimes precancerous.

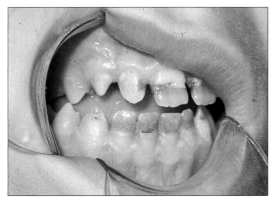

▲ Figure 4.1 Staining of the teeth due to tetracyclines given during childhood for fibrocystic disease of the lung

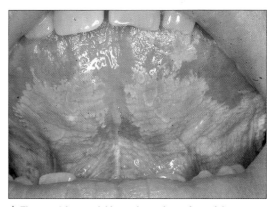

▲ Figure 4.2 Leucoplakia on the undersurface of the tongue

It is characterized by white and sometimes thickened patches in the mucosa (Figure 4.2). Tuberculous ulceration is associated with pulmonary infection and commonly involves the tip of the tongue. With the decline in syphilis and tuberculosis, Crohn's disease has become a relatively more common cause of mouth ulcers. Swabs or sections from the ulcer may help to identify such conditions as Crohn's disease, syphilis, tuberculosis and malignant disease.

In Addison's disease, brownish areas of pigmentation may be seen in the buccal mucous membrane, a useful confirmatory sign in doubtful cases (Figure 4.4).

Buccal pigmentation can also occur in normal people, especially Negroes, and rarely in haemochromatosis. Telangiectases are seen on the lips in hereditary haemorrhagic telangiectasia, systemic sclerosis and scleroderma (Figure 4.5). Pigmentation of the lips and mouth is a cutaneous marker for the Peutz–Jegher's syndrome (Figure 4.6) in which gastrointestinal polyps may cause intussusception or bleeding. Haemorrhages are occasionally found in purpura and if accompanied by thrush may suggest leukaemia. Note will be made of the movements of the soft palate and uvula.

See also Koplik's spots, page 317.

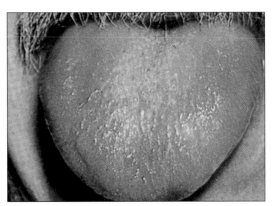

▲ **Figure 4.3 Macroglossia due to amyloid**

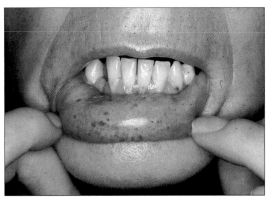

▲ **Figure 4.5 Telangiectasia of the lips in systemic sclerosis**

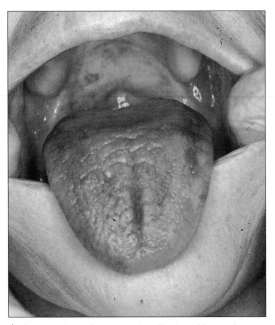

▲ **Figure 4.4 Buccal pigmentation.** Patches of brown pigment on the palate in a patient with Addison's disease

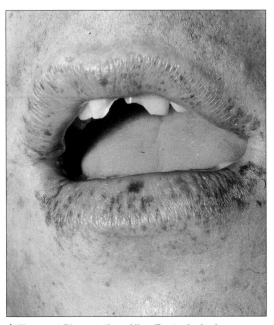

▲ **Figure 4.6 Pigmentation of lips (Peutz–Jegher's syndrome) in a patient with colonic polyps**

THE BREATH

An offensive faecal odour to the breath sometimes occurs in symptomless people due to putrefaction of food fragments retained around the teeth or the proliferation of organisms in the gums or tonsils. More rarely, a foul smell can arise from the stomach contents, as in gastric carcinoma and intestinal obstruction, or from chronic suppuration in the lung (bronchiectasis; lung abscess). A sweet smell may be imparted to the breath by acetone in cases of diabetic coma and in acidosis, especially in children. The breath in uraemia sometimes has a urinose smell, while that in hepatic coma is musty. The smell of alcohol on the breath does not always mean that it has been consumed to excess, or that it is responsible for any symptoms, but alcohol misuse should be suspected if the smell is evident before about 11.00 a.m. (see Coma, page 12).

DIAGNOSIS OF DISEASES OF THE MOUTH

Many diseases of the mouth are within the province of surgical diagnosis and oral medicine and are not described here. One which deserves mention is stomatitis.

STOMATITIS

The term embraces a number of conditions of varying aetiology, characterized by signs of inflammation, exudate and ulceration usually with increased salivation. Sometimes these are due to mechanical traumatic causes such as jagged teeth, ill-fitting dentures or burns. They may be due to local infections such as moniliasis ('thrush') which is characterized by a patchy white exudate scattered throughout the mouth but especially on the soft palate (Figure 4.7). Today this is one of the commonest forms of mouth infection and appears especially in those

receiving broad-spectrum antibiotics or corticosteroid inhalers, or in AIDS. Systemic causes of an ulcerative stomatitis include leukaemia, uraemia, metallic poisons such as mercury and, in tropical areas, kala-azar.

The term *aphthous stomatitis* is applied to a fairly common condition in which small vesicles may change to ulcers of superficial but painful nature (Figure 4.8). The cause is obscure, but it may be associated with Crohn's disease in a few cases.

Nutritional causes should be looked for, especially in tropical zones where deficiency in vitamin-B complexes are common. (See also Scurvy, page 200, and Agranulocytosis, page 193.)

Angular stomatitis (cheilosis) is a characteristic feature of nutritional deficiency (see Figure 4.8 and Chapter 8).

A number of skin conditions also have buccal mucous membrane manifestations, e.g. erythema multiforme.

THE OESOPHAGUS

SYMPTOMS
Dysphagia

Dysphagia or difficulty in swallowing is the principal symptom of oesophageal disease. Dysphagia may consist

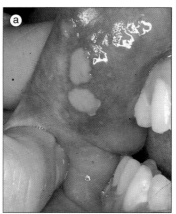
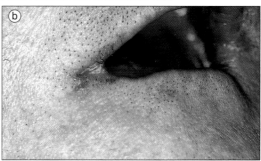

◀ Figure 4.8 (a) Aphthous ulcers; (b) angular stomatitis

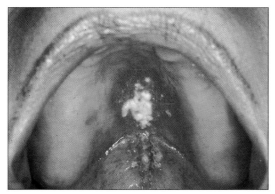

▲ Figure 4.7 White patches on the soft palate due to moniliasis in a patient with AIDS

of a difficulty in emptying the mouth because of poor salivation, paresis of the tongue or painful conditions of the mouth or pharynx. In oesophageal dysphagia, the food is felt to lodge in the throat or behind the sternum. The obstruction can sometimes be accurately localized by the patient, but a lower oesophageal obstruction can sometimes give rise to dysphagia at a higher level. The commoner causes of dysphagia are listed in Table 4.1. Of these, carcinoma and peptic stricture are the commonest. At first, the patient has difficulty only with solid foods and for a time this can be overcome by chewing food until it is of fluid consistency; later, as obstruction increases, fluids and even saliva cannot be swallowed. Dysphagia due to other causes is rarely complete and, in the case of achalasia, may be intermittent over a period of many years and affects solids and fluids equally. Dysphagia of neuromuscular origin may be accompanied by a bout of coughing due to food entering the larynx.

Pain

Pain which accompanies dysphagia is probably due to muscle contractions in the oesophagus above the obstruction. This pain is retrosternal and maximal at the site of the obstruction, but it can spread across the chest and radiate into the neck and through to the back. It may thus simulate cardiac pain, but it usually occurs immediately after swallowing and can be eased by regurgitation of food. A more persistent pain of this nature can result from rupture or perforation of the oesophagus. A lower sternal burning pain provoked by stooping and relieved by antacids suggests an oesophagitis due to reflux of acid from the stomach. This occurs particularly in hiatus hernia (see also Heartburn, page 55). Painful swallowing without obstruction (odynophagia) occurs

in oesophagitis secondary to peptic reflux or infections such as candidiasis or herpes simplex.

Regurgitation

Food and secretions may be retained behind an obstruction of the oesophagus or within a diverticulum and subsequently regurgitated. Regurgitation, as distinct from vomiting (i.e. evacuation of the gastric contents) is rarely preceded by nausea and is often effortless. The regurgitated food is undigested but it may undergo bacterial putrefaction and become foul-smelling. The inhalation of regurgitated matter during sleep is an occasional cause of nocturnal bouts of coughing and can lead to serious pulmonary infections.

Haemorrhage

Oesophageal haemorrhage presents as haematemesis or melaena (see page 54) or, more insidiously, as anaemia. The bleeding may come from peptic oesophagitis or from oesophageal varices, secondary to portal hypertension. A massive haemorrhage from ruptured varices can present as an effortless regurgitation of dark venous blood unaltered by gastric acid. Fresh blood at the conclusion of forceful vomiting suggests a traumatic tear at the gastro-oesophageal junction – a Mallory–Weiss tear.

PHYSICAL SIGNS: EXAMINATION OF THE OESOPHAGUS

DIAGNOSIS OF DISEASES OF THE OESOPHAGUS

The examination of the oesophagus is largely dependent on radiography, oesophagoscopy and biopsy. The clinician relies chiefly upon the history, but observes difficulties in swallowing and notes any glandular enlargement in the neck or evidence of mediastinal obstruction.

CARCINOMA OF OESOPHAGUS

This tumour causes pain, progressive dysphagia and regurgitation of food which may be foul and blood-stained. The exclusion of solid food and, later, of fluids from the stomach leads to thirst, wasting, dehydration, anaemia and other signs of malnutrition. Inability to swallow saliva can be a particularly distressing symptom. Rarely, the symptoms appear suddenly. The structures adjacent to the oesophagus may be invaded at a relatively early stage of the disease (see Mediastinal obstruction, page 126). If the obstruction cannot be relieved, the patient will die of starvation or from pneumonia due to the inhalation of regurgitated food. A rare inherited form of oesophageal carcinoma is

CAUSES OF DYSPHAGIA	
High	Carcinoma (pharynx or oesophagus)
	Cervical tumours (lymph nodes; goitre)
	Neuromuscular (bulbar palsy; myasthenia; psychogenic)
	Iron deficiency (see Chapter 8)
	Diverticulum (pharynx or oesophagus)
Middle	Carcinoma of oesophagus
	Mediastinal tumours (lymph nodes; aneurysm)
Low	Carcinoma (stomach or oesophagus)
	Peptic stricture (usually with hiatus hernia)
	Achalasia
	Systemic sclerosis

▲ Table 4.1

associated with tylosis, a thickening of the skin on the soles of the feet and palms of the hands (Figure 4.9).

ACHALASIA OF THE CARDIA

Achalasia is due to the failure of the lower oesophagus to relax before the oncoming bolus of food. This has been attributed to a non-coordinated peristaltic wave rather than to spasm of the cardia and results from degeneration of Auerbach's plexus. Achalasia tends to affect younger people than does carcinoma but may persist throughout life if untreated; the dysphagia is usually more variable and less relentless in its progression, and it can be temporarily relieved by drugs which relax smooth muscle. Nutrition is often well maintained.

PERFORATION AND RUPTURE

Although these are surgical emergencies, they are mentioned here because they so often present to the physician in the guise of myocardial infarction with severe retrosternal pain and signs of 'shock'. When symptoms of this kind come on after a meal containing sharp bones (e.g. fish, chicken, chop), oesophageal perforation should always be considered. Forceful vomiting after a heavy meal with a lot of alcohol can result in spontaneous rupture of the oesophagus. In either case, the diagnosis is supported by the finding of palpable crepitus in the neck (surgical emphysema) due to air tracking up from the mediastinum and, later, by the signs of a pleural effusion usually on the left side. The breach in the wall of the oesophagus is confirmed by radiographs taken after the patient has swallowed a radio-opaque material.

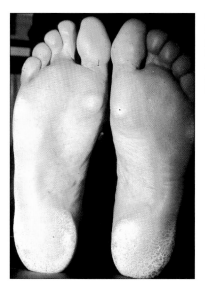

◀ **Figure 4.9
Tylosis in a
patient with an
oesophageal
carcinoma and
a positive
family history**

REFLUX OESOPHAGITIS

Reflux of the gastric contents into the lower oesophagus is particularly likely in the presence of pregnancy, obesity, raised intra-abdominal pressure or herniation of the stomach through the oesophageal hiatus (hiatus hernia). The resulting symptoms are heartburn on stooping or lying and regurgitation of bitter fluid. If severe peptic oesophagitis ensues, then pain, dysphagia and bleeding may occur. After long-standing reflux oesophagitis, there may be columnar metaplasia of the epithelium (Barrett's oesophagus) and this is a premalignant condition.

SPECIAL INVESTIGATIONS

Abnormalities in the outline of the oesophageal lumen can be demonstrated by radiological screening while the patient swallows barium sulphate, a substance opaque to X-rays. Lesions of the oesophageal mucosa can also be identified by direct vision through a flexible endoscope (fibreoptic endoscopy), by cytological examination of aspirated contents and, if indicated, a biopsy of the mucosa can be taken for histological examination.

Considerable increase in understanding of oesophageal abnormalities has been made possible by the more scientific measurements of pressure and motility, namely manometric studies. These have been particularly valuable in showing lack of co-ordination in the contraction of different segments, as in achalasia and the rarer cork-screw oesophagus of elderly persons.

Acid perfusion of the oesophagus may induce the pain of oesophageal regurgitation and may thus be helpful in the differential diagnosis of retrosternal pain.

GENERAL SYMPTOMS OF ABDOMINAL DISEASE

ABDOMINAL PAIN

Pain has been considered on page 5, and special characteristics in relation to individual abdominal viscera will be described later. Abdominal pain of organic origin falls into two classes:

1   *Visceral pain,* due to increased tension on the splanchnic nerve endings in the muscular wall of the affected viscus. This pain is deeply situated, sometimes colicky in type, and is found most commonly in obstructive lesions of the intestines and bile ducts. A similar pain is found in obstruction of other tubes, particularly the ureter in cases of renal colic. When an organ is inflamed, the threshold to visceral pain is lowered, and it may then be induced by a variety of

stimuli (e.g. acid secretion or local pressure in the case of peptic ulceration).

2 *Referred pain*, probably due in many cases to the irritative effects of inflammatory, haemorrhagic or neoplastic diseases of the abdominal viscera upon the parietal peritoneum. The parietal peritoneum in contact with the viscus receives its nerve supply from the same segments of the spinal cord as the overlying parts of the abdominal wall. This explains why pain and tenderness are experienced in many cases over the viscus, although the pain is referred. In other cases, as in the instance of shouldertip pain, the area of skin is situated remotely from the irritated peritoneum. Here irritation of the peritoneum (or pleura) covering the central portions of the diaphragm, which receives its nerve supply from the phrenic nerve (3rd, 4th and 5th cervical segments), causes the pain to be felt in an area supplied by other somatic nerves arising at the same level, over the tip of the shoulder. The pain of peritoneal irritation is mainly associated with deep tenderness and often with muscular rigidity. More constant than visceral pain, it is usually stabbing, cutting or burning in character.

Special features to be noted (Table 4.2)

An accurate description by the patient of his pain is of the greatest value in the diagnosis of digestive diseases. The following points should be ascertained in every case:

1 *The situation.* From the preceding sections it follows that when pain is due to peritoneal irritation it is usually experienced over the affected viscus, but when truly visceral it may be more vaguely situated; in the case of gastrointestinal pain it is usually central. Visceral pain, as already pointed out, depends for its position on the embryological origin of the viscus. More detail is given in dealing with individual viscera.

2 *The character.* This includes the severity, which varies from the slight discomfort of gastric flatulence to the agonizing pain of a perforated ulcer. The description of the type of pain – 'griping', 'gnawing', 'stabbing', 'cutting' and so forth – depends a good deal upon the intelligence and descriptive ability of the patient; so too much stress cannot be laid upon it as a point in diagnosis. The distinction between visceral and somatic pain may be recognized from the patient's description.

3 *Conditions aggravating the pain.* Abdominal pain so frequently arises from the stomach, intestines or organs which modify the function of these that it naturally bears a close relationship to meals. Inquiry should be made whether the pain occurs after meals; if so, for how long and whether it is relieved by taking more food. The patient should also be asked whether any particular kind of food disagrees with him and precipitates pain.

4 *Conditions relieving the pain.* The effect of starvation should be noted, or whether abstention from particular foods gives relief. Relief given by medicines, particularly antacids, may also be diagnostic. Comfort produced by evacuation of the bladder or rectum may suggest these organs as the source of pain.

5 *Duration.* If the pain comes on after meals, the patient should be asked whether it disappears before the next meal or whether it is continuous. In apparently continuous pain there are often spells in which the patient is comparatively comfortable. Intervals of freedom from the attacks of pain should also be noted. It is characteristic, for example, in gastric and duodenal ulcer to find periods of some weeks in which the patient is entirely free from discomfort. On the contrary, pain due to gastric and other visceral carcinomas often starts gradually and becomes more severe and continuous as time goes on. Pain of short duration is more likely to be due to obstructive causes such as renal or biliary colic than to inflammation or neoplasm.

6 *Associated phenomena.* Indications of the severity of the pain and its reflex effects are often seen in the association of vomiting, sweating and collapse. Severe pain, especially due to peptic ulcer, may wake the patient at night. It should be noted whether vomiting gives relief from the pain, a common history in cases of gastric disease. The association of constipation or diarrhoea with abdominal pain should focus attention on the intestinal tract. Fever suggests an inflammatory lesion such as appendicitis, cholecystitis or cholangitis complicating bile duct obstruction by stone. The combination of fever with rigors, jaundice and abdominal pain is characteristic of ascending cholangitis (Charcot's triad) usually caused by a bile duct stone.

VOMITING

Vomiting is another symptom common to so many diseases of the digestive and other systems that it is convenient to describe it before proceeding further. It is a reflex act induced through the vomiting centre of the medulla and may be caused by central or peripheral stimulation. Central stimulation of the vomiting centre may occur from external causes such as disgusting smells or sights or from increased intracranial pressure as in cerebral tumour. It may arise reflexly from labyrinthine disturbances, e.g. in seasickness and Menière's disease. It is also a fairly constant symptom in the early months of pregnancy and may arise from metabolic causes such as uraemia and hypercalcaemia.

However, in this chapter we are concerned with vomiting due to primary disorders of the digestive system. It is common as a result of indiscretions in diet, it may occur in organic disease of the stomach such as ulcer or cancer, in reflex disturbance of the stomach from disease of the gallbladder, appendix or other viscera, and when the pylorus or small intestine is obstructed. In pyloric stenosis there may be food remnants recognizable as several days old and in intestinal obstruction the vomitus may be faeculent due to bacterial invasion.

Vomiting must be distinguished from the regurgitation of food into the mouth (see Regurgitation, page 50). True vomiting implies the ejection of appreciable quantities of the stomach contents, sometimes consisting of undigested food, sometimes of partially digested food to which the gastric secretions have been added.

ANALYSIS OF SEVERE ABDOMINAL PAIN							
	Perforation	Appendicitis	Acute haemorrhagic pancreatitis	Gallbladder colic	Renal colic	Large-bowel obstruction (complete)	Small-bowel obstruction
Site	Epigastric	Umbilical	Epigastrium or right hypochondrium	Right hypochondrium and epigastrium	Loin	Hypogastric	Umbilical
Radiation	Whole abdomen and left shoulder	Right iliac fossa later	Back and whole abdomen	Right scapula	Towards groin	Flanks	Nil
Type	Sharp	Colicky, becoming constant	Constant	Colicky or continuous	Colicky	Colicky	Colicky
Severity	Very	Severe	Very severe	Very severe severe	Very severe	Severe	Severe
Onset and duration	Instant-aneous and persistent	Fairly rapid onset, many hours	Sudden and persistent hours	Sudden, lasting hours	Sudden, minutes to	Slow onset, lasting days	Fairly rapid onset, hours to days
Aggravating factors	Movement	Walking causing movement of the iliopsoas behind inflamed viscus	Nil	Nil	Jolting	Nil	Nil
Relieving factors	Nil	Nil	Nil	Nil	Nil	Nil	Nil
Associated symptoms	Shock and vomiting	Vomiting, fever	Vomiting and shock	Vomiting and sometimes fevers with rigors	Vomiting, frequency, haematuria	Constipation. Vomiting at a late stage	Vomiting
Physical signs	Board-like rigidity	Tenderness and guarding in right iliac fossa	Abdomen rigid after initial softness	Tenderness in right hypochondrium Transient jaundice	Nil	Flank distension, increased bowel sounds. Rectum ballooned and and empty	Central distension. Bowel sounds increased Rectum ballooned and empty
Investigations	Air under diaphragm seen on radiograph	Nil	Increased serum and urinary amylase	Cholecystogram or ultrasound may show calculus	Radiograph may show calculus	Intestinal fluid levels on radiograph	Intestinal fluid levels on radiograph

▲ Table 4.2

Special features

A note should be made of the following points:

1 *The relationship of the vomiting to any pain.* Note whether the pain precedes or follows the vomiting and at what interval.
2 *The time of day at which vomiting occurs.* In cases of pyloric stenosis, each meal adds to the gastric contents, and vomiting may not occur until the latter part of the day when a large quantity has accumulated. The vomiting of pregnancy and alcoholic gastritis occur characteristically in the mornings.
3 *The presence or absence of nausea.* Nausea generally precedes vomiting due to diseases of the digestive system, but in cases of increased intracranial pressure is often absent.

For details of the character of the vomitus, see page 69.

SYMPTOMS ASSOCIATED WITH INDIVIDUAL VISCERA: THE STOMACH AND DUODENUM

Both pain and vomiting are common in gastric and duodenal disease.

PAIN

In peptic ulceration pain is generally of the visceral type, localized in the epigastrium and confined to a small area irrespective of whether the ulcer is duodenal or gastric. The pain pathway is via the splanchnic nerves, but when the ulcer penetrates the mucosa and involves the peritoneum, cerebrospinal pathways may be implicated.

Muscle spasm and powerful peristaltic contractions are secondary rather than primary causes of the pain.

Tenderness on deep pressure over the ulcer may also be of direct visceral origin, but where tenderness is extreme and associated with muscular rigidity, then involvement of the parietal peritoneum should be suspected.

In cancer of the stomach, the pain is often more constant because of partial penetration of the stomach wall and involvement of the peritoneum.

Disease of other viscera, e.g. appendicitis and cholecystitis, may cause pain imitating that of a peptic ulcer (see also page 72).

VOMITING

This is a common but not invariable feature of organic disease of the stomach such as ulcer or neoplasm. Vomiting generally occurs after digestion has been in process for some time, often, also, when gastric pain is at its height. By relieving the tension of the hypertonic stomach wall it may diminish or abolish pain. Vomiting occurs especially when the pylorus is obstructed (see page 73), in which case the vomitus may be large in amount and, particularly in infants, projectile in character.

HAEMATEMESIS (VOMITING OF BLOOD)

This is most frequent in cases of peptic ulcer and is less commonly found in neoplasm of the stomach, where anaemia from chronic blood loss into the stool is more usual. A serious complication of hepatic cirrhosis is rupture of the oesophageal and gastric veins engorged as a result of portal hypertension. The amount of blood vomited varies from a mouthful to several litres. The exact amount is difficult to estimate as the blood is usually mixed with the gastric contents, which alter its colour and sometimes give the vomit a 'coffee-grounds' appearance. If the loss of blood is great, the general signs of haemorrhage will also be present. Substantial haematemesis can occur, even in patients without a chronic peptic ulcer, as a result of violent vomiting causing a breach in the gastric mucosa (Mallory–Weiss syndrome) from superficial erosions induced by a gastric irritant such as aspirin or from intestinal telangiectasia (Figure 4.10).

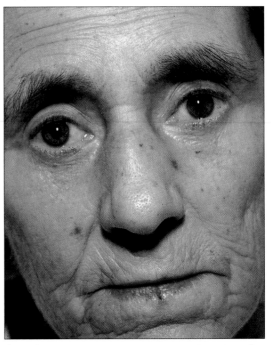

▲ Figure 4.10 Hereditary haemorrhagic telangiectasia on the face associated with intestinal lesions causing haematemesis

These three symptoms, pain, vomiting and hae-matemesis, are found usually in organic disease of the stomach, but pain and vomiting, like the symptoms now to be described, may also be found in reflex disturbances of the stomach function due to disease of other viscera, to misuse of alcohol, unsuitable diet, and to psychological causes.

NAUSEA

This is a sensation of sickness without actual vomiting, and is frequently accompanied by salivation, sweating and a feeling of faintness. It often results from psychic causes such as unpleasant sights or smells but also occurs in organic disease of the digestive system, notably carcinoma of the stomach. The possibility of drug-induced nausea should always be considered in patients receiving medicinal treatment. Vomiting of gastric origin is generally preceded by nausea.

FLATULENCE

The stomach or intestines may be distended with gas, and the patient then complains of 'wind' or 'flatulence' or in America 'gas'. The wind may be belched through the mouth or passed per rectum. Flatulence is common in many types of digestive disorder, but even more in functional than in organic disease. The gas in the great majority of cases of gastric flatulence is swallowed air (aerophagy). This may follow attempts to relieve epigastric discomfort from any cause, but frequent belching of large amounts of gas usually indicates compulsive air swallowing of psychogenic origin.

DISTURBANCE OF APPETITE

Loss of appetite or *anorexia* must be distinguished from a fear of eating because of peptic ulceration or painful conditions of the mouth or gullet. True anorexia is common as a temporary phenomenon and of little significance, but when it is persistent it is of great importance. It may then be caused by serious disease in many parts of the body, but is particularly common in local diseases of the stomach such as gastritis and carcinoma. General debilitating diseases such as tuberculosis and severe anaemias have a similar effect. Profound loss of appetite may be of psychogenic origin as in anorexia nervosa and in certain mental disorders. An aversion to particular kinds of food sometimes occurs, as in diseases of the liver and biliary system when fats are not tolerated.

Excessive appetite with compulsive eating between meals is common in certain anxiety states, especially in women, and can lead to considerable obesity (bul-laemia). Increased appetite of more moderate grade may be a feature of diseases where tissue waste is accelerated as in thyrotoxicosis and diabetes.

HEARTBURN, WATER BRASH AND ERUCTATIONS

These symptoms are often confused by the patient, who should therefore be asked to define clearly what he means by the terms.

Heartburn is a scalding or burning sensation experienced behind the sternum usually a little while after a meal or on stooping. In most cases, it is due to reflux of acid into the oesophagus especially when the pain threshold is lowered by oesophagitis (e.g. in hiatus hernia). However, it may also occur with reflux by duodenal juices containing bile and pancreatic enzymes.

Water brash consists in the filling of the mouth with a watery fluid composed of saliva. It is not necessarily a symptom of organic disease, but it may accompany the pain of duodenal ulcer or be due to reflex stimulation of saliva from gastrointestinal tract lesions.

Eructations of small amounts of the acid gastric contents along with flatus are common both in functional and organic disease of the stomach.

THE INTESTINES

Pain, constipation and diarrhoea are the most important symptoms caused by intestinal disease. Constipation and diarrhoea are even more common in temporary disturbances of health than in serious organic disease. As in the case of most gastrointestinal symptoms, persistence is a most significant point, because temporary constipation or diarrhoea rarely causes alarm except in acute abdominal disease.

PAIN

Pain is usually of the visceral type, vaguely localized and colicky in nature. It is almost certainly caused by increased tension on the intestinal musculature and exaggerated peristalsis, i.e. mechanical in origin. In gross intestinal obstruction where peristalsis is visible through the abdominal wall, the pain may be seen to coincide with the waves of peristalsis. Pain arising from the small intestine is generally situated in the centre of the abdomen. When the upper parts of the small intestine (jejunum) are affected, the pain is generally higher in the abdomen than when the lower parts are involved (ileum). Pain from the large intestine may also be experienced in the centre of the abdomen and left iliac fossa, but appears also to be common in the loins.

Possibly the latter pain is not truly visceral but due to irritant effects or dragging upon the neighbouring parietal peritoneum.

CONSTIPATION

In the average person evacuation of the bowels takes place once daily, but the event may occur twice daily or only once in 2 days in persons in good health. A sudden change in habit is significant.

The degree of constipation should be noted and precisely what the patient means by the term, e.g. less frequent evacuation or dry stools or small amounts, often pellets. In all forms of intestinal obstruction absolute constipation may take place without passage of faeces or gas. In partial intestinal obstruction incomplete constipation may occur. The patient finds he needs increasing quantities of purgatives, but the stools when passed are usually soft or liquid and may be modified in shape – e.g. the ribbon-shaped stool – if the constricted area is in the rectum. There is as a rule no difficulty in the passage of flatus in partial intestinal obstruction.

Intestinal obstruction is the most serious cause of constipation but by no means the commonest. Constipation may arise from a great variety of factors, such as improper or temporarily reduced diet, insufficient exercise, carelessness in habits and general ill health from disease in other parts of the body. It is important to distinguish between delay in the passage of faeces through the large bowel into the rectum due to a hold-up at or above the sigmoid (colonic 'spastic' constipation) and delay in emptying of the rectum itself. In the latter, the faeces may pass normally through the colon into the rectum, but, owing to neglect of the call to defaecation, they accumulate and cause distension of the rectum with loss of tone in its walls. This condition is called *dyschezia*, or rectal constipation, and as a result of it a greater amount of faeces is required to give the necessary sense of fullness which provokes the desire for defaecation. When faeces are retained in the bowel, water is absorbed so that the stool becomes hard and nodular and thus more difficult to evacuate. Rectal constipation, sometimes with impaction of faeces needing manual evacuation, is common in the elderly because of weakness of the pelvic musculature and, in some cases, difficulty in visiting the lavatory. Such patients often present with faecal incontinence due to pseudo-diarrhoea (see below).

DIARRHOEA

This symptom implies an increased frequency in evacuation of stools of liquid or semi-liquid character, not the discharge of mucus, blood or other abnormal constituents, though these may also be present. In most cases the stools are paler than normal, especially so in steatorrhoea, in which condition the stool also has a tendency to float in the pan and so is difficult to flush away.

Diarrhoea due to organic causes commonly occurs during the night and early morning as well as during the day. When diarrhoea is severe and persistent, the passage of frequent fluid stools may lead to physical exhaustion, dehydration with peripheral circulatory failure, the symptoms of potassium deficiency and protein loss (muscle weakness, oedema, etc.) and painful excoriation of the perianal skin.

The causes of diarrhoea include:

1 Those of temporary duration (a few hours to a few days), such as nervousness, allergic responses to food and drugs and acute infections, e.g. by Salmonella and other organisms.
2 More severe and prolonged infections such as bacillary and amoebic dysentery and intestinal tuberculosis which are more commonly seen in tropical zones. An acute form is exemplified by cholera with 'rice-water' stools containing enormous numbers of the vibrio.
3 Colonic diseases such as neoplasm, ulcerative colitis and irritable colon (page 76).
4 Toxic states such as poisoning with heavy metals, e.g. arsenic, or toxaemias such as uraemia.
5 The excessive use of purgatives or 'pseudo-diarrhoea' due to the liquefaction of impacted or obstructed faeces.
6 Endocrine causes including hyperthyroidism and gastrin-secreting tumours of the pancreas (Zollinger–Ellison syndrome).
7 Malabsorption syndromes such as coeliac disease and chronic pancreatitis.
8 Crohn's disease of the small or large intestine.

In separating these various causes several points must be considered, e.g. the position and character of any pain; the character of the stools; evidence of gastric, thyroid, pancreatic and malabsorption syndromes; pyrexia and exposure to infections. The presence of blood in the faeces may be noted by the patient and signifies organic rather than functional disease of the lower bowel.

TENESMUS

Tenesmus often accompanies diarrhoea and consists in straining with a desire to empty the lower bowel without evacuation taking place.

THE BILIARY TRACT

The special symptoms which need consideration in connection with the biliary tract are *pain* and *jaundice,* though many of the symptoms which have been described under the stomach may also be reflexly produced by disease in the gallbladder or bile ducts.

PAIN

A stone in the cystic or common bile duct causes pain due to the violent peristaltic movements of the wall of the duct attempting to force onwards a hard foreign body. It is not strictly a colicky pain as it is continuous rather than intermittent. It is felt in the epigastrium and right hypochondrium and is of such great intensity that the patient rolls about in agony, sweats and frequently vomits. In some cases the pain radiates to the angle of the right scapula. It is essentially visceral and lasts a few hours, but may be followed by a more localized pain in the right hypochondrium lasting several days. The latter is due to secondary cholecystitis and peritoneal involvement. This pain is associated with tenderness and rigidity on pressure and sometimes with fever or rigors.

JAUNDICE

Jaundice is a yellow pigmentation of the skin and mucous membranes caused by the presence in the blood of an excess of bile pigments. It is best seen in daylight. Jaundice may be due to increased production of bile pig-

ments, defective transport or conjugation of bilirubin within the liver cell or obstruction to the outflow of bile from the liver to the duodenum. Some knowledge of the biochemistry of bile pigments is essential for the proper understanding of jaundice.

In health *unconjugated bilirubin* (haemobilirubin) is water-insoluble and derived from the breakdown of red cells by the reticuloendothelial system. It passes, attached to plasma albumin, to the liver where it is conjugated with glucuronide and possibly other substances.

Conjugated bilirubin glucuronide (hepatobilirubin) is water-soluble and is the major constituent of bile, which passes into the intestine. There it is changed by bacterial action into urobilinogen; the major part is excreted in the faeces but some is reabsorbed to enter the liver and a small part absorbed into the general circulation to appear in the urine (Figure 4.11).

Prehepatic (haemolytic) jaundice

This form of jaundice is due to the presence in the blood of an excess of unconjugated bilirubin. Although haemolysis is the most important cause of prehepatic jaundice, it is now recognized that about 1 per cent of the population have a mild unconjugated hyperbilirubinaemia of an entirely benign nature – Gilbert's syndrome. The jaundice is often not clinically detectable, but may deepen during fasting or intercurrent illness, resulting in a mistaken diagnosis of hepatitis.

Haemolytic jaundice may result from an inherited abnormality in the red cells or from acquired causes.

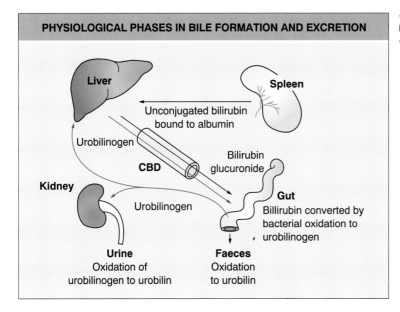

PHYSIOLOGICAL PHASES IN BILE FORMATION AND EXCRETION

Liver

Spleen

Unconjugated bilirubin bound to albumin

Urobilinogen

CBD

Bilirubin glucuronide

Kidney

Urobilinogen

Gut
Billirubin converted by bacterial oxidation to urobilinogen

Urine
Oxidation of urobilinogen to urobilin

Faeces
Oxidation to urobilin

◀ **Figure 4.11 Physiological phases in bile formation and excretion.** CBD = common bile duct

Since these forms of haemolysis are usually accompanied by anaemia, they are dealt with in Chapter 8 (page 196). Sometimes a breakdown of red cells, as in gross pulmonary infarction or incompatible blood transfusion, causes prehepatic jaundice without anaemia.

When the red cells themselves are abnormal, as in hereditary spherocytosis, thalassaemia and to a lesser extent in pernicious anaemia, the cells may become osmotically and mechanically more fragile and are thus destroyed by the reticuloendothelial system. There may be a history of previous attacks of jaundice or a family history of jaundice.

Auto-antibodies, neoplasia and certain virus infections may similarly cause acquired haemolytic jaundice.

In most forms of prehepatic jaundice, the skin and mucosae are delicately jaundiced (a lemon-yellow tint), but the urine and faeces remain normal in colour, though the urine may darken on standing due to oxidation of the excess urobilinogen.

Hepatocellular jaundice

This results from damage to the liver parenchyma interfering with the transport or conjugation of bilirubin and sometimes with its excretion through the canaliculi.

THE DIFFERENTIAL DIAGNOSIS OF JAUNDICE			
	Prehepatic (haemolytic)	**Hepatocellular**	**Posthepatic (obstructive)**
Mechanism	Increased bilirubin formation	Hepatocellular failure	Bile duct obstruction
Common cause	Haemolysis, Gilbert's syndrome	Virus hepatitis. Drugs, e.g. chlorpromazine. Chronic liver disease. Cirrhosis	Gallstones. Carcinoma of pancreas
Past history	May be previous attacks or a family history	Contact with similar case History of injections or of taking hepatotoxic drugs	May be previous attacks (stone)
Mode of development	Rapid, with anaemia and sometimes fever and rigors. Periodic attacks	After a period of anorexia and nausea; gradual onset and recovery	After an attack of pain Rapid and sometimes intermittent (stone). Insidious and progressive (carcinoma)
Pruritus (bile salt retention)	Absent	Occasional (if cholestasis). Primary biliary cirrhosis	Present
Skin colour	Faint lemon-yellow	Yellow	Brilliant or dark yellow
Urine	Colourless at first. Urobilinogenpresent; later by oxidation urobilin occurs and urine darkens slightly	Dark. (Bilirubin and urobilinogen)	Very dark. (Bilirubin; no urobilinogen)
Faeces Gallbladder	Normal Nil	Pale (if cholestasis) Nil	Pale May be palpable in carcinoma; not with stone
Enlarged spleen	Usually	Sometimes	Nil
Bilirubin	Unconjugated	Mixed	Conjugated
Serum alkaline phosphatase	Normal	Raised (if cholestasis)	Markedly raised
Tests for hepatocellular function	Normal	Grossly abnormal	Slightly abnormal
Tests for haemolysis	Positive	Negative	Negative

▲ Table 4.3

The commonest cause of hepatocellular jaundice is a virus hepatitis (see page 78), so that a history of transfusion, contact with another case or, in hospital workers, contact with the blood of a carrier may be obtained. Rarer infective causes include Weil's disease and yellow fever. The possibility of exposure to a medicinal liver toxin, such as chlorpromazine, testosterone, halothane or rifampicin, or an industrial one such as carbon tetrachloride, should always be considered. Hepatocellular jaundice also occurs in congestive cardiac failure and in the later stages of cirrhosis. When hepatic damage is accompanied by obstruction to the bile canaliculi *(cholestatic jaundice)*, the characteristics of the jaundice itself are similar to those described under post-hepatic obstruction (see below). The history of events preceding the jaundice, notably the prodromal period of anorexia and nausea in virus hepatitis, helps to differentiate the hepatocellular and posthepatic varieties (see Table 4.3). Liver function tests may also be helpful (see page 60).

Posthepatic (obstructive) jaundice

This form of jaundice results from obstruction to the bile ducts outside the liver. The common causes include gallstones, primary carcinoma of the head of pancreas or bile ducts, and secondary carcinomatous masses in the porta hepatis. When the obstruction is due to gallstones the jaundice is usually preceded by biliary colic and may be intermittent. Jaundice due to carcinoma tends to be insidious in onset and progressive in its course, and the gallbladder is sometimes palpable (see Figure 4.21, page 66). Obstructive jaundice varies in intensity from a slight yellowish tinge in the skin and mucous membranes to a pronounced canary yellow, or, in long-standing cases, a dark greenish-yellow discoloration. It affects the skin of the whole body (Figure 4.12), but is most marked on the trunk and proximal parts of the limbs. Even before the skin is affected, the yellowing is seen in the mucous membranes and should be sought in the conjunctivae and soft palate. Intolerable itching is common and is probably due to bile salts, as it may precede the actual pigmentation of the skin and mucosae. The excess of bile pigments (conjugated bilirubin) in the blood leads to their appearance in the urine, which may be visibly bile-stained or in which bile may be detected by special tests (see page 60). The lack of the normal flow of bile into the duodenum deprives the faeces of one of their colouring constituents and further interferes with the digestion and absorption of fats because of the lack of bile salts. As a result, the faeces have a lighter colour than normal and are often clay-coloured. In complete obstruction, urobilinogen is absent from the urine.

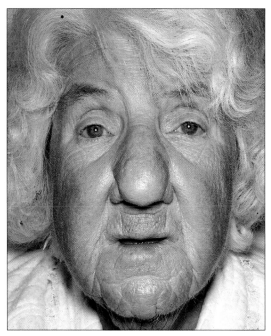

▲ **Figure 4.12 Yellow pigmentation of the skin and greenish yellow sclerae due to carcinoma of the bile ducts**

In conclusion, it must be stressed that more than one of the three types of jaundice can exist in the same patient. It has already been said that intrahepatic obstruction is common in hepatocellular jaundice, and obstruction due to pigment stones may also occur in haemolytic jaundice. Moreover, liver-cell dysfunction can result from the damming back of bile and ascending infection in obstructive jaundice. Laboratory investigations are therefore needed for the precise diagnosis of jaundice and for the differentiation of the three types.

BIOCHEMICAL TESTS

Biochemical tests of the blood and urine differentiate between the three types of jaundice (Table 4.4).

In prehepatic or haemolytic jaundice an excess of unconjugated bilirubin is formed in the blood but cannot pass into the urine as, unlike bilirubin glucuronide, it is unable to cross the glomerular membrane. However, the urine does contain an excess of urobilinogen derived from the increased quantity of bile pigments entering the bowel (see Table 4.3).

In posthepatic and hepatocellular jaundice bilirubin glucuronide is formed normally in the liver but seeps back into the blood because it cannot generally reach the bowel. It is then excreted in the urine, while the faeces are deprived of bile pigments.

URINE TESTING IN NORMAL AND JAUNDICED PATIENTS				
	Normal	**Prehepatic**	**Posthepatic**	**Hepatocellular**
Bilirubin	–	–	++	++
Urobilin	+	+++	–	++

◀ **Table 4.4**

In hepatocellular jaundice, *some* bile pigment will reach the intestine and be absorbed into the bloodstream, but the damaged liver cells cannot cope with it all and urobilinogen may then appear to excess in the urine which must be examined fresh.

The presence of jaundice, especially when doubtful or, in subclinical forms, can be confirmed by the finding of a raised *total serum bilirubin*, i.e. bilirubin and bilirubin glucuronide (see page 57). The relative proportions of these two forms of bilirubin may help to distinguish haemolytic from obstructive forms of jaundice.

Other tests used in the differential diagnosis of jaundice include measurement of the *serum alkaline phosphatase* which is generally higher in obstructive than hepatocellular jaundice and *tests for hepatocellular function* (see below) may be abnormal chiefly in hepatogenous jaundice. They are therefore useful in detection of liver damage in hepatitis, hepatic necrosis or cirrhosis.

The tests most commonly used today are dependent upon a derangement in those functions of the liver that relate to the metabolism of protein, the cellular enzymes and the excretion of foreign substances in the bile. Tests based upon the metabolism of proteins include measurement of the *serum albumin,* which may be decreased in liver disease, and the *serum globulin,* which is usually increased in active liver disease; the particular fraction of globulin which is increased can be identified by *electrophoresis.* The enzyme tests include the *serum alkaline phosphatase* (elevation of which indicates biliary obstruction rather than hepatocellular damage, see below), and the serum levels of the *transferases* and *dehydrogenases.* An increase in the serum levels of these two enzymes indicates that cell damage is permitting their leakage into the bloodstream. This increase is not specific to liver damage, since it also occurs in myocardial infarction, but a relatively greater increase in *ALT* (alanine-amino transferase) than in *AST* (aspartate-amino transferase) favours a hepatic cause. The gammaglutamyl transpeptidase (γGT) enzyme mirrors the alkaline phosphatase in cholestasis but does not rise in bone disease, it is therefore useful in distinguishing an elevated alkaline phosphatase of liver and bone origin. The γGT is also elevated by enzyme-inducing agents, particularly by alcohol; it is a useful guide to alcohol abuse even in the absence of hepatic damage. In this context the average size of circulating red cells (MCV) is valuable, being commonly elevated in alcoholism quite independent of folate or B_{12} deficiency.

ANATOMICAL CONSIDERATIONS

Before proceeding to the detailed examination of the abdomen, certain anatomical facts may be recalled. It is customary for purposes of clinical description to divide the abdomen into nine regions by two vertical and two horizontal lines. Each vertical line may be taken from the midclavicle to the midinguinal region. The upper horizontal line passes across the abdomen at the lowest point of the 10th costal arches. The lower horizontal line joins the two anterior superior spines of the ilia. The 'regions' thus marked out (Figure 4.13) are:

In the upper abdomen – the right hypochondrium, epigastrium and left hypochondrium.

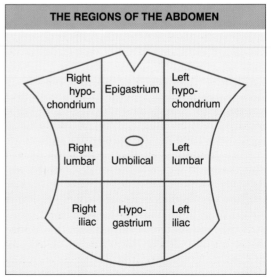

THE REGIONS OF THE ABDOMEN

Right hypo-chondrium	Epigastrium	Left hypo-chondrium
Right lumbar	Umbilical	Left lumbar
Right iliac	Hypo-gastrium	Left iliac

▲ **Figure 4.13 The regions of the abdomen**

In the middle – the right lumbar, umbilical and left lumbar.

In the lower abdomen – the right iliac fossa, hypogastrium and left iliac fossa.

Other lines are also in use, and it matters little which the student employs, as the division of the abdomen into regions is purely arbitrary and is of more clinical than anatomical value.

It must be emphasized that the main value of the regions is to describe the position of pain, tenderness, rigidity, tumours, etc. Lists of viscera contained in these regions are fallacious. The stomach, intestines and kidneys (and other viscera to a lesser extent) are so mobile that they are not constantly found in the same regions, even in the same individual, and in different normal individuals differ widely in position.

Some organs, however, are more or less fixed. The gallbladder is generally found in the right hypochondrium, the liver in the right hypochondrium and epigastrium, the spleen in the left hypochondrium. The hypogastrium contains the full bladder or pregnant uterus. Posture and respiration have a profound effect on the position of the viscera.

PHYSICAL SIGNS: EXAMINATION OF THE ABDOMEN

Examination of the abdomen should follow the routine described under the respiratory and cardiovascular systems – inspection, palpation, percussion and auscultation – though inspection and palpation are by far the most important methods of approach.

Inspection shows the condition of the abdominal wall, the size of the abdomen and any irregularity in its contour caused by enlargement of viscera or the presence of abnormal swellings in the abdominal cavity. It also shows certain motile phenomena such as the movement of the abdominal wall with respiration, the presence of visible peristalsis in the stomach or intestines and the pulsations of the aorta or an engorged liver. The external genitalia may be inspected at the same time (see page 89).

Palpation determines the presence of superficial or deep tenderness and of undue rigidity or laxity of the abdominal wall. It is the principal method by which the enlargement of viscera such as the liver, spleen and kidneys, and the presence of tumours and herniae, are detected.

Percussion may add confirmatory information in the case of enlarged viscera or tumours, and may help in recognizing the presence of free fluid in the peritoneal cavity. In cases of tympanites (gastrointestinal distension) the note on percussion is drum-like.

Auscultation is of special value in distinguishing between paralytic ileus, in which the abdomen is silent, and intestinal obstruction, in which the bowel sounds are increased.

INSPECTION

Inspection of the abdomen must be carried out in a good light and if possible with the patient both in the erect and recumbent postures.

Condition of the abdominal wall

The skin of the abdomen should first be observed for scars. Traditional surgical scars indicate the likely type of surgery (Figure 4.14) but minimal access laparoscopic scars (Figure 4.15) should lead to specific enquiry as to the type of surgery performed which may be much more extensive than is evident. When abdominal distension is present from any cause, the skin is stretched, smooth and shiny, and the umbilicus may be flattened or even everted (Figure 4.16). In obese subjects the abdomen may appear distended, but the umbilical cleft is deeper than normal. Undue laxity of the abdominal wall, causing wrinkling of the skin, is found when intra-abdominal pressure is suddenly

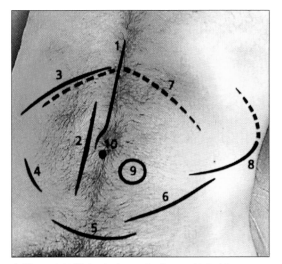

▲ **Figure 4.14 Abdominal incisions.** (Reproduced from *Clinical Examination of the Patient* by John Lumley and Pierre-Marc G. Bouloux, Butterworth–Heinemann, 1994)

1 Upper midline
2 Right paramedian
3 Kocher's incision
4 Appendicular grid iron incision
5 Suprapubic incision
6 Left iliac muscle cutting incision
7 Roof-top incision
8 Nephrectomy incision
9 Incision for terminal colostomy
10 Entry point for laparoscopic telescope

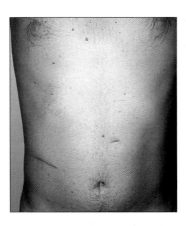

◀ **Figure 4.15 Laparoscopic scars**

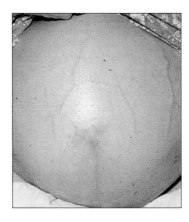

◀ **Figure 4.16 Ascites.** Note eversion of umbilicus

decreased, as after childbirth (especially in multi-parae), and after removal of fluid from the peritoneal cavity. After repeated pregnancies or loss of weight in a previously obese subject, broad silvery lines or 'stretch marks' appear on the abdominal wall. Similar marks, often purple in colour, are also seen in Cushing's syndrome (see Chapter 12).

Enlarged veins are useful evidence of obstruction in the inferior vena caval or portal systems. The greater the distension and the more numerous the veins, the greater the obstruction is likely to be.

Obstruction in the inferior vena cava or common iliac veins usually causes veins to appear at the sides of the abdomen (Figure 4.17), and when the veins are emptied by pressure with the fingers, they will be seen to fill again from below. The blood bypasses the inferior vena cava, travelling from the lower limbs (and certain viscera) to the thorax via the veins of the abdominal wall. These superficial veins are arranged longitudinally. Thrombosis of the inferior vena cava, owing to its completeness in obstructing the circulation, will cause the

most pronounced collateral circulation to become apparent on the abdominal wall, but any increase in the intra-abdominal pressure (e.g. ascites) will have a similar though less striking result.

If the obstruction is in the portal system (cirrhosis of the liver, or more rarely thrombosis of the portal vein), the engorged veins are centrally placed and may form a little cluster around the umbilicus (caput medusae). The blood in these veins flows in all directions away from the umbilicus. The direction of the blood flow should always be tested.

A section of vein can be emptied by 'milking' it with the fingers, and each end of the emptied part is sealed with the pressure of a finger. One finger can then be removed and the rate at which the vein fills is noted. The performance is repeated, removing the finger at the other end. The blood enters more rapidly from the direction of the blood flow.

Secondary nodules may be found in the skin in certain types of malignant disease (Figure 4.18). Oedema of the abdominal wall may be demonstrated by the usual

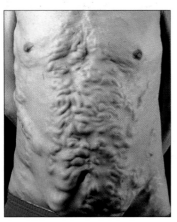

◀ **Figure 4.17 Enlarged abdominal veins in inferior venal caval obstruction**

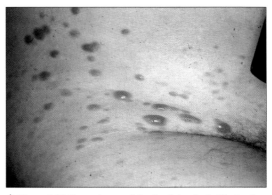

▲ **Figure 4.18 Secondary nodules in abdominal skin due to carcinoma of the gallbladder**

phenomenon of pitting (best elicited by pinching a fold of the abdominal wall), and has the same origin as oedema elsewhere. It is not to be confused with the presence of fluid in the peritoneal cavity itself (ascites). Small herniae due to extrusion of pieces of extraperitoneal fat are not uncommonly seen in the midline of the upper abdomen. They are usually symptomless. Larger herniae may be seen at or near the umbilicus or protruding through abdominal scars.

Movements of the abdominal wall

The movements of the abdominal wall should be carefully watched. In men with the abdominal type of respiration the movement should be free and equal on the two sides. In women the movement is often restricted owing to the costal type of breathing. An absolute fixation of the whole or greater part of the abdominal wall is a most important sign of generalized peritonitis. Unequal movement of the two sides of the abdomen may be seen in cases of phrenic paralysis.

Contour of the abdomen

The contour of the abdomen should next be noted. When abnormal swelling is present it is important to observe whether it is uniform or asymmetrical. Uniform swelling may be caused by obesity, by distension of the abdomen by gas in the gastrointestinal tract or by fluid in the peritoneal cavity. Large abdominal tumours such as an overfilled bladder, pregnant uterus or large ovarian cyst (Figure 4.19) cause swelling of the abdomen which at first glance may appear uniform, but which closer inspection shows to be limited to the contour of the enlarged viscus or tumour.

Irregularities in the contour of the abdomen may be caused by enlargement of viscera such as the liver, spleen, kidneys, or gallbladder, or by tumours arising from these and other organs, e.g. the stomach, intestines, pancreas or peritoneum (Figure 4.20). Distension of one portion of the alimentary tract may also produce irregularity in the abdominal contour, e.g. gastric distension producing a bulge in the epigastrium or colonic distension causing a fullness in the flanks. The type and degree of irregularity in the contour of the abdominal wall will depend upon the size, shape and irregularity of the underlying swelling.

Movements beneath the abdominal wall

Visible pulsation of the abdominal aorta is frequent in nervous individuals, especially in those with a thin abdominal wall, and must be distinguished from aneurysm of the abdominal aorta. In this condition the pulsation is usually more marked, and it is generally possible by palpation to define the outline of an enlarged expansile arterial swelling. Often aortic pulsation is transmitted through an overlying viscus or tumour. For example, the aorta may cause pulsation of a carcinoma of the stomach, which must then be differentiated from aneurysm. In these cases of transmitted pulsation the pulsating tumour is usually irregular, and its pulsations may cease if the patient is examined in the knee–elbow position, so that the tumour falls away from the underlying aorta. The enlargement of mobile organs such as the liver and spleen or a tumour in the stomach may be revealed as a downward-moving ripple beneath the skin when the patient breathes in.

Peristalsis may be visible in cases of obstruction in the gastrointestinal tract. Obstruction at the pylorus causes increased peristaltic movements of the stomach, seen through the abdominal wall as a slow wave moving from left to right across the upper abdomen. Obstruction in the large intestine may also be accom-

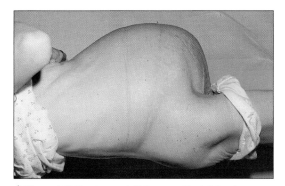

▲ **Figure 4.19 Ovarian cyst.** Note generalized distension apparently arising from the pelvis

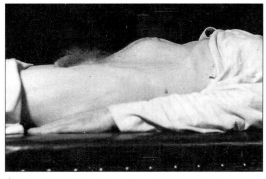

▲ **Figure 4.20 Abdominal swelling due to mesenteric cyst.** The curve of the swelling has a fairly steep rise at the pubis and in the epigastrium, and obviously occupies chiefly the central abdomen. (See for comparison Figure 5.4, page 89, Distended bladder)

panied by peristaltic waves in the upper abdomen, in this case moving from right to left. In obstruction of the small intestine the peristaltic waves may be seen in a ladder pattern down the centre of the abdomen. Such movements can be induced by gentle kneading of the abdomen, by applying a cold stimulus to the skin or by giving the patient soda-water to drink.

Intestinal peristalsis may be observed especially in elderly women with a lax abdominal wall but no organic disease.

PALPATION

Successful palpation needs much practice. The most favourable posture for the patient is lying flat on his back with the head slightly raised (one pillow), the arms to the side, and the knees extended. When the abdominal muscles are held tense it may be helpful to draw up the patient's knees. The blankets should be folded well out of the way and the edge of the sheet drawn across the groins to cover the genitalia until they are examined. The patient should be asked to breathe quietly and rather more deeply than normal, keeping the mouth open to encourage the abdominal type of respiration. When the examiner is satisfied that the abdomen is moving freely, palpation may begin, using the flat hand but exerting pressure with the fingers. The fingertips should be used only after the flat hand has first been employed, and then only under special circumstances, as the discomfort caused by their use leads to reflex spasm of the abdominal wall, which prevents satisfactory examination. Each region of the abdomen is examined in turn, very light palpation being used first to locate areas of tenderness or guarding. The following points should be systematically observed:

Tenderness

Tenderness means pain on pressure. Deep tenderness is most commonly found in inflammatory lesions of the viscera and their surrounding peritoneum. Tenderness, for example, in the right iliac fossa is frequently found in appendicitis, tenderness in the right hypochondrium in cholecystitis, and epigastric tenderness in peptic ulceration with peritoneal involvement, while purely visceral pain such as gastric or intestinal colic is not associated with any tenderness. Occasionally pressure in one region of the abdomen may cause pain in another. For example, pressure in the left iliac fossa sometimes causes pain in the right, in cases of appendicitis. This is the exception rather than the rule and is probably explained by transmission of the pressure to the right iliac fossa, e.g. through the colon. Tenderness is usually found over the region where the inflamed viscus is lying. If an area of

tenderness is expected, the palpating hand should first be placed on the abdomen in some region distant from the suspected area. In appendicitis, for example, palpation should begin in the left iliac fossa, which, being normal, will form a contrast to the tenderness in the right iliac fossa.

Closely allied to deep tenderness are *cutaneous hyperaesthesia* and *tenderness in the superficial tissues* of the abdominal wall.

All forms of tenderness may be found in neurotic individuals who have no local abdominal disease. As a temporary phenomenon *tympanites* (distension of the gastrointestinal tract with gas) may also give rise to tenderness.

Guarding and rigidity

Abdominal guarding is due to muscular contraction, which often occurs reflexly as a part of a defence mechanism over an inflamed organ. This has already been discussed.

Some patients hold the abdominal wall so tightly that examination is difficult or impossible, but in the majority, if the patient is put in a comfortable position and his mind set at rest by explaining that no undue pain will be caused by the examination, the abdominal muscles gradually relax. Nervous guarding of this type generally affects the whole abdominal wall. So also does the contraction of the abdominal muscles if the patient raises his head to satisfy his curiosity about the examination. Localized guarding is therefore more suggestive of disease. The notable exception to this is the case of acute generalized peritonitis in which there occurs a true generalized rigidity of the abdominal wall which cannot be relaxed ('board-like' rigidity).

As in the examination for tenderness, the palpating hand should first test the abdominal muscles in some part away from the suspected lesion. For example, if cholecystitis is suspected, palpation should begin in the left hypochondrium, which then forms a standard of control to the rigidity in the right hypochondrium. The bellies of the rectus muscles sometimes cause difficulty in the examination of the abdomen. Portions of them may be so prominent as to simulate a lump beneath the abdominal wall, and it is important to compare carefully the two recti. If the rectus muscles are brought into use, such a 'tumour' becomes more pronounced. In some patients, on the other hand, the rectus muscles are so poorly developed and toneless that the hand can palpate through them with the same ease as through other portions of the abdominal wall. In perfectly healthy individuals it is not uncommon to find separation of the rectus muscles producing a wide gap in which the abdominal wall is so thin that the viscera beneath can be palpated more distinctly than normal (divarication of the recti).

Enlargement of viscera

The liver

Palpation of the liver is made by resting the flat of one or both hands on the abdomen with the tips of the fingers gently inserted beneath the costal margin. To avoid overlooking gross enlargement it is advisable to move the hand from the right iliac fossa gradually upwards until any increased sense of resistance is noted. At this point the fingertips may be used to locate the liver edge accurately (Figure 4.21(a)). The liver in a healthy subject may sometimes be felt 1–2 cm below the costal margin during inspiration but in certain diseases can extend well into the right iliac fossa. For this method of palpation, the examiner has to sit on the edge of the bed. An alternative method is to place the right hand across the abdomen and to seek the liver edge with the radial border of the index finger (Figure 4.21(b)).

The *character of the edge* should be recorded. When palpable in health it is sharp, firm and regular, gradually passing upwards as it crosses the epigastrium into the left hypochondrium. Deformities of the chest (e.g. kyphoscoliosis; emphysema) are sometimes responsible for displacing the liver downwards so that it appears to be enlarged. In infants also the liver is relatively large and may be palpable in health.

An unusual tongue of liver substance, Riedel's lobe, may occasionally give rise to difficulty. It is sometimes freely mobile and may be mistaken for a movable kidney, or, if situated nearer the middle line, for a gallbladder swelling. It is almost invariably in the right upper quadrant of the abdomen.

When the liver is enlarged from fatty changes, its edge is soft and difficult to feel, especially in an obese person. Fortunately, this type of enlargement, though common. is rarely an important point in the diagnosis. In most other forms of liver enlargement the edge is firm or even harder than normal. Thus in passive congestion of the liver due

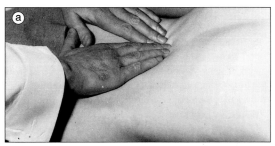

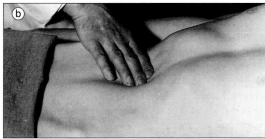

▲ **Figure 4.21 Palpation of liver.** (a) Both hands are placed flat on the abdomen with the fingers directed towards the costal margin and gradually moved upwards until resistance is encountered. The patient then takes a deep breath and the edge of the liver rides over the fingers. (b) An alternative method

CAUSES OF HEPATIC ENLARGEMENT	
Tender enlargement	**Painless enlargement**
Rapid distension from any cause (e.g venous congestion in cardiac failure)	Biliary obstruction (e.g. stone, carcinoma, cholestatic hepatitis)
Acute inflammation (e.g. virus and amoebic hepatitis)	Cirrhosis (e.g. posthepatitis, billiary, cardiac)
Hepatic abscess (e.g. portal pyaemia and virus and amoebic hepatitis)	Malignant disease (e.g. secondary carcinoma, primary hepatoma) Haemopoietic disease (e.g. Hodgkin's disease, leukaemia) Chronic infections (e.g. malaria) Amyloidosis (e.g. chronic suppuration, rheumatoid arthritis) Infiltrations (e.g. fatty liver, lipoidoses, sarcoidosis)

▲ **Table 4.5**

to cardiac failure the edge is firmer than normal, while in malignant disease it may be very hard and irregular.

The *surface of the liver* should next be palpated. In cancerous infiltration it may be grossly irregular owing to the presence of large nodules. The nodularity is clinically less obvious, however, in micronodular cirrhosis. Gross nodularity of the liver in a patient with cirrhosis suggests hepatoma. In most other forms of liver enlargement (see Table 4.5) the surface of the organ is quite smooth.

The *degree of enlargement* also gives useful information. In the congestion of heart failure, for example, the size of the liver is often roughly proportional to the degree of cardiac failure, and its shrinkage is a useful indication of the response to treatment. In moderate degrees of heart failure the liver edge extends 5–8 cm below the costal margin, but in tricuspid incompetence it may reach the level of the umbilicus or lower. Such gross enlargement of the liver is also common in cancer, amyloidosis, amoebic abscess and certain blood diseases. Moderate enlargement of the liver occurs in obstruction of the common bile duct (e.g. with gallstones) and in infective hepatitis. In cirrhosis, the liver is usually enlarged but later shrinks in advanced cirrhosis, especially in the macronodular variety.

It should be noted whether the liver is tender or painless on palpation. Tenderness is often found in the congested liver of heart failure and in inflammatory lesions, e.g. hepatitis and liver abscess, while the gross enlargements of cancer and other diseases may remain quite painless. (See Table 4.5.)

Finally, the presence of pulsation should be sought, especially in patients with signs of congestive cardiac failure. Pulsation of the liver suggests incompetence of the tricuspid valve (see page 143).

The gallbladder

In obstruction of the cystic duct, commonly by stone, or of the common bile duct, particularly by growth of the head of the pancreas, enlargement of the gallbladder may be found. The organ is felt as a smooth tense swelling projecting beneath the right costal margin in the direction of the umbilicus. If the enlargement is great, the swelling may be mistaken for another viscus – for example an enlarged right kidney. Moderate degrees of enlargement may be obscured if the gallbladder is covered by the liver. A distended gallbladder in the presence of jaundice is due to some cause other than gallstones (generally to carcinoma of the head of the pancreas). This is known as Courvoisier's law (Figure 4.22), but, as with all 'laws' in medicine, exceptions do occur. It is explained by the fact that gallstones, if present for a considerable time, cause fibrosis of the gallbladder. Thus when a stone is later impacted in the common bile duct, jaundice results, but the gallbladder is less likely to expand than in the case of a healthy gallbladder proximal to a malignant obstruction.

The colon

The colon may be palpable as a sausage-shaped tumour when distended with gas or faeces. In normal subjects the descending colon can often be felt as a firm tube in the left iliac fossa and sometimes the caecum can also be palpated (the characteristics of colonic tumour are described below).

The palpation of other enlarged abdominal viscera, e.g. the kidneys and spleen, not directly connected with the digestive tract, will be dealt with under the appropriate system.

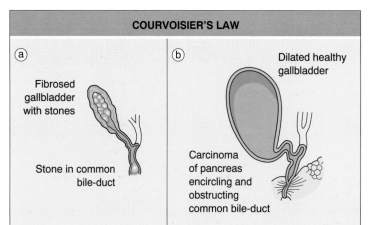

COURVOISIER'S LAW

(a) Fibrosed gallbladder with stones

Stone in common bile-duct

(b) Dilated healthy gallbladder

Carcinoma of pancreas encircling and obstructing common bile-duct

◀ **Figure 4.22 Courvoisier's law.** (a) Jaundice caused by a gallstone in the common duct. The gallbladder cannot dilate as it is fibrosed from cholecystitis due to stones within it. (b) Jaundice due to obstruction of the common bile duct by carcinoma of the head of the pancreas. The gallbladder is dilated owing to the back-pressure of the bile

Abdominal tumour

On detection of a tumour in the abdomen the following points should be observed.

Position

An accurate description of the position often helps to decide the organ from which the tumour is growing, and when its outline has been defined, the observer should consider what organs and tissues lie in this region of the abdomen. The localization of tumours is sometimes difficult owing to the fact that only a small portion may present at the abdominal wall, and the bulk of the tumour may be impalpable because of its deep situation. When a tumour does not lie in the region of a particular viscus, the possibility of a peritoneal origin should be considered. Malignant or inflammatory masses may, for example, be distributed irregularly in the omentum or mesentery, and in the latter cysts also occur. Care should be taken also to exclude the possibility of the tumour arising from the abdominal wall. In this case modifications of the shape and size of the tumour can be produced by making the patient move the abdominal muscles.

Size

The larger the tumour, the more difficult it is to determine the tissue from which it is growing, but certain tumours by their very size (e.g. an ovarian cyst, which forms a large round swelling in the lower abdomen) give a valuable clue to their nature (see Figure 4.19).

Consistency

Some organs and tissues, e.g. the stomach, intestines and bladder, are normally impalpable unless they are distended respectively by gas, intestinal contents or urine. The consistency of organs such as the liver and spleen may help to distinguish a simple enlargement of these viscera from enlargement due to neoplastic infiltration. Most malignant tumours are hard and irregular.

Shape

In the early stages a tumour may correspond in shape with the viscus from which it is arising. This is especially so in the case of the kidney and spleen. As the tumour grows larger, the characteristic shape is often lost and therefore gives no information as to its origin.

Mobility

Tumours of the stomach, transverse colon, liver, gallbladder, kidneys and spleen generally move downwards with the diaphragm during inspiration, but tumours of the pancreas, the para-aortic lymph nodes and the viscera in the lower abdomen (bladder, uterus, descending colon, caecum, etc.), upon which respiratory movements have little effect, are usually immobile.

Ability to get above or below the tumour

It is sometimes possible to define the upper border of an enlarged kidney or a pyloric tumour, but not in the case of an enlarged liver or spleen. Likewise in the pelvis, the hand may reach below a tumour of the colon but not below an enlarged uterus or bladder.

Masses in the upper abdomen are at times partially obscured by the costal margins and lie in the hollows of the diaphragmatic domes. They may be more accurately delineated by putting the patient (after suitable explanation) over a 'bridge' made by placing a pillow in the concavity of the lumbar spine. This manoeuvre may enable one 'to get above' a tumour.

Fluid in the peritoneal cavity

When free fluid is present in the peritoneal cavity, palpation of enlarged viscera is difficult, but the edge of the enlarged organ, e.g. the liver or spleen, may be felt by dipping or ballotting. This method of palpation is performed by a quick pressure of the tips of the fingers over the region where the edge of the viscus is expected. The pressure displaces the fluid temporarily and allows the fingers to come in contact with the enlarged viscus (Figure 4.23).

The *fluid thrill* is also used to detect the presence of free fluid. The observer places one hand flat on one flank and with the fingers of the other hand gives a sharp tap

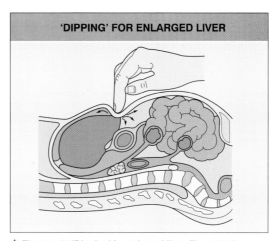

'DIPPING' FOR ENLARGED LIVER

▲ **Figure 4.23 'Dipping' for enlarged liver.** The palpating fingers prod sharply over the expected enlarged viscus, the fluid is displaced as shown by the arrows, and the fingers strike the surface or edge of the organ. Note also the gas-containing intestines which float to the surface and give a central area of resonance on percussion

on the opposite flank. This produces a wave in the fluid which is detectable by the palpating hand. A similar sensation may be obtained if the abdominal wall is very fat, and to avoid this a second person should place the edge of his hand along the linea alba, exerting firm pressure so as to damp out any vibrations in the abdominal wall itself (Figure 4.24). (See also Percussion, below.)

The hernial rings

The superficial inguinal rings should be examined in every case and evidence of herniation should also be sought in the epigastric and umbilical areas. This is particularly necessary in any case that suggests intestinal obstruction, of which strangulation of an inguinal or femoral hernia is quite a common cause. In the male, when no hernia is visible on standing, a finger should be inserted through the invaginated scrotum into the external abdominal ring and the patient asked to cough. Small herniae can be detected in this way as they give a forcible impulse to the palpating finger.

RECTAL EXAMINATION AND PROCTOSCOPY

Examination of the rectum is employed for many purposes and is mentioned more fully in Chapter 5. In the examination of the digestive tract it is used to determine the tone of the anal sphincter, the presence of any haemorrhoids, the condition of emptiness or fullness of the rectum, and, above all, the presence of any new growth in the rectum itself or any tumour of the surrounding

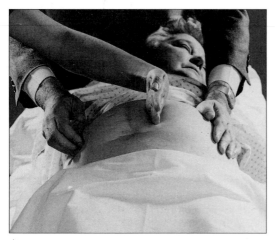

▲ **Figure 4.24 The fluid thrill.** The nurse's hand is placed firmly along the linea alba. The observer places one hand flat on the flank, while the fingers of the other percuss on the opposite flank

tissues which may press on or obstruct the rectum. 'Ballooning' of the rectum suggests obstruction at the junction of the sigmoid colon and rectum.

The small amount of faeces obtained on the glove or fingerstall after rectal examination may be enough to provide for certain quick observations. The colour may confirm pale stools in steatorrhoea, bright blood in rectal haemorrhage or melaena from higher intestinal bleeding. Tests for occult blood, microscopy for ova, and examination under ultraviolet light in cases of porphyria variegata are examples.

Fuller details of faecal characteristics are given later (pages 70–2).

PERCUSSION

Percussion has only a limited use in the examination of the alimentary system. However, it is important in delineating the upper border of the liver, usually at the level of the fifth or sixth right intercostal spaces in the midclavicular line, thus distinguishing an enlarged liver from one that is merely displaced downwards by overinflated lungs. Light percussion as a rule gives more information than heavy and is of most value in helping to elucidate the cause of abdominal enlargement. Uniform enlargement caused by gastrointestinal distension with gas yields a tympanitic note, whilst a similar enlargement caused by fluid yields a dull note, which may be present all over the abdomen if the fluid is large in amount, or only in the flanks if the fluid is insufficient to cover the centrally placed coils of intestine (Figure 4.23). When fluid is suspected, percussion should be performed first with the patient lying on his back and then lying alternately on each side. This movement will lead to a displacement of the fluid into the flank nearest the bed, over which a dull note will be obtained, whilst the empty upper flank will yield a tympanitic note. This phenomenon is known as shifting dullness. Care must be taken to percuss a strictly comparable site on each side of the abdomen: with the patient recumbent the percussion may start centrally and continue laterally until dullness appears. Percussion must take place with the finger running the length of the abdomen parallel to the level present in the flank (Figure 4.25).

Percussion may be used as an accessory method to palpation in defining the outline of enlarged viscera or abdominal tumours. The nearer the viscus or tumour lies to the abdominal wall, the more definite will be the results of percussion. An enlarged spleen, over which the percussion note is dull, can thus be distinguished from an enlarged left kidney over which the percussion note is resonant because of intervening colon. The lower edge of the liver can also be detected by percussing the

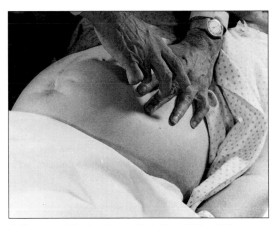

▲ **Figure 4.25 Ascites demonstrated by shifting dullness.** Note how the struck finger is parallel to the long axis of the abdomen and hence the fluid level

abdomen from the right iliac fossa up towards the costal margin. When the liver is either enlarged or displaced downwards, a dull note is elicited at some point below the costal margin. In the case of downward displacement, the upper border of liver dullness will be lower than normal.

AUSCULTATION

In cases of paralytic ileus due to peritonitis or other causes, the absence of the normal sounds due to peristaltic activity may be a suggestive sign, but it may be necessary to listen for several minutes. In peritonitis, the sounds disappear first in the neighbourhood of the lesion. On the other hand, in obstructive lesions of the gastrointestinal tract the sounds may be greatly exaggerated *(borborygmi)* and sometimes have a high-pitched tinkling note. Their intensity corresponds with waves of pain.

When the pylorus is obstructed gastric contents are retained for longer than 3 or 4 hours after a meal. A 'succussion splash' can then be elicited by palpation over the stomach or by gently rolling the patient from side to side.

Auscultation of the abdomen may also reveal sounds of vascular origin. A systolic murmur suggests narrowing of an artery by atheroma or, more rarely, by tumour (e.g. pancreatic carcinoma invading the splenic artery to give a systolic murmur radiating towards the left side). Systolic murmurs in the lower abdomen or groins usually originate in the aorta or iliac arteries; those in the upper abdomen may indicate narrowing of superior mesenteric vessels but can be referred from the heart. More continuous murmurs are sometimes heard, especially in the upper abdomen. These can arise from vas-

cular tumours such as hepatoma or hypernephroma. They may also occur in the form of a venous hum, increasing on inspiration, over porto-systemic anastomoses in patients with portal obstruction.

EXAMINATION OF THE GASTROINTESTINAL CONTENTS

The naked-eye inspection of vomited material or of the gastric contents removed by the stomach tube, and of the stools, often helps in the diagnosis of gastrointestinal diseases. The more detailed analyses of the gastric contents and of the faeces by microscopical and chemical tests are mentioned later, under Special investigations.

VOMITUS

Instruction should be given to the nurse or whoever is in charge of the patient to save any vomited material. This should be examined for its quantity, odour, colour and reaction, and for the presence of normal and abnormal constituents.

QUANTITY

The vomit may be large in quantity if there is delay in the passage of the food through the pylorus, especially when this is due to pyloric carcinoma, and the gastric contents increase throughout the day to be vomited in the afternoon or evening. In organic lesions causing pyloric obstruction the food is frequently undigested, and the nature of the last meal should always be ascertained so that undigested articles of diet may be recognized.

ODOUR

Most vomit possesses a sour odour due to the acid present, but offensiveness usually indicates serious disease, e.g. malignant disease of the pylorus due to excessive fermentation in the retained gastric contents. It occurs late in intestinal obstruction, when the vomit may have a faeculent odour.

COLOUR AND CONSTITUENTS

The colour of the vomit varies considerably with the length of time the food has been in the stomach, with the amount of duodenal regurgitation, and with the presence of abnormal constituents. *Blood* may give it a bright-red appearance if vomiting occurs soon after the haemorrhage, but usually the blood remains in the stomach sufficiently long to be altered to a dark brown colour – 'coffee-grounds' due to acid haematin (see

Haematemesis, page 54). *Bile* is a normal constituent, giving a yellowish or greenish appearance to the vomit, but it may be excessive in disease such as intestinal obstruction and absent in pyloric stenosis. In certain phases of intestinal obstruction the vomit may consist very largely of bile, later being replaced by a thin brownish fluid derived from the small intestine and recognized only by a faeculent odour. *Mucus* is identified by its jelly-like appearance and is present in small amounts in most vomit. In large amounts it suggests inflammation of the gastric mucosa – chronic gastritis. Rarer constituents of vomit are *pus*, which may be swallowed or derived from some extrinsic abscess, pieces of new growth, and various parasites and ova. These constituents usually require microscopy for their recognition. The presence of food items ingested days earlier is diagnostic of pyloric stenosis.

THE FAECES

A simple examination of the stools should never be omitted when the patient has symptoms of alimentary disease.

The faeces are made up of voluminous soap gels, residues of intestinal secretions, excretions and innumerable bacteria, many of them dead. Normally the only food residues are remnants of muscle fibre and the rough debris of vegetables, for practically all the food is digested and absorbed by the time it reaches the ileocaecal valve.

The *quantity, odour, colour, consistency and presence or absence of abnormal constituents* should be systematically noted.

QUANTITY
This varies considerably in different individuals and by type of diet; it is usually about 100–200 g daily in one or two motions. It may be considerably increased by undigested food, as in the bulky stools of certain types of pancreatic disease and malabsorption syndromes as well as a high residue diet (see Table 4.6, page 74).

ODOUR
A certain degree of offensiveness is normal, due to the presence of indol and skatol, constituents which are more plentiful when the diet contains much meat. When offensiveness is excessive some derangement of digestion or absorption should be suspected, though it may only be temporary and have no serious significance. Putrefaction of protein, such as may occur in pancreatic disease, gives a musty smell; carbohydrate fermentation produces 'acids of fermentation' and the rancid smell of butyric acid.

COLOUR
The colour also varies with the type of diet. In persons on a milk diet the stools are canary yellow in colour; in those taking much meat they are dark. In an average mixed diet the stools are usually of a light brown colour. Certain articles of diet, such as wines, fruit and stout, may cause darkening of the stools, as may medicinal preparations, especially those containing iron or bismuth. When peristalsis is excessive and the intestinal contents are hurried downwards, bile gives a yellowish-green or greenish appearance to the faeces. When bile pigments do not reach the intestine, the stools become clay coloured. In steatorrhoea the stools are pale and yellow owing to increased fat content. Blood is found in the stools in two forms: first, bright-red blood in small or large amounts derived from the large intestine, especially in its lower parts (e.g. haemorrhoids, cancer and polyps of the lower bowel); secondly, altered blood originating from the stomach or small intestine and partially digested on its way down, so that it gives the stool a dark tarry appearance – melaena (e.g. from gastric and duodenal ulcer). Small amounts of blood may not be visible on inspection but can be shown by tests for occult blood. The combination of melaena and steatorrhoea, as caused by a bleeding carcinoma of the ampulla of Vater, produces a characteristic 'silver stool' known as a 'flash in the pan'!

CONSISTENCY
The normal stool has a pultaceous consistency. It should be sufficiently soft for it to be moulded by the intestinal tube, the shape of which it retains. If too soft it may have the liquid or semi-liquid consistency of a diarrhoeic stool (see Diarrhoea, page 56). If the stool is unusually hard it may form rounded masses called *scybala*. In extreme cases of constipation these scybalous masses may be very dry owing to the great absorption of water from them during their prolonged stay in the large intestine.

ABNORMAL CONSTITUENTS
Many of these are more easily recognized by microscopical examination and may cause considerable difficulty to the inexperienced observer.

Faeces may be abnormal either because normal constituents are absent (e.g. stercobilin, derived from bile pigments) or because abnormal constituents are present (e.g. undigested food constituents, blood, serum, pus, mucus, parasites). *Mucus* occurs in two forms: as small flakes, intimately mixed with the faeces (usually due to inflammation), and as jelly-like masses either coating the surface of a hard faecal mass, or appearing separately as a cast or membrane (irritable colon). The recognition of *blood* has already been mentioned in describing colour of the stools, but unaltered blood may be passed without any faecal material. Excess of translucent *starch granules,* which stain blue with iodine, suggests failure of carbohydrate digestion. Excess of *fats* is recognized by the light, greasy nature of the stool and generally indicates failure of fat digestion through insufficiency of bile or pancreatic secretion or impaired absorption from the small intestine. This type of stool may be associated with visible grease or fat floating in the lavatory. However, it should be noted that 20 per cent of normal people have colonic bacterial flora producing sufficient hydrogen and methane to cause the stool to float. Failure of protein digestion may lead to the presence of undigested *meat fibres,* which, though generally recognized through the microscope, may appear as light brown threads in the stool (see also Table 4.6, page 74). *Pus* may appear in masses separate from the faeces, especially when it is derived from an extrinsic abscess bursting into the intestine. It is more intimately mixed with the stool in ulcerative conditions of the bowel such as malignant disease and ulcerative colitis.

Foreign constituents such as gallstones, rarely enteroliths, but many types of worms and ova may establish or give valuable clues to the diagnosis.

In Europe and North America the commonest types of worm to infest the bowel are tapeworms, roundworms and threadworms. Tapeworms *(Taenia saginata or solium)* can be recognized by their great length, segmented body and a head surmounted by hooks and suckers. Roundworms *(Ascaris lumbricoides)* are usually several centimetres in length and resemble the common earthworm. Threadworms *(Enterobius vermicularis)* appear like minute strands of white cotton. In tropical countries many other helminths are causative of disease. Among those seen in the faeces examples are hookworms *(Ancylostoma duodenale),* both worms and their ova, *Schistosoma mansoni* and numerous others, which affect many people, but with a light infestation may cause little or no ill health. An example of the last group is giardiasis, although this has now become quite a common cause of mild but persistent diarrhoea in European countries. (See also Chapter 13). Stool porphyrin analysis will help to characterize a particular type of porphyria but cannot be used as a screening test.

DIAGNOSIS OF DISEASES OF THE STOMACH

When the symptoms suggest a lesion of the stomach it is to be remembered that the organic lesions of this organ are few. The more important are described below.

GASTRITIS

Acute gastritis is most commonly the result of alcohol or anti-inflammatory agents such as aspirin, and presents with gastrointestinal bleeding. Very rarely, acute phlegmonous gastritis may occur as a result of intramural infection with alpha-haemolytic streptococci or gas-forming organisms. Chronic gastritis is either related to an immunological disturbance (when pernicious anaemia frequently ensues) or is part of the spectrum of peptic ulceration and is related to damage by agents such as bile and alcohol. In this condition morning vomiting, pain and sometimes fever with epigastric tenderness are found. The diagnosis is confirmed at endoscopy. *Helicobacter pylori* infection is the commonest cause of chronic non-autoimmune gastritis.

ULCER

Peptic ulcer may arise in the stomach or duodenum, and more rarely in the oesophagus or jejunum. Except for those caused by non-steroid anti-inflammatory drugs, gastric and duodenal ulcers are now thought to be due to *Helicobacter pylori* infection; eradication of the infection speeds ulcer healing and prevents relapse.

Both gastric (Figure 4.26, see also Figure 4.31) and duodenal ulcers (Figure 4.27, see also Figure 4.32) are characterized by periodic attacks of epigastric pain, often in the spring or autumn months, separated by symptom-free intervals. The pain usually occurs in a steady fashion from 30 minutes to 3 hours after meals and is relieved by antacids and by certain foods, milk especially.

Duodenal ulcer is more common and has a more recognizable clinical pattern. The pain tends to occur some hours after a meal or shortly before the next; hence the term 'hunger pains', which are generally relieved by food. A similar picture may occur in gastric and other forms of peptic ulceration, and sometimes in oesophagitis. Associated symptoms include heartburn, waterbrash, vomiting (which may relieve the pain), and in gastric ulcer there may be loss of appetite and weight confusing the diagnosis with carcinoma. Tenderness in the epigastrium during exacerbations is the only constant physical sign. In differential diagnosis neoplasm must always be considered, but in tropical areas and sometimes in the immigrant population hookworm disease *(Ancylostoma duodenale)* may cause a very similar syndrome to that of duodenal ulcer.

Inquiry should be made as to whether the patient is taking drugs which may favour or exacerbate ulceration, e.g. aspirin, steroids or other anti-inflammatory drugs.

Peptic ulcer may be complicated by haemorrhage (Figure 4.28), pyloric stenosis or perforation. Pain in the back may be due to penetration of posterior abdominal

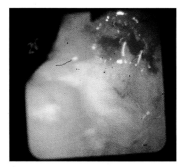

▲ **Figure 4.26 Benign gastric ulcer**

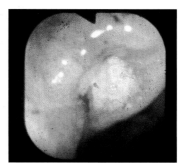

▲ **Figure 4.27 Duodenal ulcer**

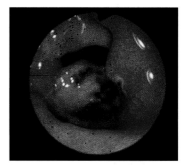

▲ **Figure 4.28 Bleeding duodenal ulcer showing vessel**

structures, sometimes the pancreas, or possibly to radiation from the main site.

NEOPLASM

Carcinoma of the stomach causes symptoms similar to those of gastric ulcer but as the tumour progresses the pain is less regular, remissions do not occur, the appetite disappears, and there is progressive loss of weight. The diagnosis should be suspected in any patient complaining of persistent indigestion for the first time in middle or later life. Physical examination may reveal evidence of weight-loss, a lump in the epigastrium or signs of spread to other parts (e.g. a hard nodular enlargement of the liver or malignant nodes in the left supraclavicular fossa – Virchow's node, Figure 4.29). Early diagnosis depends upon a careful history, radiological studies and endoscopic inspection and biopsy of the gastric mucosa (Figure 4.30, see also Figure 4.33).

MECHANICAL DEFORMITIES

These often result from ulcer or neoplasm. The most important is pyloric stenosis, an obstruction at the pylorus interfering with the normal onward passage of the gastric contents. The digesting food is retained in the stomach and periodically vomited in large quantities in which food eaten many hours previously may be recognized. Pyloric stenosis may also be congenital, manifesting itself early in infancy, when the vomiting is often projectile in character.

The chief physical signs of pyloric stenosis are visible peristalsis and succussion splash. The loss of gastric contents by vomiting may lead to alkalosis and disturbance of electrolytes.

Other deformities of the stomach may be demonstrated in radiographs but are not necessarily associated with symptoms. These include herniation of the stomach into the thorax (hiatus hernia, see page 51), 'hourglass' stomach and other deformities consequent upon the healing by fibrosis of a gastric ulcer, and displacement or distortion of the stomach from extrinsic masses such as a pancreatic cyst or enlarged spleen.

MISCELLANEOUS DISORDERS

There are certain gastric symptoms for which an organic lesion of some other tissue is responsible. Appendicitis, cholecystitis and pancreatic disease are

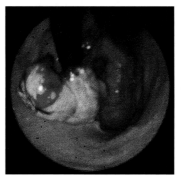

◄ **Figure 4.30 Polypoid gastric carcinoma**

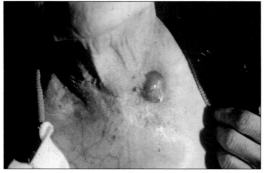

▲ **Figure 4.29 Virchow's node.** Malignant lymph node in the left supraclavicular fossa due to carcinoma of the stomach

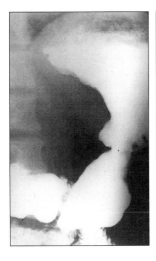

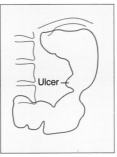

◀ **Figure 4.31 Barium meal showing large penetrating ulcer on lesser curvature of the stomach**

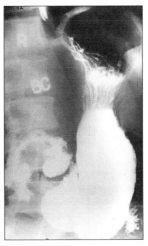

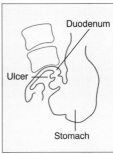

◀ **Figure 4.32 Barium meal showing large duodenal ulcer**

examples of diseases in this category, but the cause is not always to be found in a lesion of the abdominal viscera. Familiar examples of remote causes are bronchial carcinoma, pulmonary tuberculosis, uraemia and cerebral tumour.

Lastly, there remain many cases of indigestion or dyspepsia of a functional nature, that is in which no organic lesion is to be found in the stomach or other related organ. For these some cause will usually be found in the general health and habits of the patient. Examples of such causes are anxiety states, dietary indiscretion, and excessive smoking.

SPECIAL INVESTIGATIONS

Diseases of the stomach which alter the internal outline or peristaltic activity of the viscus (e.g. ulcer, carcinoma) can be demonstrated by radiological examination using a radio-opaque meal such as barium (see Figures 4.31–4.33).

The flexible fibreoptic endoscope allows direct inspection of the upper gastrointestinal tract. The oesophagus and the whole of the stomach and duodenum can be repeatedly examined under local anaesthesia with relatively little discomfort to the patient. A biopsy specimen may be taken from any visible abnormality for histological examination.

Cytological examination may also give valuable information, particularly in distinguishing between gastric carcinoma or ulcer.

Helicobacter infection is readily diagnosed at endoscopy by taking antral biopsies for histological examination. The organisms are visible on standard H & E stains, but are best visualized with a Giemsa stain. The biopsy may also be used to give an 'instant' result by determining its urease activity in a colorimetric assay. *Helicobacter pylori* may also be detected non-invasively either by the detection of serum antibodies or by the administration of ^{13}C- or ^{14}C-urea by mouth and detection of labelled CO_2 in breath. This latter test again depends on the urease activity of the organism.

Chemical investigation of the vomitus is only of value in cases of poisoning.

The maximum hydrochloric acid output is obtained over a 1-hour period after injection of the gastrin analogue pentagastrin. The aspiration should preferably be preceded by checking the position of the tube by X-ray screening and should be carried out by an experienced person so as to ensure that the gastric secretions are removed uninterruptedly and completely.

Gastric acid analysis is now not often performed, but after administration of the gastrin, a very high acid production with a high ratio of basal to maximal output suggests a gastrin-producing tumour of the pancreas (Zollinger–Ellison syndrome).

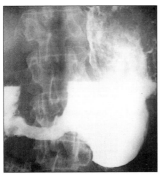

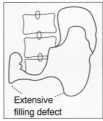

◀ **Figure 4.33 Extensive carcinoma of the lower third of the body of stomach**

◄ **Table 4.6**

THE MALABSORPTION SYNDROME	
Symptoms and signs	
Symptoms and signs	*Element not absorbed*
Pale, bulky, greasy stools	Fat
Distended abdomen; frothy stools	Carbohydrate
Wasting, failure of growth, oedema	Protein
Anaemia	Iron; folic acid; vitamin B_{12}
Pellagroid lesions of skin; ulceration of mouth; peripheral neuropathy	Vitamin-B group
Bone pains, fractures and deformities; tetany	Calcium
Haemorrhage	Vitamin K
Watery diarrhoea	Bile acids
Finger-clubbing	Cause unknown
Causes	
Due to small intestine disease	*Due to inadequate digestive enzymes*
1 Reduced mucosal surface area: extensive bowel resection is a common cause in Western countries	1 Lack of bile: obstructive jaundice
2 Diffuse mucosal damage: gluten enteropathy (coeliac disease); intestinal ischaemia	2 Lack of pancreatic enzymes: chronic pancreatitis; cystic fibrosis; carcinoma
3 Diffuse mucosal infiltration: amyloid disease; lymphoma; Crohn's disease	3 Poor mixing of enzymes: after gastrectomy
4 Abnormal bacterial flora and infestations: 'blind loops'; tropical sprue; internal fistulae; after antibiotics	
5 Impaired lymphatic drainage: intestinal lymphangiectasia	

DIAGNOSIS OF DISEASES OF THE SMALL INTESTINE

ENTERITIS

Whether due to infected food usually with salmonella organisms, occasionally with staphylococci, or dysentery caused by shigella or unusual micro-organisms in immunosuppressed patients with AIDS, all forms of enteritis (inflammation of the intestine) have colic and diarrhoea as their cardinal symptoms, with a few or no physical signs. The term colic, as applied to the intestine, means a pain of griping or twisting character lasting only some seconds at a time and corresponding with waves of peristalsis. Microbiological examination of the stools is necessary for a complete diagnosis.

Typhoid fever deserves special mention as an example of an enteritis, affecting chiefly the ileum. In addition to local symptoms such as diarrhoea (pea-soup stools) or constipation, there are well-developed constitutional symptoms and signs due to bloodstream infection. Notable points are the pyrexia, sometimes with bradycardia, the splenic enlargement and positive blood culture, the rash and positive agglutination reactions (Widal).

THE MALABSORPTION SYNDROME

Defective absorption may be confined to one particular constituent of food, for example vitamin B_{12} in pernicious anaemia. The term 'malabsorption syndrome' is usually reserved for those cases with multiple defects of absorption. It results either from diseases of the small intestine or from an inadequate supply of digestive enzymes (see Table 4.6). Coeliac disease is the commonest form of generalized malabsorption and is due to the flattening of the small intestinal villi brought about by contact with dietary gluten (gluten enteropathy). The clinical features include steatorrhoea (fatty stools) due to failure of fat absorption; anaemia resulting from inadequate absorption of iron, folic acid or vitamin B_{12}; osteomalacia and tetany due to calcium deficiency; wasting and oedema due to loss of protein; and various lesions of the skin, mucosae and nervous system resulting from a lack of vitamin B (Figure 4.34). Finger-clubbing may also occur (see Table 4.6).

CROHN'S DISEASE

This is a chronic granulomatous process that most commonly affects the lower ileum ('regional ileitis') and colon (Crohn's colitis), but may appear in any part of the alimentary tract from the mouth (see Figure 4.35) to the anus. There is diffuse infiltration and thickening of the bowel wall with narrowing of the lumen. Penetrating mucosal ulcers may lead to fistulae between loops of bowel, the pelvic viscera and the skin.

Symptoms and signs depend on the site of the lesion. Localized disease of the ileum may simulate appendicitis and present with colicky abdominal pain, fever and a tender mass in the right iliac fossa. More diffuse involvement of the small bowel or an entero-colic fistula can give rise to a malabsorption syndrome. Colonic disease may resemble ulcerative colitis with blood and mucus in the stools. Intestinal obstruction, fever and mucocutaneous ulceration or fistulae (especially perianal) are other typical features of the disease. The diagnosis may be established by demonstrating characteristic radiological changes in the small bowel and by the appearance in a biopsy specimen of non-caseating granulomas with giant cells.

DIAGNOSIS OF DISEASES OF THE LARGE INTESTINE

ULCERATIVE COLITIS

This is a non-specific inflammatory condition in which there is recurrent ulceration of the colonic and rectal mucosa. Unlike Crohn's disease, ulcerative colitis usually involves the rectum, spares the small bowel and does not produce fistulae. The complications include perforation, haemorrhage, stricture and, in some long-standing cases, carcinoma. There may also be systemic manifestations such as erythema nodosum, pyoderma gangrenosum (Figure 4.36), iritis, arthritis or finger-clubbing.

Ulcerative colitis may present insidiously with loose stools and abdominal discomfort or with an acute attack of fever, pain and bloody diarrhoea. The subsequent course is characterized by remissions and exacerbations which are sometimes related to emotional stress. In the established case, there are frequent loose stools with blood, mucus and pus, especially on waking, but often disturbing sleep. Rectal involvement results in tenesmus and the passage of blood and mucus alone, sometimes with constipation rather than diarrhoea. Physical signs may be lacking, but in patients with chronic extensive disease there is often anaemia and wasting and, rarely, the systemic features already listed. On proctoscopy, the rectal mucosa appears inflamed, bleeds easily and ulcers may be seen. The diagnosis is established and carcinoma excluded by endoscopy and a barium enema.

CARCINOMA

The colon and rectum are among the commonest sites for carcinoma. Symptoms and signs depend upon the position and malignancy of the tumour and whether it

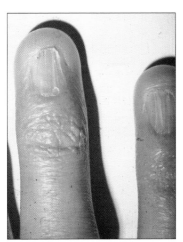

◀ **Figure 4.34 Ribbing of the nails associated with the malabsorption syndrome**

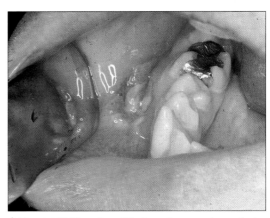

▲ **Figure 4.35 Ulceration of the buccal mucosa in a patient with Crohn's disease**

consists mainly of an ulcerative lesion or a stricture. Rectal carcinoma usually presents with blood, mucus and sometimes pus in the stool and can often be felt with the finger or seen through the proctoscope. Blood from an ulcerating carcinoma of the colon or caecum may not be visible in the stool, and in these cases the first symptoms are often anaemia and loss of weight. An abdominal tumour may be felt, but it must be remembered that the sigmoid colon, a common site for carcinoma, is not accessible to palpation. Alteration in bowel habit is an important symptom of the carcinoma especially when there is a stricture. Increasing constipation, sometimes alternating with diarrhoea, may be followed by colicky pains due to intestinal obstruction. Highly malignant or neglected lesions may first present with signs of peritoneal invasion or distant metastases. Radiography following a barium enema and endoscopy with biopsy are used to confirm the diagnosis.

DIVERTICULITIS

Diverticula are balloon-like protrusions of the colonic mucosa through parts of the wall where the muscle layers are weakened or absent. Diverticulosis is a common condition in elderly obese subjects, particularly in those who suffer from chronic constipation. Symptoms occur only if the diverticula are inflamed (diverticulitis) and include fever, colicky pain, constipation sometimes alternating with diarrhoea, haemorrhage and symptoms of cystitis if inflammation spreads to the bladder. A tender mass can sometimes be palpated, usually in the left iliac fossa.

IRRITABLE COLON

This is the commonest gastrointestinal complaint in developed countries and is the result of a poorly under-

stood disorder of motility that often affects not only the colon but also other parts of the gastrointestinal tract. Symptoms include constipation with fragmented pellet-like stools, diarrhoea (often alternating with constipation), abdominal pain, bloating. flatulence and the passage of mucus. The diagnosis is easy when symptoms are classical and of long-standing. However, it is important, particularly when symptoms are of recent onset, to exclude more serious causes such as carcinoma or inflammatory bowel disease. Furthermore, there are other less serious causes, such as intolerance to certain foods. Apart from coeliac disease (page 74), the most important of these is hypolactasia, an inability to split the disaccharide lactose in cow's milk which results in diarrhoea and flatulence.

INTESTINAL OBSTRUCTION

The small as well as the large intestine may be involved. When the cause is mechanical, as in strangulated hernia, mural growths or volvulus, constipation and colic are the initial symptoms. Soon, however, vomiting follows as a distinguishing feature in cases of acute obstruction. At first the vomitus consists of the stomach contents, later of bile regurgitated from the duodenum, and later still of the faeculent contents of the small intestine. In chronic cases of obstruction, especially of the large bowel, this characteristic vomiting is not present and the diagnosis must depend upon the history of constipation and colic and special methods of examination. It must be emphasized again that the symptoms assume a special importance when they are persistent, for colic may arise from trivial disorders such as irritant food, temporary constipation or purgatives, but as a rule it passes away in such cases within a few days.

Paralytic ileus (adynamic ileus) is most common in cases of peritonitis but may occur in many painful thoracic and abdominal lesions. Constipation is associated with progressive gaseous abdominal distension, but colicky pain is uncommon and the abdomen is silent on auscultation. More rarely, vascular insufficiency (ischaemia) may give a similar clinical picture.

SPECIAL INVESTIGATIONS

A plain X-ray of the abdomen may reveal distended loops of bowel with fluid levels in cases of intestinal obstruction. Abnormalities in the structure or activity of the intestines can be studied by radiographs taken over a 24-hour period after a barium meal (barium follow-through). If small intestinal disease is suspected, a special barium preparation can be introduced in controlled amounts directly into the small bowel via a nasoduodenal tube (small bowel enema). The outline of the large

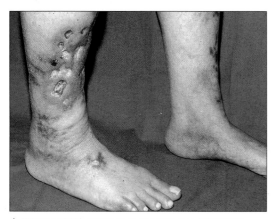

▲ **Figure 4.36 Pyoderma gangrenosum in a patient with ulcerative colitis**

intestine is better demonstrated by injection of barium via the anus (barium enema). The rectum and lower reaches of the sigmoid colon are poorly visualized in radiographs and such lesions as carcinoma, polyps, ulceration and haemorrhoids may be overlooked. Endoscopic methods are therefore employed for examination of the anal canal (proctoscopy) and for the lower sigmoid and rectum (sigmoidoscopy). The flexible fibreoptic endoscope permits inspection of the mucosa throughout the whole length of the colon (colonoscopy).

Examination of the faeces plays an important part in the diagnosis of intestinal diseases. *Inspection of the faeces* with the naked eye is described on page 70. When foreign bodies such as gallstones and intestinal worms are anticipated, the stool should be washed repeatedly through muslin or a fine sieve. The most important chemical test applicable in the clinic room is that for occult blood. This is of great value in the detection of slight continual bleeding from ulceration or carcinoma of the stomach or intestines. Occult blood is recognized by smearing a little stool on a guiac-impregnated filter paper inside a plastic or cardboard wallet. A blue colour indicates a positive reaction produced by the pseudo-peroxidase activity of haemoglobin. *Microscopy of the faeces* may reveal pus cells, red cells, bacteria, ova and parasites such as *Entamoeba histolytica*. *Culture of the faeces* permits a more precise identification of pathogenic bacteria. These methods are used for the recognition of infections and infestations of the bowel and are thus essential to the investigation of diarrhoea. *Faecal fat excretion* is measured by chemical analysis of the total amount of faeces passed over a period of 3–5 days while the patient is taking a normal ward diet. An amount greater than 5 g daily indicates malabsorption of fat from the small intestine. Because of the unaesthetic nature of the laboratory analysis of faecal fats, there are continuing attempts to develop alternative tests for fat malabsorption, such as the ^{14}C-triolein breath test. A useful qualitative side-room test is to add a lipophilic dye to a faecal smear and examine this microscopically for stained fat globules.

Failure to absorb other constituents of the diet can be detected by measuring their levels in the blood (e.g. *serum iron, vitamin B$_{12}$, folate, protein, calcium*) or the amount excreted in the urine after ingestion of the appropriate substance (e.g. *xylose excretion test, Schilling test*). In a patient with intestinal malabsorption, vitamin B$_{12}$ deficiency suggests a lesion in the lower ileum (where the vitamin is absorbed) or a blind loop syndrome. A normal xylose excretion test helps to distinguish pancreatic disease, in which only fat absorption is impaired, from intestinal causes of malabsorption.

A fragment of jejunal mucosa can also be obtained by means of a biopsy device which consists of a knife actuated within a small capsule at the end of a flexible tube (Crosbie capsule). Histological examination of the jejunal mucosa is of particular value in the diagnosis of adult coeliac disease (gluten enteropathy), in which there is marked atrophy of the villi.

DIAGNOSIS OF DISEASES OF THE PERITONEUM

It is convenient to consider the peritoneum at this stage in view of its close association with the alimentary tract. In the description of abdominal pain it has already been pointed out that the peritoneum plays a great part in the production of pain in disease of individual viscera, and it is preferable to envisage such diseases as appendicitis and cholecystitis as diseases affecting the appendix and gallbladder with their enveloping visceral and neighbouring parietal peritoneum.

In some instances the involvement of the peritoneum is the most important aspect of the case. This is so in acute generalized peritonitis and in certain forms of chronic peritonitis.

ACUTE GENERALIZED PERITONITIS

The examination of the 'acute abdomen' more frequently falls to the family doctor or surgeon than to the physician, but acute abdominal accidents are not infrequent in medical wards, and the condition therefore warrants some attention here. The symptoms are similar whatever the cause of the acute peritonitis (e.g. perforated ulcer, ruptured appendix abscess, acute pancreatitis). Intense, agonizing abdominal pain and circulatory collapse are the notable features. Other points of distinction are familiar to the surgeon, such as the less severe pain of a perforation into the lesser sac of the peritoneum, but only general features will be described here.

Inspection shows the abdomen to be fixed, exhibiting little if any movement with respiration. Breathing is of a thoracic type. The anxious distressed facies leaves no doubts as to the severity of the symptoms.

Palpation shows extreme abdominal tenderness and board-like rigidity of the abdominal muscles. The tenderness is often accompanied by hyperaesthesia of the skin. 'Rebound tenderness', a characteristic sign of acute peritonitis, can be elicited by gentle pressure on the abdominal wall followed by sudden withdrawal of the palpating hand.

Percussion – which, if employed, should be practised gently – may demonstrate tympanites due to the paresis of the intestinal musculature and the accumulation of gas in the intestines. Free gas may also be present in the peritoneal cavity, causing tympany in place of the usual liver dullness, and free fluid can sometimes be detected.

Auscultation. Bowel sounds may disappear completely in the later stages due to paresis of the intestinal musculature.

Several conditions may simulate peritonitis quite closely, and when the signs are at all indefinite particular care should be taken to examine other systems. Severe abdominal pain may be caused by myocardial infarction, ketoacidosis in diabetes, aortic aneurysm, mesenteric arterial occlusion, diaphragmatic pleurisy, nerve root irritation, tabes dorsalis and acute porphyria, to mention only the more important lesions.

CHRONIC PERITONITIS

Several types of chronic peritonitis are described but the most important is the *tuberculous form,* though even this has become rare in Western countries. Causes of chronic peritonitis include the carcinoid syndrome and certain drugs such as the beta-blocking agent practolol and methysergide used in the treatment of migraine but there are now effective alternatives to these drugs. Chronic fibrosis of the peritoneum, especially of its posterior parts, can also occur without any evident precipitating cause. Chronic peritonitis is less common than peritoneal neoplasia, but the symptoms and signs are similar and the prognosis much more favourable in the former condition. This diagnosis should therefore always be considered in any patient presenting with the clinical features of chronic peritoneal disease.

The symptoms are indefinite and depend more upon mechanical interference with the stomach and intestines than upon the disease of the peritoneum itself. Thus colic, constipation and diarrhoea may occur. Constitutional symptoms of the causative disease are added, e.g. loss of weight, anaemia, and fever, in the case of tuberculosis. Peritoneal fibrosis can also lead to the symptoms and signs of chronic renal failure due to bilateral ureteric obstruction.

Inspection may show enlargement of the abdomen due to the presence of ascites (see Figure 4.22) or of infiltrating masses in the peritoneum. The signs of ascites have been described. Peritoneal masses are most commonly seen in the upper abdomen lying in a transverse manner so that they may resemble an enlarged liver or a loaded transverse colon. Their contour, however, is more irregular and does not conform to the shape and size expected from these viscera.

Palpation helps to define a 'rolled omentum' of this kind from the liver and transverse colon.

SPECIAL INVESTIGATIONS

The main investigations of value in the diagnosis of peritoneal diseases are paracentesis and peritoneoscopy. *Paracentesis* (needle aspiration of the peritoneal cavity) is sometimes used for the relief of ascites, and microscopic examination or culture of the ascitic fluid can be helpful in identifying the organism responsible for a chronic peritonitis (e.g. tuberculosis) and for demonstrating carcinoma cells in malignant cases. *Peritoneoscopy* (inspection of the peritoneal cavity through an illuminated tube) is sometimes used to determine the cause of ascites or liver enlargement when it is desirable to avoid laparotomy. *Peritoneal biopsy* may help to distinguish inflammatory from neoplastic disease.

DIAGNOSIS OF DISEASES OF THE LIVER

Serious disease of the liver may be present without abnormal physical signs, as quite a small amount of liver tissue appears able to carry on the functions of the diseased portions.

A suspicion of liver disease may be aroused by enlargement of the organ especially if it is hard or irregular in outline; more rarely by diminution in size suspected by increased resonance over right lower ribs. Portal hypertension and hepatocellular failure also produce characteristic signs (see Table 4.7).

Many of the causes of liver enlargement and jaundice are not primarily those of liver disease and necessitate the examination of other systems for the discovery of their cause (see Chapter 8).

Three primary diseases of the liver need mention, namely infective hepatitis, cirrhosis and abscess.

INFECTIVE HEPATITIS

This is due to a virus infection of the liver. The onset is characterized by marked anorexia, nausea, vomiting and depression, associated with evidence of general toxicity, e.g. fever and malaise. After a few days the nausea and toxicity lessen, but the patient then becomes jaundiced, the liver enlarges and some pain may occur in the right hypochondrium. Darkness of the urine and pallor of the faeces may be noticed before any change in the colour of the skin. The jaundice fades over the next week to ten days; complete recovery in a few weeks is the rule. In some rare fulminating cases an acute necrosis of the liver cells (acute hepatic necrosis) leads to *hepatic coma* in which the patient is usually deeply jaundiced, the liver decreases in size, and there is a characteristic foetor hepaticus. Hepatic cirrhosis may be a late complication of type B or C hepatitis, but type A infection produces no chronic sequelae.

PRODUCTION OF SYMPTOMS AND SIGNS IN LIVER DISEASE		
Pathological changes	**Functional disturbance**	**Symptoms and signs**
Mechanical factors (e.g. cirrhosis or congestive cardiac failure)	1 Change in consistency and size 2 Rapid stretching or involvement of capsule	The liver may be enlarged or smaller, smooth or irregular, soft, firm or hard Pain in right hypochondrium, intense nausea and vomitting
Portal hypertension	1 Rise in portal vein pressure 2 Congestion of splanchnic vessels 3 Development of collateral circulation 4 Intoxication of brain by crude nitrogen products from gut which have bypassed the liver filter in anastomatic channels	Splenomegaly Anorexia, nausea, flatulence and abdominal discomfort Oesphageal varices and haematemesis; internal haemorrhoids and caput medusae (Figure 4.36) Hepatic encephalopathy manifested by personality changes progressing through stupor to coma. Also motor changes including a flapping tremor

Hepatocellular failure	1 Reduction in serum albumin with resultant lowering of colloid osmotic pressure
	2 Failure to excrete bilirubin glucuronide
	3 Failure to store certain vitamins, e.g. vitamin K
	4 Impaired detoxication of various metabolites may lead to a raised blood level and toxic symptoms:
	   Oestrogens
	
	   Aldosterone
	   Crude nitrogenous products from the gut
	   Morphine and barbiturates
		Ascites and generalized oedema (Figure 4.37)
		
		Jaundice (Figure 4.38)
		Bleeding tendency
		
		Spider naevi (Figure 4.39), palmar erythema, gynaecomastia, loss of body hair and testicular atrophy (see Figures 4.40 and 4.41)
		Aggravation of oedema
		Hepatic encephalopathy
		
		Dangerous sensitivy to these drugs

▲ Table 4.7

CIRRHOSIS OF THE LIVER

This condition is characterized by necrosis of hepatic cells followed later by fibrosis, nodular regeneration and abnormalities of the hepatic circulation. The commoner causes are as follows:

1 *Toxins:* These include alcohol and certain drugs (e.g. methyldopa). Alcohol probably accounts for most cases of cirrhosis in Western countries.

2 *Infections:* Hepatic cirrhosis occasionally follows severe or repeated attacks of viral hepatitis *(see above)*.

3 *Auto-immune reaction* may take the form of primary biliary cirrhosis or chronic active hepatitis. *Primary biliary cirrhosis* is mainly a disease of middle-aged women and usually presents as an obstructive type of jaundice

with troublesome pruritus. *Chronic active hepatitis* can occur at any age and in either sex and may simulate the clinical picture of a persistent or recurrent viral hepatitis (see above). In these forms of cirrhosis, auto-antibodies are usually present in the blood.

4 *Metabolic* causes of cirrhosis are rare but also important because effective treatment is available. *Haemochromatosis*, although it most often presents in middle-aged or elderly men, is probably a genetic abnormality of iron absorption. This results in iron deposition in the liver, pancreas, skin, gonads and joints to cause cirrhosis, diabetes, pigmentation, testicular atrophy and arthropathy. The condition can also result from excessive intake of iron from repeated blood

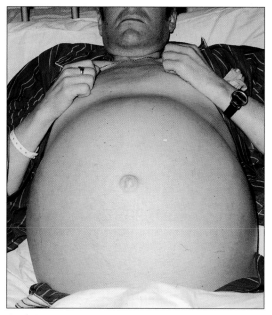

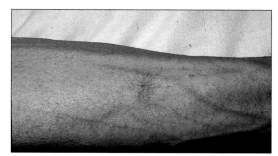

▲ **Figure 4.40 Spider naevus on the forearm of a patient with hepatic cirrhosis**

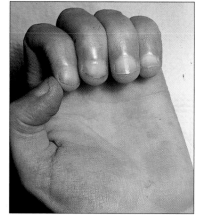

◀ **Figure 4.41 Cirrhosis of the liver:** palmar erythema and white nails

▲ **Figure 4.37 Ascites and caput medusae**

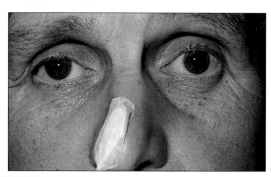

▲ **Figure 4.38 Jaundice**

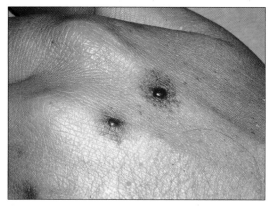

▲ **Figure 4.39 Giant spider naevi on dorsum of hand**

transfusion and may respond to regular venesection. *Wilson's disease* (hepatolenticular degeneration) is also a congenital metabolic defect. Copper is deposited in the liver, brain and cornea. It usually shows itself in childhood with extrapyramidal or psychiatric features as well as cirrhosis, and may be recognized by the presence of Kayser–Fleischer rings in the cornea (see page 30). Another rare metabolic cause for juvenile cirrhosis of the liver is congenital deficiency of α_1-antitrypsin.

5 *Congestive changes* in the liver from chronic cholestasis ('biliary cirrhosis') or right-heart failure ('cardiac cirrhosis') are usually reversible if the cause is removed and rarely lead to true cirrhosis as defined in the first paragraph of this section.

The chief symptoms and signs of cirrhosis can be attributed to three main causes:

1 Enlargement of the liver, followed by shrinkage in the later stages – the surface is finely granular, but this can rarely be detected except through a very thin abdominal wall.
2 Portal hypertension.
3 Hepatocellular failure.

The symptoms and signs attributable to these last two causes are listed in Table 4.7 (see also Figures 4.39–4.41). Nail changes of uncertain cause also occur in hepatic cirrhosis; these include clubbing and leukonychia.

LIVER ABSCESS

Multiple abscesses of the liver may result from systemic infection, but, more commonly, from spread of suppurative processes through the portal system from some other part of the alimentary tract – e.g. the appendix. The latter condition is known as portal pyaemia and the liver symptoms are essentially secondary; it has become relatively rare since the introduction of broad-spectrum antibiotics. Diverticulitis and biliary tract sepsis are now the usual causes.

Amoebic abscess of the liver, although strictly speaking secondary to amoebic infection of the intestine, forms such a separate entity that it is considered here as a primary disease of the liver. Pain over the liver, toxaemia and fever are the characteristic symptoms. The liver is enlarged and tender, and irregularities in the surface of the organ are occasionally found. Examination of the stools may show the presence of *Entamoeba histolytica,* and a puncture of the liver itself through the abdominal wall or intercostal space enables the typical 'anchovy sauce' pus to be withdrawn (see also Chapter 13). The diagnosis may be made reliably by a serological fluorescent antibody test.

A rarer cause of liver abscess is actinomycosis, which is secondary to a focus elsewhere in the alimentary tract, usually in the ileocaecal region.

SPECIAL INVESTIGATIONS
Radiology

The liver cannot be displayed by conventional radiological techniques but is well shown by both ultrasound examination and computed tomography (CT scanning). These are useful for detecting filling defects in the liver substance (e.g. cysts, abscesses, tumours) and for diagnosing dilated hepatic ducts in extrahepatic obstruction and are therefore valuable in establishing the cause of jaundice. As well as showing the presence of extrahepatic obstruction, they may show the level and nature of the block (e.g. carcinoma of the pancreas), but usually direct cholangiography will be needed to confirm this (see below).

A radionuclide scan of the liver is useful in showing filling defects greater than 2 cm in diameter, such as metastases, cysts and abscesses. Characteristic patterns of uptake may be seen in hepatocellular disease such as cirrhosis.

Portal hypertension may be diagnosed by the finding of oesophageal varices on barium swallow (Figure 4.42) or at endoscopy which may show gastric varices (Figure 4.43) . The site of the obstruction can be identified by the injection of contrast medium into the spleen or, via the aorta, into the splenic artery, whence it fills the splenic and portal veins (Figure 4.44).

Magnetic resonance imaging gives high quality images of the liver although it has not yet replaced computed tomography.

Histology

Histological examination of the liver may be of value in the diagnosis of cirrhosis, tumours, infiltrations and infections of the liver, and for assessing the activity of a chronic hepatitis as in certain auto-immune disorders. A fragment of liver tissue can be obtained for this purpose by percutaneous needle biopsy and may be used for immunological tests, chemical estimations and enzymology.

DIAGNOSIS OF DISEASES OF THE GALLBLADDER AND BILE DUCTS

CHOLECYSTITIS

Inflammation of the gallbladder commonly results from gallstones, and its symptoms are often combined with those due to calculi. Occasionally acute cholecystitis may occur without stones – acute acalculous cholecystitis.

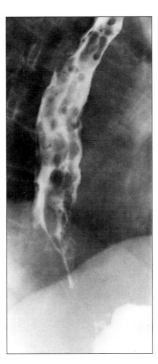

◀ **Figure 4.42 Oesophageal varices.** Note the rounded filling defects displacing the barium in the oesophagus

This is usually a surgical emergency terminating in gall-bladder gangrene, and may be a complication of severe burns or follow major surgery.

Pain in the right hypochondrium and at the inferior angle of the right scapula is common. If the patient takes a slow, deep breath whilst the examiner's fingers are pressed firmly but gently over the right hypochondrium, there may be momentary interruption of breathing because of pain (Murphy's sign). Acute cholecystitis is accompanied by constitutional disturbances such as fever and leucocytosis, and on palpation there may be marked tenderness and guarding. The significance of the classical gallbladder symptoms of fat intolerance, flatulent dyspepsia and abdominal discomfort is now doubtful.

In acute cases greater constitutional disturbances such as pyrexia and leucocytosis are present together with more pronounced tenderness and guarding.

GALLSTONES

These may produce the symptoms of cholecystitis just described. If a stone lodges in the neck of the gallblad-

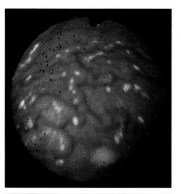

◀ **Figure 4.43 Gastric varices showing mucosal irregularity**

der or passes into the cystic or common bile duct, a characteristic attack of *biliary colic* results (see page 57). Obstruction of the common bile duct gives rise to jaundice (see page 57). Although gallbladder carcinoma is rare, when it is seen it is almost always in a gallbladder containing calculi.

SPECIAL INVESTIGATIONS

The diagnosis of calculous gallbladder disease is made either by ultrasonography or cholecystography. About 20 per cent of calculi are calcified and will therefore show up on a plain abdominal radiograph (Figure 4.45). If a stone is occluding the cystic duct, contrast material in bile cannot enter the gallbladder and it will be reported on oral cholecystography to be 'non-functioning'. Other causes of failing to opacify the gallbladder are poor hepatic function or jaundice and failure to swallow or absorb the cholecystogram tablets.

The bile ducts may be seen on ultrasound or CT scan but direct cholangiography is often necessary, and three methods are available. *Intravenous cholangiography* rarely gives a clear diagnosis, and is unsuccessful if there is more than minimal jaundice. *Endoscopic retrograde cholangiography* (ERCP) (Figures 4.46 and 4.47) and *percutaneous cholangiography* (PTC) give excellent visualization of the biliary system, although PTC may be difficult if the ducts are not dilated.

DIAGNOSIS OF DISEASES OF THE PANCREAS

Three lesions may be mentioned as illustrative types of pancreatic disease.

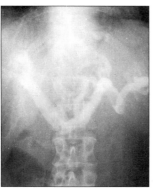
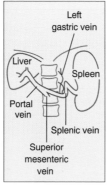

Left
gastric vein

Liver

Spleen

Portal
vein

Splenic vein

Superior
mesenteric
vein

▲ **Figure 4.44 Porto-splenogram. A direct injection into the spleen demonstrating the dilated gastric veins in portal hypertension**

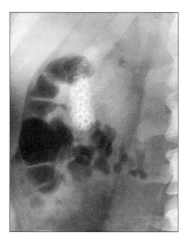

◀ **Figure 4.45 Radio-opaque stones filling the gallbladder and cystic duct**

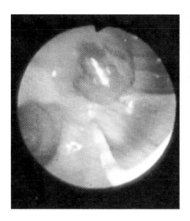

◀ Figure 4.46
Impacted stone in
common bile duct
showing ERCP
catheter entering
the ampulla

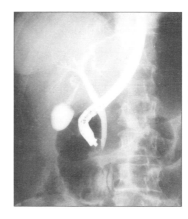

◀ Figure 4.47
ERCP via the
duodenoscope
outlining normal
common bile duct,
gallbladder and
cystic duct, and
hepatic duct

PANCREATITIS

In acute pancreatitis there is intense agonizing upper abdominal pain with shock due to extravasation of blood and pancreatic secretions into the peritoneal cavity. An abdominal catastrophe is confirmed by the findings of severe tenderness and muscular rigidity and the diagnosis suggested by a raised serum amylase.

Chronic pancreatitis is nearly always alcohol-induced. The cardinal features are pain, exocrine insufficiency (protein malnutrition and steatorrhoea) and endocrine insufficiency (diabetes mellitus). The pain may be particularly severe and unrelenting, situated in the central abdomen, often radiating through to the back and eased by leaning forward.

CANCER OF THE PANCREAS

The early symptoms are those common to many dyspepsias; pain, loss of appetite and flatulence. The pain is usually of a persistent boring type which radiates to the back and disturbs the patient's sleep. Just as in chronic pancreatitis it is sometimes partially relieved by bending forwards over a chair or bed, a posture not infrequently adopted by the patient. There are also symptoms of malignant disease, namely loss of weight, loss of strength and the development of cachexia. An important sign when present is *jaundice* of a persistent and increasing nature, due to the increasing constriction of the common bile duct by the growth. The tumour may be palpable in the epigastrium, especially if the patient is examined in the knee–elbow position. Painless jaundice and enlargement of the gallbladder may occur when the head of the pancreas is involved. It is more difficult to diagnose lesions in other parts of the gland.

Evidence of pancreatic insufficiency is often only slight until the late stages of the disease, and in many cases sufficient pancreatic tissue is left to carry on the functions of the organ. Because local functional and structural evidence of pancreatic carcinoma is often scanty, the tumour may first present with systemic manifestations of cancer such as unexplained weight loss, metastatic spread (e.g. lymphangitis carcinomatosa of the lung) or recurrent venous thromboses (thrombophlebitis migrans).

FIBROCYSTIC DISEASE OF THE PANCREAS (CYSTIC FIBROSIS)

This congenital abnormality of the pancreas is one manifestation of a diffuse disorder of exocrine glands and their secretions. The mucous glands of the bronchi, the sweat glands and the testes are also involved. The disease usually presents in infancy with recurrent bronchial infections associated with bronchiectasis and bulky fatty offensive stools due to steatorrhoea of pancreatic origin. Some victims die in childhood or adolescence, usually from respiratory infection, but with modern broad spectrum antibiotics an increasing proportion now survive to adult life. The males are usually infertile because of impaired testicular function. A diagnostic feature of the disease is the high salt content of the sweat.

ENDOCRINE DISORDERS

Abnormalities of endocrine secretion relating to the pancreas are mentioned elsewhere and include diabetes mellitus, insulin-secreting tumour of the islet cells causing spontaneous hypoglycaemia (Chapter 12) and peptic ulcer with diarrhoea due to a gastrin-secreting adenoma (see page 56).

SPECIAL INVESTIGATIONS

Diseases of the pancreas, especially alcoholic chronic pancreatitis, are sometimes associated with calcification and this can be demonstrated in a plain radiograph of the abdomen. A barium meal may reveal widening of the duodenal loop in cases of carcinoma of the head of the pancreas. Other techniques for delineating the physical contours of the pancreas include the use of ultrasound, computerized axial tomography and coeliac axis angiography. The anatomy of the pancreatic duct system can be demonstrated by cannulation of the ampulla of Vater and introduction of contrast medium at the time of fibreoptic duodenoscopy (retrograde pancreatography, Figure 4.48). In diseases of the pancreas, there may be a deficiency of enzymes in the bowel as a result of obstruction to the pancreatic duct (e.g. in carcinoma) or an excess of enzymes, e.g. amylase or lipase, in the blood and urine due to leakage from pancreatic cells (e.g. in acute pancreatitis). A lack of lipase in the bowel leads to steatorrhoea due to excess of neutral fats in the stool, while lack of trypsin causes deficient protein digestion with the appearance in the stool of striated muscle fibres. Normally only small amounts of pancreatic digestive

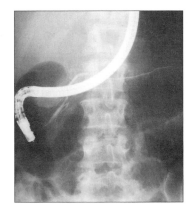

◀ Figure 4.48 Retrograde pancreatography via the duodenoscope illustrating normal pancreatic duct systems

enzymes find their way into the bloodstream and appear in the urine. Pancreatic secretion can also be obtained for analysis by aspirating the duodenal contents after the injection of a pancreatic stimulant (e.g. secretin).

Renal, urinary and genital systems

Symptoms suggesting diseases of the kidney and urinary tract include:

1 Disturbances in the act of micturition, including frequency, retention, incontinence and dysuria.
2 Alteration in the amount of urine.
3 Alteration in the appearance of the urine.
4 Pain: renal, ureteric, vesical or urethral.
5 General symptoms of abnormal renal function.

DISTURBANCES IN THE ACT OF MICTURITION

Frequency (without increase in the amount of urine) results from irritation of the bladder by infection, stone, tumour or blood; or from a reduction in the capacity of the bladder by fibrotic contraction or pressure from a pelvic tumour. In all these conditions, the patient's sleep is disturbed by the need to micturate (*nocturia*), whereas frequency due to emotional causes or cold is usually confined to the waking hours. Polyuria may also lead to frequency (see below).

Retention occurs in obstructive lesions of the urethra such as stricture and prostatic hypertrophy, in diseases of the spinal cord or sacral nerve roots and in coma due to various causes. Complete retention may be heralded by a phase of *hesitancy* (delay in starting micturition), by a poor or intermittent stream and by terminal dribbling.

Incontinence of urine is common when the mental faculties are impaired, especially in the elderly and those with cerebrovascular lesions. In spinal cord diseases retention of urine is often followed by incontinence due either to overflow or to reflex evacuations of the bladder. Among the commoner neurological diseases resulting in incontinence are paraplegia, especially traumatic, and multiple sclerosis. Incontinence can also result from disease or deformity of the lower urinary tract such as a vesicovaginal fistula, a prolapsed uterus with cystocele, or muscular weakness in parous women. In these circumstances it is usually provoked by coughing or sneezing ('stress incontinence'). In men prostatic enlargement, benign or malignant, has the same result, which also occurs (fortunately rarely now) after prostatectomy. Precipitancy, the sudden onset of micturition without warning, is another cause of occasional incontinence, especially in neurological disorders.

Dysuria means difficulty in micturition and may thus include some of the symptoms already discussed. More commonly, however, the term is used to describe pain or discomfort during the act of micturition which usually results from disease of the bladder, prostate or urethra (see below).

ALTERATION IN THE AMOUNT OF URINE

The urine volume may be increased (*polyuria*) or diminished (*oliguria*) or negligible (*anuria*).

POLYURIA
Large quantities of urine will be passed if the reabsorption of water from the tubular fluid is impaired in any way. Normally fluid is delivered to the tubules from the glomerular capillaries at a rate of 120 ml/min; 99 per cent of the water delivered to the tubules is reabsorbed secondarily to the reabsorption of sodium, chloride and other solutes. The formation of normal urine depends on the concentration gradient between the cortex, medulla and the papillae of the kidney; this gradient is determined by the functional anatomy of the loop of Henle, the secretion of antidiuretic hormone (vasopressin) by the posterior pituitary and the sensitivity of the tubular cells to vasopressin.

The urine volume is increased normally following the ingestion of large quantities of fluid, especially when this contains substances with a diuretic action (e.g. alcohol, tea, coffee). Polyuria may also result from nervousness (e.g. during medical examination). Diseases causing polyuria include the following:

1 Chronic renal failure: the solute load filtered and excreted by each of the few remaining nephrons is greatly increased, and there are not enough nephrons to maintain an effective medullary concentration gradient.
2 Diabetes mellitus: the osmotic effect of the unreabsorbed glucose prevents reabsorption of water from the tubular fluid.
3 Neurohypophysial diabetes insipidus: the secretion of vasopressin is impaired e.g. following trauma to the head.
4 Nephrogenic diabetes insipidus: where the tubules are insensitive to the action of vasopressin. This occurs

primarily in a rare familial condition and secondarily in hyperparathyroidism and potassium depletion.

5 Oedematous states, such as cardiac failure, cirrhosis and the nephrotic syndrome treated with diuretics that primarily impair the tubular reabsorption of sodium chloride and thence the reabsorption of water.

In chronic renal failure, diabetes mellitus, and diabetes insipidus, thirst and *polydipsia* result from the abnormal losses of water and are often the presenting symptoms of the underlying disorder.

OLIGURIA AND ANURIA

The urine volume is diminished physiologically under conditions of water deprivation. In a healthy subject the functions of the kidney can be maintained with the passage of as little as 500 ml of urine daily.

Oliguria may be defined as the passage of less than 500 ml of urine daily. This may occur in pre-renal conditions, such as shock, haemorrhage, dehydration and cardiac failure, when the kidney is not damaged but the renal blood flow and glomerular filtration rate are diminished. Oliguria is also found in established acute renal failure from primary renal disease such as acute glomerulonephritis.

Anuria can result from infarction of a single kidney or of both kidneys through massive embolization or dissecting aneurysm of the abdominal aorta with occlusion of the renal arteries. Other causes include bilateral cortical necrosis, which may follow severe postpartum haemorrhage, and complete obstruction of the ureters from bilateral stone or retroperitoneal fibrosis. Care must be taken to prove that failure to pass urine is due to anuria and not retention of urine. The lower abdomen must always be examined for a distended bladder and catheterization may be necessary to exclude obstruction of the urethra.

ALTERATION IN THE APPEARANCE OF THE URINE

This is considered more fully under the examination of the urine (page 91). It is only necessary here to point out that the patient may first suspect urinary disease by noticing alteration in the colour and general appearance of the urine, e.g. red or smoky brown in haematuria, cloudy with an offensive smell when infected, frothy with proteinuria and dark orange or brown in obstructive jaundice. Various drugs may colour the urine, causing alarm or sometimes delight if the patient thinks it reflects the efficacy of treatment.

PAIN

In acute glomerulonephritis there may be a dull ache in the lumbar regions. Pain is common in acute pyelonephritis and is usually localized to the renal angle on the side of the affected kidney. Pain is particularly associated with any obstruction of the ureter, either at its origin in the pelvis of the kidney, during its course in the abdomen or at its entrance into the bladder. Obstruction may be caused by stones or by solid material such as blood or pus in urinary infections. An obstruction of uncertain nature is sometimes present in hydronephrosis; hence pain is also common in this condition. Only rarely is the obstruction caused by stricture or kinking of the ureter (e.g. by an aberrant renal artery). In some of these instances the characteristic pain of *renal colic* may be present (Figure 5.1). This consists of intense sharp pain generally referred in the first place to the lumbar region, i.e. at the renal angle (outer edge of erector spinae and the lower border of the 12th rib). It radiates forwards into the abdomen and downwards into the groin, the testis or the thigh. This spread is due to *ureteric colic*. Vomiting, sweating and great prostration generally accompany these attacks, which may last for several hours, especially when calculus is the cause of the obstruction. Although certain movements may aggravate the pain, the patient is often restless and rolls from side to side in an effort to gain relief. In this regard, the pain of renal colic differs from that of peritonitis in which the patient prefers to lie still. Between attacks of renal colic a dull ache may be present in the loin.

Pain arising from the bladder or urethra may be due to the passage of solid material such as pus, blood or stone and will then be similar in character to renal colic. Such pain is usually referred to the lower abdomen, the perineum and in the male to the glans penis. The term

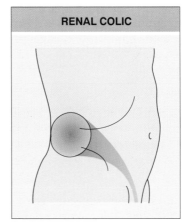

RENAL COLIC

◀ **Figure 5.1**
Renal colic. Pain starts in the loin and radiates to the groin, and sometimes into the genitalia and thigh

strangury is sometimes used if the urine is passed painfully, drop by drop. A burning or scalding discomfort is felt when there is inflammation of the lower urinary passages (e.g. cystitis or urethritis), especially if the urine is excessively acid. These pains generally occur during or at the end of micturition (see also Dysuria).

GENERAL SYMPTOMS
Renal oedema
In acute glomerulonephritis the oedema may be slight and short-lived, chiefly occurring in the face, though sometimes in dependent parts. In the nephrotic syndrome the oedema may be generalized, extreme and long-standing. In severe chronic renal failure the development of oedema indicates that the failing kidney can no longer maintain homeostasis with respect to sodium and water and that the terminal stage of the illness is not far away. In all cases, renal oedema results from the inappropriate retention by the kidney of sodium chloride and water. In acute glomerulonephritis, the reduction in glomerular filtration rate with continued reabsorption of sodium and water by the tubules is probably to blame. In the nephrotic syndrome the massive loss of proteins in the urine results in a fall in their plasma concentration. This leads to a reduction in the colloid osmotic pressure of the plasma and so to increased transudation of fluid into the tissues. The plasma volume is thus reduced, and in compensation the renal tubules reabsorb sodium chloride and water to expand the extracellular fluid volume until the plasma volume is restored. In chronic renal failure the tubular reabsorption of sodium is proportionately increased, but the glomerular filtration rate and the filtered load of sodium are reduced. Oedema often develops when more than 95 per cent of nephron function is lost and the glomerular filtration rate expressed as creatinine clearance falls below 5 ml/min. Renal oedema is not confined to the dependent parts as in heart disease and may be generalized (see Figure 5.13, page 97). In most patients the effect of gravity is apparent, ankle oedema developing at the end of the day in the ambulant patient and sacral oedema in the patient who rests in bed.

Symptoms due to high blood pressure
Many of the clinical features of renal disease are due to associated hypertension, which may lead to disturbance of the cerebral circulation. In most patients the rise in blood pressure is caused by the retention of sodium chloride and water with an increase in plasma volume and not by an increased secretion of renin.

In acute nephritis there is often a sharp rise in blood pressure during the early stages so that convulsions and

signs of cardiac failure may appear, but these are often indistinguishable from the effects of salt and water retention. Hypertension in chronic renal disease may be associated with headaches, vomiting and left ventricular failure.

Renal failure
The clinical features of renal failure are as varied as the functions carried out by the normal kidney. The kidney has a considerable functional reserve, and the body has a surprising tolerance of the nitrogenous waste metabolites normally excreted in the urine. In most patients the failing kidney can maintain homeostasis with respect to body water and ionic concentrations of electrolytes as the glomerular filtration rate declines over a tenfold range from 100 ml/min to only 10 ml/min. When more than 90–95 per cent of nephron function has been lost, or when the system is stressed by trauma or by intercurrent illness, the manifold features of the *uraemic syndrome* appear. These have defied explanation in terms of a single identifiable uraemic toxin. Many can be attributed to the imbalance in fluid and electrolyte metabolism. Generally, the patient feels tired, listless and breathless on exertion. These features can often but not always be explained by anaemia which is frequently present and which reflects a decrease in erythropoietin secretion by the kidney. There may be purpura and bleeding from the gastrointestinal tract due to defective platelet function.

Urogenital symptoms include thirst, polydipsia, polyuria and nocturia. In both sexes there is loss of libido and infertility, with impotence in men and secondary amenorrhoea in women.

Cardiovascular symptoms include precordial pain from pericarditis, ankle swelling, breathlessness on exertion and paroxysmal nocturnal dyspnoea from hypertension, with salt and water retention.

The *alimentary* system is disturbed by anorexia, nausea, vomiting and sometimes diarrhoea. The breath has an ammoniacal odour from the breakdown in the mouth of urea to ammonium carbonate under the influence of bacterial urease. The patient loses weight.

The *respiratory* system is implicated in the hyperventilation that results from metabolic acidosis, and which the patient often does not notice (Kussmaul's breathing).

Central, peripheral and *autonomic nervous* system involvement leads to an inability to concentrate, muscle twitching, restlessness of the legs, paraesthesiae and pareses due to peripheral neuropathy and autonomic neuropathy with hypohidrosis, impotence and postural syncope due to hypotension.

The skeleton is affected in patients with long-standing renal disease even when renal function is only moderately impaired. Bone pain and pathological fractures indicate defective mineralization and secondary hyperparathyroidism. These may result from a failure of the kidneys to synthesize the active metabolite of vitamin D and from their failure to excrete phosphate. Both may depress the plasma concentration of ionized calcium and thus stimulate increased secretion of parathyroid hormone and hypertrophy of the parathyroid glands.

Ultimately there is extreme prostration, drowsiness, mental confusion, convulsions and coma, gastrointestinal haemorrhage and haemorrhagic pericarditis with cardiac tamponade. Death may also result from hyperkalaemia or severe acidosis.

PHYSICAL SIGNS: EXAMINATION OF THE RENAL, URINARY AND GENITAL SYSTEMS

Examination comprises the following routine procedure:

1 *General examination* of the patient, with particular attention to the cardiovascular system, nervous system and retinae.
2 *Examination of the abdomen* to detect any enlargement of the kidneys or any tenderness over these or over the ureters or bladder. Occasionally it may be possible to palpate a thickened ureter or tumours arising from the bladder.
3 *The external genitalia* should also be examined especially for evidence of enlargement, neoplastic or inflammatory signs in the testis or epididymis and abnormalities in the urethra.
4 *Examination of the pelvic organs* through the rectum or vagina.
5 *Examination of the urine* by chemical and microscopical methods.

GENERAL EXAMINATION

The presence or absence of oedema should be noted in every case. The colour of the patient is important, as anaemia is a common secondary effect of nephritis. Undue dryness of the skin and haemorrhages should also be noted, as they are common in uraemia. In these cases the skin often has a dirty brownish appearance like fading sunburn. This may be due to the retention of urinary pigments or to the failure of the kidney to degrade melanocyte-stimulating hormone from the pituitary.

Systematic examination should include measurement of blood pressure and a search for signs attributable to hypertension such as a thrusting left ventricular impulse, crackles at the lung bases, evidence of cerebrovascular disease and retinal vascular changes (Figure 5.2) (see also Chapter 10, page 220). Signs of uraemia may be found in the respiratory system (Kussmaul's breathing), heart (pericardial friction rub), nervous system (twitching, drowsiness, peripheral neuropathy) and alimentary tract (dry coated tongue, bloody diarrhoea).

EXAMINATION OF THE ABDOMEN

THE KIDNEYS

Palpation of the kidneys is best carried out with the patient in the recumbent position and the head slightly raised on a pillow. One hand is placed under the loin with the tips of the fingers resting against the erector spinae, while the other is placed flat on the abdomen with fingers pointing upwards towards the costal margin (Figure 5.3). The patient is then instructed to take a deep breath, and firm pressure is exerted by both hands at the height of inspiration, so that if the kidney is palpable it moves down into the space between the examining hands and is 'trapped'. When the organ can be felt in this way it is recognized as a swelling with a rounded lower pole. The consistency of the swelling should be firm without hardness. It is not uncommon to feel the right kidney in women, and in some cases both kidneys may be freely movable and can be manipulated into different parts of the abdomen (floating kidney).

'Tumours' of the kidney when of moderate size retain the characteristic kidney shape, but with experience can be recognized as larger than normal. Those commonly recognized on abdominal examination are hypernephromas and polycystic kidneys; the former may be unduly hard and somewhat irregular, while in the latter cystic swellings may be palpable as characteristic bosses.

Inspection and percussion are of lesser importance, but tumours may show as a bulge in the loin which is dull on percussion and is best seen with the patient sitting up. Colonic resonance occurs in front of a renal tumour on the left side, thus distinguishing it from a splenic tumour. The character of the skin in the loin should also be noticed, as redness and oedema may be present in perinephric infection.

THE BLADDER

If distended with urine the bladder can be seen as a rounded or pyriform swelling arising from the pelvis (Figure 5.4) and extending upwards, sometimes as far

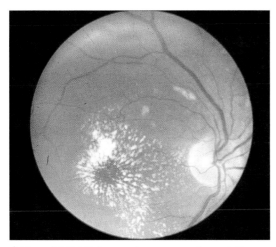

▲ **Figure 5.2 Ophthalmoscopic appearance in renal disease showing hard retinal exudates and the 'macular fan'**

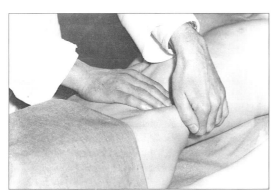

▲ **Figure 5.3 Palpation of the kidney.** One hand is placed on the abdomen with the fingers pointing towards the costal margin, the other is pressed firmly against the loin. If the kidney is enlarged or mobile it moves downwards on inspiration and is sandwiched between the two hands

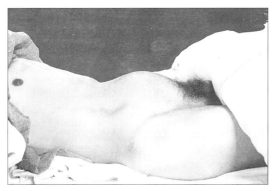

▲ **Figure 5.4 Distended bladder**

as the umbilicus. Its outline is confirmed by palpation and percussion and its lower margin cannot be felt. A distended bladder must be distinguished from a pregnant uterus or an ovarian cyst which may be of similar consistency. Proof that it is the bladder is obtained by catheterization, but voluntary evacuation should always be attempted first.

THE EXTERNAL GENITALIA

The external genitalia may provide some important clues to the diagnosis (see also Chapter 3, page 41).

MALE
Meatal ulcer is a common cause of painful micturition, haematuria and retention in babies and infants. It is a sequel to circumcision and may lead to meatal stenosis. A purulent discharge in the adult is diagnostic of urethritis and in company with swelling and tenderness of the epididymis suggests gonorrhoea, but infection with *Escherichia coli* is now at least as common. Strictures can be palpated in the penile urethra. The epididymis which is moderately enlarged, craggy and only slightly tender suggests genito-urinary tuberculosis, while tethering of the scrotal skin posteriorly and sinus formation are diagnostic. The ductus deferens (vas) is frequently thickened, but beading is uncommon. Swellings of the testis itself are more likely to be neoplastic, though orchitis occurs in mumps, and gummas are still occasionally seen. Hydrocele may be a sign of some other disease, inflammatory or neoplastic, involving the tunica vaginalis.

FEMALE
Vulvovaginitis due to monilial, trichomonal or gonococcal infection will explain scalding in the adult and urethral caruncle, scalding and tenderness in the elderly. A cystocele large enough to protrude from the vulva can cause retention; smaller cystoceles are often associated with stress incontinence. Vulval itching (pruritus vulvae) is an important early symptom of diabetes mellitus.

EXAMINATION OF THE PELVIC ORGANS

MALE
Rectal examination is necessary in all cases of suspected urinary disease. The left lateral or dorsal positions are used, the latter permitting bimanual examination, though the former is more commonly employed. When it is used, and the finger has been inserted with its dorsum towards the bladder, it should be gently rotated,

so that the more sensitive pulp of the finger palpates tissues and organs anterior to it (Figure 5.5).

The prostate (Figure 5.6) can normally be felt as an elastic swelling with a median groove terminating in a notch at the top. Gross adenomatous enlargement of the gland makes it more difficult to feel the upper surface or the notch, but the consistency is rubbery or even spongy. The apparent size of the gland is often exaggerated by a distended bladder. The malignant prostate has lateral infiltration so that it is difficult to identify the lateral margins. There is no 'give' when the finger pushes the prostate forwards. Irregularity and hardness in the prostate suggest malignant disease or occasionally prostatic calculi. Prostatic massage may give smears which are useful in the diagnosis of prostatitis and occasionally in malignant prostate.

The seminal vesicles lie above the prostate, running upwards from its outer margins, but can only be felt if they are full. Thickening due to tuberculous infiltration is sometimes an important diagnostic point in suspected urinary tuberculosis.

FEMALE

Inspection of the vulva (Figures 5.7 and 5.8) should first be made. Such common conditions as vaginal discharge, prolapse or urethral caruncle may at once be apparent. The vagina and cervix can then be inspected with a bivalve speculum in the dorsal position or a duck-bill speculum in the left lateral position. Differentiation between the types of vulvovaginitis will be facilitated, and urethral, vaginal and cervical swabs taken for bacteriological confirmation. Cystocele may be disclosed as a cause of frequency (Figure 5.8). An advanced cervical carcinoma might explain uraemia, due to ureteric obstruction, or incontinence if a vesical fistula is demonstrated. Obstruction to the passage of the speculum by

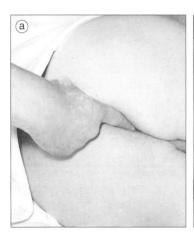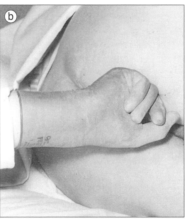

◀ **Figure 5.5 Rectal examination.**
The finger is inserted as shown in (a) and then gently rotated to define the prostate (b)

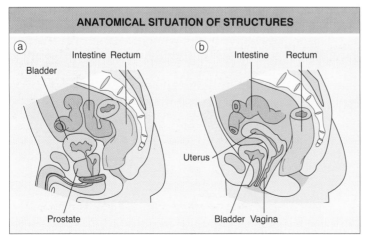

ANATOMICAL SITUATION OF STRUCTURES

(a) Bladder, Intestine, Rectum, Prostate

(b) Intestine, Rectum, Uterus, Bladder, Vagina

◀ **Figure 5.6 Shows the anatomical situation of structures which can be palpated per rectum or per vaginam**

a complete vaginal septum (frequently miscalled an 'imperforate hymen') will explain acute retention in the adolescent due to haematocolpos. Diverticulum of the urethra or paraurethral abscess may explain dysuria and dribbling incontinence.

Vaginal examination in the dorsal position permits bimanual assessment of the uterus and its appendages. Softening of the cervix and body of the uterus and enlargement of the latter, due to pregnancy, may explain urinary frequency without scalding. Tenderness in the renal angles during the second half of pregnancy, especially when accompanied by fever and vomiting, suggests pyelitis. Acute retention is uncommon in women, but with the exception of hysteria is due to intrapelvic masses, such as an impacted retroverted gravid uterus, uterine fibroids, ovarian cyst or haematocele due to ectopic gestation. In contrast to the male, genital tuberculosis is not usually accompanied by urinary tuberculosis. Calculi in the terminal portion of the ureter are palpable per vaginam.

EXAMINATION OF THE URINE

Examination of the urine is pre-eminently the method by which the diagnosis of urinary diseases is established.

INSPECTION
Inspection shows the colour of the urine and any deposit (Figure 5.9).

Colour
Highly concentrated urine usually has a dark amber colour inclining to orange. It frequently results from loss of fluid through other channels, as by sweating or diarrhoea. It also occurs in heart failure. These conditions lead to increased concentration of the urine, but a deeper colour may also result from changes in diet as increased proteins and purines favour the excretion of uric acid derivatives. Pale urine, on the contrary, is found when the concentration of solids diminishes and the urine is of large amount and usually of low specific gravity. It therefore occurs after excessive intake of fluids, alcohol and other diuretics, and in certain types of chronic renal disease; also in diabetes insipidus, in which the volume of urine is increased and its concentration diminished. A pale urine of high specific gravity (owing to the presence of sugar) occurs in diabetes mellitus.

Abnormal constituents may produce a complete change in the colour of the urine. Bile gives it a dark greenish-orange appearance, blood a red, reddish-brown or smoky colour, haemoglobin a deep red, and melanin

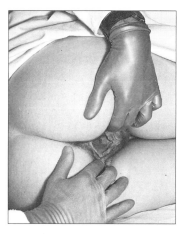

◀ Figure 5.7
Inspection of vulva and vaginal entrance

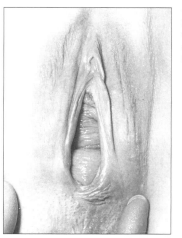

◀ Figure 5.8
Inspection of vulva showing cystocele and rectocele

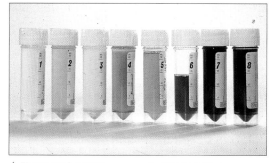

▲ **Figure 5.9 Coloured urines**

1 Yellow, normal
2 Pink, phenolphthalein or rhubarb
3 Orange, rifampicin
4 Red, haematuria
5 Orange, obstructive jaundice
6 Claret red, porphyria
7 Black, alkaptonuria
8 Black, melanuria

and alkapton a very dark appearance, sometimes black. Red urine or one which darkens on standing may suggest the rare but important condition of porphyria. The possibility of excreted drugs modifying the colour of urine has been mentioned, among them riboflavin, rifampicin and phenindione (Dindevan), an orange to orange-pink colour, while brighter pink may result from santonin or phenolphthalein. Even food and drink may cause a similar colour, e.g. beetroot and rhubarb.

Deposit

Fresh urine rarely has much deposit if it is normal, but on standing deposits of phosphates or urates may produce a cloudiness or even a thick heavy layer. Phosphates are usually a white or light buff colour and disappear if the urine is acidified, whilst urates vary from a buff colour to a pink or brick-red disappearing on heating. These constituents have no pathological significance. A fainter cloudiness may be produced by bacteria, giving the urine an opalescent or shimmering appearance. Pathological constituents such as pus and blood also produce turbidity, increasing in some cases to a thick deposit.

Specific Gravity (Relative Density)

The normal specific gravity of urine is generally about 1.015 to 1.025 (conveniently styled 1015 or 1025), but wide variations are found in health, according to the quantity of fluid ingested and the amount lost through the skin and bowels. A persistently low specific gravity (1010 or rather less) suggests chronic renal disease if rarer causes such as diabetes insipidus can be excluded. Very high specific gravities (1030–1060) are rarely found except in the presence of large amounts of sugar in the urine in diabetes mellitus. When a specific gravity of over 1050 is found, the possibility of artefact must be excluded.

Reaction

The urine may be acid or slightly alkaline in health. It is frequently alkaline for a short period during the digestion of food, the so-called 'alkaline tide'. Decomposition on standing and the liberation of free ammonia also render it alkaline, especially when the urine is heavily charged with bacteria. The type of diet may also alter the reaction, vegetables and fruit tending to make it alkaline, meat acid.

Smell

A strong ammoniacal smell is frequently found in infants and after decomposition when the urine has been left standing. Infection with *Escherichia coli* imparts a fishy odour, while certain foods, notably asparagus, also give rise to a characteristic smell.

Quantity

The amount of urine passed in 24 hours should be recorded. In health it averages 1500 ml.

Chemical Examination

Rapid and simple tests for the presence in the urine of protein, glucose, ketones, bilirubin, urobilinogen and blood are available. These tests can be carried out at the bedside and should be regarded as a part of the physical examination of the patients rather than as a special investigation. Each test is based upon a colour change in a strip of stiff absorbent cellulose which has been impregnated with the appropriate reagent. A fresh specimen of urine is collected in a clean test-tube free of contaminants (especially detergents and acids). The change in colour of the strip after contact with urine is compared with a colour chart in a bright white light. Single strips for the simultaneous detection of a number of abnormal urine constituents are available for routine urine testing (Figure 5.10).

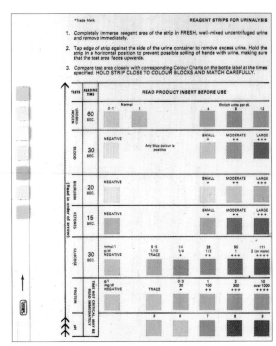

▲ **Figure 5.10 The detection of abnormal urinary constituents, by colour reaction.** The strip carrying seven different reagents (left of picture) is immersed in the urine and any colour changes are compared with those in the control chart after the appropriate time interval. (Reproduced by courtesy of Ames Company, Division of Miles Laboratories Ltd, Slough, UK)

The chemical principles underlying the colour reactions illustrated in Figure 5.10 are as follows:

pH test: This test is based on a double indicator principle which gives a broad range of colours covering the entire urinary pH range. Colours range from orange through yellow and green to blue.

Protein test: This test is based on the protein error of indicators principle which means that at a constant buffered pH, the development of any green colour is due to the presence of protein. Colours range from green–yellow for 'negative' through yellow–green and green to green–blue for 'positive' reactions.

Glucose test: This is a double sequential enzyme reaction. The reaction utilizes the enzyme glucose oxidase to catalyse the formation of glucuronic acid and hydrogen peroxide from the oxidation of glucose. In turn, a second enzyme, peroxidase, catalyses the reaction of hydrogen peroxide with a potassium iodide chromogen to oxidize the chromogen to a green-brown colour.

Ketone test: This reaction is based on the purple colour developed with aceto-acetic acid or acetone and nitroprusside. The components are stabilized in a dry reagent containing glycine as the nitrogen source and a strongly alkaline buffer.

Bilirubin test: This reaction is based on the coupling of bilirubin with diazotized dichloraniline in a strong acid medium. The colour developed is a tan-to-purple shade.

Blood test: The detection of occult blood is based on the peroxidase-like activity of haemoglobin which catalyses the reaction of peroxide and the chromogen ortho-tolidine to form blue oxidized orthotolidine.

Urobilinogen test: This test area is based on the Ehrlich reaction in which paradimethylaminobenzaldehyde reacts with urobilinogen in a strongly acid medium to form a red colour.

False-positive results for protein may occur with alkaline highly buffered urine, for ketones if the urine contains L-dopa metabolites and for bilirubin in patients taking chlorpromazine. A false-negative result for blood may occur with infected samples of urine and those of high specific gravity and also in the presence of ascorbic acid.

It is important that the instructions which accompany the reagents should be followed exactly. The information given here is intended only as a general guide; the details are not necessarily applicable to all the available reagents.

The common abnormal constituents indicating the presence of urinary tract disease are protein, blood and pus.

Proteinuria

The presence of protein in the urine may vary from a trace to 10 g per litre or more. Very small amounts may be derived accidentally from the urinary passages, particularly from the vagina and prepuce. Protein derived from these sources is inconstant and has no pathological significance. Diseases of the kidney, the bladder and the urethra, in which pus or blood is produced, are also accompanied by proteinuria, and the possibility of these should be considered before attributing proteinuria to nephritis.

Protein excreted into the urine by the kidneys otherwise falls into two classes:

1. Physiological proteinuria.
2. Pathological proteinuria.

The distinction between these two is not always easy.

Physiological proteinuria

This generally occurs in children or young adults, and the amount of protein is usually small, though occasionally considerable. It appears in the urine in significant circumstances. Usually it is absent in the early morning specimen, but appears after the patient has been up for an hour or two; sometimes it appears only after exercise. Various names have been applied to the different types of physiological proteinuria, such as orthostatic or postural when it seems to be dependent upon change in posture of the individual.

It is thought that this harmless form of proteinuria is due to venous congestion of the kidneys chiefly from altered posture, especially with lordosis. Repeated examination is often necessary before proteinuria can be called 'physiological'. Its inconstancy is an important point, and also the fact that it usually disappears after 24 hours' rest in bed. It is not accompanied by other evidence of nephritis, as is shown by good response to the renal efficiency tests and the absence of casts (occasionally a few hyaline casts may occur) in the urine.

Pathological proteinuria

Although heavy proteinuria suggests organic renal disease, the amount of protein may be quite small even when the kidneys are badly damaged and functioning poorly. The persistent presence of more than 1 g/l of protein in the urine generally indicates the presence of nephritis, unless pus or blood is responsible. In chronic pyelonephritis proteinuria is generally mild, whereas in the nephrotic syndrome the loss of protein in the urine usually exceeds 5 g per 24 h and can reach 20–30 g in severe cases. Proteinuria may occur as a manifestation of systemic disease affecting the kidneys. Thus in cardiac failure and febrile states, small amounts of protein (up to 1 g per 24 h) may be lost in the urine without any real kidney disease, but this disappears if treatment is successful. Proteinuria occurs in eclampsia, amyloidosis and diabetes mellitus and also following the ingestion of certain chemical poisons. Bence Jones protein, consisting of fragments of light chains of the immunoglobulin molecule, is found in the urine in certain cases of multiple myelomatosis. It can be demonstrated by heating a specimen of urine, acidified with acetic acid, in a tube to which a thermometer is attached. The protein is precipitated between temperatures of 40 and 60 °C, almost disappears as boiling point is approached, and reappears on cooling.

Microalbuminuria is increased urinary albumin excretion without detectable proteinuria. It may last for years and is found in the course of diabetic kidney disease.

Haematuria

Blood in the urine may vary in amount from large quantities visible to the naked eye to a few red corpuscles detectable only by microscopical examination. The blood may be derived from any part of the urinary tract – the kidneys, rarely the ureters, the bladder or the urethra. When derived from the kidney it has an opportunity to become intimately mixed with the urine, which is correspondingly reddish-brown in colour ('smoky') or evenly pink, but when derived from the bladder or urethra it may remain separate from the urine, and have the bright-red appearance of pure blood. Clots may appear, sometimes stringy if casts of the ureter are caused by excessive bleeding from the kidney. Blood from the urethra may be dislodged by the urinary stream and thus precedes the urine. The reverse is the case when the bleeding is taking place in the bladder.

Haematuria may be due to haemorrhagic conditions, to disease of the kidney itself or to lesions in the lower urinary tract. Haemorrhagic conditions can cause bleeding from the kidney as one part of a generalized disorder of the blood (e.g. thrombocytopenia, prothrombin deficiency) or the blood vessels (e.g. scurvy, allergic purpura, certain acute fevers). The renal diseases producing haematuria include the acute forms of nephritis, trauma, infarction, malignant hypertension, congenital cystic kidney, nephrotoxic drugs (e.g. sulphonamides), calculus, neoplasm, tuberculosis and acute bacterial infection. These last four conditions are also the main causes of bleeding from the bladder and, less commonly, from the ureters or urethra.

Pyuria

A few pus cells in the urine have little significance, especially in women, as they may derive from the vagina. Larger quantities of pus usually indicate an inflammatory lesion of the urinary tract, and in most cases organisms are to be found on microscopical examination and on culture. Quantitative estimations of the number of pus cells passed per hour can vary from a few hundred in normal persons to 1,000,000 or more in heavy urinary infections. In all cases in which pus is found, therefore, a specimen of urine collected aseptically is a necessity both to establish the presence and nature of the organisms and the fact that the pus has a urinary origin. The urethral meatus is swabbed with a weak antiseptic and a midstream specimen of urine is then collected in a sterile receptacle. A catheter should be used only if, for any reason, this procedure is impracticable (e.g. in the unconscious patient).

Cystitis, pyelitis and suppuration in the kidney substance are important causes of pyuria, but smaller amounts of pus may occur from prostatitis and urethritis in men. While protein and blood are the usual abnormal constituents in cases of nephritis, pus cells are not uncommonly found, especially in acute nephritis. Pus may also be derived from extrinsic causes such as diverticulitis of the colon or the rupture of an appendix abscess into the bladder.

Pneumaturia

Gas is rarely expelled with the urine, but pneumaturia may occasionally prove of considerable diagnostic value, suggesting a communication between the urinary tract (usually the bladder) and the alimentary tract (the colon). It is occasionally found, for example, in cases of diverticulitis in which the diverticulum has become adherent to the bladder. Carcinoma of the colon is the next most common cause. Rarely, faeces may be passed with the urine.

MICROSCOPICAL EXAMINATION

The urine should always be examined microscopically. Apart from the presence of small numbers of red corpuscles and pus cells which may not be recognizable by chemical tests, microscopical examination may show the presence of casts, crystals, foreign bodies, micro-organisms and parasites. Phase contrast microscopy can help define the site of origin of red cells. Dysmorphic or irregularly shaped forms suggest nephritis whereas normally shaped red cells are more often associated with lower urinary tract lesions such as bladder tumours.

Casts (cylinduria) in appreciable numbers are most commonly found in cases of nephritis. They are formed by protein being precipitated in the tubules and moulded into cylindrical shape with the incorporation of any cellular elements or debris that may also be present. Red cells in the tubular lumen can only have come from the glomerular capillaries. Their presence in casts is thus pathognomonic of glomerulonephritis, and the recognition of red cell casts in the urine provides an important contribution to the differential diagnosis of patients with haematuria. Their reddish-brown colour may be lost, but they can still be recognized by comparison with free red cells elsewhere in the urinary sediment. A fresh specimen must be examined since red cell casts degenerate rapidly if the urine is left to stand. Leucocyte casts are found in chronic pyelonephritis, and epithelial cell casts are produced by desquamation of the renal tubular epithelium from any cause. Granular casts may result from the degeneration of cellular casts or from the incorporation of debris. Hyaline casts reflect the severity of proteinuria and are found most commonly when the urine contains few cells.

Crystals are often found in the urine but are rarely of diagnostic importance. It is important to recognize the hexagonal crystals of cystine which are found in patients with a rare congenital metabolic defect (cystinuria) associated with recurrent stone formation.

Bacteria need to be sampled. As catheterization is now avoided, when possible, to prevent trauma and consequent risk of urinary infection, the midstream technique is used to provide a suitable specimen of urine for all purposes.

This may be handled in any hospital laboratory to ascertain the bacterial count, but in domiciliary practice a simple 'dip-inoculum' enables the doctor to send the specimen through the post to a laboratory. High bacterial counts (100,000 per ml or more) may be found as the only urinary tract abnormality.

Parasites in the urine are rare in Great Britain, but *Trichomonas vaginalis* is sometimes found even in catheter or midstream specimens. Of the more exotic parasites, *Bilharzia haematobia* is the most important; the large ova are easily recognized under low magnification (see Chapter 13)

Many other bodies may be seen in urine, and some of these need experience for their recognition. They are rarely indicative of urinary or any other form of disease. They include vaginal epithelium, spermatozoa, urates, phosphates and all manner of foreign bodies.

SPECIAL INVESTIGATIONS

Special investigations of value in the elucidation of urinary-tract disease include radiography, cystoscopy, chemical examination of blood and urine, tests of renal function and renal biopsy.

Radiography

A direct radiograph of the abdomen will usually reveal the size and contour of the kidneys. The urinary conduit including the renal pelvis, ureters and the bladder, are best outlined by the intravenous injection of a radio-opaque dye which is excreted in the urine–intravenous pyelography (IVP) or intravenous urography (IVU) (Figure 5.11). If the dye cannot be excreted because of poor renal function, it may be injected through a ureteric catheter inserted at cystoscopy (retrograde pyelography). Alternatively, when the ureteric orifice is blocked, a needle may be inserted percutaneously into a dilated renal pelvis under ultrasound guidance (antegrade pyelography). Ultrasound examination is a safe, non-invasive technique to estimate the shape, size and consistency of the kidneys and is particularly useful in distinguishing a benign cyst from a solid and probably malignant swelling (Figure 5.12). CT scanning may demonstrate the spread of a renal tumour into the renal veins and para-aortic lymph nodes as well as perinephric swellings. Renal angiography outlines abnormalities of the renal arteries and arterial, capillary and venous changes in the kidney itself.

Cystoscopy

This is mainly of value in the diagnosis of bladder disease (e.g. tumours) by direct vision and by biopsy. Cystoscopy also permits catheterization of the two ureters for pyelography or for studies of differential renal function.

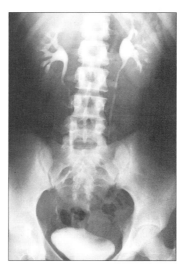

◀ **Figure 5.11 Intravenous pyelogram**. Normal appearance of renal pelves, ureters and bladder

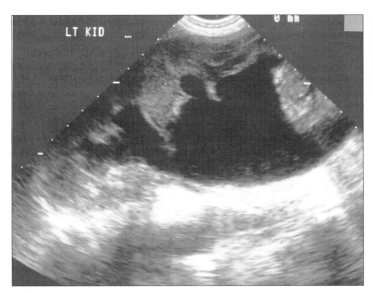

◀ **Figure 5.12 A longitudinal section through the left kidney demonstrating marked dilation of the calyces renal pelvis and proximal ureter due to hydronephrosis.** Note the distal enhancement (white echoes) on this ultrasound scan

Blood and urine chemistry

Disordered renal function is most simply assessed by measurement of urea, creatinine and electrolyte (sodium, potassium and bicarbonate) concentrations in plasma and urine. The commonest abnormality is an increase in plasma urea and creatinine concentrations, but as renal function deteriorates metabolic acidosis results in a fall in plasma bicarbonate, and ultimately there is a rise in plasma potassium which can be fatal. The plasma sodium concentration reflects a change in body water as often as a change in sodium balance, being increased in dehydration and decreased in water intoxication. The additional measurement of plasma calcium, phosphorus and alkaline phosphatase concentrations in patients with moderately severe renal failure provides useful information on the response of the skeleton to disordered vitamin D metabolism and to changes in parathyroid hormone concentrations.

Three main aspects of renal function and disease can be studied: glomerular filtration, the control of renal tubular reabsorption and the differential function of the two kidneys.

Glomerular filtration rate can be assessed most conveniently in terms of the creatinine clearance, using a timed collection of urine which is usually made over a 24-hour period. The creatinine clearance is derived by dividing the excretion rate of creatinine by the plasma creatinine concentration. The quantity of protein excreted per day can be measured on the same 24-hour sample of urine. In patients with glomerulonephritis the differential clearance of two proteins of high and low molecular weight is measured to obtain an index of selectivity of the proteinuria. In some cases, only proteins of low molecular weight such as albumin and transferrin escape the glomerular filter. In others, larger quantities of proteins of high molecular weight, such as the immunoglobulins and fibrinogen, pass through the glomerular basement membrane and the proteinuria is termed 'unselective'.

Tubular reabsorption of water is assessed in terms of the ability of the kidney to alter the specific gravity or osmolality of the urine in response to water deprivation and loading. Defective tubular reabsorption of sodium, potassium or magnesium can be revealed by limiting the oral intake of these substances and measuring the ability of the kidney to compensate in terms of reducing their urinary excretion rates.

The differential function of the two kidneys was assessed at one time by comparing the composition of urine samples obtained from the two sides by ureteric catheterization. Such information can now be obtained non-invasively from intravenous pyelography or by scanning the two kidneys with an external counter following the intravenous injection of a radio-isotope which is excreted in the urine (isotope renography).

Renal biopsy

The histological diagnosis of diffuse renal disease can often be established by needle biopsy. This method is of particular value in determining the cause of a nephrotic syndrome.

THE DIAGNOSIS OF RENAL AND URINARY TRACT DISEASES

Sometimes the symptoms already enumerated – frequency, dysuria, pain, oedema and so forth – attract attention to the urinary system, but not infrequently, especially in cases of nephritis, the onset is insidious and silent, and routine examination of the urine may first throw light on the cause of a patient's poor health. This is one of a number of reasons for making the examination of the urine a necessary part of every medical examination, a measure often throwing unexpected light on an obscure case and saving the examiner from making serious mistakes in diagnosis.

The more common diseases of the urinary system follow. Some of them fall more frequently within the province of the surgeon but are discussed briefly as they may overlap into that of the physician.

DISEASES OF THE KIDNEYS

Many renal disorders ultimately result in total renal failure with the clinical features of uraemia already described. Common causes of chronic renal failure are listed in Table 5.1. The development of techniques to replace renal function by mechanical means or by kidney transplantation, and the limited availability of these dramatic measures, means that accurate diagnosis is essential. This has been facilitated by a greater understanding of pathophysiological mechanisms and by classifications based on analysis of renal biopsy material.

Diseases affecting the glomeruli, whether primary or secondary to systemic disorders, account for well over half of all patients developing chronic renal failure, as well as for many patients with self-limiting conditions. Renal biopsy, used in conjunction with laboratory indices of disordered immunological function, has helped to identify distinct patterns of disease in a field which was previously greatly confused. Five distinct clinical syndromes can be recognized.

ACUTE GLOMERULONEPHRITIS

Acute glomerulonephritis (or acute nephritic syndrome) was common in children but, like rheumatic fever, is now seen infrequently. Both are apparently immunological responses to streptococcal infections, generally of the throat in Western countries but sometimes of the skin in the tropics or where living standards are poor.

An acute nephritic syndrome may also complicate systemic lupus erythematosus, Henoch–Schönlein purpura and subacute bacterial endocarditis. The glomeruli are congested with cellular proliferation and deposition of immune complexes of antigen, antibody and complement in the capillary walls. The clinical picture consists of haematuria, albuminuria, casts, oedema (especially facial, Figure 5.13), with associated hypertension and sometimes uraemic symptoms. The course of the illness is usually benign leading to full recovery within a few months. A few cases are fulminating, leading to death within months.

RECURRENT HAEMATURIA

Recurrent haematuria with insignificant proteinuria, normal blood pressure and normal renal function, often within 1–3 days of an upper respiratory tract infection, can develop in some patients. The condition is commoner in children, resolves spontaneously within a week, and in most cases carries a good prognosis. Renal biopsy reveals focal proliferation of mesangial cells in some of the glomeruli, with mesangial deposition of immunoglobulins, especially IgA. This association was recognized by Berger in 1968, and the condition now bears his name.

CAUSES OF CHRONIC RENAL FAILURE
Glomerulonephritis (primary and secondary)
Chronic pyelonephritis
Renal vascular disease
Polycystic kidneys
Chronic obstructive uropathy (e.g. prostatic)
Congenital nephropathies
Analgesic nephropathy
Diabetes mellitus

▲ **Table 5.1**

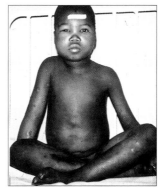

◀ **Figure 5.13 Acute glomerulonephritis.** Note facial oedema causing narrowed palpebral fissures, oedema of legs and septic skin lesions

RAPIDLY PROGRESSIVE GLOMERULONEPHRITIS

A small but significant number of patients develop proteinuria, oedema, mild hypertension and progress to end-stage renal failure within weeks or months of their presentation. Some cases follow a viral or bacterial infection. Occasionally the lungs are involved with haemoptysis from alveolar haemorrhage, an association recognized by Goodpasture in 1919. In the kidney the glomerular capillaries are compressed and eventually obliterated by a crescent of proliferating epithelial cells which line Bowman's capsule. In Goodpasture's syndrome the glomerular damage is caused by a circulating antibody formed against a protein in the capillary wall, possibly shared by the alveolar capillaries. In other patients, circulating immune complexes are to blame.

ASYMPTOMATIC PROTEINURIA

Many patients have no symptoms but are found to have proteinuria or an increased blood pressure on routine medical examination. Renal function may be normal or variably impaired, and the glomeruli may show proliferation of cells or fibrosis. In some patients the proteinuria continues with no deterioration in renal function, whereas others slowly progress to fatal renal failure.

NEPHROTIC SYNDROME

The triad of oedema, hypoalbuminaemia and heavy proteinuria can arise from a variety of diseases affecting the glomeruli. The common pathogenetic factor is the magnitude of the protein loss. This is usually greater than 5 g daily in adults or 0.1 g/kg in children, and this amount exceeds the capacity of the liver to compensate by increased synthesis. An increased plasma cholesterol is also found. Patients present with the insidious onset of oedema and some notice frothy urine. Some primary and secondary causes of the nephrotic syndrome are listed in Table 5.2. In minimal lesion glomerulonephritis the glomeruli appear normal on light microscopy, although with the electron microscope loss of pedicle structure can be seen. The condition occurs more commonly in children, the proteinuria is highly selective, and most cases respond to treatment with corticosteroids. In membranous, proliferative and mesangiocapillary glomerulonephritis there is deposition of immunoglobulins and complement in the glomeruli, with thickening of the basement membrane or proliferation of cells, or a combination of the two. Hypertension is more common and remissions less frequent than in the minimal lesion type and many patients progress slowly to chronic renal failure. Among conditions in which glomerular damage occurs

secondarily, quartan malaria deserves mention as possibly the commonest cause of nephrotic syndrome in the world.

RENAL VASCULAR DISEASES

The most important of these is *malignant* or *accelerated hypertension*. This may complicate either essential or renal forms of hypertension (see also Chapter 7) and generally develops rapidly over a matter of months presenting with albuminuria, casts, high blood pressure readings and papilloedema.

The renal changes in the malignant phase are due to a necrotizing arteriolitis, and the end result (apart from vascular complications) is renal failure. At this stage it is difficult to be sure of the origin of the condition, whether in fact the hypertension is primary or secondary.

Acute tubular necrosis

This condition may be regarded as vascular in origin resulting from shock, especially in association with crush injuries or postpartum haemorrhage. Acute failure of renal function occurs with oliguria, anuria and uraemic symptoms. Spontaneous recovery may occur in a few weeks: if the patient is maintained by dialysis, function may be restored in about 10 days.

Renal artery stenosis

Renal artery stenosis (Figure 5.16) is occasionally responsible for hypertension and, if proved by arteriography, may offer chances for surgical relief.

CAUSES OF NEPHROTIC SYNDROME
A *Primary or idiopathic glomerulonephritis*
(minimal lesion, membranous, proliferative, mesangiocapillary)
B *Secondary*
(a) Infections or disordered immunity: quartan malaria, infective endocarditis, systemic lupus erythematosus (Figure 5.14), Henoch–Schönlein purpura (Figure 5.15)
(b) Drugs and other chemicals: mercury, gold, penicillamine, probenecid
(c) Glomerular infiltrations: amyloidosis, diabetes mellitus, myelomatosis
(d) Tumours: myelomatosis, lymphomas, bronchogenic and other solid tumours

▲ Table 5.2

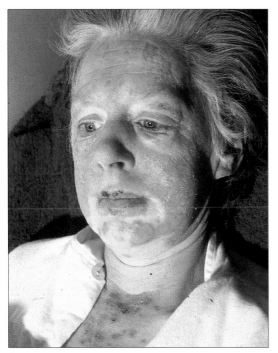

▲ **Figure 5.14 Systemic lupus erythematosus.** This patient developed nephrotic syndrome

Renal vein occlusion

Thrombosis of the leg veins may extend through the inferior vena cava to involve the renal veins. The ensuing clinical picture is usually that of the nephrotic syndrome (page 98) or acute renal failure.

PYELONEPHRITIS

This is the most serious manifestation of urinary-tract infection. The organism commonly responsible is *Escherichia coli,* as in the case of cystitis (see page 101).

In the acute form the classic syndrome includes pain in the loin, on one or both sides, marked loin tenderness, with high fever, rigors and frequency of micturition. There may be recurrent attacks of this kind and the disease may become chronic. In such cases radiological changes due to cortical scars and clubbing of the calices may be found. The urine generally shows a high content of the infecting organism (100,000 per ml or more), pus cells and granular or leucocyte casts. An increase in antibody titres against the O antigen of *Escherichia coli* may also be found.

Pyelonephritis is particularly common during pregnancy and may have been preceded by a high bacteriuria, possibly dating back to childhood. It is now

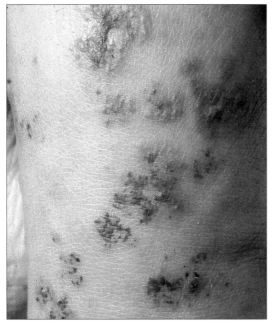

▲ **Figure 5.15 Henoch-Schönlein purpura on the leg of a patient passing 10 g protein a day**

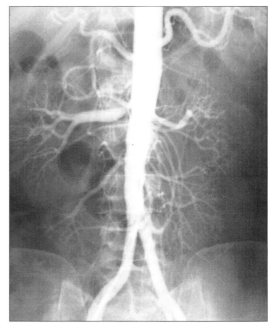

▲ **Figure 5.16 An aortogram carried out by catheterization of the femoral artery showing stenosis of the mouth and proximal end of the right renal artery**

considered that chronic pyelonephritis may exist without clinical symptoms; this may result in a pathological kidney which is difficult to distinguish from other forms of renal disease and indeed may terminate in renal failure.

ANALGESIC NEPHROPATHY

The regular consumption over many years of mild analgesics containing phenacetin and aspirin can result in necrosis of the renal papillae (papillary necrosis) and interstitial nephritis with ultimately the development of chronic renal failure. The condition is common in Australia where the endemic consumption of analgesics is high while the hot climate encourages the formation of small volumes of highly concentrated urine.

RENAL TUBERCULOSIS

The primary lesion is cortical and remains subclinical until the calices and pelvis are affected, when symptoms begin to appear. It is often associated with tuberculous lesions in other parts of the urinary system, e.g. the bladder or epididymis. A tuberculous focus may be found elsewhere, as in the chest or spine.

Constitutional symptoms are rare and the patient remains in good condition. Of the local symptoms, frequency of micturition is most important and progressive; it may be accompanied by pain on micturition. Haematuria may also be a presenting sign. Pyuria is generally recognized if microscopic examination of the urine is made, but special methods of investigation, particularly examination and culture for tubercle bacilli in the urine, cystoscopy and pyelography, may be necessary to establish the diagnosis.

RENAL CALCULUS

Stones may be present in the kidneys without symptoms. Sometimes a dull ache may occur, and if the stone becomes dislodged and passes down the ureter, an attack of colic results (see Pain, page 86).

The traumatic effects of the stone, especially when in movement, often result in haematuria, and the urine should be examined microscopically for red corpuscles.

Calculi may lead to infection of the kidney, affecting the pelvis (pyelitis) or kidney substance (pyelonephritis). A stone impacted at the junction of the pelvis and ureter may cause hydronephrosis or pyonephrosis (Figure 5.17). The impaction of a stone may also cause temporary anuria.

A tendency to form renal calculi may reflect a disturbance in calcium, uric acid or, more rarely, cystine metabolism. Symptoms and signs of hyperparathyroidism (page 312) should especially be sought.

'TUMOURS' OF THE KIDNEY

Kidney 'tumours', i.e. swellings or enlargement, generally have the shape of the normal organ (see page 88), but if very large may fill the whole loin or spread into other parts of the abdomen. They vary in consistency from that of normal renal tissue to the extreme hardness of some malignant growths. The more important tumours are hydronephrosis, polycystic disease and hypernephroma. It should be remembered that a normal right kidney is quite commonly palpable, especially in women.

Hydronephrosis is a ballooning of the kidney calices and pelvis by retained urine, due to intermittent or partial obstruction of the ureter, in some cases idiopathic and due to neuromuscular disturbance, in some due to calculus. The kidney retains its normal shape but is occasionally large enough to be palpable. Bilateral hydronephrosis results from obstruction to the urethra by a stricture or prostatic enlargement.

Polycystic disease is characterized by the development of numerous cysts in the kidney which destroy its substance (Figure 5.18). It is generally bilateral, and the kidneys are palpable as large 'bossed' reniform tumours. Other symptoms suggest the presence of chronic renal disease (polyuria, proteinuria, high blood pressure, etc.). Haematuria is sometimes a symptom. The condition is often familial, and if it is not recognized in infancy, symptoms may be delayed until middle life.

Hypernephroma, the commonest malignant tumour of the kidney, is generally recognized by the presence of a renal tumour with haematuria which is often painless, thus distinguishing it from calculus. It may also show itself by metastases in bone or lungs, and

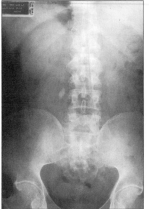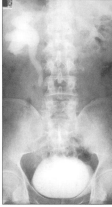

▲ **Figure 5.17 Right hydronephrosis due to obstruction of ureter by stone illustrated on plain radiograph and intravenous pyelogram**

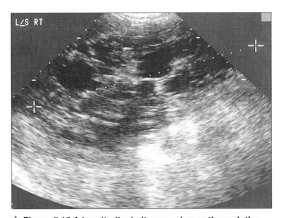

▲ **Figure 5.18 A longitudinal ultrasound scan through the right kidney.** The round black areas are fluid filled spaces consistent with adult polycystic kidney disease

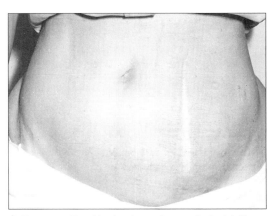

▲ **Figure 5.19 Renal implant beneath a scar in the left iliac fossa**

corresponding symptoms such as pain or cough, or by malignant ascites.

DIALYSIS AND TRANSPLANTATION

Chronic renal failure is fatal, but many patients can now be treated successfully by dialysis and by transplantation. These therapeutic activities have created a new range of extraordinary physical signs to replace the traditional features of severe uraemia.

The patient with a functioning transplant will not usually be anaemic but may show features of mild Cushing's syndrome from taking corticosteroid drugs to prevent graft rejection. There will be an easily palpable, firm, non-tender kidney in either the right or left iliac fossa under the scar of a healed surgical wound (Figure 5.19). During rejection there will be fever and hypertension; the graft will enlarge and become tender, the urine volume falls and renal function deteriorates.

Patients on haemodialysis are more commonly anaemic and pass little or no urine. They usually have an arteriovenous fistula (Figure 5.20) in one arm or forearm with distension of the proximal veins, scars from frequent venepuncture and a palpable thrill with audible bruit over the anastomosis. In some patients the veins may become greatly distended over the years (Figure 5.21). A few patients may have indwelling central venous cannulae. Some patients are maintained on long-term peritoneal dialysis. In these cases an indwelling soft silastic cannula will be found emerging from the anterior abdominal wall below the umbilicus, usually slightly to one side of the midline.

DISEASES OF THE BLADDER

CYSTITIS

Frequency of micturition and dysuria are the characteristic symptoms of cystitis. Fever is rarely marked. The diagnosis is completed by the finding of pyuria, by

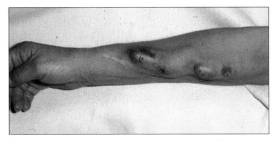

▲ **Figure 5.20 The swellings on the forearm are dilated veins showing puncture sites created for access for haemodialysis**

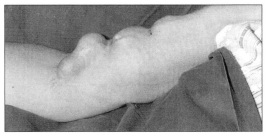

▲ **Figure 5.21 Gross venous distension in the upper arm resulting from a long-standing arteriovenous fistula**

the discovery of some causal factor such as prostatic enlargement or vesical calculus and sometimes by cystoscopic examination, which may be necessary to determine the essential nature of the cystitis. Special forms of cystitis causing severe symptoms, especially in women, include Hunner's ulcer (interstitial cystitis) and urethro-trigonitis. Symptoms of recurrent apparent cystitis are common in women and may be due to a chronic urethritis, the so-called 'urethral syndrome'. The aetiology is obscure but is probably multifactorial and includes trauma and prolapse, bacterial infection and hormonal factors.

CALCULUS

Calculus in the bladder may cause dysuria and haematuria. Its presence generally requires instrumental (cystoscopy) or radiological methods for its recognition. As it is nearly always secondary, a decision must be made as to whether it has come down from the kidney, or whether it complicates prostatic enlargement or a diverticulum of the bladder.

TUMOURS

Tumours (papillomas and carcinomas) usually cause haematuria, and require cystoscopy for their diagnosis. Adenomatous or carcinomatous enlargements of the prostate may project as tumours into the bladder and cause urinary obstruction. This may be recognized by rectal examination. Enlargement of the prostate should always be considered as a cause of urinary symptoms in elderly men, especially when the symptoms resemble those of chronic renal disease (nocturia and slight proteinuria).

The respiratory system

SYMPTOMS OF RESPIRATORY DISEASE

COUGH

Cough may be either a voluntary act or a reflex response to irritation of the respiratory mucosa mediated through a centre in the medulla. It consists of a forceful expiratory effort with the glottis closed, followed by the sudden explosive release of the pent-up air along with sputum or other irritant matter.

The student must note whether a cough is dry or productive of sputum, whether it is short or paroxysmal, the times at which it tends to occur and finally the character of the sound. A dry cough occurs when the mucous membrane of the larynx, trachea or bronchi is congested with little or no exudate, as in the early stages of respiratory infections and following the inhalation of irritant dusts or fumes, e.g. tobacco smoke. A 'loose' or productive cough indicates free exudate in the respiratory passages, as in chronic bronchitis and bronchiectasis.

A short cough is usual in upper respiratory infections such as the common cold and when respiratory movements are suppressed by pleuritic pain.

Prolonged or paroxysmal coughing is characteristic of chronic bronchitis and also of whooping-cough, in which a rapid series of coughs is followed by a deep inspiration through a partially closed glottis. A foreign body may be responsible for the abrupt onset of paroxysmal cough, and this possibility must always be considered, especially in children, from whom no history may be forthcoming. A severe paroxysm may be followed by vomiting or by syncope, the latter being due to the raised intrathoracic pressure interfering with venous return to the heart and thus diminishing cardiac output.

Any tendency for cough to occur at particular times should be noted. Cough and expectoration of sputum are often most troublesome on rising in the morning and going to bed at night, especially in chronic bronchitis and bronchiectasis. This may be due to the change in posture moving secretions from damaged insensitive areas of mucosa to more sensitive parts. A change of temperature, as in moving from a warm room to the cold outside air, also provokes cough in patients with chronic bronchitis. For this reason, and also because of the greater frequency of respiratory infections, the cough is worse in winter than in summer. Cough waking the patient at night, although quite common in chronic bronchitis, should always suggest the possibility of pulmonary oedema due to left heart failure or mitral stenosis (see page 172). Other causes of nocturnal cough include asthma (especially in children), secretions running down the larynx from the posterior nares in patients with chronic infections of the nose or sinuses and the inhalation of oesophageal or gastric contents due to oesophageal obstruction or hiatus hernia with reflux.

Finally, the character of the actual sound produced by the cough should be noted. Intrathoracic tumours, especially aneurysm, can press on the trachea and cause cough with a metallic, hard quality described as 'brassy'. If a tumour involves the recurrent laryngeal branch of the vagus and interferes with the normal movements of the vocal cords, the cough loses its explosive character and becomes prolonged and wheezing, like that of a cow; it is then known as a 'bovine' cough. Diseases of the larynx responsible for cough (e.g. neoplasm) are sometimes identified by the hoarseness of the cough and the accompanying stridor.

SPUTUM

Quite apart from the laboratory examination of sputum, much important information can be gained by naked-eye inspection. The patient should be instructed to expectorate into a sputum cup, and the amount measured after 24 hours. The student should note the amount, consistency and colour of the sputum. Large amounts may be found in bronchiectasis and pulmonary abscess or when an empyema ruptures into a bronchus. The expectoration of large quantities of sputum on change of posture is particularly characteristic of bronchiectasis and pulmonary abscess, and in these conditions the sputum may sometimes have an offensive smell due to infection by anaerobic organisms. A large amount of thin, colourless sputum is sometimes seen in the relatively rare alveolar cell carcinoma of the lung; in such cases the taste may be salty.

The consistency and colour of the sputum may be of diagnostic value. Thick, viscid sputum, which sometimes takes the shape of bronchial casts, occurs in asthma, especially the kind associated with bronchopulmonary aspergillosis (Figure 6.1). Thin, watery sputum suggests pulmonary oedema. Green coloration indicates pus while a yellow colour may be due to pus or to a high eosinophil content. Blood in the sputum may give a rusty appearance in pneumonia, a diffuse pink staining in pulmonary oedema or it may appear as streaks or clots (see below).

HAEMOPTYSIS

Expectoration of blood is known as haemoptysis. The amount may vary from streaks to several pints and may consist of pure blood or be mixed with sputum or salivary secretions. From the patient's history it is not always easy to determine whether the blood has been coughed up or vomited. The important differences between haemoptysis and haematemesis are summarized in Table 6.1.

The staining of the sputum for some days after the haemorrhage is perhaps the most convincing point of distinction between haemoptysis and haematemesis.

If it is definitely established that the blood has been spat up, the mouth and throat should be examined for any local cause, such as epistaxis, bleeding gums or a congested pharynx, which may cause small amounts of blood to appear in the mouth. However, haemoptysis

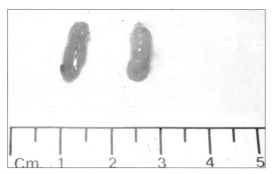

▲ **Figure 6.1 Bronchial casts consisting of viscid sputum and fungal mycelia from a patient with asthma associated with bronchopulmonary aspergillosis**

DIAGNOSIS OF HAEMOPTYSIS AND HAEMATEMESIS	
Haemoptysis	**Haematemesis**
Cough precedes haemorrhage	Nausea and vomiting precede haemorrhage
Blood frothy from admixture with air	Generally airless
Sputum bright red in colour and may be stained for days	Blood often altered in colour by admixture with gastric contents, usually dark red or brown
History suggests respiratory disease	Previous history of indigestion
Confirmed by bronchoscopy	Confirmed by gastroscopy

▲ **Table 6.1**

must never be attributed to these causes until a chest radiograph has been proved normal.

The most serious common causes of haemoptysis are bronchial carcinoma, bronchiectasis, mitral valve disease, tuberculosis and pulmonary infarction.

DYSPNOEA
Physiological aspects

Dyspnoea, or breathlessness, may be defined as an undue awareness of respiratory effort or of the need to increase this effort.

The awareness of respiratory effort has been related to the force used to ventilate the lungs. This force is increased when the thoracic cage or pleura is abnormally rigid, the pleural cavity filled with fluid or air, airways resistance increased, or the lungs less distensible than normal; this also occurs when there is an increased demand for breathing as a result of hypoxia, anaemia, acidosis or thyrotoxicosis. Dyspnoea may also take the form of an awareness of the need to increase respiratory effort, as in breath-holding and paralysis of the respiratory muscles (e.g. poliomyelitis).

The sensation of dyspnoea is probably derived from two main sources: receptors sensitive to stretch and deflation in the thoracic cage and lungs, and chemoreceptors in the aorta and carotid arteries and in the reticular substance of the medulla which are sensitive to oxygen lack, carbon dioxide excess or changes in pH. The relative importance of these thoracic and central sources of dyspnoea is not known, but experimental work suggests that stimuli arising from receptors in the respiratory muscles themselves are the main immediate cause of dyspnoea even when there is no increase in respiratory movements.

Clinical aspects

An attempt should be made to assess the severity of the dyspnoea by noting whether it is present at rest, with gentle activity such as undressing or walking on level ground, during moderate exertion, such as climbing stairs, or only on more strenuous exercise. The ability of the patient to carry out routine tasks at work or in the home should also be recorded.

Dyspnoea may be due to disease of the bronchi, lungs, pleura or thoracic cage, to cardiac failure, to an increased central demand for respiration or to psychogenic causes.

1 Dyspnoea due to *disease* of the *bronchi*, *lungs*, *pleura* or *thoracic cage* is usually brought on by exertion. Dyspnoea which develops suddenly at rest suggests pulmonary embolism or pneumothorax.

2 The dyspnoea of *cardiac failure* is due to an increased stiffness of the lungs resulting from engorgement with blood when the mitral valve is diseased or the left ventricle fails. The dyspnoea is provoked by exertion and relieved by rest, but it is also influenced by posture. When the patient lies flat, gravitational effects increase the congestion of the lungs. This causes dyspnoea when the patient lies down ('orthopnoea', or 'upright breathing'), and sometimes a violent attack of breathlessness may waken him from his sleep ('paroxysmal nocturnal dyspnoea'). These attacks may be accompanied by cyanosis and the expectoration of large amounts of thin, frothy sputum stained pink with blood due to pulmonary oedema. Attacks of cardiac dyspnoea unassociated with effort or changes in posture can also result from myocardial infarction or a rapid dysrhythmia (see also Cardiovascular system, Chapter 7).

3 Dyspnoea can result from an *increased demand* for respiration even when the heart, lungs and thoracic cage are healthy. This increased demand arises from stimulation of central receptors by hypoxia (e.g. high altitudes, anaemia), acidosis (e.g. diabetes, uraemia), or when metabolism is increased (e.g. fever, thyrotoxicosis). Other signs of the disease causing the dyspnoea will usually be apparent; the pallor of anaemia should especially be looked for in all patients complaining of breathlessness.

4 *Psychogenic dyspnoea* should never be diagnosed until all possible organic causes have been excluded. This form of dyspnoea is quite common because any discomfort in the chest may be interpreted as breathlessness by the nervous patient. Such discomfort may be due to anxiety about the heart or lungs, ectopic beats, muscular symptoms such as a 'stitch' or gastric flatulence. These relatively innocent conditions in an apprehensive patient may result in sighing respirations and a desire to take frequent deep breaths; the dyspnoea occurs as often at rest as on exertion and especially while talking. These patients may ventilate in excess of metabolic requirements, thus lowering the arterial tension of carbon dioxide to produce such symptoms as dizziness, paraesthesiae and tetanic cramps in the hands due to respiratory alkalosis (see also page 311).

PAIN

Lung tissue is insensitive and pain (see also page 5) in the chest is always the result of conditions which affect the surrounding structures. When the pleura is involved, pain is a prominent feature. The pain is usually described as 'cutting', 'stabbing' or 'tearing' on deep breathing or coughing. Most commonly it is felt in the axillae and beneath the breasts, but it may occur in regions remote from the chest and cause difficulty in diagnosis. The parietal pleura, including that covering the outer portion of the diaphragm, is innervated through the thoracic roots (intercostal nerves), the lower six of which are responsible for the supply of skin areas on the abdominal wall and back. Pleural pain is therefore frequently referred to the abdomen and lumbar regions, and has given rise to a mistaken diagnosis of acute abdominal lesions.

The innervation of the central portion of the diaphragm by the phrenic nerve (3rd and 4th cervical) occasionally leads to referred pain in the neck and shouldertip in diaphragmatic pleurisy.

In lesions of the apex of the lung such as Pancoast's syndrome (bronchial carcinoma causing Horner's syndrome with involvement of the 8th cervical and 1st dorsal nerve roots), all the pain may be referred to the arm (Figure 6.2).

Finally, it must be mentioned that many pains that occur in the chest are not associated with respiratory disease. These include pains due to disease of the heart (see Chapter 7), oesophagus and upper abdominal viscera (e.g. hiatus hernia), osteoarthritis of the spine, lesions of the ribs, sternum and intercostal muscles, herpes zoster and diseases of the breast.

UPPER RESPIRATORY TRACT SYMPTOMS

These include sneezing, a 'sniffly' nose, nasal obstruction and discharges, facial pain due to disease of the nose or paranasal sinuses, and hoarseness or aphonia resulting from laryngeal disease.

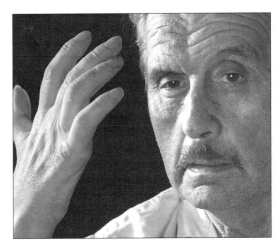

▲ Figure 6.2 Right Pancoast's syndrome showing Horner's syndrome and wasting of small muscles of the hand

EXTRATHORACIC SYMPTOMS OF RESPIRATORY DISEASES

Diseases of the respiratory system can produce symptoms in other parts of the body:

1 'Constitutional' symptoms such as loss of appetite and weight, lassitude, sweats and dyspepsia, as in tuberculosis and carcinoma.
2 Symptoms of hypoxia and carbon dioxide retention ('hypercapnia'), including mental disturbances, headaches, sweats, tremors, convulsions and coma (see also Bronchitis, page 121).
3 Evidence of pulmonary heart disease ('cor pulmonale'): oedema, jugular venous engorgement, liver distension and ascites (see also page 172).
4 Finger clubbing and painful swellings in the limbs due to pulmonary osteoarthropathy, as in bronchial carcinoma and bronchiectasis (see page 121).
5 Distal manifestations of bronchial carcinoma also include the symptoms of metastases in other organs and, more rarely, various forms of myoneuropathy and endocrine disorder (see also Bronchial carcinoma, page 122).

PHYSICAL SIGNS: EXAMINATION OF THE RESPIRATORY SYSTEM

Certain signs may be noted before the systematic examination of the chest is made, namely, the character of any sputum (page 127), the presence of cyanosis or clubbing of the fingers and the condition of the neck.

CYANOSIS
Physiological aspects

Cyanosis, a blue coloration of the skin or mucosae, occurs when there is an excess of desaturated haemoglobin or of certain abnormal haemoglobins in the capillaries. Desaturated haemoglobin rarely causes cyanosis until it amounts to more than about 5 g/dl (30 per cent of the total amount of haemoglobin in the capillaries), and even then there is great variation in the ability of different observers to recognize cyanosis. Moreover, desaturation does not happen until there is already considerable hypoxia because haemoglobin only gives up its oxygen when the tension in the blood has fallen below about 10.6 kPa (80 mmHg) (normal 13.3 kPa, 100 mmHg). It is apparent, therefore, that cyanosis is usually a sign of severe oxygen deficiency.

Cyanosis may be classified according to its cause:

1 *Peripheral cyanosis.* This is due to a diminished capillary blood flow allowing more time for the removal of oxygen by the tissues. There are two types of peripheral cyanosis:
(a) Cyanosis due to a reduced cardiac output (e.g. mitral stenosis, shock, etc.).
(b) Cyanosis due to local vasoconstriction (e.g. cold).
2 *Central cyanosis.* In this form of cyanosis there is an excess of desaturated haemoglobin in the blood leaving the aorta. There are three types of central cyanosis:
(a) Cyanosis due to deficient oxygenation of the blood in the lungs resulting from inadequate ventilation of perfused areas of lung (e.g. pneumonia; chronic bronchitis), from a reduction in the total amount of air ventilating the lungs as a whole (e.g. poliomyelitis); or from impaired oxygen transfer across the alveolar capillary membrane (e.g. fibrosing alveolitis).
(b) Cyanosis due to a right-to-left shunt of blood bypassing the lungs through a septal defect in the heart (e.g. Fallot's tetralogy) or between a pulmonary artery and vein (arteriovenous aneurysm) (page 184). A shunt effect may also occur through a lobe or segment of lung of which the bronchus is occluded (e.g. bronchial carcinoma).
(c) Cyanosis due to an absolute excess of desaturated haemoglobin, the percentage saturation being normal. This occurs in primary polycythaemia.
3 *Cyanosis due to abnormal pigments (Enterogenous cyanosis).* This form of cyanosis, which results from the presence in the red cells of an excess of either sulph-haemoglobin or methaemoglobin, sometimes imparts a mauve or brownish tinge to the skin. It is unaccompanied by dyspnoea or other respiratory symptoms, but headache, lassitude and constipation are common. Enterogenous cyanosis is usually due to the ingestion of substances that favour the combination of haemoglobin and sulphur absorbed from the bowel or the reduction of haemoglobin to methaemoglobin (e.g. sulphonamides, phenacetin and other analgesic drugs). These abnormal haemoglobins can be identified by spectroscopic examination of the blood.

Clinical aspects

The patient or a relative may report that cyanosis is present all the time or only during exertion or exposure to cold. Cyanosis must be looked for in the extremities (the fingers and toes, nose, lips and ears) and also in the oral mucosa. If there is doubt, cyanosis can be brought to light by exercise, which increases the removal of oxygen by the tissues. Peripheral and central cyanosis can be distinguished by warming the hands in a bowl of hot water or by inspection of a naturally warm part such as the oral mucosa: heat increases capillary flow and thus abolishes peripheral cyanosis. If cyanosis persists in a warm part, then it must be either central or enterogenous. The effect of breathing pure oxygen for 10 minutes should then be observed: cyanosis due to lung disease or polycythaemia will disappear while cyanosis due either to a right-to-left shunt bypassing the lungs or to abnormal pigments will remain (see Table 6.2).

CLUBBING OF THE FINGERS

Clubbing (Figure 6.3) is an important sign of certain diseases of the lungs and also of the heart and alimentary system; rarely it may be congenital in origin. It can be recognized by a bulbousness of the soft terminal portion of the fingers and by an excessive curvature of the nail in both the longitudinal and lateral planes. An early sign of clubbing is loss of the normal angle at the base of the nail, seen best in the lateral view. Later the nail may become loose in its bed so that movement can be elicited when light pressure is exerted over the nail base ('fluctuation'). Sometimes, the finger ends are also cyanotic and the nails abnormally shiny.

Finger clubbing may be associated with similar changes in the toes and, in bronchial carcinoma especially, with a painful swelling over the ends of the long bones. This last condition is known as 'hypertrophic pulmonary osteoarthropathy' and must always be considered when a patient with finger clubbing complains of symptoms that suggest arthritis in the wrists and ankles. The exact cause of clubbing and osteoarthropathy remains uncertain, but the local changes are probably due to an overgrowth of the soft tissues and subjacent periosteum associated with an increased peripheral blood flow (Figure 6.4). These changes will sometimes regress if the primary cause is removed.

THE EFFECTS OF LOCAL HEAT AND BREATHING OXYGEN ON THE DIFFERENT TYPES CYANOSIS		
Cause of cyanosis	**Local heat**	**Breathing oxygen (for 10 min)**
Peripheral	Abolished	Remains
Central		
• Pulmonary	Remains	Abolished
• Polycythaemic	Remains	Abolished
• Right-to-left shunt	Remains	Remains
Enterogenous	Remains	Remains

▲ Table 6.2

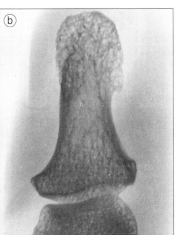

▲ Figure 6.3 Finger clubbing due to bronchial carcinoma

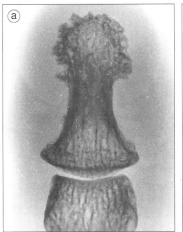

◀ Figure 6.4 Radiograph of a clubbed finger (a) compared with the normal (b). Note soft tissue swelling and overgrowth of subperiosteal bone

THE NOSE

Examination of the nose with a nasal speculum (see Figure 6.5) may reveal a nasal discharge from chronic sinus infection which is commonly associated with bronchiectasis. Rhinitis may be associated with hay fever and indicates a potential asthmatic which may also be linked with nasal polyps. Nasal granulomata often accompany similar lesions in the lung caused by sarcoidosis or Wegener's granulomatosis.

THE NECK

Examination of the neck may reveal important signs of respiratory system disease. The student should inspect the neck for scars of phrenic crush, lymph node excision and mediastinoscopy (see Figure 6.6) as well as engorged jugular veins and accessory respiratory movements. The trachea and lymph nodes should then be palpated.

The jugular veins

These may be overfilled, not only in congestive cardiac failure (pages 142, 172) but in superior mediastinal obstruction due, for example, to bronchial carcinoma (Figure 6.7).

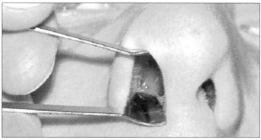

▲ **Figure 6.5 Nasal speculum – note the anteroposterior position to avoid stimulating the sensitive nasal septum** (reproduced from *Clinical Examination of the Patient* by John Lumley and Pierre-Marc G. Bouloux, Butterworth–Heinemann, 1994)

These two causes can be distinguished by the presence of pulsation in cardiac failure and its absence in mediastinal obstruction (page 126). Filling of the jugular veins during expiration and emptying during inspiration may result from raised intrathoracic pressure in patients with expiratory airways obstruction (e.g. asthma).

Accessory respiratory movements

Inspiratory contraction of the sternomastoid muscles may occur with respiratory distress of any kind, but is particularly associated with overinflation of the lungs due to chronic airways obstruction. The sternomastoids are best examined by drawing them backwards between thumb and forefinger to see if they become taut with inspiration. Abnormal recession of the suprasternal and supraclavicular fossae may also be observed during inspiration in these patients.

The trachea

This is palpated in the suprasternal notch for lateral displacement (page 113). The length of trachea which can be felt between the cricoid cartilage and sternal notch (normal: 3–4 fingerbreadths) may be reduced by elevation of the sternum in patients with chronic overinflation of the lungs. Also in these patients, the downwards pull of the diaphragm can cause descent of the trachea and larynx during inspiration; this can be detected by resting the tip of the index finger on the thyroid cartilage. A downwards pull on the larynx may also occur during systole in patients with aortic aneurysm ('tracheal tug').

Lymph nodes

These may be enlarged from secondary bronchial carcinoma, lymphoma, tuberculosis or sarcoidosis. Careful palpation of the supraclavicular fossae is especially

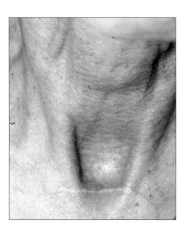

◀ **Figure 6.6 Subtle scar of mediastinoscopy to obtain lymph nodes in a patient treated for non-Hodgkin's lymphoma**

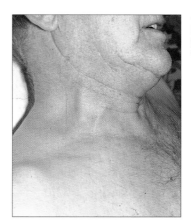

◀ **Figure 6.7 Mediastinal tumour. Engorged veins in the neck**

important in cases of lung disease since the scalene nodes are the most commonly affected and also because carcinoma of the lung apex (Pancoast tumour) may be felt at this site (Figure 6.8).

THE LARYNX

Examination of this structure should be made in all cases of chronic respiratory disease. Changes in the voice and special types of cough should be noted. The laryngoscope may show tuberculous ulceration in association with the pulmonary disease or vocal cord paralysis, especially in cases of mediastinal tumour and malignant disease of the lung.

INSPECTION OF THE CHEST

The skin over the chest wall should be noted as in the inspection of any part of the body. Particular attention should be directed to the presence of engorged veins (Figure 6.9), subcutaneous nodules and surgical scars. Common thoracic scars include left and right thoracotomy (Figure 6.10), median sternotomy and drainage scares of an empyema (Figure 6.11). Modern 'keyhole' surgical scars may be unobtrusive (Figure 6.12).

POSITION OF THE APEX BEAT AND TRACHEA

Except in very thin patients, the trachea can rarely be seen, and obesity may also mask the impulse of the heart apex; palpation is therefore necessary to confirm their position. The heart and trachea may be displaced to the opposite side by pleural effusion or pneumothorax, or drawn to the same side by pulmonary fibrosis. Displacement of the heart towards the left axilla may give a false suggestion of cardiac enlargement. Displacement

to the right causes the cardiac impulse to appear well within the nipple line, and the maximal pulsation may even be to the right of the sternum.

CHARACTER OF RESPIRATORY MOVEMENTS
Expansion of the chest

The degree of the expansion of the chest may be measured by placing a tape measure just below the nipples, with its zero mark at the middle of the sternum, and instructing the patient to breathe in and out as deeply as possible. In women mammary tissue should be avoided by making the measurements above or below the breasts. It is important that several readings should be taken, as the initial respiratory efforts are often shallower than subsequent ones.

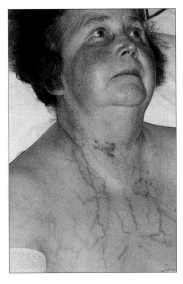

◄ **Figure 6.9 Superior mediastinal obstruction.** Note swelling of neck, dilated veins on the chest and dusky tint of face

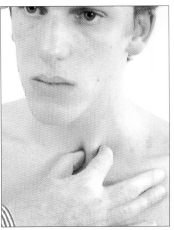

◄ **Figure 6.8 Palpating the left scalene node behind the lower end of the relaxed sternomastoid** (reproduced from *Clinical Examination of the Patient* by John Lumley and Pierre-Marc G. Bouloux, Butterworth–Heinemann, 1994)

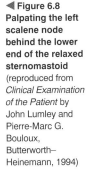

▲ **Figure 6.10 Right thoracotomy and drainage scars performed for right pleurectomy for recurrent pneumothorax in identical twins**

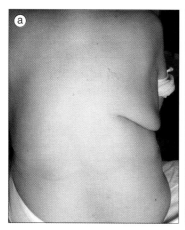

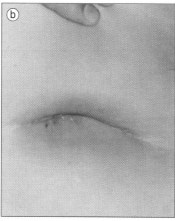

Figure 6.11 Right empyema scar revealed when the flesh of the posterior chest wall is elevated

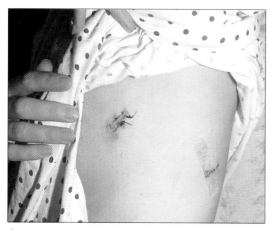

Figure 6.12 Recent left pleurectomy using keyhole surgical approach. Compare Figure 6.10

Particular note should also be made of the equality of expansion of the two sides. In the absence of muscle or skeletal changes, such as scoliosis, a definite inequality signifies disease of the bronchi, lungs or pleurae. The affected side, whatever the pathology, usually moves less than the sound side. Generalized restriction of expansion is more commonly seen in emphysema, though it occurs in extensive bilateral disease and in ankylosing spondylitis.

Manner of breathing

The manner of breathing should next be noted. In men the diaphragm is more freely used than the intercostal muscles, and its downward excursion with inspiration leads to free movements of the abdominal wall–abdominal respiration. Similar breathing is characteristic of children.

In women, on the other hand, the movements of the chest are greater than those of the abdomen, because respiration is chiefly accomplished by use of the intercostal muscles–thoracic respiration. Various mixtures of these two types of breathing – diaphragmatic and costal – are found in health, but a sudden change in the type of breathing may be significant of disease. Thus, acute peritonitis by limiting the abdominal movements produces a costal type of breathing, while pain from pleurisy or other cause may lead to restriction of the chest movements. When the diaphragm is paralysed, the upper part of the abdomen may be drawn in during inspiration.

The rate and depth of respiration

The rate and depth of respiration should be observed without the patient's knowledge, as consciousness of the act of breathing tends to make it irregular. The rate varies in normal individuals between 16 and 20/min at rest, but is faster in children and slower in old age. It bears a definite ratio to the pulse rate of about 1:4, which is usually constant in the same individual. The depth of breathing, or tidal ventilation, is about 500 ml at rest, but some form of spirometer is needed to make this measurement (see Pulmonary function tests, page 127).

The rate and depth of breathing are regulated by the respiratory centre through reflexes deriving from receptors in the thorax and great vessels (see also Dyspnoea, page 104). They usually increase or decrease together, but rate may increase at the expense of depth when deep breathing is inhibited by a pleuritic pain or by gross reduction of the vital capacity (e.g. extensive pulmonary fibrosis, poliomyelitis). Conversely, slow deep breathing is sometimes seen in airflow obstruction and cerebral conditions associated with coma. An increased rate ('tachypnoea') and depth ('hyperpnoea') occur when there is an increased demand for ventilation, as in exercise, fever, thyrotoxicosis, acidosis and diseases of the heart or lungs associated with hypoxia or hypercapnia (see also Dyspnoea, page 104). A decrease takes place during sleep and when the respiratory centre is depressed by cerebral disease or narcotic drugs.

Abnormal types of breathing

When there is great dyspnoea the accessory muscles of respiration may be called into play. During inspiration, the sternomastoid and other neck muscles contract, the nares are dilated by the alae nasi (especially in children) and there are often gasping movements of the mouth. During expiration the abdominal muscles contract and patients with airways obstruction may purse their lips; this probably serves to prevent collapse of the airways during expiration by raising the intrabronchial pressure (Figure 6.13) (see also Emphysema, page 125). In-drawing of the intercostal spaces during inspiration may be seen in patients, children especially, with severe airways obstruction. Multiple fractures of the ribs or sternum can result in a flail chest with paradoxical breathing, the unsupported chest wall being drawn in by the negative intrathoracic pressure during inspiration.

A special variety of breathing known as Cheyne–Stokes respiration consists of a temporary cessation of breathing (apnoea) followed by respirations which gradually increase in magnitude to a maximum and then diminish until apnoea occurs once more. This phenomenon is usually found in illnesses which interfere with the function of the respiratory centre, such as hypoxia, raised intracranial pressure, uraemia and advanced heart disease (see also Chapter 7). In nervous subjects, breathing may be irregular in rate and depth and interspersed with deep sighing breaths.

The partner may report snoring interspersed with silence by night and day in the sleep–apnoea syndrome.

CHEST DEFORMITIES

Abnormalities of the chest wall are not infrequently present without disease of the thoracic contents. The softness of the bones in childhood renders the chest liable to deformities if the normal relationship between intrathoracic pressure and that of the atmosphere is disturbed. For example, nasal obstruction due to adenoids and bronchial narrowing due to asthma or bronchitis may produce gross alteration in the configuration of the chest. Many types of chest deformity exist, amongst which may be mentioned:

1 *Harrison's sulcus,* a groove running horizontally from the sternum outwards in the lower part of the chest.
2 *Pigeon-chest,* in which there is marked bulging of the sternum; this is an occasional sequel to asthma in childhood (see Figure 6.35, page 121).
3 *Funnel breast,* an exaggeration of the normal depression seen at the lower end of the sternum. This is often congenital in origin (Figure 6.14). Combinations of these three are sometimes present. Rickets favours their production by making the bones abnormally soft, and sometimes leaves further traces as a 'rickety rosary', a series of knob-like projections on the chest wall at the junction of the ribs with the costal cartilages. Deformities of the thoracic cage can also result from osteomalacia due to malabsorption from the bowel (see Malabsorption syndrome, page 73).

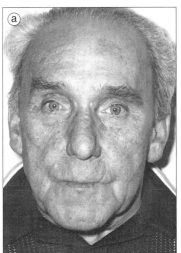
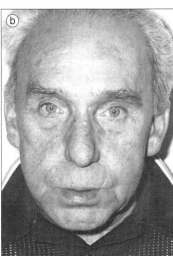

◀ **Figure 6.13 Lip pursing in a patient with emphysema.** (a) Lips tightly apposed at height of inspiration. (b) Lips held narrowly apart during expiration

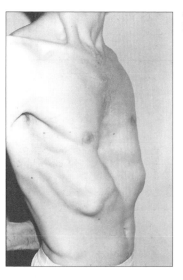

◀ **Figure 6.14**
Funnel sternum

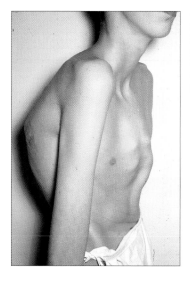

◀ **Figure 6.15**
Congenital
kyphoscoliosis
and sternal
deformity
(Marfan's
syndrome)

4 The *barrel-shaped chest,* in which the chest is fixed in the inspiratory position. This deformity may occur in emphysema but is not a constant or diagnostic sign of this disease.

5 *Spinal deformities:* ankylosing spondylitis restricts the expansion of the chest by immobilizing the costovertebral joints, while kyphoscoliosis (Figure 6.15) may so diminish the volume of the lungs as to cause cardiac and respiratory failure in middle life.

6 Localized bulging or recession of the chest wall may result from aneurysm, empyema, cardiac hypertrophy, local disease of the ribs or sternum and fibrotic changes in the lungs and pleura.

ANATOMICAL LANDMARKS

It will be convenient before leaving the examination of the chest by inspection to recall a few important facts in thoracic anatomy (Figures 6.16 and 6.17).

The *sternal angle* is formed by the junction of the manubrium with the body of the sternum, and corresponds with the attachment of the second costal cartilage to the sternum. It is a convenient bony point from which to count the ribs and intercostal spaces. It serves as a guide to the position of the thoracic viscera by marking the level of the bifurcation of the trachea, the meeting of the lung borders and the upper limit of the atria.

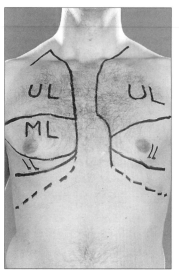

◀ **Figure 6.16**
Anatomical
landmarks of the
lungs and pleurae
as seen from the
front. The lobes of the lungs are marked out by plain black lines. The lower limit of the pleura is marked by the dotted line. UL, upper lobe; ML, middle lobe; LL, lower lobe

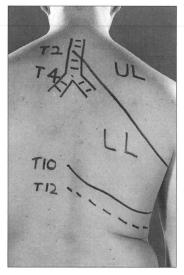

◀ **Figure 6.17**
Anatomical
landmarks of the
lungs and pleurae
as seen from the
back. The right side only is marked. The plain lines indicate the upper and lower boundaries of the lower lobe of the lung. The dotted line indicates the lower limit of the pleura. The trachea and its bifurcation and the positions of the spines of the 4th, 10th and 12th dorsal vertebrae are shown. UL, upper lobe; LL, lower lobe

Posteriorly, the *scapulae* cover a large area of the chest which is relatively inaccessible to examination. The spine of the scapula is usually at the level of the 2nd thoracic vertebra, its angle reaching to the 7th vertebra. The roots of the lungs lie in the interscapular region at the level of the spines of the 4th, 5th and 6th thoracic vertebrae.

The *lobes of the lung* are separated by the oblique fissure, above which lies the upper lobe (and the middle lobe on the right side), and below it the lower lobes.

The fissure runs roughly in the line of the fifth rib, being slightly above at the back and a little below in the front. The upper margin of the right middle lobe is defined by a line from the 4th costal cartilage to the fifth rib in the mid-axilla: the lingula of the left upper lobe is a little higher in front but extends to a similar point in the axilla.

It will be recognized that the upper lobes are principally accessible from the front, and the lower lobes from the back: in the axillae important segments of all lobes are open to examination. Further, it will be appreciated that there are five bronchopulmonary segments above the fifth rib, and on the right side at least, five below. The radiological identification of these segments is important in defining more accurately the site of a pulmonary lesion within a lobe (Figures 6.18 and 6.19).

The apices of the upper lobes rise about 2–3 cm above the clavicles. From this point the inner margins of the lungs and their covering pleurae slant towards the sternum, meeting each other in the midline at the sternal angle. On the right side this margin of the lung continues down the sternum as far as the sixth costal cartilage, where it turns outwards and downwards to meet the midaxillary line about the eighth rib, the scapular line at the tenth rib, and the paravertebral line at the spine of the 10th thoracic vertebra. On the left side the landmarks are the same, with the exception that the lung border turns away from the sternum at the fourth instead of the sixth costal cartilage, owing to the position of the heart, which lies closely in contact with the chest wall over this region. At the apices, and along the inner margins of the lungs, the pleura lies so close to the lungs as to follow the same surface markings, but at the lower borders of the lungs the pleura extends farther, lying 4–5 cm below the lung borders anteriorly and posteriorly, and as much as 9–10 cm below in the axillae. These costodiaphragmatic recesses of the pleural cavity may be filled up with lung substance during deep inspiration.

PALPATION

For successful palpation the hands must be warm and used as gently as possible. They should be placed over the two apices, and by looking over the patient's shoulders, with his chin dropped on the chest, the movement of the upper lobes can be compared. The lower lobes may similarly be examined by placing the hands around the costal margins, in the lower parts of the axillae or over the bases of the lungs at the back (Figures 6.20 and 6.21).

Examination of the vocal fremitus may then be made at the same areas (see below).

The position of the apex beat and of the trachea should be confirmed by palpation (Figure 6.22). To determine the position of the trachea the finger should

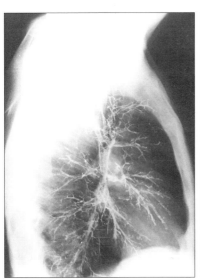

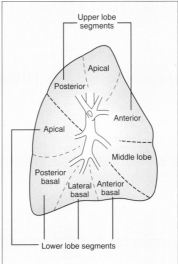

Upper lobe segments

Apical

Posterior

Anterior

Apical

Middle lobe

Posterior basal

Lateral basal

Anterior basal

Lower lobe segments

◀ **Figure 6.18 Bronchogram and diagram of bronchopulmonary segments of right lung.** The middle lobe embraces a medial and a lateral segment. The lower lobe also has a medial basal segment which lies on the mediastinal aspect of the lobe and is therefore not shown in this lateral view

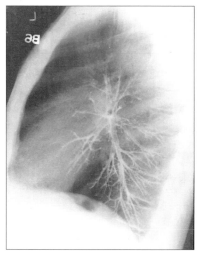

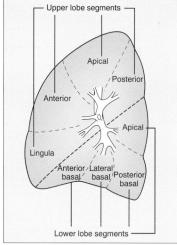

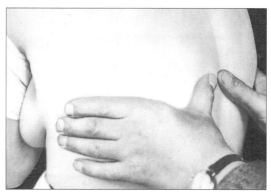

◀ **Figure 6.19 Bronchogram and diagram of bronchopulmonary segments of left lung.** Note that the apical and posterior segments of the left upper lobe arise from a common bronchus so that they are usually described together as the 'apicoposterior segment'

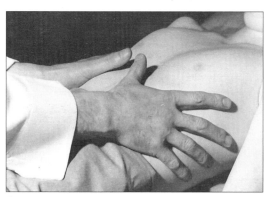

▲ **Figure 6.20 Method of comparing expansion of the two sides of the chest.**

▲ **Figure 6.21 Palpation of the bases behind.** The thumbs meet at the vertebral spines during expiration and the fingers extend towards the axillae

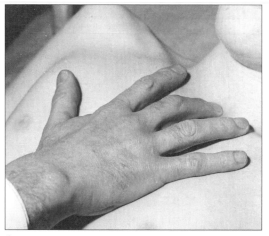

▲ **Figure 6.22 Tracheal position: method of palpation**

be inserted above the suprasternal notch. The finger will slip to one side if the trachea is deviated.

The axillae and supraclavicular fossae should be examined for hard lymph nodes which may be the only evidence of malignancy. Palpation also detects subcutaneous emphysema, which has a characteristic spongy feeling and usually results from injury to the lung due to fracture of the ribs, drainage of a pneumothorax or rupture of the oesophagus. If it is overlooked and the area auscultated, crepitations may be wrongly diagnosed. The sternum, ribs and intercostal spaces should be palpated for abnormal swellings or tenderness.

VOCAL FREMITUS

This special sign consists in detecting vibrations transmitted to the hand from the larynx through the bronchi, lungs and chest wall. The patient is asked to say 'ninety-nine', or 'one, one, one', and the same hand is placed on the chest in identical places on the two sides in turn. The flat of the hand may be used, or for more accurate localization the ulnar border of the hand, which is more sensitive (Figure 6.23).

An increase or decrease in vocal fremitus has the same significance as the corresponding change in vocal resonance (see below).

PERCUSSION

Percussion consists in setting up artificial vibrations in a tissue by means of a sharp tap, usually with the fingers. The middle finger of the left hand is placed in close contact with the tissues, in this case the chest wall. A blow is then made on the second phalanx of this finger with the middle finger of the right hand. The striking finger must be kept at right-angles to the other finger as it falls, and the blow must be made by movements of the wrist only; no movement of the shoulder is necessary (Figures 6.24–6.27). The striking finger must be lifted clear immediately after the blow to avoid damping the resulting vibrations. If the organ or tissue to be percussed lies superficially, percussion should be light, but if it lies deep or should it be desired to set into vibration a large mass of tissue such as the base of one lung, heavy percussion must be employed. Light percussion on the clavicles (Figure 6.28) is a useful method of determining changes in the character of the lung substance at the apices. Heavy percussion may be accomplished by using two fingers instead of one, or by using several fingers without any intermediate finger (Figure 6.29).

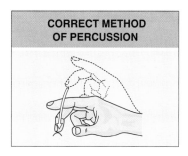

CORRECT METHOD OF PERCUSSION

◀ **Figure 6.24 Correct method of percussion.** Note the movement of the wrist and the vertical position of the terminal phalanx of the percussion finger as it strikes the other

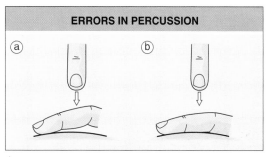

ERRORS IN PERCUSSION

(a) (b)

▲ **Figure 6.25 Errors in percussion.** (a) Incorrect – the striking finger is not making close contact with the tissue to be percussed. (b) Correct position

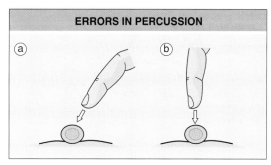

ERRORS IN PERCUSSION

(a) (b)

▲ **Figure 6.26 Errors in percussion.** (a) Incorrect – the finger is not vertical as it strikes the other. (b) Correct method

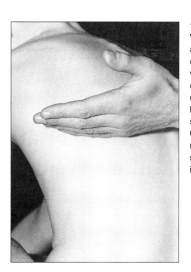

◀ **Figure 6.23 Vocal fremitus.** For accurate comparison of the vocal fremitus in different parts of the chest the ulnar border of the hand should be used. Compare ribs with ribs, and intercostal spaces with intercostal spaces

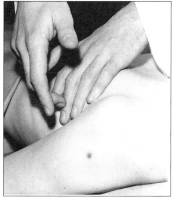

◀ **Figure 6.27 Percussion of the axilla**

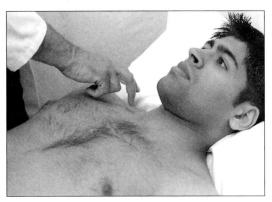

▲ **Figure 6.28 Percussion on the clavicle.** Sometimes changes in the character of the lung tissue at one apex, e g. consolidation, produce a change of note on percussion over the corresponding clavicle

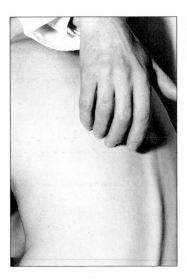

◀ **Figure 6.29 Heavy percussion.** The fingers are used direct

The percussion note is altered by change in the structure of the underlying tissues. Thus hyper-resonance is found when air fills the pleural cavity (pneumothorax), or is contained unloculated in a large lung cyst. Dullness may be found when the normal air-containing lung tissue becomes solidified, as in pneumonia, tumour and fibrosis, while absolute or stony dullness is present over pleural effusions or occasionally over solid lung if the bronchus is blocked. Overinflation of the lungs, as in emphysema, may abolish the normal liver and cardiac dullness. The student should familiarize himself with these various notes by percussing the appropriate parts of his body (lung for normal resonance, lower abdomen for hyper-resonance or tympany, liver for dullness and thigh for stony dullness).

AUSCULTATION

Before using the stethoscope the student should listen carefully to the patient's breathing. The breathing of a healthy resting subject cannot be heard at a distance of more than a few inches from the face. Audible breathing at rest can be an important early sign of airways disease. It may be caused by vibrations of airways tissues or secretions, or by turbulent airflow due either to increased velocity of flow or to airways narrowing.

A variety of breathing sounds of diagnostic relevance can be detected by the unaided ear.

1 *Stertorous breathing.* This is due to vibrations of the soft tissues of the nasopharynx, larynx and cheeks resulting from loss of muscle tone. It may occur in coma from any cause and in some subjects during sleep (snoring).

2 *Rattling breathing* due to vibration of mucus retained in the main airways. This indicates ineffectual cough due to suppression of the cough reflex or to general weakness.

3 *Gasping, grunting and sighing.* These sounds are mainly due to increased velocity of airflow and can be normal responses to a variety of physical and emotional stimuli: exercise, pain, cold, fear and grief. When persistent, however, they may reflect some form of chronic anxiety state.

4 *Hissing* (Kussmaul's) breathing is produced by the patient taking deep breaths through a nearly closed mouth. This probably signifies hyperventilation without dyspnoea and therefore without reflex opening of the mouth during inspiration. It is a sign of severe acidosis, as in diabetic ketosis, uraemia and salicylate poisoning.

5 *Wheezing* is usually louder on expiration than on inspiration and denotes narrowing of the bronchi as in asthma. As already mentioned, airways narrowing of lesser degree can lead to audible breathing without wheeze.

6 *Stridor* is of lower pitch than wheeze and more closely resembles a voice sound. It can be simulated by partial closure of the vocal cords while breathing deeply. Unlike wheeze, stridor is at least as loud in inspiration as in expiration for two reasons: first, because it usually results from narrowing of the extrathoracic airways (trachea or larynx), which are not subject to intrathoracic pressure changes; secondly, because the narrowing is often due to a rigid lesion such as tumour, which prevents fluctuation in airways diameter during the respiratory cycle.

USE OF THE STETHOSCOPE

Quietness is essential for good auscultation, and some experience is necessary in learning to disregard noises which come through the stethoscope but which are not the direct result of respiration or cardiac contraction. Hair on the chest produces crackling noises which may be mistaken for lung sounds. Unless all clothes are removed from the chest, sounds will inevitably be heard from their friction against the chest wall or on stethoscope tubing, and care should be taken to see that blankets put around the shoulders are not allowed to move. If the patient is nervous or cold, shivering will produce sounds similar to those heard over a contracting muscle. In general, low pitched sounds are best heard with the bell resting lightly on the skin and high pitched sounds with firm pressure from the diaphragm.

As in other methods by which the chest is examined, identical points on the two sides must be compared, particularly beneath the clavicles and in the supraspinous fossa to examine the upper lobes, and over the lower ribs (seventh to tenth) at the back for auscultation of the lower lobes, and in the axillae where there is access to parts of all the lobes.

Auscultation must be carried out with definite objectives in mind:

1 To determine whether the breath sounds are equal on the two sides.
2 To ascertain the character of the breath sounds.
3 To detect any added sounds and decide their nature, and whether they are intra- or extrapulmonary.
4 To compare the voice sounds over different parts of the lungs.

BREATH SOUNDS

Breath sounds (Figures 6.30 and 6.31) are due to fluctuations in intraluminal pressure and oscillation of solid tissues which result from turbulent gas flow in the trachea and proximal bronchi. In the small peripheral airways and alveoli, gas flow is of lower velocity and laminar in type and is therefore silent.

The type and intensity of breath sounds are modified by the filtering effect of tissues between source and stethoscope. Breath sounds from which high frequencies have been filtered by normally inflated alveoli are described as *vesicular* (the vesicles, or alveoli, acting as the filter, not the source, of the sound). This is a rustling noise, louder and more prolonged in inspiration than in expiration (Figure 6.32). The less the filtering, the more closely will the sound approximate to its source in the trachea and bronchi, i.e. to *bronchial* breathing. This is a higher pitched clearer sound than vesicular breathing, inspiration and expiration are of equal length and there is a distinct gap between them. When this type of breathing is found over the lungs themselves it is invariably abnormal, although a modified form *(bronchovesicular)* may be heard when the stethoscope is placed near to the trachea in the midline of the chest.

Abnormal breath sounds

Thoracic diseases may either diminish the intensity of breath sounds or alter their quality to give bronchial breathing.

A generalized reduction in the intensity of the sound may result from obesity or overinflation of the lung and also from hypoventilation. A localized reduction in breath sounds occurs when there is diminution of air

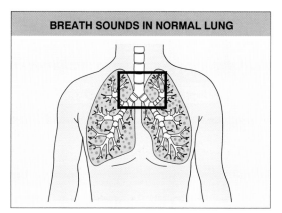

▲ **Figure 6.30 Breath sounds in normal lung, anterior aspect.** The square marks the area of broncho-vesicular breathing, which is found also over the corresponding part of the back. Over other areas normal vesicular breath sounds are heard

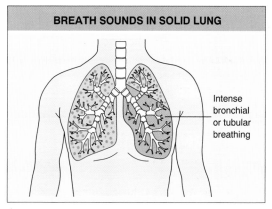

▲ **Figure 6.31 Breath sounds in solid lung, such as occurs in pneumonia.** Lung alveoli airless, bronchi patent, breath sounds bronchial or tubular. Lower lobe only shown as affected

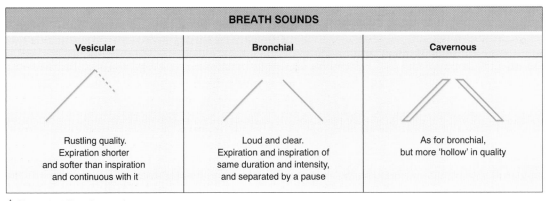

▲ Figure 6.32 Breath sounds

entry (e.g. bronchial occlusion) or when the bronchial source of the sound is deflected at interfaces between media with different acoustic properties, as in the case of pleural effusion and pneumothorax.

Bronchial breathing is heard when the medium interposed between the bronchi and stethoscope is a good conductor of sound and, unlike normal alveoli, permits the passage of high frequencies. This occurs when the alveoli contain fluid instead of air (consolidation), when there is collapse or fibrosis of the lung with patent bronchi and sometimes over a thin layer of pleural fluid (e.g. at the top of a pleural effusion). Bronchial breathing may also occur when for any reason the trachea or main bronchi are so displaced as to be physically nearer to the stethoscope.

Rarely, a bronchus may communicate directly with a large abnormal air space either in the lung (cavity) or pleural space (pneumothorax). This can give rise to a hollow resonating breath sound known as *cavernous* or *amphoric* breathing.

VOICE SOUNDS

Normal lung filters out high frequency vowel sounds so that speech (e.g. 'ninety-nine') is heard through the stethoscope as a low-pitched mumble. When the lung is airless as in consolidation, fibrosis or collapse with a patent airway, the vowel sounds come through to produce intelligible, syllabic speech. This sound is termed bronchophony and its acoustic basis is the same as for bronchial breathing.

Whispering is a high frequency sound produced by turbulent airflow in upper airways. This sound is therefore filtered out by normal lung and, like bronchophony, can be heard through the stethoscope only when the lung is airless and the airways patent – *whispering pectoriloquy*.

At the upper limit of a pleural effusion, where the fluid layer is thin, the voice sounds are reflected with loss of the low frequency elements. This gives rise to a high-pitched sound with a nasal bleating quality – *aegophony*.

ADDED SOUNDS

Chest diseases can give rise to three kinds of added sound: wheezes, crackles and pleural friction (Figure 6.33). Wheezes are due to the oscillation of airways and other tissues set into motion by an impediment to airflow.

Fixed monophonic wheeze

This is a single note of constant pitch, timing and site. It results from air passing at high velocity through a localized narrowing of one airway. Bronchial carcinoma is the commonest cause. *Stridor* (see page 116) is a special example of this sound.

Random monophonic wheezes

These are random single notes which may be scattered and overlapping throughout inspiration and expiration and are of varying duration, timing and pitch. They signify widespread airflow obstruction, as in asthma or bronchitis.

Expiratory polyphonic wheeze

This is a complex musical sound with all its component parts starting together and continuing to the end of expiration. It is probably due to expiratory dynamic compression of large central airways and is therefore audible at the mouth. When unaccompanied by inspiratory wheezes, it usually indicates emphysema in which the central airways are narrowed by the positive pressure which has to be exerted to empty the inelastic lungs.

Sequential inspiratory wheezes ('squawks')

A series of sequential (not overlapping) inspiratory sounds or sometimes a single sound (Figure 6.33(e)), due to the opening of airways which had become abnormally apposed during the previous expiration. These tend to occur in deflated areas of lung and are therefore heard in various forms of pulmonary fibrosis, especially fibrosing alveolitis. The mechanism is similar to that of crackles and these often precede the squawk.

Crackles

Crackles (Figure 6.34) result from the explosive equalization of gas pressure between two airway compartments when a closed section between them suddenly opens. Expiratory closure of airways is gravity-dependent, so that crackles are mainly basal in site.

Early inspiratory and expiratory crackles signify abnormal expiratory closure of proximal intrapulmonary airways with re-opening later in expiration or early in inspiration. They tend to be scanty, low-pitched, audible at the mouth and unaffected by posture. Those that disappear after a few deep breaths are common in the elderly and of little pathological significance. Otherwise, they are usually indicative of bronchitis.

Late inspiratory crackles are generally due to restrictive conditions of the lung itself, resulting in expiratory closure of the small peripheral airways with re-opening at the end of inspiration. In contrast to early inspiratory crackles, they are usually fine, profuse, high-pitched, inaudible at the mouth and may vary with posture. They are heard especially in patients with fibrosing alveolitis, pneumonia and pulmonary oedema.

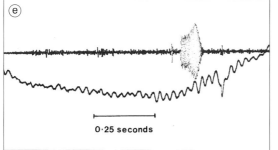

▲ **Figure 6.33 Added sounds.** (a) Fixed monophonic wheeze. (b) Random monophonic wheezes. (c) Expiratory polyphonic wheeze. (d) Sequential inspiratory wheezes (squawks). (e) Pneumograph of a squawk (immediately preceded by a crackle). The lower curved line indicates the rate of inspiratory airflow. ((a)–(d) reproduced from Lung Sounds, by kind permission of Dr Paul Forgacs and Ballière Tindall; (e) by kind permission of Dr John Earis)

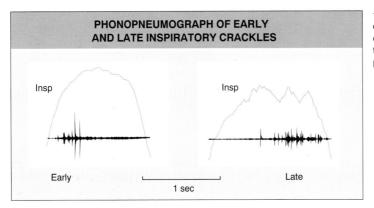

◄ Figure 6.34 Phonopneumograph of early (left) and late (right) inspiratory crackles. (The upper curved lines indicate the rate of air flow.) (Redrawn with the kind permission of Dr Leslie Capel and *Thorax*)

Coarse crackles are heard as easily in expiration as in inspiration. They are often altered by coughing and can be heard over segments and lobes affected by bronchiectasis. They may also be heard at the mouth without the aid of the stethoscope, and are usually caused by air bubbling through collections of mucus or pus in areas of bronchiectasis. They should be distinguished easily from the audible gurgling noises arising in the larynx, trachea or major bronchi characteristic of the dying or unconscious patient who has failed to clear such secretions due to inadequate coughing. In the past, this noise was known as the Hippocratic rattle.

Pleural friction

Oscillations arising from frictional resistance between two layers of inflamed or roughened pleura produce a creaking sound: the pleural friction rub. This tends to recur in the same part or parts of each respiratory cycle. The intensity of the sound may be increased by firm pressure of the stethoscope.

EXAMINATION AFTER EXERCISE

Examination of the patient after exercise is essential to the assessment of the respiratory system. Exercise may take the form of running, in the case of younger patients, climbing flights of stairs or, if the equipment is available, riding a static bicycle or walking on a treadmill. The following observations should be made after exercise:

1 The amount of exercise needed to induce dyspnoea, or the distance walked in a given time.
2 The respiratory and heart rate and the time needed for these to return to the pre-exercise level.
3 Whether cyanosis appears during exercise.
4 Whether wheeze develops after exercise (see page 121).

THE DIAGNOSIS OF RESPIRATORY DISEASES

For convenience in describing their symptoms and signs, the common diseases of the respiratory organs may be grouped under the following headings – those affecting:

1 The bronchi.
2 The lungs.
3 The pleura.
4 The mediastinum.

THE BRONCHI

The symptoms and signs of bronchial disease can be attributed to:

1 Irritation of the bronchial mucosa with increased secretions causing cough and expectoration.
2 Narrowing of the bronchial lumen, which results in dyspnoea, wheeze, early inspiratory and expiratory crackles and the signs of overinflation of the lungs (see also Emphysema, page 125).
3 Complete occlusion of the lumen causing the symptoms and signs of collapse of the lung (see page 124). The bronchi may be narrowed or occluded by exudate or foreign bodies in the lumen, by mucosal oedema, tumour or spasm arising in the bronchial wall, or by pressure from without by enlarged lymph nodes.

It is convenient to consider diseases of the bronchi according to whether they affect the whole of the bronchial tree or are localized to one part of it. Generalized bronchial disease includes asthma and bronchitis and usually reveals itself by auscultatory signs with few changes in the radiograph. In localized disease, such as bronchiectasis and bronchial carcinoma, physical signs are often lacking so that radiography or bronchoscopy are needed to make a diagnosis.

BRONCHIAL ASTHMA

Bronchial asthma usually starts in childhood, but may not appear until middle age ('late-onset asthma'). It is characterized by attacks of wheezing dyspnoea due to narrowing of the bronchi by spasm, mucosal oedema or mucous secretions. These attacks are brought on by a variety of factors including allergy to certain inhaled dusts (e.g. house dust or pollens), respiratory infections, emotional upsets, physical exertion (exercise induced asthma) or occupational exposure (e.g. glutaraldehyde in nursing staff). A history of other 'allergic' manifestations, such as hay fever and infantile eczema, or a family history of these conditions, is common in those with an early onset of the disease.

The patient may be quite free of symptoms and abnormal signs between the attacks, but the illness can become continuous. Cough usually occurs only during the attacks, when it may be associated with the expectoration of viscid mucoid sputum; nocturnal cough is a characteristic presenting symptom of asthma in childhood.

Physical examination reveals laboured breathing associated with a prolonged expiratory wheeze, activity of the accessory muscles of respiration, signs of overinflation of the lung due to trapping of air during expiration (see also Emphysema, page 125) and, in a severe attack, cyanosis may also be seen often in association with sinus tachycardia and sometimes with pulsus paradoxus. In children, there may be permanent deformity of the chest wall (pigeon chest, Figure 6.35). Bronchial asthma must be differentiated from the paroxysmal dyspnoea of left heart failure (see Chapter 7) and from localized wheezing due to partial bronchial obstruction by neoplasm or foreign body.

BRONCHITIS

Acute bronchitis usually complicates an acute infection of the upper respiratory tract. Chronic bronchitis may be associated with chronic respiratory infections, but more often it can be related to cigarette smoking or to environmental causes such as air pollution. The principal symptom is cough, with mucoid sputum, which is worse in the morning and during the winter months. Acute exacerbations are provoked by adverse climatic conditions such as fog, and also by respiratory infection, when fever, purulent sputum and wheezing dyspnoea are additional symptoms. The main physical signs are expiratory wheeze and early inspiratory crackles. The signs

in acute cases are similar to those of asthma. Chronic bronchitis in men is often complicated by emphysema in middle life (see page 125). Other important complications in severe chronic cases are respiratory and cardiac failure, the combination of cyanosis and oedema producing the 'blue-bloater' syndrome (see also the 'pink-puffer' syndrome of emphysema, page 125).

BRONCHIECTASIS

This most commonly results from tenacious plugs of mucus formed during an attack of pneumonia or acute bronchitis (often associated with measles, whooping-cough or cystic fibrosis) in early childhood (Figure 6.36); bronchiectasis will occur if the lung collapses and irreversible damage is done to the bronchi before the plug has been dissolved or expelled. Bronchiectasis may also complicate bronchopulmonary aspergillosis and auto-immune

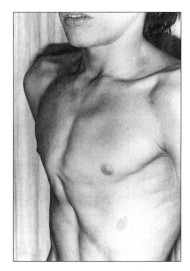

◀ **Figure 6.35 Pigeon chest** in a 15-year-old boy with asthma since infancy

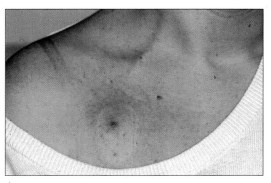

▲ **Figure 6.36 Portacath and intravenous line positioned subcutaneously for self-administration of intravenous antibiotics in a patient with bronchiectasis**

disorders in adult life. The dilatation of the bronchi, and the loss of ciliary action and cough reflex due to damage to their mucosa, causes retention and infection of secretions. These secretions are responsible for the chief symptom of bronchiectasis which is the expectoration of large amounts of purulent sputum, sometimes stained with blood. The main physical sign is coarse crackles, usually over the lower lobes of the lungs. In the absence of active infection (as in the treated case), however, there may be no abnormal signs, and then the diagnosis must depend upon radiological examination, including CT scanning or bronchography (see Figure 6.25). Finger clubbing and, rarely, amyloidosis occur in the more advanced cases and the disease may also be complicated by recurrent pleurisy, pneumonic consolidation and by fibrosis in the surrounding lung (see below and page 124).

BRONCHIAL CARCINOMA

Carcinoma of the bronchus is the commonest form of malignant tumour in men. Heavy cigarette smoking is an important causative factor.

The most frequent early symptoms are cough and haemoptysis, although it may present with a feverish pneumonic illness which tends to persist or relapse, pleuritic pain, dyspnoea on exertion or with various manifestations outside the chest (see below). As in other forms of malignant disease, there is progressive wasting leading to cachexia and death within a few months to a year in the untreated case.

The commonest signs are those of collapse, consolidation and effusion, or a combination of all three. The finding of pleural effusion without mediastinal displacement suggests either that there is also an underlying collapse of the lung or that the mediastinum has been invaded and fixed by tumour. This disease is often associated, and may even present, with signs outside the chest. These include anaemia and loss of weight, the signs of metastases to other organs (e.g. bone or brain), finger clubbing and painful swellings of the hands and feet due to osteoarthropathy, engorgement of the face due to mediastinal obstruction, and, more rarely, various forms of myoneuropathy and endocrine disorder due to peptides secreted by the tumour.

THE LUNGS

The more important pathological changes which may take place in the lungs include oedema, consolidation, cavitation, collapse, fibrosis and emphysema (see Table 6.3). These changes are found in various combinations in different lung diseases.

OEDEMA

Pulmonary oedema results from engorgement of pulmonary veins and capillaries and consists of transudation of fluid into the walls and lumina of the smaller air spaces in the lungs. The commonest causes of congestion and oedema are left ventricular failure and mitral stenosis (see Chapter 7, page 172), but more rarely it can be due to acute inflammation of the lung (e.g. influenza) or to the inhalation of an irritant gas (e.g. phosgene, nitric oxide).

The main symptoms of pulmonary oedema are dyspnoea, which in the cardiac case is worse when the patient lies flat ('orthopnoea'), cough and the expectoration of pink frothy sputum which may become copious and frankly blood stained. Fine inspiratory crackles may become coarse and accompanied by wheeze.

CONSOLIDATION AND PNEUMONIA
Consolidation

This is a condition in which the alveoli are filled with an exudate from the blood, either inflammatory (e.g. pneumonia) or haemorrhagic (e.g. infarction due to occlusion of a pulmonary artery).

The symptoms are those of the cause. Pneumonia is characterized by dry cough, sometimes with rusty sputum, pleuritic pain, fever with rigors and, if consolidation is extensive, dyspnoea and cyanosis. The symptoms of infarction are similar, but the onset is usually more sudden, fever of lesser degree and frank haemoptysis is common.

The physical signs of consolidation are diminished expansion (especially when there is pleuritic pain), moderate impairment of percussion note (less than in effusion), increased vocal fremitus, bronchial breathing, bronchophony, whispering pectoriloquy and late inspiratory crackles. An overlying pleural friction rub is common. The mediastinum remains central.

Pneumonia

In community acquired pneumonia (Figure 6.37) it is important to establish whether the patient had pre-existing lung disease and whether or not there had been contact with pigeons (psittacosis), air-conditioning units (Legionnaire's disease), other animals (Q fever), or whether there has been contact with a known epidemic of mycoplasma pneumonia. It should also be established whether there has been close contact with an open case of pulmonary tuberculosis.

Pneumonia may also be acquired in a patient in hospital or recently discharged within the previous two weeks when the condition is known as nosocomial pneumonia. It should be established whether other cases have

PHYSICAL SIGNS IN CHEST DISEASES						
	Consolidation	**Collapse**	**Fibrosis**	**Emphysema**	**Effusion**	**Pneumothorax**
Mediastinal shift	None	Towards	Towards (with chest wall retraction)	None	Away	Away
Vocal fremitus	Increased	Usually diminished	Diminished	Diminished	Diminished	Diminished
Percussion note	Dull	Dull	Dull	Hyperresonance. Loss of liver and heart dullness	Flat or stony	Tympany
Breath sounds	Bronchial	Absent or bronchial	Diminished or bronchial	Diminished. Prolonged expiration	Diminished (bronchial above)	Diminished or amphoric
Voice sounds	Bronchophony. Whispering pectoriloquy	Diminished or bronchophony	Diminished or bronchophony	Diminished	Diminished (aegophony above)	Diminished
Added sounds	Fine inspiratory crackles (in the early stages and during resolution)	None	Coarse crackles (if bronchiectatic)	Expiratory wheeze	Friction rub (in early stages)	'Metallic' crackles Succussion (if fluid present)

*It must be noted that two or more of these conditions often occur together, e.g. consolidation and collapse. The signs of both conditions may then be found.

▲ Table 6.3

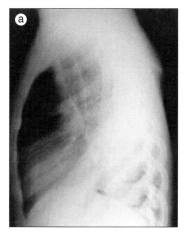
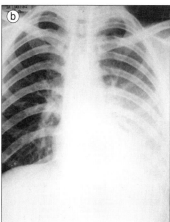

◀ **Figure 6.37 The chest, showing lobar pneumonia of the lower left lobe.** (a) Left lateral radiograph. (b) Posteroanterior radiograph

been reported from the same ward with a similar infecting organism.

In addition to community acquired and nosocomial pneumonia, the condition may be recognized in the community or in hospital in association with infection with the AIDS virus. Patients at risk such as homosexual men, haemophiliacs or intravenous drug abusers or their sexual partners may present with a pneumonia-like illness as the first manifestation of the acquired immune deficiency syndrome. Such patients may or may not have previously been recognized as suffering from AIDS, and pneumonia is often the first AIDS defining illness. Under these circumstances, the protozoon *Pneumocystis pneumonii* is the common infecting organism. There may be associated features such as oropharyngeal candidiasis, generalized lymphadenopathy, or the purplish skin lesions of Kaposi's sarcoma which may also be found in the oropharynx. Examination of the chest in a case of *Pneumocystis pneumonii* may be relatively normal, although bilateral basal crackles may be heard. It would also be important to seek involvement of the central nervous system and the gastrointestinal tract when diarrhoea may be a feature. If AIDS is suspected, it is essential to obtain an HIV test with the patient's consent and adequate counselling facilities.

COLLAPSE

Pulmonary collapse or atelectasis may occur as a congenital abnormality but will be discussed here only in its acquired form.

Collapse results from bronchial obstruction preventing air from entering the lung, so that the air which remains is absorbed into the bloodstream. The symptoms vary in intensity according to the rapidity with which the collapse occurs. Breathlessness is the principal symptom and, in cases of sudden collapse, e.g. bronchial occlusion by a foreign body, it is extreme (Figure 6.38). In the more gradual collapse from bronchial carcinoma, dyspnoea may be noticed only on effort.

Inspection may reveal some flattening and reduced expansion over the affected part, but gross retraction of chest wall structures suggests fibrosis. In upper lobe collapse the trachea is displaced to the affected side (Figure 6.39) and in lower lobe collapse, the heart. The percussion note is dull because the lung is airless. Breath sounds and voice sounds are diminished or absent because the bronchus is occluded. However, the lung may remain collapsed and perhaps consolidated after the obstruction has been relieved (e.g. after the expectoration of a mucus plug). In such cases, bronchial breathing and bronchophony will be heard. These signs may also occur if, as a result of the collapse, the trachea or a main bronchus has been drawn over to one side and thus lies nearer to the stethoscope.

FIBROSIS

Pulmonary fibrosis may be the result of many inflammatory diseases of the lung. Localized fibrosis is most often due to tuberculosis, bronchiectasis or to a destructive form of pneumonia (e.g. staphylococcal).

The eventual results of localized fibrosis of the lung are in some ways comparable to those of pulmonary collapse, for the lung becomes shrunken in volume, contains little air and draws in the chest wall on the affected

side and the mediastinum from the opposite side. The results are, however, produced in a much more gradual manner, and, although the chief symptom is again breathlessness, it is rarely so urgent as in acute forms of pulmonary collapse. Cough and expectoration occur if the fibrosis is associated with bronchiectasis.

The signs of fibrosis (Figure 6.40) depend on the shrinkage of the lung and its consequent drag on surrounding tissues, and on the diminished amount of air entering and contained in the lung. The chest is retracted and smaller in volume, and the heart and trachea are pulled towards the affected side. The ribs are often closer together, and expansion is limited or absent. The percussion note is dull because of the relatively airless state of the lung. The breath sounds are faint and may be bronchial, as in the case of pulmonary collapse when the bronchus is patent or drawn nearer to the stethoscope. Added sounds when present are generally due to associated changes, e.g. bronchitis, tuberculosis or bronchiectasis.

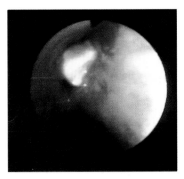

◀ **Figure 6.38 Obstruction of the right upper lobe bronchus which caused collapse due to the inhalation of peanut subsequently remove at bronchoscopy**

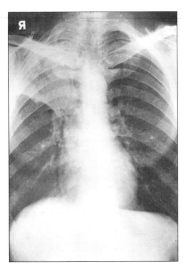

◀ **Figure 6.39 Pulmonary collapse. Note that the right upper lobe is airless.** The trachea is deviated to the right and the fissure between the upper and middle lobe is elevated

A more generalized form of fibrosis can result from sarcoidosis and from the inhalation of irritant dusts such as silica or asbestos. A special form of generalized fibrosis known as *fibrosing alveolitis* may be due to the inhalation of an allergen, as in the case of farmer's lung ('extrinsic allergic alveolitis'), or to some intrinsic process of unknown cause ('cryptogenic fibrosing alveolitis'). The clinical features are dyspnoea, cyanosis, rapid shallow breathing and fine late inspiratory crackles. Finger clubbing is common in cryptogenic alveolitis but rare in the extrinsic type.

EMPHYSEMA

This is a condition characterized by permanent overinflation of the distal air spaces of the lung with disruption of their walls. These changes are associated with expiratory airflow obstruction and loss of elasticity of the lungs. Emphysema is seen most often in middle-aged men who have suffered for many years from chronic bronchitis, but it may develop without any preceding respiratory illness. Rarely, emphysema is associated with an inherited deficiency of α_1-antitrypsin. It presents with increasing breathlessness on exertion, with more severe disability provoked by respiratory infection in the winter months.

Inspection may reveal a distended chest fixed in the inspiratory position ('barrel chest'): the sternum is displaced outwards and the ribs and clavicles are more horizontal than normal. However, the barrel chest is not evident in all cases and may be found in healthy subjects. Expansion is limited and inspiration can only be achieved with the aid of the accessory muscles of the neck elevating the clavicles. Expiration is greatly prolonged and is often accompanied by pursing of the lips (Figure 6.13).

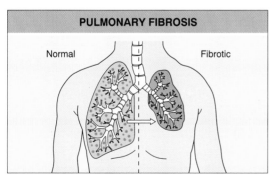

▲ Figure 6.40 Pulmonary fibrosis. The shoulder is lower and the chest wall retracted on the affected side. The lung is shrunken and the bronchi compressed. The signs are therefore: limited movement; diminished vocal fremitus and vocal resonance (variable); percussion note impaired; breath sounds faint (sometimes bronchial); mediastinal contents (trachea, heart etc.) displaced in direction of the arrow

On percussion, the note is hyper-resonant and the normal areas of dullness over the heart and liver are obliterated by the distended lung. On auscultation, the breath sounds are diminished, and expiration is prolonged and wheezing, but the wheeze may only be apparent during a forced expiration when there is passive collapse of proximal airways.

The disease may be complicated by the formation of bullae on the surface of the lung, which sometimes rupture to form a pneumothorax (see page 126).

The resulting disturbance in respiratory function is responsible for the chief symptom, dyspnoea, and also for various extrathoracic manifestations in the later stages of the disease. These include the symptoms and signs of hypoxia, of carbon dioxide retention (see page 106) and of right heart failure, the last being due in part to hypoxic constriction of the pulmonary arterioles and in part to obliteration of the capillaries surrounding the overinflated alveoli. In the non-bronchitic forms of emphysema, these signs of respiratory and cardiac failure are relatively uncommon, the patients remaining well oxygenated at the cost of considerable hyperventilation and dyspnoea. This is known as the 'pink-puffer' syndrome (see also the 'blue-bloater' syndrome of chronic bronchitis, page 121).

THE PLEURA

PLEURISY

Inflammation of the pleura can result from various diseases of the underlying lung, especially pneumonia, infarction or neoplasm, and more rarely from diseases in other sites (e.g. oesophagus; subphrenic abscess). In the early stages, friction between the two layers of the pleura gives rise to pleuritic pain and an audible friction rub. Later, if fluid forms between the two layers of the pleura, the pain and rub may be replaced by the features of pleural effusion (Figure 6.41).

Pleural effusion may take the form of an exudate from the causes already mentioned. The fluid has a high protein content, may contain inflammatory cells or blood and sometimes consists of pus (empyema). In cases of cardiac failure, or hypoproteinaemia due to renal disease, the fluid is a clear, watery transudate with a low protein and cell content and usually forms without preceding pleural friction. A rare form of pleural effusion is that which results from impaired lymphatic drainage. Obstruction to the thoracic duct causes a fatty or 'chylous' effusion. In congenital hypoplasia of the lymphatics, pleural effusion is accompanied by a yellow discoloration of the finger nails (Figure 6.42). Patients with pleural effusion complain of

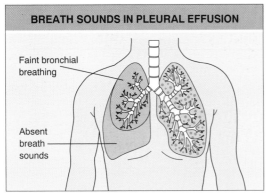

BREATH SOUNDS IN PLEURAL EFFUSION

Faint bronchial breathing

Absent breath sounds

▲ **Figure 6.41 Breath sounds in pleural effusion.** Lung compressed, therefore relatively solid. Bronchi narrowed by compression. (See also Figure 6.39 for other signs of pulmonary collapse)

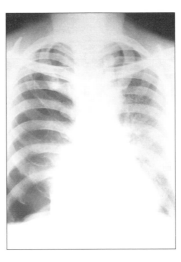

◀ **Figure 6.43 Air fills the right pleural cavity.** Note the lack of lung markings compared with the normal side. The edge of the partly deflated lung can be seen as a thin white line

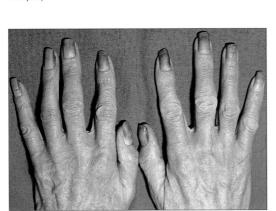

▲ **Figure 6.42 Yellow nails**

gradually increasing dyspnoea and the signs consist of mediastinal shift towards the opposite side and stony dull percussion note with diminished vocal fremitus, breath sounds and voice sounds at the affected lung base. Bronchophony and aegophony may be heard over the upper part of the effusion.

Pneumothorax

Air in the pleural cavity is known as pneumothorax (Figure 6.43). The air generally enters through a communication between the lung and the pleural cavity.

Spontaneous pneumothorax is usually due to the rupture of a subpleural bulla of congenital or inflammatory origin and is commonest in young men, especially those who are tall and thin. A rare form of pneumothorax in women tends to present at the onset of a menstrual period (catamenal pneumothorax). It also occurs as a serious complication of generalized emphysema in older patients.

The condition usually develops suddenly with the production of dyspnoea and pain which may resemble that of myocardial infarction (see page 164) when the pneumothorax is large, or it may be pleuritic in type. If the air leaks gradually, the symptoms may be unnoticed and the condition discovered only by radiography.

The mediastinum is displaced towards the opposite side when the pneumothorax is large. The most characteristic sign is impairment of breath and voice sounds in the presence of a well-preserved or even hyper-resonant percussion note. Rarely, the breath sounds have a hollow 'amphoric' quality due to the resonating properties of the pneumothorax. In cases of left-sided pneumothorax, the displacement of air trapped in the mediastinal pleural space can cause a clicking sound, synchronous with each heart beat.

THE MEDIASTINUM

MEDIASTINAL OBSTRUCTION

This may be caused by inflammatory and neoplastic processes of which the commonest is bronchial carcinoma invading the mediastinum directly or by metastatic involvement of lymph nodes. There may be pressure effects upon the superior vena cava, the sympathetic, recurrent laryngeal and phrenic nerves, and sometimes on the trachea, main bronchi and oesophagus (Figure 6.44, see Figure 6.7, page 108).

The resulting symptoms and signs thus include engorgement of veins in the neck, arms and chest with suffusion and oedema of the face and 'bursting' headaches on lying or bending, Horner's syndrome (see page 226), hoarseness, dyspnoea, stridor and dysphagia.

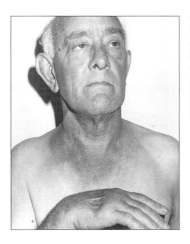

◀ **Figure 6.44 Mediastinal obstruction from bronchial carcinoma.** Note pitting oedema of hand, engorged neck veins and right-sided ptosis

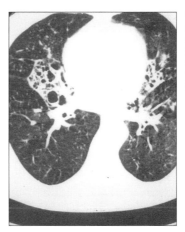

◀ **Figure 6.45 CT scan outlining widened bronchi with thickened walls in both lower lobes due to bronchiectasis**

SPECIAL INVESTIGATIONS

RADIOGRAPHY

A radiograph of the chest must be regarded as routine in all patients complaining of persistent respiratory symptoms. Special radiological investigations include fluoroscopy (or screening) of the lung and diaphragmatic movements; lateral, oblique and apical views; X-rays focused at different depths in the lung (tomography) to detect local lesions, such as a cavity or tumour; and the introduction of a radio-opaque medium into the bronchial tree (bronchography) to demonstrate bronchiectasis or bronchial narrowing, or into the pulmonary artery (angiography) to demonstrate arterial occlusions by embolism. Computerized axial tomography (the CT scan) may be used to define the precise size, site and consistency of an intrathoracic lesion (Figure 6.45).

EXAMINATION OF SPUTUM AND PLEURAL FLUID

Microscopy of the sputum may reveal cells and organisms of various kinds. These include tubercle bacilli, appearing as red rods when stained by Ziehl–Neelsen's method, malignant cells or an excess of eosinophil leucocytes, suggesting an allergic state. More rarely, evidence of the inhalation of a noxious dust may be found, e.g. asbestos bodies. Patients producing little sputum may be helped to do so by the inhalation of nebulized saline or water. Such induced sputum may be stained with silver salts to identify pneumocystis carinii so commonly found in immunosuppressed patients such as those with AIDS.

Culture of the sputum is of value in detecting the dominant infecting organism and its sensitivity to the available antibiotics, but special techniques are needed to grow tubercle bacilli. These observations on the sputum apply also to the pleural fluid, but in this case additional help can be obtained by a cell count and by measuring the specific gravity and protein content of the fluid. A high value for any of these three suggests an exudate (e.g. tuberculosis) rather than a transudate (e.g. congestive cardiac failure). The type of cell in a pleural exudate should also be noted: a predominance of red cells is commonest in carcinoma, pus cells indicate empyema, while a lymphocytic effusion favours a chronic infection such as tuberculosis. Fat globules may be seen in the chylous effusion of thoracic duct obstruction. The glucose level may be low and the rheumatoid factor concentration high in the pleural effusion associated with rheumatoid arthritis.

PULMONARY FUNCTION TESTS

The commonly used tests of respiratory function can be considered under two headings: ventilation of the lungs and gas exchange in the lungs. Tests in the first category include measurements of lung size (e.g. vital capacity, VC), the patency of the airways (e.g. forced expiratory volume, FEV, and peak expiratory flow, PEF), and the amount of air used to ventilate the lungs during normal breathing at rest and on exercise (minute and alveolar ventilation). These tests can all be made by simple spirometric methods. Many patients with asthma or obstructive bronchitis have their own peak flow meters with which they are able to make consecutive measurements to monitor the progress of their airflow obstruction (Figure 6.46). Gas exchange is examined by measuring the tensions of oxygen and carbon dioxide in arterial blood and by calculating the gas transfer factor or diffusing capacity using a carbon monoxide uptake technique (see Table 6.4).

COMMONLY USED TESTS OF LUNG FUNCTION		
Test	**Definition**	**Conditions in which it is most commonly used**
1 Spirometric tests of ventilation		
Vital capacity (VC)	The volume of air which can be expelled after a maximal inspiration Normal: 3–5 l	Decreased in conditions restricting the expansion of the lungs (e.g. deformities of thoracic cage, pleural thickening or effusion, lung fibrosis)
Peak expiratory flow (PEF)	The maximum flow rate during expiration Normal: 400–600 l per min	Decreased in diffuse airways obstruction (e.g. asthma, bronchitis, emphysema)
Forced expiratory volume in 1 s (FEV$_1$)	The amount of air which can be expelled in 1 s after a maximal inspiration. Normal: 75 per cent of vital capacity	Decreased in diffuse airways obstruction (e.g. asthma, bronchitis, emphysema)
Minute and alveolar ventilation	Minute ventilation The amount of air breathed in 1 min during normal respiration, i.e. tidal volume × respiratory rate. Normal at rest: 6–8 l per min Alveolar ventilation The amount of air ventilating the alveoli in 1 min during normal respiration, i.e. (tidal volume minus anatomical dead space*) × respiratory rate. Normal at rest: 4–6 l per min	Increased in many lung diseases (e.g. pneumonia) and metabolic disorders (e.g. acidosis, thyrotoxicosis) Decreased in cerebral and neuromuscular diseases (e.g. narcotic drugs, poliomyelitis)
2 Tests of gas exchange		
Arterial oxygen saturation (see also Cyanosis, page 106)	The oxygen content of arterial haemoglobin as a percentage of the content when blood is exposed to air. Normal: 97 per cent	Decreased in hypoventilation (e.g. cerebral and neuromuscular disorders). Continued perfusion of under ventilated parts of lung (e.g. in emphysema). Impaired diffusion (e.g. fibrosis due to dust diseases). Shunts of blood bypassing the lungs (e.g. Fallot's tetralogy)
Arterial oxygen tension (PaO$_2$)	The partial pressure of oxygen in arterial blood. Normal: 100 mmHg (14 kPa)	Increased in hypoventilation.
Arterial CO$_2$ tension (PaCO$_2$)	The partial pressure of CO$_2$ in arterial blood. Normal: 40 mmHg (5 kPa)	Reduced in hyperventilation. (Less affected by diffusion impairment or shunts because of relatively high diffusibility of CO$_2$)
* Normal (approximately): 100 ml in women, 150 ml in men.		

▲ Table 6.4

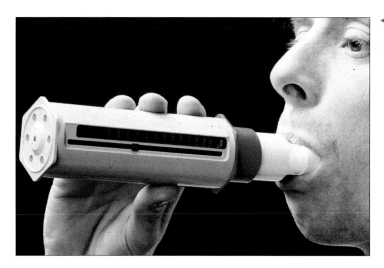

◀ **Figure 6.46 Peak flow meter**

ENDOSCOPY AND BIOPSY PROCEDURES

1. Direct inspection of the larynx (laryngoscopy) and the bronchial tree (bronchoscopy) by a rigid or flexible fibre optic instrument to detect carcinoma or other abnormality in the wall or lumen of the airways (Figure 6.47).
2. Various secretions or tissues can be procured for laboratory examination. Pleural fluid is collected by aspiration of the pleural cavity with a needle, while bronchoalveolar secretions and samples of the bronchial mucosa or lung can be obtained during bronchoscopy. Percutaneous biopsy of the pleura or of the lung can be carried out with a special needle or by means of an open surgical procedure such as video-assisted thoracoscopy or formal thoracotomy.

IMMUNOLOGICAL TESTS

Sensitivity to certain respiratory allergens may be inferred in atopic subjects by skin prick tests producing a weal and flare reaction or occasionally proved by the inhalation of the appropriate antigen. Measurement of serum IgE and RAST (radio allergo absorbent test) will confirm the atopic status of many asthmatics and measurement of IgA, IgG and IgM levels may sometimes reveal low or absent values in bronchiectasis. Specific precipitating antibodies can be detected in the sera of patients with extrinsic allergic alveolitis, such as farmer's lung and bird fancier's lung, as well as bronchopulmonary aspergillosis and aspergilloma.

The tuberculin test for tuberculosis consists of the intradermal injection of killed tubercle bacilli. A positive reaction appears within 72 hours as a raised weal in the skin indicating the body's past experience of tubercle bacilli, but it does not necessarily indicate active infection (Figure 6.48). The Kveim test for sarcoidosis must be biopsied 6 weeks after the intradermal injection of Kveim antigen and examined microscopically for characteristic granulomata.

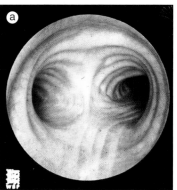
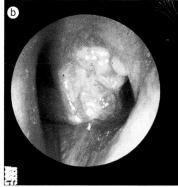

◀ **Figure 6.47 Bronchoscopic view of the bifurcation of the trachea into the two main bronchi (a) showing normal appearances and (b) carinal infiltration due to carcinoma.** (By kind permission of Dr Peter Stradling)

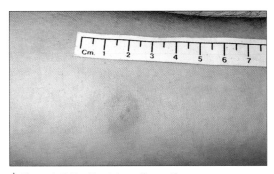

▲ **Figure 6.48 Positive tuberculin reaction**

When the white cell count shows a leucopenia, especially a low lymphocyte count characterized by a low CD4, patients with respiratory infections may be suffering from AIDS and their blood should be tested for HIV status.

Autoantibodies such as rheumatoid factor (rheumatoid arthritis), antinuclear antibody (systemic lupus erythematosus), antiScl-70 antibody (systemic sclerosis), anticentromere antibody (Crest syndrome), antiribonucleoprotein antibody (mixed connective tissue disease) and antiJO-1 (the overlap syndrome) are present in cases of fibrosing alveolitis of various causes.

The cardiovascular system

SYMPTOMS OF HEART DISEASE

The patient with heart disease may complain of many different symptoms, some of which may apparently be unconnected with the cardiovascular system. Often there are no symptoms and a cardiac lesion is found by routine examination.

Certain symptoms are, however, constantly found in cardiovascular disease, and though they may have other causes, careful attention should be paid to them in order to eliminate or confirm their cardiac origin. The patient should be encouraged to give a full and spontaneous description of his symptoms, with detailed questioning on the part of the examiner left until later.

DYSPNOEA (see also Respiratory System, page 104)

The mechanism and physiology of this symptom have been more fully considered in Chapter 6.

As it is such a common symptom of heart disease, certain special points may be noted:

Dyspnoea on effort

This generally precedes other forms of breathlessness, though there are exceptions to this rule. Serious cardiovascular disease, such as aortic incompetence or hypertension, may exist for many years without dyspnoea, yet in mitral stenosis dyspnoea is often an early feature particularly when atrial fibrillation is present.

The grade of the dyspnoea, provided that other causes mentioned in Chapter 6 are excluded, may give valuable information about the state of the cardiac reserve. For example, in valve disease for some years there may be no dyspnoea, then a patient becomes increasingly breathless with physical tasks of diminishing grade, until finally, when he reaches the stage of cardiac failure, dyspnoea will occur even on slight movement in bed.

Paroxysmal dyspnoea at rest

These attacks generally occur in bed and may follow a period of dyspnoea on exertion, but occasionally they are the first indication of a rise in pulmonary venous pressure in many types of heart disease, notably left ventricular failure and mitral stenosis. They are associated with a rise in left atrial pressure of whatever cause, as this prevents an adequate return of blood from the lungs to the left side of the heart. The attacks are often called 'cardiac asthma' as pulmonary oedema may cause airways obstruction and clinical wheezing similar to bronchial asthma. Sometimes both occur in the same patient.

Orthopnoea

Orthopnoea is said to be a later feature of cardiac failure than paroxysmal dyspnoea, though the two conditions are often found in the same patient .

Cheyne-Stokes breathing (see also page 111)

In heart disease this type of respiration, also known as periodic breathing, is commonest in similar conditions to those in which cardiac asthma occurs. The waxing and waning of the respiration, periods of hyperpnoea and apnoea, are particularly common during sleep, which they may interrupt.

Any or all of these types of dyspnoea may be found in the same patient.

PALPITATION

This term means that the patient is conscious of his heartbeats, which he may describe as 'bumping', 'throbbing', 'pounding' or 'fluttering' in the chest or peripheral vessels. Several factors may be responsible for the symptoms – namely, increased force, increased rate and irregularity of the heart – but unless the nervous system is unduly sensitive they may not result in palpitation. For this reason the symptom is more common in such conditions as hyperthyroidism and anxiety states than in organic heart disease. A placid patient with a heaving apical beat or with an abnormal rhythm or even tachycardia may be quite unaware of the heart's action.

If palpitation occurs in attacks careful attention must be paid to the patient's story. In simple sinus tachycardia, emotion or exercise generally causes the heart to beat faster, and as the precipitating cause diminishes so the heart rate and the palpitation lessen. By contrast, in abnormal rhythms, such as atrial flutter or paroxysmal tachycardia, the onset and offset of the attacks are instantaneous. The patient often states that he is conscious of the heart missing a beat or 'turning over' and then the palpitation is in full swing. Similarly, the attack passes away by a sudden consciousness of some alteration in the heartbeat. Short attacks of this character are suggestive of paroxysmal tachycardia; longer attacks, lasting many hours or days, suggest atrial flutter. Atrial fibrillation may also come in attacks, and the patient may be able to date the onset of the attack by the sudden appearance of palpitation having an irregular character. Ectopic beats are usually appreciated as occasional irregularities. The patient may be aware of a missed beat or an extra large bump corresponding with the next normal beat after the ectopic beat. This is accentuated because the post ectopic pause allows greater filling of the heart in diastole and a larger stroke volume. In most cases of palpitation the heart beats faster than normal, but occasionally, in heart block, the increased stroke volume may cause awareness of the heart's slow action.

PAIN

Pain as a symptom of heart disease is very important but sometimes difficult to evaluate. It occurs so frequently without gross evidence of cardiovascular disease that a diagnosis may have to rest on this symptom alone. For this reason an accurate and careful description of the site, character and duration of the pain is essential.

Angina pectoris

This is merely a name for pain of a particular type, namely strangling, which is experienced in the chest, generally midsternal or transternal, and often spreading to one or both arms, less commonly to the neck or jaw, and sometimes to the epigastrium or back.

It occurs under the following circumstances:

1 *Angina of effort.* In this, pain is provoked by varying degrees of physical exertion, especially walking quickly or uphill, or against a wind. It is often worse in cold weather and on walking after a meal. Similar pain may result from heightened emotion. The pain usually disappears after a few minutes of rest or relaxation.

It may be described as like a tight band, a sense of crushing or pressure, or very commonly as 'indigestion', with which it is often confused.

Its severity varies, according to the degree of myocardial ischaemia, the patient's threshold of pain and whether the provoking factor is removed.

2 *Angina at rest (unstable angina).* The pain has a similar character and distribution but may occur at rest and last longer than angina of effort. It generally occurs in the presence of severe stenosis with fluctuating thrombus altering the amount of coronary flow with or without the addition of coronary spasm. It may also occur in the presence of advanced extensive coronary disease. The term crescendo angina implies a steady worsening over a period of weeks with increasing limitation of exercise capacity.

Angina may also occur in aortic valve disease, anaemia or during disturbances of heart rhythm, especially if there is concomitant coronary artery disease.

3 *Myocardial infarction.* This usually results from occlusion of a major coronary artery (see page 164); pain may present and persist at rest.

Other forms of precordial pain

It will be useful here to mention the frequency with which pain in the chest results from non-cardiac causes which must be carefully distinguished from the type of pain just described. Pain of aching character is common in an effort syndrome, especially associated with fatigue. Aching or sharp pains occur in various rheumatic, traumatic and neuralgic affections of the chest wall. These pains are usually worse on movement of the affected parts and are sometimes associated with localized tenderness. The pain of pleurisy is generally severe, cutting or burning in character, and constantly related to breathing. All these pains tend to be mammary, axillary or dorsal in position rather than substernal. Further, they are often of long duration – hours or days. Sometimes oesophageal lesions cause a centrally placed pain like angina, as in obstructive lesions and hiatus hernia. Such pains may be related to swallowing or posture, but only occasionally to physical effort. Occasionally, hiatus hernia and reflux oesophagitis may cause a positive exercise test and the pain may be relieved by GTN.

Aneurysm

Aneurysm by erosion (Figure 7.24. page 145) may produce severe pain in the precordium, in the back or in the upper abdomen according to the site of the aortic dilatation. The pain may be due to pressure effects on bony structures and nerves. In dissection of an aortic aneurysm, the pain is caused by a tear in the aortic wall becoming further ruptured by blood being forced into the false lumen. This classically produces a tearing sensation complained of by the patient radiating between the shoulder blades up into the neck or into the abdomen, depending on the site of dissection of the aortic aneurysm.

GASTROINTESTINAL SYMPTOMS

In cases of congestive heart failure where the viscera – liver and gastrointestinal tract – are engorged with blood, dyspeptic symptoms are common. Loss of appetite, nausea, fullness after meals and distension of the abdomen are the usual features. Vomiting occurs occasionally, and the bowels are usually constipated. Such symptoms may be the result of therapy (digitalis and diuretics). Pain over the liver is common, owing to congestion of the organ and stretching of its capsule, especially if this occurs rapidly. Jaundice is rare and only in advanced cases, but some impairment of liver function may precede it.

RESPIRATORY SYMPTOMS

With the onset of pulmonary venous hypertension, the lungs are usually congested, resulting in cough, dyspnoea and not uncommonly in haemoptysis. In long-standing cases altered blood may be found in the sputum. If there is oedema of the lungs, the sputum may be plentiful and frothy, sometimes tinged pink by blood.

URINARY SYMPTOMS

Altered circulation through the kidneys leads to decrease in the secretion of urine, rarely to complete suppression. The urine passed is highly coloured owing to its great concentration, and frequently contains protein casts and red cells. 'Oliguria', as this decrease in urinary output is called, is one of the most important symptoms of severe cardiac failure (cardiogenic shock) and is a useful guide to the grade of failure and its response to treatment.

CEREBRAL SYMPTOMS

The most important of these is syncope, which is considered separately below. Dizziness, headache and psychological changes are not uncommon features in cerebral atherosclerosis and cardiac failure, but they also occur more commonly in effort syndrome in which no organic cardiovascular lesion can be found. An important cardiac cause for central nervous symptoms is embolism from the left side of the heart.

Syncope (see also Chapter 1)

Transient loss of consciousness may result from inadequacy of the cerebral blood flow. This is known as syncope and has to be distinguished from epilepsy, coma and hysteria.

The symptoms are more fully described below. A small, but important, group of cases can be classified as cardiac syncope. They include abnormalities of rhythm with very high rates, as in paroxysmal tachycardia. Unless the speed of the heart is abnormal on examination, a careful study will be necessary to avoid overlooking these possibilities. Stokes–Adams attacks are periods of ventricular asystole occurring commonly in complete heart block causing sudden syncope and resolving spontaneously in less than a minute. Typically, the patient collapses and becomes white and then cyanosed; as recovery takes place reactive hyperaemia causes extensive flushing.

Syncopal attacks are a feature of aortic stenosis. Generally, the more severe the aortic stenosis the more likely syncope becomes, but this may occur with a relatively mild gradient. The main mechanism is thought to be secondary to a baroreceptor stretch mechanism within the left ventricle with sudden changes in the force of contraction of the heart against the stenotic valve causing the left ventricle to stretch and syncope to occur. Clinically, the typical form of syncope associated with aortic stenosis is syncope on sudden effort. Dizziness is often attributed to aortic stenosis though this is rarely the sole cause.

Sudden mechanical obstruction of the circulation is rare, e.g. a ball-valve thrombus or myxoma blocking the mitral orifice, but illustrates how immediate syncope may occur and often cause death.

Lastly, local cerebral vascular changes, as in hypertension and cerebral arteriosclerosis or occurring as a result of hyperventilation or anoxia, are occasional causes of syncope.

OTHER SYMPTOMS

Finally, it should be noted that in serious heart disease a great variety of symptoms may arise owing to malnutrition of the body as a whole or of certain special organs. In children, wasting and lack of normal development are a common result, and even in adults some loss of weight is usual, though increase of weight may also occur from inactivity or as an early sign of oedema. The weight loss and cachexia in chronic heart failure is generally due to a reduction in muscle bulk, some of which is due to inactivity but much of which is due to abnormal protein metabolism and heart failure. This may be an adaptive mechanism. Fatigue has been accepted as a symptom indicating a low fixed output, especially in tricuspid valve disease.

PHYSICAL SIGNS: EXAMINATION OF THE CARDIOVASCULAR SYSTEM

The examination of the cardiovascular system comprises a study of the heart and blood vessels, but corroborative evidence of heart disease is so frequently present in other organs that certain signs should be looked for in every case. These may conveniently be discussed first.

OEDEMA

The patient may complain of swelling of the ankles or feet, but if this symptom does not enter into the history, it should be sought purposely. The pathology of oedema is not discussed here, save certain mechanical factors of clinical importance. Gravity plays an important part, especially in cardiac oedema, and the swelling is found in the most dependent parts of the body – in the feet, ankles and legs when the patient is ambulatory, over the sacrum (sacral cushion, Figure 7.1), lumbar region, genitalia, and backs of the ankles and thighs in patients who are sitting upright in bed. Looseness of the subcutaneous tissues also favours the accumulation of oedematous fluid, hence the occurrence of oedema in the genitalia and beneath the eyes in renal disease or extreme cardiac failure. Interference with the return of the blood to the heart also contributes to oedema. This is seen in cases of localized venous thrombosis, e.g. in patients with varicose veins, but there is little doubt that the more generalized obstruction to venous return which occurs in many types of heart disease acts in the same way. Much is ill-understood in the pathology of oedema and for fuller discussion textbooks of pathology and medicine should be consulted, with particular reference to the part played by sodium retention and the reduction of plasma-proteins.

Oedema is recognized by the characteristic 'pitting' on pressure and should be distinguished from the more solid swelling of myxoedema or lymphatic blockage. As a gauge of the disappearance of oedema the weight of the patient is generally reliable, for, with the dispersal of the fluid and its excretion through the kidneys, bowel and skin, there is a rapid reduction in weight; while, conversely, increase in weight suggests fluid retention. Oedema is not confined to the subcutaneous tissues, but may affect serous sacs, causing pleural and pericardial effusion and ascites.

CYANOSIS

This physical sign is fully discussed in Chapter 6, page 106, and may be of considerable diagnostic value in certain forms of heart disease: it occurs in mitral stenosis, but not always, and also in conditions where pulmonary arterial hypertension occurs together with a low cardiac output. It is seen whenever nonoxygenated blood reaches the systemic circulation, as in the reversed, or right-to-left, shunting of blood in some forms of congenital heart disease.

RESPIRATORY DISTRESS

While the patient is undressing, the physician will note the presence or absence of breathlessness and will compare this with the patient's subsequent statement. If there is no apparent breathlessness special exercises may be employed to demonstrate its presence or absence with a more severe degree of exertion. This may be accomplished by getting the patient to touch his toes a dozen times, or, while lying on a couch, to sit up and lie down quickly. Naturally such tests must be subject to the safety with which they can be employed. In all cases the lungs should be examined, for, apart from the congestion which occurs in cardiac failure, such abnormalities as chronic bronchitis or fibrosis may be responsible for the production or aggravation of the heart condition.

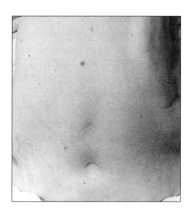

◀ **Figure 7.1 Sacral cushion of oedema.** Pitting on pressure over the sacrum is common in patients who have been bedridden in the usual sitting posture adopted in heart failure

ABDOMINAL SIGNS

The abdomen should be examined in all cases of heart disease, as there may be enlargement of the liver or ascites, suggestive of congestive failure, and enlargement of the spleen in cases of bacterial endocarditis. The hepatomegaly of congestive heart failure can be demonstrated best by palpation, which determines the presence of a firm smooth tender enlargement between the costal margin and the umbilical level. This can be confirmed by percussion. When ascites is present, an enlarged liver can often be determined easily by 'dipping' (see also page 67, Figure 4.23). Examination of the femoral pulses can be undertaken at this time (see later).

Pulsation in the epigastrium

Epigastric pulsation may be due to:

1. The contraction of the right ventricle; it is seen as a systolic retraction in the epigastrium, and may occur in normal persons; when the heart is hypertrophied it may be felt as a systolic thrust on palpation.
2. Aortic pulsation in nervous but otherwise normal persons, especially when the abdominal wall is thin; aortic pulsation follows the heartbeat by about 0.1 s.
3. Abdominal aortic aneurysm, in which an expansile swelling bigger than the normal aorta is present.
4. Pulsation of the liver; the area of pulsation extends more to the right than in the case of aortic or ventricular pulsation, and signs of congestive failure are usually present. It is generally due to tricuspid incompetence and is therefore systolic in time. It is to be noted that the enlarged liver may transmit pulsation from the heart or aorta.

AETIOLOGICAL POINTERS

The symptoms and signs of the more common causes of heart disease are listed in Table 7.1.

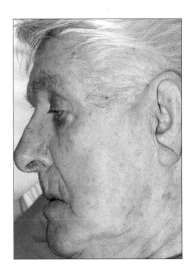

◀ Figure 7.2
Frank's sign
showing crack in
the pinna of the
ear in a man with
ischaemic heart
disease whose
siblings have both
heart disease and
a similar
appearance of the
ear

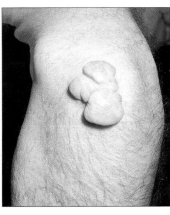

◀ Figure 7.3
Tendon
xanthomata over
elbow in 40-year-
old man admitted
with acute
myocardial
infarction

AETIOLOGICAL POINTERS	
Cause	**Clinical pointers**
Hypertension	Family history
	Raised BP
	Left ventricular failure
	Retinal vascular changes (page 182)
	Albuminuria
Atherosclerosis	Family history (Figure 7.2)
	Angina
	Myocardial infarction
	Absent peripheral pulses
	Aortic stenosis or aneurysm
	Signs of hyperlipidaemia (e.g. xanthelasma, tendon xanthelasma (see Figures 7.3 and 7.4)
	Diabetes
Pulmonary heart disease	Chronic lung disease
	Wheezing dyspnoea
	Central cyanosis
	Right ventricular failure
Thyroid disease	Signs of hyper- or hypothyroidism (Chapter 11)
	Atrial fibrillation
Congenital	Early onset
	Septal defects
	Pulmonary or aortic stenosis
	Patent ductus
	Aortic coarctation
	Mitral incompetence
	May be cyanosis and clubbing
Rheumatic disease	History of rheumatic fever or chorea
	Pericarditis
	Nodules (acute)
	Mitral or aortic valve disease (chronic)
Bacterial infection	History of mouth infection (e.g. dental)
	Mitral or aortic valve disease
	Fever
	Anaemia
	Splenomegaly
	Osler's nodes
	Petechiae
	Clubbing
Syphilis (now rare)	Venereal history
	Aortic incompetence or aneurysm
	Neurological signs (see page 262)
Certain toxic (e.g. alcohol) and infective (e.g. virus) causes	Cardiomyopathy (see page 164)

▲ Table 7.1

INVESTIGATION

We may now proceed to investigate the cardiovascular system proper. This involves examination of the peripheral vascular system (arterial and venous) and the heart.

The abnormalities to be found on examination of the cardiovascular system will be illustrated by actual recordings of *arterial and venous pulse waves*, the electrical activity of the heart (*electrocardiography*), heart sounds and murmurs (*phonocardiography*) and changes in structure and function of the heart as revealed by ultrasound (*echocardiography*). The reader will find descriptions of these recording methods on pages 173–80.

EXAMINATION OF THE PULSE

It is usual to examine the pulse before proceeding to the examination of the heart itself. This should include

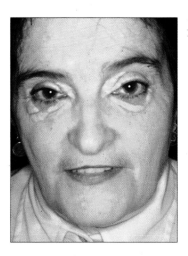

◀ **Figure 7.4**
Xanthelasma

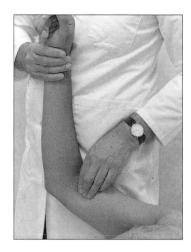

◀ **Figure 7.5**
**Palpating the
brachial pulse**

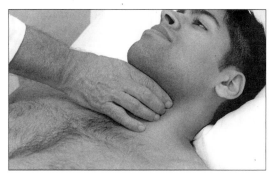

▲ **Figure 7.6 Palpating the left carotid pulse**

EXAMINATION OF THE PULSE	
Rate	Compare with heart rate (pulse deficit)
Rhythm	*Sinus arrhythmia*: quicker in inspiration
	Ectopic beats: occasional or regular
	Partial heart block: regular omissions
	Atrial fibrillation: totally irregular
Blood pressure	Systolic
Diastolic
Form	*Thready*: small volume
	Bounding: large volume
	Plateau or anacrotic: slow rise and fall (Figures 7.13 and 7.14)
	Dicrotic and bisferiens: bifid wave (Figures 7.17 and 7.19)
	Collapsing: sharp rise and fall (Figure 7.15)
	Alternans: small and large volume alternating (Figure 7.18)
	'Paradoxus': reduced volume in inspiration

▲ **Table 7.2**

inspection, palpation and auscultation of important arteries, especially the radial, brachial, carotids, temporals and the femorals and their distal branches. Information on rate and rhythm is derived from the radial artery, commonly called the pulse. The volume and nature of the pulse is checked by examination of the brachial (Figure 7.5) or carotid arteries (Figure 7.6). The most important method of examination is palpation, which will be considered first.

PALPATION

The pulse should be felt in both wrists, as variations are sometimes found on the two sides both in health and disease. Inequality suggests:

1 Abnormally placed artery.
2 Abnormal aortic arch, due either to congenital malformation or acquired disease such as aneurysm with intravascular clotting or dissection.

3 Obstruction of brachial or subclavian arteries by atheroma, thrombosis or embolism. The femoral pulses should be routinely palpated to rule out aortic defects such as coarctation. Thereafter the following points (Table 7.2) should be noted in sequence.

1 RATE

The pulse rate normally averages about 72 per minute, but in children is more rapid (90–100), and in old age may become slow (55–65). Quite trivial disturbances are sufficient to cause an acceleration in the pulse rate – for example, the emotion roused by a medical examination, or the effort of climbing stairs or hurrying to the consulting room. Due allowance must be made for these factors before attaching too much importance to a rapid pulse rate, and it is useful to take the rate at the beginning of the consultation and again before the patient leaves. The heart rate should always be compared with the pulse rate, as in some cases there is a 'pulse deficit', i.e. the pulse rate is less than the ventricular rate.

2 RHYTHM

The normal pulse waves succeed one another at regular intervals, but respiratory variations are common in health, the pulse quickening with inspiration and slow-ing with expiration. If this variation in rate is notice-able even with quiet breathing the term 'sinus arrhyth-mia' is applied (Figure 7.7). During inspiration there is a pooling of blood in the thorax reducing the amount of blood in the left ventricle, thus the heart rate increases due to stroke volume reduction. This is reversed on expiration when blood is forced into the left ventricle increasing the stroke volume and thus the pulse slows. If other forms of irregularity are present, the observer should note whether the pulse is irregular all the time or only occasionally. Finally, the effect of effort on the rhythm should be noted. Decisions as to rhythms should always be deferred until examination of the heart has been made, as the pulse alone may be deceptive.

The commonest irregularities detectable in the pulse are ectopic (premature) beats and atrial fibrillation (Figures 7.8 and 7.9), though variable heart block and atrial flutter may be suspected if the rate changes

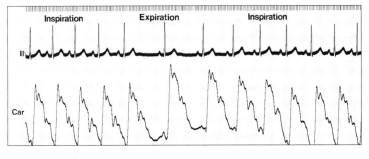

◀ **Figure 7.7 ECG and carotid pulse tracing of sinus arrhythmia.** The record was taken from a healthy young woman. (Recording speed 25 mm/s)

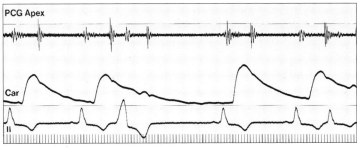

◀ **Figure 7.8 ECG, phonocardiogram (PCG) and carotid pulse of ventricular ectopic beats.** The ECG is abnormal showing a left bundle-branch block (LBBB) pattern (see Figure 7.48). (Recording speed 50 mm/s)

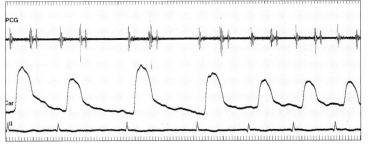

◀ **Figure 7.9 ECG, PCG and carotid pulse of atrial fibrillation; the pulse is irregular in spacing and form.** The patient had mitral stenosis and regurgitation, the PCG showing a clear opening snap and systolic murmur. (Recording speed 50 mm/s)

abruptly. Ectopic beats usually produce an occasional irregularity where a beat appears to be missed or in which a small pulse wave occurs earlier than is expected. If the ectopics are numerous, the pulse may appear to be completely irregular. In atrial fibrillation the pulse is persistently irregular, and this is usually easily recognized, though it may not be observed if the heart rate is slow, so that exercise should be employed to quicken the heart. Ectopics, on the other hand, often disappear with exercise though they may reappear with increased frequency shortly after the period of exertion.

3 BLOOD PRESSURE

Only a very rough idea of the blood pressure can be achieved by estimating the degree of digital compression necessary to obliterate the artery, and hypertension can never be detected in this way.

Instrumental estimation of blood pressure

This is accomplished by use of a sphygmomanometer. Many instruments are on the market, some with a mercury manometer and some of the aneroid type.

The inflatable bag should be about 10 cm in width (and 25 cm long), as narrower ones are known to give false readings.

The band is wrapped firmly and evenly around the arm about 8 cm above the elbow, which should be quite free to move, so that the diaphragm of the stethoscope can be placed in the cubital fossa. The arm band contains a rubber bag which is blown up until the brachial artery is occluded. At this point the radial pulse disappears.

The systolic pressure
The systolic pressure (i.e. the maximum pressure during the propagation of the pulse wave) may be estimated by:

1 *The palpatory method.* The armlet is pumped to a greater degree than is necessary to obliterate the radial pulse. The air is then slowly released until the pulse is once more palpable. The reading on the manometer at this point represents the systolic pressure.
2 *The auscultatory method.* The diaphragm of the stethoscope is placed over the brachial artery (located first by palpation) at the bend of the elbow, and the armlet pumped up until all sounds disappear (Figure 7.10). It is then gently released until a soft puffing noise is first heard. This point represents the systolic pressure (Figure 7.11*).*

It is preferable to use the auscultatory method for the systolic as well as the diastolic pressure, but the systolic should be checked by the palpatory method, by

which it may be found 5–10 mm lower. Further, in a few cases of hypertension, auscultation will show disappearance of the sounds, which reappear higher up the scale. This is known as the 'auscultatory silent gap' and will not be overlooked if the pressure is checked by palpation.

The diastolic pressure
The diastolic pressure (i.e. the constant pressure in the artery between each systole) is only roughly measurable. The auscultatory method is employed. The procedure is the same as for obtaining the systolic pressure; the

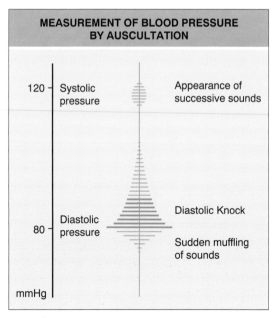

▲ **Figure 7.10 Auscultatory method of estimating blood pressure**

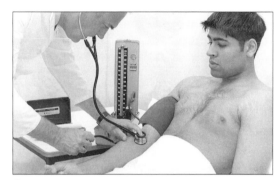

MEASUREMENT OF BLOOD PRESSURE BY AUSCULTATION

120 — Systolic pressure — Appearance of successive sounds

80 — Diastolic pressure — Diastolic Knock — Sudden muffling of sounds

mmHg

▲ **Figure 7.11 Measurement of blood pressure by auscultation.** Shows the sounds which may be audible over the brachial artery

observer listens for sounds over the brachial artery at the elbow. Following the puffing noise heard at and below the systolic reading, there occurs a knocking or thudding sound which increases in intensity and then passes suddenly into another softer sound and disappears. The sharp transition from the loud knocking to the soft blowing sound is taken as the diastolic pressure. Sometimes it is impossible to record the diastolic pressure owing to lack of any distinction between the knocking and soft sounds. In aortic incompetence the soft sounds may continue almost to zero and it is impossible to state the exact diastolic pressure.

A useful rough confirmation of the diastolic pressure is obtainable by noting that it corresponds with the sudden decrease of the maximum oscillation of the mercury column.

4 FORM

Under this heading may be considered the volume and variations in the type of the pulse wave, which can really be best appreciated by graphic methods. Considerable experience is necessary before much information can be obtained by the use of the fingers alone, but by careful comparison of a series of normal (Figures 7.12 and 7.16) and abnormal pulses the student will learn to distinguish a thin thready pulse (low volume) from a full bounding one (high volume), and with experience the slighter grades of these extremes. Low volume is found in conditions where there is a low stroke output, e.g. in mitral stenosis, and in shock, where vasoconstriction with pallor and sweating may also be present, as occasionally happens with myocardial infarction. The bounding pulse on the other hand is found in hyperkinetic circulatory states where there is vasodilatation and increased stroke output, e.g. pregnancy, thyrotoxicosis, fevers and anaemias. Special varieties of pulse form are as follows:

1   The *plateau pulse* (Figures 7.13 and 7.14) in which the summit of the pulse wave has a longer duration than normal.

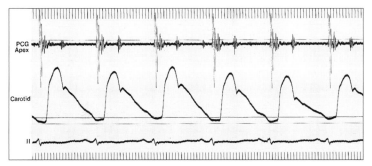

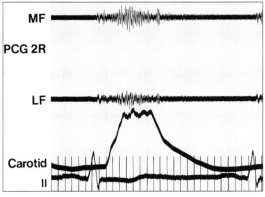

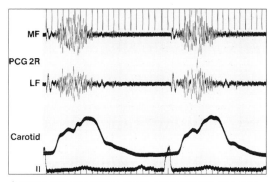

◀ **Figure 7.12 Normal carotid pulse.** The PCG and ECG in this tracing are abnormal. (Recording speed 50 mm/s)

▲ **Figure 7.13 'Plateau' pulse in aortic stenosis. The slow rising pulse has coarse summit vibrations which could be felt as a thrill.** Note the crescendo–decrescendo 'diamond' shape of the systolic murmur in the accompanying PCG. The ECG also is abnormal, with a negative T wave and a bifid P. (Recording speed 100 mm/s)

▲ **Figure 7.14 Anacrotic pulse in aortic stenosis.** The slow rise of this pulse is of the same nature as the 'plateau' pulse shown in Figure 7.13, showing a well-defined anacrotic notch on the upstroke of the pulse, and a sustained peak. The PCG shows a typical 'ejection' systolic murmur, this time followed by a much less intense decrescendo diastolic murmur, produced by an insignificant degree of aortic regurgitation. (Recording speed 100 mm/s)

2 The *collapsing pulse,* in which the peak of the pulse wave occurs early and is of very brief duration, and from which there is an equally swift descent. It is the rapid fall in pulse pressure which gives the characteristic 'collapsing' sensation, but when the stroke output of the left ventricle is very large, as in aortic regurgitation of severe degree, the rapid ascent to a high systolic pressure level contributes to the typical pulse contour. The bisferiens pulse of aortic regurgitation and stenosis has a rapid rise, a double peak and a fall not quite so rapid as in a true collapsing pulse (see Figure 7.19).

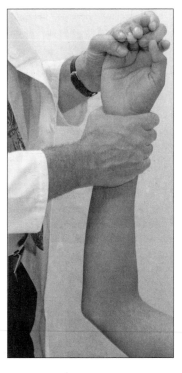

◀ **Figure 7.15 The collapsing pulse. (The water-hammer pulse.)** To elicit the collapsing pulse the patient's arm should be raised well above the head and the wrist grasped so that the palm of the examiner's hand lies over its anterior aspect. This intensifies the collapsing sensation felt in the arteries after each systole of the heart

3 The *dicrotic* or *hyperdicrotic pulse* in which the dicrotic notch and wave are so pronounced as sometimes to give the impression of two separate pulse waves, the second being smaller than the first. It is present when a low stroke output is accompanied by peripheral vasodilatation.

The plateau pulse is found in aortic stenosis where systole is more sustained than usual. The collapsing pulse, best elicited by placing the hand around the patient's wrist with his arm held vertically (Figure 7.15), is found in conditions where the diastolic pressure is so low as to produce a relative emptiness of the arteries and a flaccidity of their walls, and occurs in aortic regurgitation, arteriovenous fistula, especially patent ductus arteriosus. Generally, the collapsing pulse is obvious from inspection and palpation of the carotid pulse (Corrigan's sign).

The patient may complain of throbbing headache or pulsation in the finger tips. The collapsing or 'water-hammer' pulse derives its name from the effect of concussion of moving water against the sides of a pipe on sudden stoppage of the flow. In studying the form of the pulse invaluable knowledge may be acquired by comparing pulse tracings (Figures 7.16–7.19) with the results of palpation.

Alteration in the volume of the pulse may occur from beat to beat. In normal persons the volume was once thought to be greater with inspiration because of increased venous return to the heart. In fact this is not the case, but a fall in pulse volume during inspiration is still known as '*pulsus paradoxus*'. This may be seen physiologically if the breathing is thoracic in type or if the chest is held rigidly with the shoulders braced backwards and also in severe asthma. If these conditions have been excluded, pulsus paradoxus suggests the presence of pericardial effusion or constrictive pericarditis – conditions which interfere with the

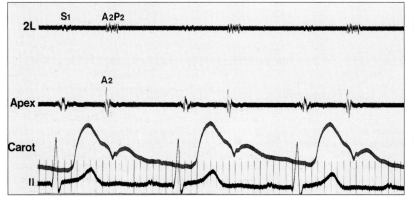

◀ **Figure 7.16 Normal carotid pulse.** The ECG is normal and the PCG, recorded by separate microphones at 2L (pulmonary area) and apex, shows normal splitting of the second sound at the pulmonary area, the aortic component first. The PCG recorded at the apex is also normal, showing a single (aortic) component of the second sound. (Recording speed 100 m/s)

normal return of blood to the heart and produce a diminished stroke output at the height of inspiration. This is not actually paradoxical but an exaggerated form of the normal pulse.

In *pulsus alternans* (Figure 7.18) there is an alternate variation in the size of the pulse wave, said to be due to a defective myocardium in which not all the fibres are capable of contracting at each heartbeat. It is often found in serious myocardial disease and is a sign of grave omen when the cardiac rhythm is normal. It is important, however, to realize that pulsus alternans may occur without serious myocardial disease if the ventricular rate is rapid, as, for example, in paroxysmal tachycardia.

The uncommon condition of hypertrophic obstructive cardiomyopathy (HOCM) produces a 'jerky' pulse with an initial sharp rise followed by prolongation, as in aortic stenosis. The shape of the recorded pulse wave is quite typical (Figure 7.20).

5 CONDITION OF THE ARTERIAL WALL

The examination of the pulse is completed by observations on the wall of the artery. An attempt should be made to roll the vessel under the index and second fingers. In many young persons the arterial wall is so compliant that with pressure of this kind it seems to merge into the surrounding tissues and to have no separate entity. In middle age it becomes distinctly palpable, and

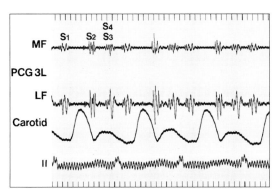

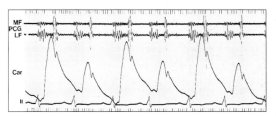

▲ **Figure 7.18 Pulsus alternans.** This patient was recovering from open heart surgery, and aortic valve replacement. The alternating volume and duration of the pulse is well shown. There are abnormalities also in the ECG and PCG. (Recording speed 50 mm/s)

▲ **Figure 7.17 Dicrotic pulse. The ECG shows marked a.c. interference**. The carotid pulse is typical of low stroke output, being an almost symmetric triangle in shape, followed by a large dicrotic wave. The PCG shows a summation gallop rhythm. The patient had congestive cardiomyopathy. (Recording speed 75 mm/s)

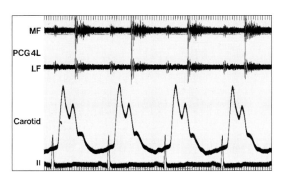

▲ **Figure 7.19 Bisferiens pulse.** This pulse has a palpable dip, resembling in some ways the dicrotic pulse, but with distinguishing features on palpation. Present when there is a combination of aortic regurgitation and stenosis, the diastolic murmur of the regurgitation is particularly well seen here. See Figure 7.38 for the pulse of aortic regurgitation without stenosis – the 'collapsing' pulse. (Recording speed 50 mm/s)

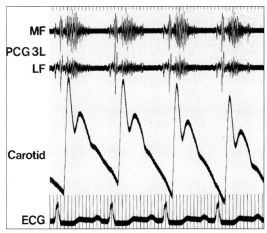

▲ **Figure 7.20 The sharp rise of the 'jerky' pulse of hypertrophic obstructive cardiomyopathy (HOCM) can be readily seen here.** The initial sharp upstroke is followed by the much slower rise to the second peak. The PCG shows a fourth heart sound immediately before the first heart sound; no ejection sound, and no diastolic murmur. (Recording speed 50 mm/s)

in the later decades can usually be felt as a cord-like structure. No hard-and-fast rule can be laid down as to what should be considered physiological and what pathological arterial thickening. Again it is only by experience that the examiner can form suitable standards for comparison.

While palpating the arterial wall note should also be made of any irregularity in its surface and of any tortuosity in its course. Irregularities are chiefly associated with those types of arteriosclerosis where calcareous material is deposited in the vessel wall, the 'pipe-stem' arteries of old age, and in certain cases hard ring-like structures can be felt along the course of the vessel, giving it a semblance to the trachea. Rarely, a localized aneurysm or inflammatory thickening of a peripheral artery may be found, as in giant-cell arteritis. Further consideration of the peripheral vessels now follows. (See also page 181.)

INSPECTION AND AUSCULTATION OF THE PERIPHERAL VESSELS

INSPECTION

Although the principal examination of the pulse is by palpation, useful information may be derived from inspection and auscultation. All the important peripheral vessels should be inspected. In those conditions in which a collapsing pulse is found, notably aortic regurgitation, the arteries pulsate vigorously and in a jerky manner (Corrigan's sign). This is well seen in the carotids, causing the head to nod or the ears to move with each systole of the heart.

Arteriosclerosis may often be recognized by the tortuosity of the superficial vessels (e.g. superficial temporal and brachial arteries) due to their lengthening while remaining more or less fixed at their proximal and distal points. In particular when the arm is flexed at the elbow to about 110°, the tortuosity of the brachial artery becomes most noticeable, and the snake-like movements of the tortuous vessel with each systole have earned for this phenomenon the name of 'locomotor brachialis'. It is important that the elbow should not be flexed beyond a right-angle, otherwise spurious tortuosity may be apparent.

The *retinal vessels* should be specially examined (see page 220).

Capillary pulsation is found where there is marked vasodilatation, particularly if there is also a big pulse pressure. It is therefore most frequently seen in aortic regurgitation but may be found in normal persons if the skin is warm and in hyperthyroidism in which the skin is usually warm. It may be observed by pressing with a glass slide on the fingernail, tongue or lip sufficiently heavily to cause partial blanching. The blanched area becomes pink with each systole of the heart.

It can also be demonstrated by shining a pen torch through the pad of the thumb and watching the pulsations in the nail bed. When there is a very big pulse pressure as in severe aortic regurgitation, capillary pulsation may be seen in the patient's forehead and face, when the alternate blanching and flushing is known as the 'lighthouse sign' for obvious reasons.

AUSCULTATION

Murmurs are not uncommonly propagated into the great vessels. The harsh systolic murmur of aortic stenosis is usually transmitted into the carotids. A systolic and diastolic murmur may be heard on pressure of the stethoscope over the great vessels (especially the femorals) in aortic regurgitation. Similarly, in this disease, the sudden output of a large quantity of blood from the left ventricle into the relatively empty arteries causes the 'pistol shot' sound to be heard. This has the same significance as the water-hammer pulse.

A systolic murmur may be heard over a stenosed peripheral artery, e.g. over the kidneys in renal artery stenosis and in the neck in carotid or vertebral stenosis.

EXAMINATION OF THE VEINS

This should include inspection and palpation of the superficial veins for evidence of engorgement, varicosity, and the presence of thombi or evidence of inflammation.

VENOUS ENGORGEMENT

Venous engorgement is most easily observed in the neck (Figure 7.21), though other veins than the jugulars may exhibit evidence of it. In judging whether veins are over-distended, it is necessary to fix a zero level. This is taken to be the sternal angle, i.e. the junction of the manubrium with the body of the sternum, for in whatever position the patient may be, sitting, standing, lying or in intermediate postures, it represents the zero position in the venous system, the level, in other words, of the blood in the mid-right atrium. Veins above this level are collapsed; veins below filled to varying degrees.

Judgement as to whether a vein is pathologically over-filled, therefore, will depend upon the height above the sternal angle at which the distension can be recognized. Normally, when the patient is supine with the head on pillows, the level of the blood in the jugular veins reaches about one-third of the way up the neck.

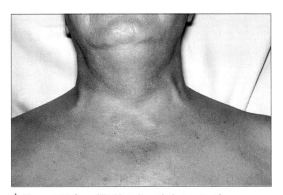

▲ **Figure 7.21 Over-filled jugular vein in a case of constrictive pericarditis.** A similar appearance is seen in congestive cardiac failure, in which, however, the veins are pulsatile. (Cf. Figure 6.7, page 108)

This level will be found to coincide with the level of the sternal angle. In early cases of congestive failure in the same position, the jugular column rises half-way to the jaw, and, in more severe cases, right to the jaw. Now if the patient sits gradually more upright, the column of blood will fall, in normal subjects, to such an extent that it can no longer be seen (it has sunk to the level of the sternal angle and is no longer filling the jugular veins). In cases of congestive failure, however, the column may still be visible above the clavicle for several centimetres or even throughout the course of the veins. Before assuming that a rise in venous pressure is due to cardiac failure (the commonest and most important cause), it must be recognized that a rise may also occur from increased intrathoracic pressure, but in this case the venous engorgement will usually disappear on deep inspiration. Obstruction to the superior vena cava is also a cause, but errors will be uncommon if search is made for supporting signs of congestive cardiac failure. (Cf. also Mediastinal obstruction, page 126.)

The filling of the veins should be bilateral and roughly equal, though the right side is more reliable as it is unaffected by aortic unfolding. A local obstruction may cause unilateral distension, often removed by turning the head. The venous engorgement should be accompanied by pulsation even when it is due to constrictive pericarditis or tamponade, but the venous pressure in these patients may be so high as to make the pulsation difficult to observe.

When more precise information about the venous pressure is required these simple clinical procedures can be checked by direct measurements. A catheter may be introduced into the right atrium from the superior vena cava or internal jugular vein for direct monitoring of central venous pressure.

PULSATION OF THE VEINS

This should be noted carefully. It often helps to localize the upper limit of jugular engorgement. In itself it is not pathological but may indicate that the level of venous distension is above the sternal angle. It must be distinguished from arterial pulsation, which is more obvious in the erect posture, while venous pulsation will diminish or disappear as the venous column falls with the assumption of an erect posture, unless the pressure is raised. It is difficult to feel normal venous pulsation, and then only with lightly placed fingers, but arterial pulsation pushes the fingers away forcibly. None the less, the distinction between the two is sometimes difficult, and when the jugular venous pressure is raised, it is readily palpable deep to the clavicular head of the sternomastoid, a fact well known to cardiographers who use very firm pressure in this area in recording the jugular pulse. It may be helpful to note that two positive waves may be identified in jugular pulsation but only one in carotid pulsation, though venous and arterial pulsations are often visible together. These two venous waves are the 'a' and 'v' waves identifiable graphically (see below).

Pulsation in the jugular veins (Figure 7.22) affects both external and internal vessels. The former is more easily recognized in the normal person, but the latter is more often found in congestive failure. When venous pulsation is not easy to identify, it may help to observe the patient in a good light, looking obliquely across the

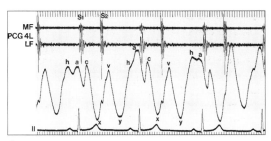

▲ **Figure 7.22 Normal jugular pulse.** Shown with a normal ECG and PCG. 'a' occurs with atrial systole. 'c' as the tricuspid valve moves into the atrial cavity with ventricular systole. Note the second, tricuspid component of the first heart sound occurs at the notch between the 'a' and 'c' waves. The 'x' descent occurs with atrial relaxation, and the rise to the 'v' peak (interrupted by a small notch coincident with the second heart sound) occurs with the passive filling of the right atrium from the great veins. After the tricuspid valve opens, the passage of blood into the relaxing ventricle corresponds with the descent of the pulse wave form from the 'v' peak to the 'y' trough, at which point the ventricle becomes more resistant to filling, the pressure in the atrium rises again, and when the heart rate is sufficiently slow, the wave form levels out at a point designated 'h'. This latter point is often summated with the next 'a' wave, as shown in the second complex here. (Recording speed 50 mm/s)

root of the neck from the front. Inspiration, by increasing venous return to the thorax, may make the venous pulse more obvious.

When the engorgement is due to non-cardiac causes such as mediastinal tumours, there is often no pulsation, as the pressure of the tumour interferes with the movement of blood between the jugular veins and right atrium. This is made more obvious by compression of the abdomen, which still further increases the jugular over-filling and pulsation in cases of congestive failure, but not when the veins are obstructed. The test also has the advantage of distinguishing carotid pulsation which is uninfluenced by abdominal pressure.

The pulsation observed in the jugular veins reflects the pressure changes in the right atrium, provided no obstruction of the vein exists. As the atrium contracts, so the pressure in the atrium rises, to force blood into the right ventricle, at the end of ventricular diastole. This rise in atrial pressure shows in the jugular veins as the 'a' wave, which begins at the peak of the 'P' wave of the ECG, immediately before the onset of the first heart sound and the carotid pulse.

As the atrium relaxes, the intra-atrial pressure falls, represented by the downstroke from the peak of the 'a' wave, but at the same time ventricular systole begins and the intraventricular pressure rises above that in the atrium, resulting in closure of the tricuspid valve. As the valve cusps balloon into the atrial cavity, there is a temporary halt in the falling intra-atrial pressure and a transient rise, shown as the 'c' wave. The onset of the 'c' wave corresponds with the tricuspid component of the first heart-sound.

As atrial relaxation continues after the 'c' wave, the pressure also falls until at the 'x' trough it reaches its lowest point, when with the inflow of blood from the great veins pressure begins to rise again to the second peak of the venous pulse, the 'v' wave. At this point, ventricular diastole has proceeded far enough for the intra-atrial pressure to exceed that in the ventricle, and the tricuspid valve opens. The intraventricular pressure is still falling and blood flows through the valve into the ventricle, with a resultant fall in the intra-atrial pressure also, until at the 'y' trough the ventricle is filled, and the pressure in ventricle and atrium begins to rise again, to even out until the onset of the next 'a' wave (Figure 7.22).

Any rise in right atrial pressure will cause an increase in the height of the 'a' wave. Thus, if tricuspid stenosis is present, very large 'a' waves are seen in the neck. If the intraventricular pressure is high at the end of diastole, as will occur in pulmonary arterial hypertension and pulmonary stenosis, and in other conditions where there is right ventricle hypertrophy and loss of compliance, the right atrial contraction must be correspondingly more vigorous if it is to force blood into the ventricle, and the 'a' wave will again be high (Figure 7.23).

If the ventricle contracts before or at the same time as the atrium because of complete heart block then the atrium will contract on to a closed tricuspid valve, resulting in a very high intra-atrial pressure, reflected in the jugular pulse as 'cannon' waves.

Rapid regular atrial contraction in atrial flutter can be seen in the jugular pulse, as 'a' waves interspersed with 'cannon' waves.

When atrial fibrillation is present, the 'a' wave disappears, and the 'x' descent is also obliterated as no significant atrial relaxation occurs, so that the jugular pulse is seen as a single positive wave, the 'v' wave.

With tricuspid incompetence, atrial fibrillation is frequently present. Since the intraventricular pressure is transmitted to the atrium, the jugular pulse in these circumstances shows a tall systolic wave only, the 'x' descent being totally obliterated. With the cessation of ventricular contraction, the pressure quickly falls and blood flows rapidly back through the tricuspid valve, shown in the jugular pulse as a rapid descent to the 'y' trough. In these circumstances the 'y' collapse after the tall 'v' wave is easily seen.

The clinical analysis of jugular pulsations needs some practice and skill, and rapid action of the heart tends to

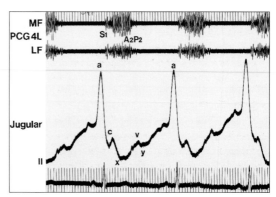

▲ **Figure 7.23 Tall jugular 'a' waves in pulmonary stenosis.** The PCG shows a characteristic systolic murmur extending through the position of the aortic component of the second sound, to end before the small pulmonary component of this sound. The tall 'a' wave occurs because of right ventricle hypertrophy, making a rise in right atrial pressure necessary to produce late diastolic ventricular filling properly. The 'a' wave begins at about the peak of the P wave in the ECG, is followed by a normal 'c' wave and 'x' descent, but the descent to the 'y' trough after the 'v' peak is slow. (Recording speed 50 mm/s)

fusion of the waves. Graphic methods of recording these pulsations can be of great value.

EXAMINATION OF THE HEART

The examination of the heart should follow the usual routine of inspection, palpation, percussion and auscultation.

Inspection enables the examiner to see the position and extent of the cardiac impulse and its rhythm. The presence of abnormal pulsation is noted over the precordium, over the great vessels in the neck and in the epigastrium. Some of these points have been considered under the Examination of the pulse, page 135.

Palpation confirms the position of the apex beat and gives more information about the force, duration and character of the cardiac impulse. Thrills (palpable murmurs) are felt in severe valve lesions. Expansile pulsation may be detected in cases of aneurysm.

Percussion has been discredited as a method of examining the heart because of the greater accuracy of radiology and will not be considered in detail. It may have some value when the patient is too ill to move by showing the increased dullness due to pericardial effusion. Occasionally it may demonstrate the basal dullness, especially to the right of the sternum, in cases of aortic aneurysm.

Auscultation is of great value in the detection of abnormalities of the valves which commonly produce both changes in the heart-sounds and added sounds called *murmurs*. It is also of importance in other diseases which alter the character of the heart sounds and in pericarditis where a friction sound is present. The rhythm of the heart is determined by examination of the pulse and auscultation of the heart.

These points will now be considered more fully.

fingers should be placed systematically over the apex beat and over the base of the heart. The extent of the cardiac impulse already defined by inspection should be confirmed; the force and character of the cardiac thrust can also be appreciated. The palm of the hand should then be placed on all areas of the precordium in order to detect any abnormal pulsations or vibrations.

As the cardiac impulse is normally circumscribed at the apex beat, the palm of the hand is too large for accurate palpation, and the information gained by it should be supplemented by the use of two fingers allowed to rest lightly over the cardiac thrust (see Figure 7.30, page 152). In this way the area of the cardiac impulse and its quality can be defined more carefully.

Apart from radiology, palpation is the most reliable method of estimating the size of the heart. The apex beat is the lowermost, outermost easily palpable cardiac impulse and is normally in the fifth intercostal space in the mid-clavicular line. Deviation from this position should be noted and the rib spaces counted from the sterno-manubrial angle.

It should be noted that in the normal adult little or no pulsation is communicated to the hand from the heart base or great vessels. Undue pulsation in this region is suggestive of aneurysmal enlargement of the great vessels, especially of the ascending part or arch of the aorta, more rarely of the pulmonary artery. Pulsation in the second left intercostal space may, however, be seen normally in children. Left parasternal pulsation may be caused by right ventricle hypertrophy, but it may also be the result of transmitted pulsation from an enlarged left atrium due to severe mitral regurgitation (see also page 154). Occasionally, a right parasternal impulse may be felt when the right atrium is enlarged in severe tricuspid incompetence.

INSPECTION

This method of examination is of greatest value in studying the position, character and rhythm of the cardiac impulse. Abnormal pulsations especially of cardiac hypertrophy and aneurysms, may also be visible (Figure 7.24). The patient should be in a good light, and the cardiac and other pulsations examined both in the erect and recumbent posture.

PALPATION

Palpation also should be carried out with the patient first in the recumbent and then in the erect posture. The

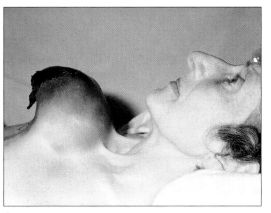

▲ **Figure 7.24 Aortic aneurysm bulging through chest**

The student should make it a practice to place the hand on each side of the chest in turn, especially when the apex beat is not easily palpated in its normal position on the left side. In this way he will avoid overlooking *dextrocardia*.

THE CARDIAC IMPULSE

The cardiac thrust is maximal normally at the apex beat and can be examined by inspection and palpation. Two separate aspects must receive attention, the position and the character.

Position

The normal impulse (apex beat) is sometimes visible and usually palpable 7.5–10.5 cm (3–4 in) from the midline and generally in the fifth intercostal space. It is circumscribed and almost invariably within the nipple line except occasionally in children and adolescents. In women this landmark for obvious reasons is of no value, but in men it is useful, as the nipple is generally further from the midline in asthenic individuals whose hearts are also proportionally larger. The systolic thrust is caused by the contracting left ventricle lifting the chest wall before retracting medially. Thus the period of time during which the normal apex beat is felt is shorter than the duration of the ventricular systole. Internal to the thrust may be seen an area of systolic retraction caused by movements of the right ventricle, and it is necessary that this systolic retraction should not be confused with that of pathological origin. With changes of posture (lying on one side) the apex beat may move as much as 1.5–2 cm. If the impulse is abnormal in position, particular care should be taken to look for causes of cardiac displacement such as scoliosis and funnel sternum; also pleural and pulmonary diseases (e.g. pleural effusion and pulmonary fibrosis). When these causes have been eliminated, an abnormal position generally signifies cardiac enlargement.

Left ventricular hypertrophy initially causes an increased duration of the apex beat and later results in a minimally displaced but more forceful impulse.

Right ventricular hypertrophy causes strong pulsation in the left parasternal region and often movement of the sternum and ribs (see above).

Character

In normal persons the apex beat gently raises the palpating fingers. The strength of this thrust can only be judged by experience. It is diminished in health by a thick chest wall (muscle or fat) or by emphysema, and is more noticeable in thin persons.

If the impulse is feeble, less significance can be attached to it, unless it has been watched from day to day and is known to have changed. In this case a feeble diffuse impulse, combined with change in position towards the axilla, may suggest dilatation. Diffuseness alone or sometimes with temporary increased forcibility often results from simple overaction of the heart as in nervous persons, after exercise or in hyperthyroidism. Certain special types of cardiac impulse are recognizable to the experienced fingers, such as the tap or shock of mitral stenosis (actually a palpable first heart sound). If the thrust is forcible, hypertrophy is suggested. When great cardiac enlargement is present there may be a diffuse markedly displaced heave.

The position and character of the cardiac impulse thus give valuable information as to the presence of cardiac enlargement and whether this is due to hypertrophy or dilatation. It will be convenient here to consider briefly the clinical significance of these phenomena.

HYPERTROPHY

The presence of hypertrophy indicates that the heart is working under a pressure overload. The clinical examination is therefore directed primarily to the discovery of this load, which may include systemic hypertension, aortic valve disease, pulmonary hypertension and primary diseases of heart muscle. The degree of the hypertrophy is also a rough indication of the extent of the load, i.e. the seriousness of the condition causing hypertrophy. Left and right ventricular hypertrophy can generally be recognized clinically, but enlargement of the atria cannot easily be detected except radiologically, although systolic left atrial expansion may be suspected when there is systolic pulsation in the left parasternal area in patients with mitral regurgitation.

DILATATION

Dilatation of the left ventricle causes displacement of the apex beat due to a volume overload. This may be physiological as in exercise, when the cardiac output increases with increased venous input because of the stretch on the ventricular muscle fibres at the end of diastole.

Pathological changes in the heart muscle may alter the response to the stretch, so that although the heart dilates, its output falls.

This is commonly seen in aortic or mitral incompetence and after myocardial infarction; it may also be found in various cardiac muscle disorders, and as a temporary response when the ventricles beat at a high speed as in atrial flutter.

Dilatation is not easy to recognize, though in acute cases displacement of the apex beat may be apparent, and radiology will demonstrate enlargement of the cardiac shadow.

It is often accompanied by hypertrophy as in mixed aortic valve disease, heart block and sometimes in athletes, where the stroke output of the ventricle is increased.

Atrial dilatation, usually with hypertrophy, is seen in some types of valvular and congenital heart disease. A good example is the enlargement of the left atrium in mitral stenosis although this is not clinically detectable.

THRILLS

When vibrations are communicated to the palpating hand from the heart or its great vessels, they are spoken of as thrills. They are usually detected best when the breath is held in expiration. A thrill is a palpable murmur and is produced in the same way, though as a rule the conditions necessary for its production must be more exaggerated than in the case of a murmur. Of these conditions the main ones are obstruction to the passage of blood from the chambers of the heart through a narrowed valve, and the abnormal blood flow in certain congenital defects, but the thrill will be more readily palpable if the chest wall is thin, if the blood flow is rapid, and if the site of production is comparatively near the surface. Like murmurs, thrills may be systolic or diastolic in time, or, more rarely, may occur continuously throughout the cardiac cycle. For the novice it is often difficult to time a thrill accurately, and it is justifiable to consider the timing in conjunction with that of the murmur which always accompanies it. The presence of a thrill is more certain evidence of organic disease of the heart than the presence of a murmur.

At the base of the heart thrills are more commonly systolic. In aortic stenosis and in aneurysm of the great vessels at the root of the neck a powerful systolic thrill may be palpable over the second right interspace, usually spreading upwards towards the neck. To the left of the sternum in the second interspace pulmonary stenosis gives rise to a similar type of thrill. Lower down the sternum, usually in the second interspace, systolic thrills are occasionally felt due to congenital lesions of the heart, particularly patency of the interventricular septum. Occasionally systolic thrills are found at the apex alone, due to mitral regurgitation, but it is not uncommon for a thrill arising at the other areas mentioned to extend into the region of the apex.

By contrast, diastolic thrills at the apex are uncommon and usually due to mitral stenosis. They correspond in time with the murmur, and if this is presystolic, the thrill may end with a systolic shock at the apex synchronizing with an abrupt first sound.

The combination of a systolic and diastolic thrill is rare. It sometimes occurs over the base of the heart in patients with patent ductus arteriosus. If such a thrill exists care should be taken not to overlook the possibility of other vascular abnormalities, such as an enlarged overactive thyroid gland, a vascular mediastinal tumour, or still more rarely an arteriovenous aneurysm.

AUSCULTATION

Auscultation ranks with inspection and palpation as a most important method of examining the cardiovascular system. A suitable stethoscope is one that has a bell chest piece for low-pitched sounds, e.g. the diastolic murmur of mitral stenosis, and a flat diaphragm-like chest piece which is more suitable for high-pitched sounds such as the murmur of aortic regurgitation. By means of auscultation the rate and rhythm of the heart may be confirmed and compared with those of the pulse, but its main value is in the information it yields concerning the functions of the heart valves and to a lesser extent of the state of the myocardium and pericardium. The student should learn to concentrate first on the auscultation of the heart sounds before turning his attention to any additional sounds or *murmurs* which may be present. He should also pay attention to each heart sound separately, ignoring the others for a while, and at each separate area ask himself the following questions:

1   Can I hear the first sound, and is it normal? If it is not normal, how does it differ from the usual?
2   Can I hear the second sound, and is it normal? Can I hear splitting of the second sound, and if so, does it vary normally with respiration?
3   Can I hear any added sounds? If so, where in the cardiac cycle do they occur, and what character do they have?
4   Are any murmurs present? If so, where in the cardiac cycle do they occur, what relationship do they have to the sounds and added sounds, what is their character and to where are they propagated?

THE HEART SOUNDS

Even in perfect health considerable differences exist in the intensity and character of the heart sounds in different individuals. To form some idea of the limits of these variations the beginner should examine as many normal hearts as possible. In obese persons, in emphysema or in those with well-developed musculature, the sounds are diminished in intensity. Conversely, thin coverings of muscle or fat on the chest wall allow the sounds to be conducted more clearly and loudly to the stethoscope. Therefore, it is usually easy to define the heart sounds at all areas of the precordium in children.

Auscultation of the heart should be made over a large area of the precordium, but especially over the apex and base of the heart, i.e. a little distance from the anatomical position of the valves. The apex is sometimes called the 'mitral' area, and the base is divided into 'aortic' and 'pulmonary' areas. The 'tricuspid' area at the lower end of the sternum is of less importance. These areas are chosen for auscultation because of the variability of the heart sounds over them and also because murmurs associated with valve disease may be heard most commonly at one of them, e.g. the diastolic murmur of mitral stenosis at the mitral area. However, auscultation must not be confined to these named areas, and the site of any abnormality heard should be recorded in terms of intercostal level and distance from the sternum (to left or right). It must be clearly understood that sounds produced in the heart have a common origin, though their component elements may be heard with a different intensity over different parts of the chest. The first sound, associated with closure of the mitral and tricuspid valves, is heard best at the apex, and as the mitral element is louder than the tricuspid, this is the most easily heard component of the first sound. The second sound is associated with closure of the aortic and pulmonary valves. Normally the aortic component of the second sound is best heard over the aortic area and is transmitted to the apex. The pulmonary component, on the other hand, is generally heard best over the pulmonary area and in the region of the second and third left interspaces. Both components of the second sound may normally be heard, the aortic component preceding the pulmonary. The intensity of the components varies with age, the aortic element dominating in the older age groups and the pulmonary element in the young.

A third sound is sometimes heard, particularly in childhood and adolescence, and may cause confusion in deciding whether or not a mitral diastolic murmur is present. It is associated with rapid distension of the ventricle in early diastole, although its exact mode of production is not clear. It occurs at the nadir of the trough in the appropriate venous pulse, shortly after the second heart sound, and is best heard at the apex and left sternal border, with the patient recumbent.

If atrial systole is abnormally vigorous it may produce a fourth heart sound, occurring before the first sound. This occurs when atrial augmentation of ventricular filling in late diastole takes place with a 'non-compliant' ventricle, i.e. one not easily distended.

The heart sounds are often likened to the syllables 'lub-dup' and have definition which helps to distinguish them from additional sounds such as murmurs. It is important to be aware of the notable variation of the heart sounds in health which makes difficult any precise imitation of the sounds.

Just as the pulse rate and the blood pressure should be examined at the end of the consultation as well as at the beginning, in order to exclude the effects of emotion or exercise, so the heart sounds should be compared at the beginning and end of the examination. If this is done systematically the student will learn that a considerable modification of the sounds may take place as the result of excitement or physical effort – both of which tend to make the heart sounds sharper and louder than normal, though the relative intensity of the sounds remains the same, the first sound being louder at the apex and the second sound at the base.

NORMAL RHYTHM OF THE HEART SOUNDS

In a normal heart the first and second sounds are quite close together, but the interval following the second sound is relatively long. The sequence is thus lub-dup-pause, lub-dup-pause (Figure 7.25).

EXAGGERATION OF THE SOUNDS

The heart sounds become louder in conditions which increase the activity of the heart, e.g. nervousness, exercise and hyperthyroidism. The increase is most obvious in the first sound at the apex and to a lesser extent in the second sound at the base. The first sound is also louder and abrupt in mitral stenosis, particularly at the apex. The second sound (aortic component) is increased at the aortic area in systemic hypertension. At the pulmonary area the pulmonary component of the second sound is increased when the pulmonary arterial pressure rises, as may occur in mitral stenosis, in certain forms of congenital heart disease and in some pulmonary diseases.

DIMINUTION OF THE SOUNDS

Diminution in the heart sounds is more often due to extracardiac than to cardiac causes. Of these, emphysema is one of the most important, as the air-containing lung spreads over the area where the heart normally comes in contact with the chest wall. Similarly, fluid or air in the pleural or pericardial cavities may form a layer preventing the heart sounds from reaching the surface normally. Until these causes and the physiological ones mentioned earlier have been considered, feebleness of the heart sounds does not rank as an important sign; but if the patient has been examined previously and was

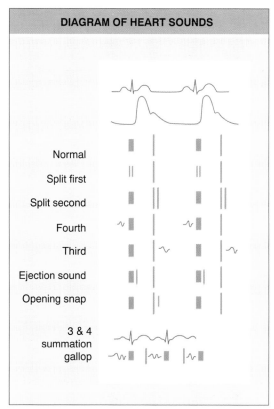

DIAGRAM OF HEART SOUNDS

Normal

Split first

Split second

Fourth

Third

Ejection sound

Opening snap

3 & 4
summation
gallop

▲ **Figure 7.25 Diagram of heart sounds**. Note: the diagrammatic representation of the fourth and third heart sounds is to indicate that they have a lower frequency than the first and second sounds

known to have well-defined heart sounds which have become feeble, the sign is of more significance and may suggest cardiac failure.

SPLITTING OF SOUNDS

Splitting of the first or second sound may be audible, the two elements being very close together. This closeness is an essential character of splitting, and distinguishes it from various forms of gallop rhythm in which three sounds are present but at considerable intervals one from the other. Splitting may be imitated by the syllables 'l-lub' and 'd-dub'. When affecting the *first sound* it is usually heard best at the apex, and is probably due to an asynchronous closure of the mitral and tricuspid valves. It is not pathological but the inexperienced may confuse it with an ejection click or even a short presystolic murmur.

Splitting of the second sound due to asynchronous closure of the aortic and pulmonary valves varies with

respiration, is common and is often physiological. When the splitting is wide and fixed, i.e. not varying with respiration, it is more likely to be pathological. Normal splitting of the second sound is recognized by a widening of the interval between the aortic and pulmonary components during normal inspiration, and narrowing with expiration. This is caused by a temporary increase in venous return to the right heart, with prolongation of right ventricular systole, and consequent delay in pulmonary valve closure. Abnormalities of conduction, e.g. bundle-branch block, will alter the normal pattern of ventricle contraction, and in the case of left bundle-branch block may so delay left ventricle contraction as to cause the aortic component of the second sound to follow the pulmonary, when normal inspiration will then cause the splitting of the sound to narrow – the phenomenon of 'reversed splitting' of the second sound.

THE OPENING SNAP

This has considerable importance in the clinical appraisal of mitral stenosis. It is associated with the sudden movement of the valve as it opens in early diastole and is of a relatively sharp character. Its intensity probably depends upon the mobility of the mitral valve and the severity of the stenosis, but when it is present it should indicate that at least part of the valve is still mobile (Figure 7.26).

With lessening mobility of the valve, as happens commonly in mitral incompetence, the opening snap is less well heard, and, of course, calcification and fibrosis may make it totally inaudible.

It is often heard over a wide area of the precordium, but usually best over an area from the apex to the left sternal edge.

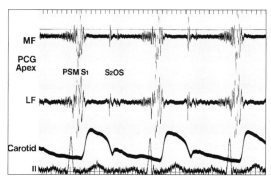

▲ **Figure 7.26 The sound records show a presystolic murmur (PSM) rising to a crescendo to meet the loud first heart sound (S1). S2 (the second heart sound) is followed by a clear opening snap (OS)**. The S2–OS interval is about 0.06 s. The carotid pulse is normal. (Recording speed 100 mm/s)

EJECTION CLICKS

These are sharp sounds, and occur coincidentally with the onset of the arterial pulse tracing, immediately after the first heart sound. They occur with the sudden opening of the appropriate semilunar valves, in conditions where this opening is delayed, e.g. in aortic valve stenosis, hypertension, pulmonary valve stenosis, or where the opening of the valve is abnormally rapid. In a similar way to the opening snap of the mitral valve, the ejection sound is an indication of the mobility of the appropriate semilunar valve.

Thus if aortic valvular stenosis is congenital with no calcification, an ejection click will be present. When the valve becomes calcified and immobile, the ejection click is absent or very much diminished.

It is often difficult to distinguish the first sound from an ejection sound, but phonocardiography will be of help in this distinction (see Figure 7.37, page 158).

GALLOP RHYTHM

This term is applied to *triple rhythms* produced by the addition of the third or fourth heart sounds to the normal first and second. As mentioned before, a normal third sound is often heard in youth, but over the age of 40 years any triple rhythm should be regarded with suspicion.

The *third sound gallop rhythm* (formerly called *protodiastolic*) is a sign of serious myocardial disease, and is thought to be produced by distension of a diseased myocardium in early diastole after the atrioventricular valves open. Arising from the right ventricle, it is best heard parasternally or in the epigastrium. From the left ventricle it is loudest at and internal to the apex.

The *fourth sound* or '*atrial*' gallop is produced by an abnormally loud fourth sound, which occurs when atrial contraction is forcing blood into a ventricle where the end diastolic pressure is abnormally high. This may occur in the early stages of ventricular failure but also when the ventricle is 'non-compliant', e.g. with severe ventricular hypertrophy, as in aortic stenosis, when the cavity of the ventricle is small, and atrial contraction has to produce a considerable pressure rise to augment ventricular filling.

The fourth sound disappears, of course, in atrial fibrillation. Its areas of maximal intensity are similar to those of the third sound.

True gallop rhythm has a fancied resemblance to the noise of a galloping horse and only occurs with a rapid heart rate, arbitrarily stated to be 100 per minute or over. In these cases the third and fourth sounds occur together and are said to be 'summated'. This summation gallop rhythm is of even greater seriousness than the third or fourth sound triple rhythm alone (Figure 7.27).

MIDSYSTOLIC CLICKS

These sounds were thought to be of no significance, produced by pericardial adhesions, but recent studies have shown them to be produced by abnormalities of the atrioventricular valve mechanism, usually the mitral valve. They are caused by abnormal prolapse of the valve into the atrial cavity and are often accompanied by a systolic murmur of mitral regurgitation. They are readily identified by phonocardiography and demonstrated as being associated with valve prolapse by echocardiography (Figure 7.28).

The more common abnormal heart sound are summarised in Table 7.3.

ADDITIONAL SOUNDS

These include the class of sounds known as murmurs, originating at the valves or in the great vessels, and friction sounds produced in the pericardial layers and in the pleura which lies in close contact with the heart. Peculiar sounds are also heard occasionally due to impact of the

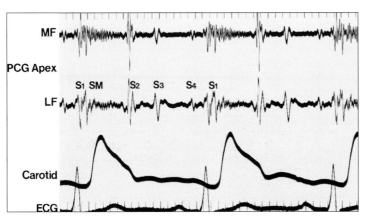

◀ **Figure 7.27 Illustrates the third (S3) and fourth (S4) heart sounds, in a patient with myocardial pathology of unknown aetiology.** The carotid pulse and ECG are normal. Also present is wide splitting of the first heart sound (S1) and an early systolic murmur (SM). The second heart sound (S2) is normal. When S1, S2, S3 and S4 are audible it represents an unusual quadruple rhythm, a variety of so-called 'gallop' rhythm. See Figure 7.25. (Recording speed 100 mm/s)

heart against surrounding tissues – for example, against fluid or air in the pleural cavity, or through the diaphragm against the air- and fluid-containing viscera. These sounds have little importance, and, although their origin is often uncertain, they are rarely confused with the murmurs and pericardial sounds to be described.

Pericardial friction sounds (Figure 7.29)

A friction sound or rub is heard in cases of acute pericarditis and is comparable with a pleural rub. It is produced by the movement of the two layers of pericardium over one another in the presence of an exudate. The sound may be heard over any part of the precordium, and sometimes over so small an area as to be overlooked, while at other times it is so extensive as to be present over every part of the heart. The rub has a peculiar superficial quality and is sometimes rough and grating in character, sometimes scratchy, and at other times soft and blowing, so that it may be confused with the to-and-fro murmur so frequently heard in aortic regurgitation. Its intensity may be increased by heavier pressure with the stethoscope. Not uncommonly pericarditis is associated with pleurisy, and the pericardial friction

rub may become continuous with the pleural rub and extend outside the limits of the precordium. Classically 'tripartite', the friction over the ventricle is heard during ventricular systole; in diastole when early filling of the ventricle is happening, and in late diastole when atrial augmentation of ventricular filling occurs.

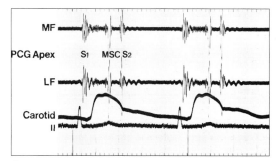

▲ **Figure 7.28 The ECG and carotid pulses are normal, but the sound records show a clear midsystolic click (MSC) between a normal S1 and S2, and after a low intensity short systolic murmur.** This is an unusual variety of triple rhythm, most often associated with an abnormal mitral subvalvar mechanism. (Recording speed 75 mm/s)

ABNORMAL HEART SOUNDS			
Timing	**Abnormal sound**	**Mechanism**	**Significance**
1st sound	Accentuation (normal with increased cardiac activity e.g. exercise)	?Abrupt closure of mitral valve	Mitral stenosis
Systole	Ejection click	Delayed opening of semilunar valves	Aortic or pulmonary stenosis with mobile valve
	Mid-systolic click	Mitral valve prolapse into atrium	Congenital anomaly of mitral valve mechanism
2nd sound	Accentuation	Abrupt closure of semilunar valves	Systemic or pulmonary arterial hypertension
	Splitting (normal if widening on inspiration)	Asynchronous closure or aortic and pulmonary valves	Left or right bundle branch block
Diastole	Opening snap	Sudden opening of abnormal mitral valve	Mitral stenosis with mobile valve
	3rd heart sound (normal in youth)	Diastolic distension of diseased myocardium	Left or right ventricular failure
	4th heart sound	Forceful atrial contraction against raised ventricular pressure	Left or right ventricular failure or hypertrophy

▲ Table 7.3

MURMURS

Once the position and character of the heart sounds have been determined, the student is then in a position to pay attention to any murmurs which may be present.

The following points should be ascertained whenever a murmur is present.

1 THE TIME RELATIONSHIP

This implies not only whether the murmur occurs in systole or diastole but also whether it occupies a part or the whole of these. Great care is often necessary to time a murmur successfully. If the cardiac impulse is sufficiently great to lift the stethoscope during systole, or to be palpable with the finger, this forms an easy way of timing the first sound of the heart and thus of the murmur (Figure 7.30). If the impulse is feeble, reliance must be placed on the pulsation of the carotid artery and allowance made for the fact that this occurs about one-tenth of a second later than the actual contraction of the ventricles. Many systolic murmurs follow the first sound immediately, although some are mid or late systolic. Diastolic murmurs may appear immediately after the second sound or only after an appreciable interval and, in case of presystolic murmurs, just precede the first sound. It is sometimes very difficult to time a murmur with certainty, and its position in the cardiac cycle may then be suggested by its character, to which close attention should be paid. Phonocardiography may be needed, but even without

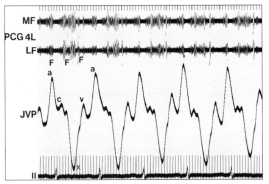

▲ Figure 7.29 Pericardial friction occurring where **tuberculous pericarditis was later shown to be present.** The high-frequency friction sounds (F) have been recorded at the left sternal edge and, by comparing with the simultaneous carotid, jugular and ECG traces, can be seen to be present when there is movement associated with atrial contraction (and ventricular filling), with ventricular contraction during systole, and during ventricular relaxation and rapid passive filling of the ventricle in early diastole. The friction noise is recorded at times when there is rapid movement of the cardiac chambers, with changes in volume. (Recording speed 50 mm/s)

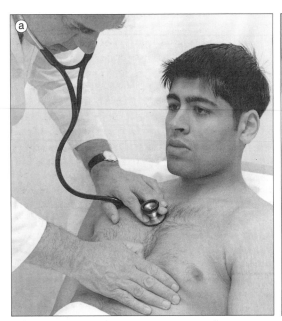

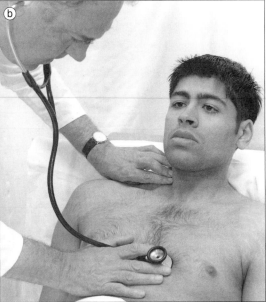

▲ Figure 7.30 Timing murmurs. (a) In this illustration the stethoscope is placed so as to time an aortic murmur. The fingers are lifted with each systole of the heart corresponding with the first heart sound. (b) When the apex beat cannot be felt reliance must be placed on palpation of the carotid artery in which the palpation follows that of the apex beat by 0.1 s

this aid, identification of the second heart sound should have been decisive in showing the division between systole and diastole.

2 The Character of the Murmur

Murmurs may vary from a soft blowing sound to a harsh rasping one. Loud and especially rough murmurs are more commonly associated with organic valvular and congenital lesions. Soft murmurs are often harmless, though some, e.g. that of aortic incompetence, may be conclusive of pathological changes. It must be emphasized, however, that there is no correlation between the loudness of a murmur and the haemodynamic severity of the lesion producing the noise.

3 Distribution

A careful record should be made, preferably in the form of a diagram, of the area over which the murmur is heard and of the point of maximum intensity. A record of this kind constitutes a valuable method of assessing the significance of a murmur and its place of production. Associated with this observation there should be noted:

4 Direction of Spread

When the maximum intensity of the murmur has been noted, the stethoscope should be moved radially from this point in different directions to observe whether the murmur is circumscribed or conducted to other parts of the chest wall. The direction of conduction, or, on the contrary, the absence of conduction, is characteristic of certain murmurs.

5 Relation to Respiration, Posture and Exercise

Many murmurs, especially innocent ones, are modified by respiration, often disappearing at the height of inspiration. This is particularly true of pulmonary systolic murmurs, but may occur in the case of mitral systolic murmurs. Aortic diastolic murmurs can best be heard on expiration, tricuspid murmurs on inspiration.

The effect of posture should be observed, as some murmurs – e.g. an aortic diastolic – are best heard in the erect posture with the patient leaning forwards, while others – e.g. a mitral diastolic – are heard most clearly when the patient is recumbent, especially in the left lateral position.

Again, exercise modifies murmurs, and when there is no contraindication (e.g. active carditis or heart failure) the patient should be exercised to increase the cardiac output and hence the rate of flow across the valves. Presystolic mitral murmurs are often intensified by such exercise. However, the rapid heart rate induced by exercise may make murmurs more difficult to time.

Causes of Murmurs

The ultimate cause of many murmurs is uncertain and our views are changing in the light of the information now available from operations on the heart and from direct sound recordings via a cardiac catheter. In general, the factors which are responsible include turbulence and eddy currents resulting from modification in the size of the valve opening, irregularities and deformities in the valve itself and in surrounding parts, such as the chordae tendineae. In many cases, especially where there is obstruction at a valve, the production of the murmur depends upon the relative disproportion of the orifice, which is narrowed, and the chamber beyond.

The velocity of the blood flow also plays a considerable part, and this is well seen in the increase of the diastolic murmur of mitral stenosis by exercise. Increased velocity of the blood flow may also be responsible for murmurs which occur even when the valves and their rings are normal, e.g. in thyrotoxicosis and anaemia. The regurgitant murmur in aortic incompetence is again due to the blood passing through a relatively narrow orifice at high velocity and possibly setting up vibration in structures upon which it impinges.

From a clinical point of view it is useful to divide murmurs into *innocent* or *insignificant* on the one hand, and *organic* or *significant* on the other. From the brief description of the causation it will be appreciated that very minor variations in the anatomical proportions of the valve orifices and the heart chambers may give rise to insignificant murmurs. These are always systolic in time, usually faint in character, though increased by exercise, and quite commonly found over the pulmonary area and to a lesser extent over the cardiac apex. These characteristics, together with the complete absence of any other signs of cardiac disease (in particular any abnormal heart sounds) or of any past aetiological factors which might produce such disease, will often justify the dismissal of the murmur as insignificant. These murmurs are commonly 'ejection' in type, i.e. occurring only at an interval after the first sound and ceasing before the second sound. There are, however, certain systolic murmurs which, while they do not indicate permanent valve or congenital heart disease, may be significant. Such is the murmur of mitral incompetence due to papillary muscle–chordal dysfunction produced by dilatation of the left ventricle from causes such as hypertension or aortic disease without any involvement of the mitral valve. It is possible for such a murmur to disappear, though this is uncommon, but when the murmur results from deformed cusps it will remain permanent. The murmur equally persists when it is due to obstruction or a congenital lesion which remains stationary, though alteration in the dynamics of the heart may modify the murmur from time to time.

Careful judgement is necessary to determine the significance of many murmurs. This is particularly so in the case of systolic murmurs, which are often harmless, but may raise suspicion of organic disease when there is a history of rheumatic fever or associated signs of heart disease.

The decision as to the seriousness of these murmurs is important, for on the one hand the patient may be unnecessarily alarmed, or on the other an early valve lesion may be overlooked, and the patient will go untreated.

Diastolic murmurs are more simple. Sometimes, as in the case of mitral stenosis, the murmur alone suffices to make the diagnosis probable. Similarly the diastolic murmur of aortic incompetence is rare except in that disease, though corroborative vascular phenomena help to complete the picture. The signs which support a diagnosis of valve disease are considered elsewhere.

Special details relating to murmurs may now be discussed under the headings of the areas of the heart where they are found, again remembering that loudness does not necessarily correlate with severity.

MURMURS AT THE CARDIAC APEX
Systolic murmurs
Systolic murmurs at the cardiac apex are common, and may be difficult to evaluate as indications of organic disease. The murmurs are often soft in character, but if sufficiently loud and caused by a posteriorly directed flow of regurgitant blood through the mitral valve, they are conducted in a characteristic manner towards the axilla and often through to the back at the inferior angle of the left scapula (Figure 7.31). The murmur alone gives limited indication of the degree of leakage.

Some of the conditions which produce papillary muscle–chordal dysfunction to a greater or lesser degree are susceptible of improvement, with a corresponding disappearance of the mitral regurgitation and the systolic murmur. The murmur therefore may be described as 'functional'. The diagnosis of the true value of the murmur is made by looking for the causal disease, and by watching the patient to see if the murmur disappears or changes. If the murmur does not disappear, as may happen for example in dilatation of the left ventricle due to cardiomyopathy, the mitral regurgitation remains as a permanent feature of the illness, and the murmur may then be regarded as no less important than if there were damage to the valve cusps.

Systolic murmurs dependent on abnormality of the cusps of the mitral valve from rheumatic or other causes may be similar to the so-called innocent or insignificant murmurs. In assigning to them their correct importance, attention should be paid to a history of rheumatic illness, the size of the heart and the presence of any other valve lesion; but it must be admitted that it is sometimes impossible to decide whether or not a systolic apical murmur indicates the presence of organic disease of the mitral valve cusps, though the course of the disease and the subsequent development of other evidence of rheumatic damage to the myocardium or valves may establish a correct diagnosis. When it is suspected that a systolic murmur indicates rheumatic mitral regurgitation, a persistent search must be made for the diastolic murmur of mitral stenosis which so commonly accompanies the disease in this form.

Since rheumatic fever has become a much less common disease from the year 1950 and onwards, so the incidence of rheumatic valve disease has decreased, at least in Western Europe and North America. Rheumatic mitral regurgitation is still a common cause of an incompetent mitral valve, but other abnormalities of the mitral valve mechanism producing regurgitation are now more easily recognized, and in particular the

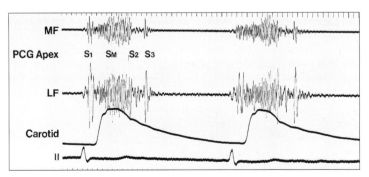

◄ Figure 7.31 Mitral regurgitation. The carotid pulse is normal, the ECG shows no atrial activity, i.e. atrial fibrillation is probably present. The murmur is pansystolic (SM) extending from S1 to S2. A short diastolic murmur envelops a loud third sound (S3). The pansystolic murmur should be compared with the midsystolic murmur of aortic stenosis (cf. Figures 7.13, 7.14, 7 37). (Recording speed 100 mm/s)

prolapsing cusp in the midsystolic click – late systolic murmur syndrome – has been shown to be relatively common by phono- and echocardiography. The stream of regurgitant blood through the valve may be directed other than posteriorly, and if this direction is superior and medial, the systolic murmur may be propagated in the same direction and be best heard parasternally rather than in the axilla, and thus be easily confused with the murmur of aortic stenosis (Figure 7.32).

It only remains to add that murmurs originating at other areas of the heart may be conducted to the apex and imitate those due to mitral insufficiency. An example of this is sometimes seen in aortic stenosis. In determining the origin of the murmur it is helpful if a distinction can be made between a pansystolic murmur, usual in mitral incompetence and ventricular septal defects, and the midsystolic murmur which characterizes aortic and pulmonary stenosis (Figures 7.31 and 7.37).

Correct timing is of great importance, though sometimes difficult without a phonocardiogram. Pansystolic murmurs in mitral incompetence and ventricular septal defects start with the first sound and continue to, or even through the second sound, whereas ejection murmurs, as in aortic stenosis and pulmonary stenosis, cannot be heard immediately after the first sound but are easier to time as ending before the second sound. Timing of the murmur can only be achieved by recognition of the heart sounds, hence the emphasis on these signs.

Diastolic murmurs

When a diastolic murmur is heard only at the mitral area it is nearly always due to mitral stenosis, in which the valve cusps are fused together and the orifice from the left atrium into the ventricle is narrowed. Only rarely is a diastolic murmur heard when the mitral valve is normal, and in such cases there is increased velocity and volume of the blood flow across the mitral valve, as in ventricular septal defects and other types of left-to-right shunting 'downstream' from the mitral valve. The same cause may be at work in mitral and aortic regurgitation, though in the latter it is possible that the diastolic and presystolic murmur, called, after its describer, the 'Austin

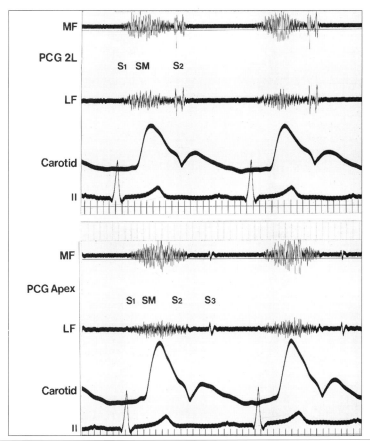

◀ **Figure 7.32 Mitral regurgitation.** These phonocardiograms from 2L (pulmonary area) and apex were recorded from a man with mitral regurgitation in sinus rhythm, and no aortic valve disease. Both illustrations show the pansystolic murmur starting with a low intensity S1, and passing up to S2 – the latter being widely split in the 2L position. A third sound (S3) is recorded at the apex. The systolic murmur is crescendo–decrescendo in shape, as in aortic stenosis, but is shown to be pansystolic in timing and position. Compare with Figure 7.31, where atrial fibrillation is present. (Recording speed 100 mm/s)

Flint', is due to impingement of the regurgitation jet on the anterior mitral valve leaflet. This causes a functional partial obstruction at the mitral orifice, and the regurgitant jet may also cause the anterior leaflet of the mitral valve to vibrate (Figures 7.33 and 7.34).

The mitral diastolic murmur of mitral stenosis is nearly always of low pitch and rumbling in character. It is often appreciated with difficulty by the unpractised ear, and to avoid overlooking it the student should examine the patient in the recumbent posture, when it may easily be audible in cases in which it was not apparent with the patient erect. The murmur is often intensified when the patient lies on the left side so that the

cardiac apex is brought into closer contact with the chest wall. Exercise may also bring out a murmur which is otherwise difficult to hear, and the stethoscope should be applied immediately the patient lies down after the effort, so that the first few heart beats will not be missed, for it is in these, when the blood velocity is high, that the murmur is generally heard. Diastolic murmurs, in contrast with systolic, are circumscribed and often localized to an area of a few square centimetres around the apex beat. The murmur is separated from the second sound by a short pause, but may then fill the remainder of diastole (Figures 7.35 and 7.36). If it is chiefly late diastolic and becomes continuous with an accentuated

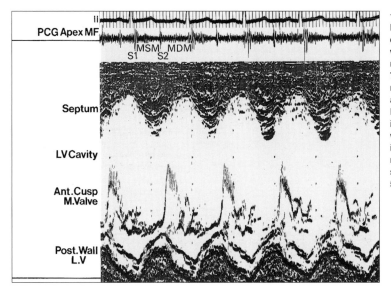

◀ **Figure 7.33 This combined ECG, PCG and echocardiogram shows the diastolic murmur (MDM) at the apex, with an appearance similar to that of mitral stenosis (cf. Figures 7.25, 7.35, 7.36).** The echocardiogram of the mitral valve shows the vibration of the anterior cusp associated with an Austin Flint murmur, and the valve movement is otherwise normal. The left ventricle wall movement and that of the interventricular septum is in excess of normal, as is the left ventricular cavity size (cf. Figure 7.34). (Recording speed 50 mm/s)

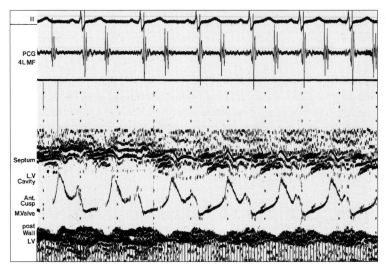

◀ **Figure 7.34 Normal ECG, PCG and echocardiogram of a patient aged 26 without heart disease.** Note the normal second sound splitting on the PCG. Movement of the anterior cusp of the mitral valve is normal, in diastole and systole (cf. Figure 7.33). Ventricular cavity size is normal, as is movement of the interventricular septum and left ventricle posterior wall. (Recording speed 50 mm/s)

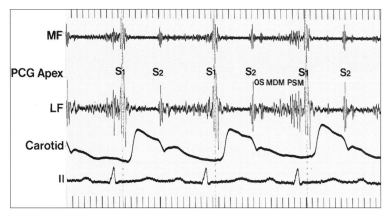

▶ **Figure 7.35 The long diastolic murmur of mitral stenosis, ending before the accentuated S1 with presystolic accentuation (MDM and PSM). S2 is the position of the second sound, and OS the opening snap**. The carotid pulse and ECG are both normal. (Recording speed 75 mm/s)

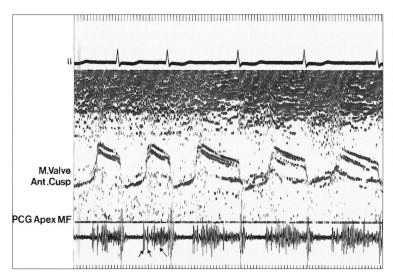

▶ **Figure 7.36 Echocardiogram, ECG and PCG of mitral stenosis with atrial fibrillation**. The echogram shows thickening of the cusp, but normal early diastolic movement coincident with the opening snap (OS) of the PCG. The long diastolic murmur is shown in conjunction with the shallow diastolic (E–F) slope of the anterior cusp of the mitral valve, demonstrating how the valve is held down into the ventricular cavity. (Recording speed 50 mm/s.) See Figure 7.34 for comparison

first sound, it has an apparently crescendo character and is often called a *presystolic murmur*, though in reality it is usually only a part of a longer diastolic murmur. This is present only in patients in sinus rhythm as it is due to active atrial contraction. Before making a diagnosis of mitral stenosis on the presence of a presystolic murmur the observer should listen most carefully for the low-toned rumble which is generally present in other parts of diastole, and for the characteristic abnormalities of the heart sounds.

MURMURS AT THE AORTIC AREA
Systolic murmurs

Systolic murmurs are very common at the aortic area and may be associated with increased cardiac output as in anaemias or with increased stroke output as in aortic incompetence. The murmur of increased output is often soft and blowing, but where stroke output is increased in aortic incompetence there is also valve deformity and the murmur may be very loud.

A similar murmur may be heard with dilatation of the aorta and calcification at the root of the aorta, but its loudness is not an indication of valve narrowing.

The systolic murmur of *aortic stenosis* (Figure 7.37) is harsh in character, conducted upwards into the carotid arteries, and usually accompanied by a thrill. The position of the murmur, as mentioned, is roughly midsystolic, but being often preceded by an ejection click this latter may be mistaken for a first heart sound, and the murmur for one of pansystolic timing. The murmur may also be heard at the apex and the student should be cautious in making a diagnosis of aortic stenosis unless other evidence of obstruction is present, as systolic murmurs at the aortic area may be due to the

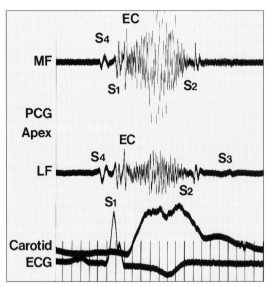

▲ **Figure 7.37 Aortic stenosis**. The murmur is recorded as having a characteristic diamond-shape, crescendo–decrescendo, starting with the ejection click (EC) and ending before the second sound (S2). Both 3rd and 4th sounds are present, there is a plateau or anacrotic pulse, and the ECG (lead II) is abnormal. (Recording speed 100mm/s)

alternative causes mentioned. If the stenosis produces much narrowing of the valve opening, a plateau type of pulse will be present (Figure 7.37), an important confirmatory sign in diagnosis.

Diastolic murmurs

These are rarely found at the aortic area except in *aortic regurgitation*. The murmur is usually soft and blowing in character and is heard over a large area of the chest wall. It is propagated characteristically down the sternum and towards the apex beat. In the aortic area itself it is often faint and difficult to hear, and it reaches its maximum intensity about the middle of the sternum at its left border. It may be well heard over the apex or even in the axilla but can generally be distinguished from a diastolic murmur of mitral origin by its higher pitch and by the fact that it follows immediately after the second sound, except when it is faint. In listening for this murmur the student should have the patient in an erect posture, leaning forwards and holding his breath in expiration, and should auscultate systematically from the second right costal cartilage down the sternum and towards the apex beat (see also Figure 7.38).

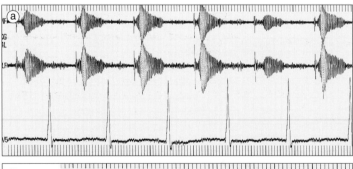

◀ **Figure 7.38 Aortic regurgitation**. The murmur in this patient is intense, and the regularity of the vibrations is unusual. When this characteristic is recorded the sound has a musical quality when heard with a stethoscope. This patient has a valve cusp perforated by infective endocarditis. The carotid pulse is abnormal, showing the characteristic 'collapsing' quality of aortic regurgitation. (Both illustrations, recording speeds 50 mm/s.) (cf. Figures 7.5 and Table 7.2)

Murmurs at the Pulmonary Area
Systolic murmurs

Systolic murmurs over the pulmonary area may be soft and blowing like those sometimes found over the aortic zone. They occur with great frequency in perfectly healthy individuals, and are probably due to turbulence being produced by rapid blood flow through a normal valve (Figure 7.39). The murmur of *congenital pulmonary stenosis* (Figure 7.40) is comparable with the murmur of aortic stenosis, as it is loud, rasping and usually accompanied by a thrill, with the difference that in the more severe grades of pulmonary valve stenosis the crescendo part of the murmur is later than is the case in aortic stenosis. There is delay in the appearance of the soft pulmonary component of the second sound (Figure 7.40).

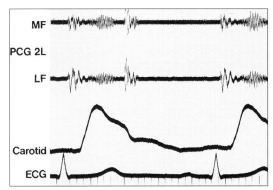

▲ **Figure 7.39 Functional or innocent systolic murmur.** The ECG and carotid pulse are normal. The heart sounds are normal, with no added sounds. The murmur is midsystolic, seen to be of low frequency and, when heard, has a 'buzzing' quality, most easily detected along the left sternal border. (Recording speed 100 mm/s)

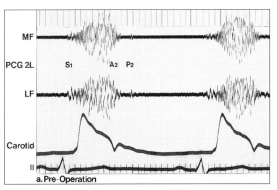

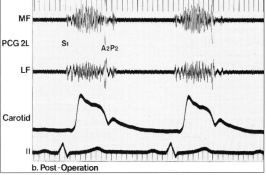

▲ **Figure 7.40 Congenital pulmonary valve stenosis.** The systolic murmur is similar in shape to that of aortic stenosis, but reaches the crescendo later in systole, to end before the delayed pulmonary component (P2) of the second sound. The distance from the aortic second sound (A2) to P2 is a measure of the severity of the obstruction at the pulmonary valve, and the shortening of this interval after surgery (compare the pre-operation with the post-operation records) is a measure of the success of the operation

	Timing	Character	Site	Radiation	Accentuation
COMMON ORGANIC MURMURS					
Mitral stenosis	Mid to late diastolic	Rumbling	Apex	Nil	On left side after exercise
Mitral incompetence	Pansystolic	Loud, blowing	Apex	Axilla and back	In all postures
Aortic stenosis	Midsystolic	Harsh	Right parasternal	Neck	Leaning forward. Expiration
Aortic incompetence	Early diastolic	Soft, blowing	Left parasternal	Apex (Austin Flint)	Leaning forward. Expiration

▲ **Table 7.4**

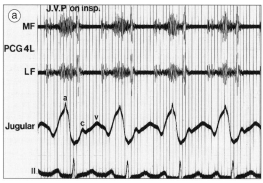

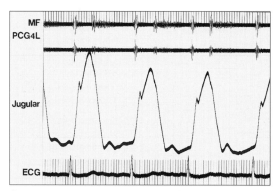

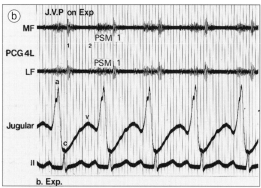

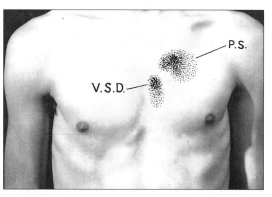

▲ **Figure 7.42 Tricuspid regurgitation with jugular pulse recording. The phonocardiogram shows little systolic murmur, and a short diastolic murmur.** The jugular pulse has almost the appearance of a collapsing arterial pulse, and indeed the pressure was high enough to move the earlobes. The patient had gross tricuspid regurgitation, with a pulsatile liver also. Atrial fibrillation is present, so that no 'a' wave is recorded. The 'c' notch is followed by a huge 'v' wave which is followed by a precipitate fall to the 'y' trough, both the rise to the 'v' peak and the fall to the 'y' trough being typical of this condition

▲ **Figure 7.41 Tricuspid stenosis with jugular pulse recordings. Record (a) is taken during inspiration, (b) during expiration.** Both records show prolongation of the P–R interval of the ECG, and both show a presystolic murmur of crescendo–decrescendo shape, ending before the first heart sound. This is a true atrial systolic ejection murmur, ending before S1 because of the early atrial contraction. The increased venous return produced by inspiration raises the right atrial–right ventricle pressure gradient in diastole, flow across the stenosed valve increases and the murmur is louder. The jugular pulse, recorded most easily in expiration, shows a tall 'a' wave, small delayed 'c' wave and marked delay in descent from the 'v' wave. These findings are typical of tricuspid stenosis. The smaller 'a' during inspiration is artefactual, caused by difficulty in recording the pulse beyond a tense sternomastoid muscle

▲ **Figure 7.43 Murmurs of congenital heart disease. PS = pulmonary stenosis; VSD = ventricular septal defect.** These murmurs are systolic in time

Diastolic murmurs

At the pulmonary area diastolic murmurs are uncommon and in many cases sound exactly the same as those of aortic regurgitation. A pulmonary diastolic murmur due to regurgitation will occasionally occur in pulmonary arterial hypertension, or dilatation of the pulmonary artery (Graham Steell murmur); this is most commonly due to mitral valve disease or congenital lesions with an Eisenmenger reaction.

MURMURS AT THE TRICUSPID AREA

Murmurs at the tricuspid area are commonly associated and confused with those arising from mitral disease.

Systolic murmurs may be present at the lower end of the sternum in tricuspid regurgitation, and diastolic murmurs of a low rumbling type may occur in tricuspid stenosis, but diagnosis is always difficult, although both these murmurs may be increased by deep inspiration, sometimes a useful manoeuvre in distinguishing them from murmurs arising at the mitral valve. Examination of the venous pulse may reveal other clues in the diagnosis of tricuspid valve disease (Figure 7.41 and 7.42).

OTHER MURMURS

Sometimes murmurs are found which do not correspond with any of the 'valvular' areas. In these cases the possi-

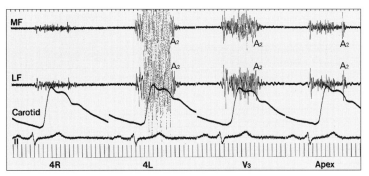

◀ **Figure 7.44 Ventricular septal defect. PCG recorded across 4R, 4L, V3 and apex position, with the carotid pulse**. This shows the murmur to be loudest at the left sternal edge, to begin with the first sound and extend throughout systole, to 'spill over' the position of A2, and end before or with P2. The murmur is very loud, but it should be remembered that loudness does not equate with severity of the left-to-right shunt

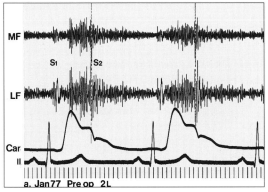

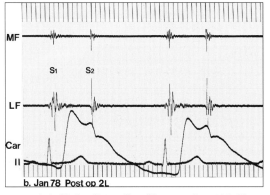

▲ **Figure 7.45 Patent ductus arteriosus. Pre- and post-operation records from the same patient, after surgical obliteration of the ductus**. The typical murmur rises to a crescendo just before the position of the second sound, but is seen to be continuous throughout systole and diastole

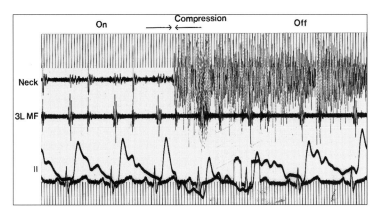

◀ **Figure 7.46 Bruit de diable**. This continuous venous hum could be heard over both internal jugular veins in a healthy girl. Compression of the veins readily abolished the hum

bility of congenital heart disease always arises. Systolic murmurs midway between the pulmonary and mitral areas, i.e. over third and fourth left interspaces, may be present in cases of pulmonary stenosis when the obstruction is near the origin of the artery from the right ventricle, infundibular stenosis, and in cases of patency of the interventricular septum (Figures 7.43 and 7.44). These murmurs are nearly always rough, and generally accompanied by a thrill. A murmur occupying both systole and diastole, present over the base of the heart, and maximal over the pulmonary area, is characteristic of a *patent ductus arteriosus* (Figure 7.45). Usually the murmur has a typical quality described by Gibson as 'machinery-like'. It is almost continuous but waxes and wanes; it is most pronounced in late systole. Similar murmurs may be heard in some forms of arteriovenous fistula, but these are rare.

Systolic murmurs may also be found over the base of the heart in coarctation of the aorta and atrial septal defects, but the murmur is not the main feature in the diagnosis.

Murmurs which have a vascular as opposed to a cardiac origin are usually systolic in time and blowing in character and may be heard over a toxic thyroid gland, over vascular tumours in the thorax and over aneurysm of the aorta or other large vessels. The *bruit de diable* is the name given to a continuous venous hum sometimes heard over the neck in profound anaemias and is thought to be caused by the associated hyperdynamic circulatory state with blood flowing very rapidly through the great veins to the heart. A venous hum is occasionally heard over the jugular veins or even over the chest, in health, but disappears in recumbency or pressure over the neck veins (Figure 7.46).

THE DIAGNOSIS OF HEART DISEASES

It is convenient to deal with the diagnosis of heart disease under two headings:
1 Structural defects.
2 Derangements of function.
These are commonly found together, but one may occur without the other.

STRUCTURAL DEFECTS

Diseases of the heart resulting from anatomical changes may involve the pericardium, the heart muscle and the endocardium and valves. Congenital defects may affect any or all of these structures. The majority of diseases result from inflammatory or degenerative processes, and the signs by which they may be recognized overlap to a considerable extent.

THE PERICARDIUM
Pericarditis
Inflammation of the pericardium is recognized in its acute stage by the friction rub (see page 151). This may appear during the course of an acute illness, especially rheumatic fever, but also in pneumonia, tuberculosis and virus infections. It is a common feature of myocardial infarction and of uraemia. The rub is usually discovered as a result of routine examination in these conditions, rather than by any special complaint of the patient, though in some cases there may be pain. The electrocardiogram characteristically shows convex ST elevation and sometimes T-wave inversion over the affected area.

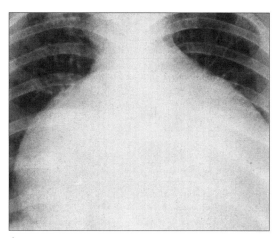

▲ **Figure 7.47 Radiograph of pericardial effusion**. The 'heart' shadow is enlarged, the enlargement being greater in the transverse diameter than the longitudinal. There is obliteration of the normal notches on the heart's outline so that the shadow becomes globular or pear-shaped with a short vascular pedicle, but these minor changes in the shape of the cardiac outline should not be overstressed

Pericardial effusion
Some increase in pericardial fluid occurs in most cases of acute pericarditis but may only be discovered on routine examination and may not cause symptoms. If the intrapericardial tension is high, resulting in restricted venous return and lowered cardiac output (tamponade), severe dyspnoea may occur, but the usual pattern is one of a lowered blood pressure with peripheral cyanosis, sweating and signs of right-heart failure, depending upon the acuteness with which the effusion occurs.
The most important signs are:

1 Feebleness of the cardiac impulse and faintness of the heart sounds because of the separation of the impulse from the chest wall by the fluid.
2 The first heart sound may be soft because of reduced late diastolic filling and the second sound soft because the blood pressure is low.
3 An early diastolic added sound, dull in character, representing restriction of ventricular filling.
4 Pulsus paradoxus (see page 140).
5 Persistence of pericardial friction.

Radiology confirms the heart and fluid outlines (Figure 7.47) but the effusion can best be shown by echocardiography. Special techniques with cardiac catheterization are occasionally necessary. Paracentesis may be justifiable.

Constrictive pericarditis

This is generally post-infective and often tuberculous in origin. It is insidious in development and may be associated with pleurisy.

The most important signs are elevated venous pressure with liver enlargement and ascites, in a patient in whom no valve disease or other cause of cardiac failure is found. The degree of dyspnoea may be relatively slight. The heart is often not enlarged, but the chest radiograph may show calcification. Pulsus paradoxus may be present.

THE MYOCARDIUM

There are no conclusive symptoms or signs of myocardial disease, though the electrocardiogram may reveal evidence of this (Figure 7.48), especially when conduction disorders of any kind are present. It is possible,

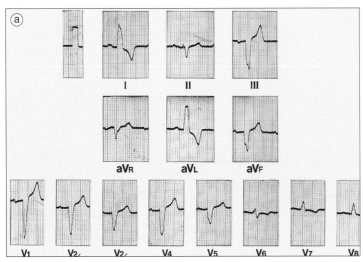

◀ **Figure 7.48 Left bundle-branch block (LBBB).** (a) This patient had aortic stenosis, with extensive calcification extending from the valve into the interventricular septum. Note QRS spread with dominant positive QRS defection in lead I, negative in lead III. The left axis deviation is pathological, and represents a conduction defect in the left anterior division of the left bundle, in addition to the main left bundle. This ECG therefore represents LBBB and left anterior hemiblock. (b) This patient had ischaemic heart disease. The QRS spread again shows LBBB, but without the same degree of left axis deviation – the main deflection being positive in lead II, there being no conduction defect in the left anterior division, i.e. there is no left anterior hemiblock

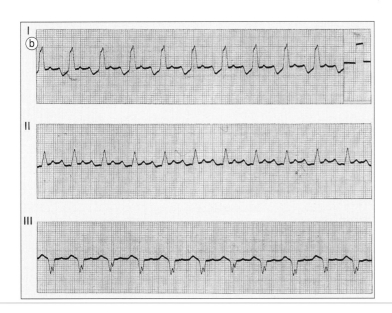

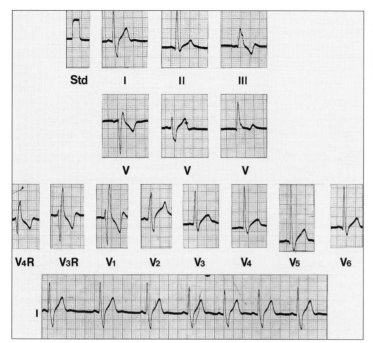

◀ **Figure 7.49 Right bundle-branch block.** This patient had an atrial septal defect. The deep S waves in leads I, aVL, and the left chest leads are well shown, as is the QRS spreading, and the RSR complexes in V4R, V3R and V1. The continuous recording of lead I shows sinus arrhythmia

however, to suspect that the myocardium is involved when there is cardiac enlargement due to unexplained hypertrophy or dilatation or both, or when the heart shows signs of failure which cannot easily be attributed to any extra burden it is carrying. Suggestions of myocardial weakness (whether due to myocardial disease or increased load) are to be found in the presence of pulsus alternans and gallop rhythm, which sooner or later are associated with clear evidence of heart failure.

Echocardiography (see Figure 7.34) is of great value in assessment of myocardial contractility and shows particularly well the impaired movements of the ventricle in cardiomyopathies.

Myocardial ischaemia and *infarction* are the commonest disorders affecting the cardiac muscle and the cardinal symptom of this condition – anginal pain – has already been considered (page 132). It only remains to add that while the pain is usually severe, it may be slight or even absent, especially in the elderly. It is of variable duration but, when infarction is present, the pain lasts generally a number of hours and nearly always is longer than in other forms of angina. It may be accompanied by collapse, shown by pallor, sweating, faintness, a feeble pulse, and falling blood pressure, and commonly by vomiting. Disorders of conduction and of rhythm may occur.

The infarct in contact with the pericardium may result in an area of pericarditis with its sign - a friction rub - and the necrotic processes in the myocardium may

be evidenced by pyrexia and leucocytosis, and by a rise in sedimentation rate and serum cardiac enzyme levels. These signs are usually maximal 2–3 days after myocardial infarction. If the infarct is extensive and involves the endocardium, a mural thrombus may form and result in systemic embolism, usually a week or two later.

In some instances cardiac failure, especially of the left ventricular type, results, and sometimes a papillary muscle ruptures or the weakened area of heart muscle bulges to form an aneurysm which can be recognized by observation and palpation and confirmed by echocardiography. The diagnosis of myocardial infarction is usually established by characteristic ECG changes (Figures 7.50–7.52) and subsequent enzyme rise. The timing of the complications of myocardial infarction are shown in Table 7.5.

Acute cardiomyopathy

During the course of rheumatic fever and certain infections, viral or bacterial, involvement of the myocardium may be suspected by the onset of precordial oppression, a rapid feeble pulse with a fall of blood pressure, and cardiac dilatation. When the conducting system is involved in the myopathic process, bradycardia can occur, and the ECG may show evidence of heart block. Other disturbances of cardiac rhythm may happen.

A number of rare diseases of the myocardium, including endomyocardial fibrosis, various collagen diseases and the toxic effect of drugs or alcohol may give a similar

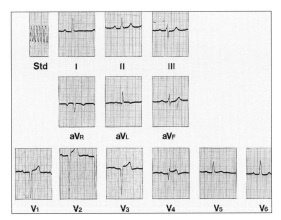

▲ **Figure 7.50 Anteroseptal myocardial infarction shown in the precordial leads and aVL only.** The P–R interval is at the upper limits of normal, the Q wave in aVL is abnormal, as it is in leads V1 to V4, with RS–T segment elevation in V3, V4 and inversion of the T wave in aVL

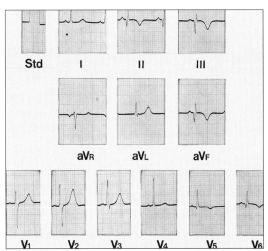

▲ **Figure 7.51 Anteroseptal infarction.** Note the RS–T arching in leads I, aVL, V2 to V6. Abnormal Q waves are present in I, aVL, V2 to V5, and T-wave inversion is present in the same leads. Abnormal left axis deviation, with S greater than R in lead II, indicates the presence of conduction deficiency in the left anterior division of the left bundle-branch

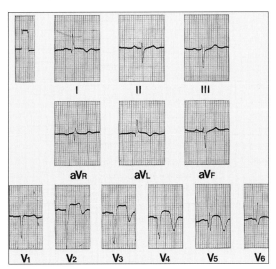

▲ **Figure 7.52 Inferolateral infarct.** Note here the abnormal Q waves in leads II, III, aVF and V5 and V6 with RS–T arching and negative T waves in the same leads

COMPLICATIONS OF MYOCOCARDIAL INFARCTION	
Immediate	Pallor, sweating, small pulse, hypotension (i.e. shock)
2–3 days	Fever, pericardial rub (raised ESR and transaminase levels)
1–2 weeks	Systemic embolism from mural infarct. LV aneurysm
At any time	Arrhythmia; heart block; LV failure (displaced apex, triple rhythm, pulmonary oedema). Acute mitral incompetence (ruptured papillary muscle), VSD

▲ **Table 7.5**

picture. Diagnosis, which is difficult, may be made more certain by the development of signs of cardiac failure.

In *rheumatic endocarditis* it may be difficult to recognize the signs of myocardial failure because they are masked by pericardial or valvular signs. This disease, once very common, is now seen much less frequently.

THE VALVES

Endocarditis, or inflammation of the endocardium, results in deformities of the valves, causing incompetence of the valve or narrowing (stenosis) of the orifice guarded by the valve. Incompetence causes regurgitation of blood through an orifice which should be closed. Stenosis impedes the passage of blood through the affected valve. Any of the valves may become incompetent or stenosed, but especially the mitral and aortic valves.

The diagnosis of valve disease can usually be made by the clinical features. While auscultation is often useful in defining which valve is diseased, a systematic examination of the pulse, the JVP and the apex beat should give a strong indication of specific valve disorders prior to auscultation. For instance, the nature of the pulse in aortic stenosis or aortic regurgitation; the position of the apex beat in mitral regurgitation or aortic regurgitation and the presence of left ventricular hypertrophy in aortic stenosis; or features of a tapping apex beat and atrial fibrillation in mitral stenosis. All these factors give a likely indication of what may be heard on auscultation and, certainly in the case of diastolic murmurs, non-auscultatory physical signs are often easier to define.

The most important valve lesions are:

1 Mitral stenosis.
2 Mitral incompetence.
3 Aortic incompetence.
4 Aortic stenosis.

The principal features of these lesions and those of tricuspid incompetence are listed in Table 7.6.

Mitral stenosis (Figures 7.26, 7.35, 7.36)

Diagnosed by the presence of a mitral diastolic murmur with accentuation of the mitral first sound and an open-ing snap. Confirmatory signs are the enlargement of the right ventricle, and, when there is pulmonary arterial hypertension, the pulmonary second sound is accentuated. The radiograph may show enlargement of the left atrium, and prominence of the pulmonary arc if there is pulmonary arterial hypertension, when recognizable changes in the vascular pattern of the lungs will also be present.

The commonest ECG change is an alteration in the P waves (Figure 7.53). They are often bifid because of left atrial hypertrophy, though sometimes tall and sharp, because of right atrial hypertrophy when there is high pulmonary vascular resistance, and when there will also be evidence of right ventricular hypertrophy.

These graphic signs may be helpful when present, but the auscultatory findings remain the most certain diagnostic signs, though are sometimes difficult to hear. The length of the murmur is the best clinical measure of severity of mitral stenosis.

COMMON VALVE LESIONS					
	Aetiology	Pulse	Heart sounds	Murmurs	Ventricular impulse
Mitral stenosis	Rheumatic	May be atrial fibrillation Small volume	Loud 1st sound Opening snap	Mid–late apical diastolic	RV+
Mitral incompetence	Rheumatic Ischaemic (ruptured papillary muscle) Congenital (floppy valve) Bacterial	May be atrial fibrillation	Soft 1st sound May be 3rd sound	Pan-systolic apex to axilla	LV+ RV+
Aortic stenosis	Rheumatic Atherosclerotic Congenital	Plateau	4th sound	Mid-systolic R 2nd inter-space to neck	LV+
Aortic incompetence	Rheumatic Syphilitic Bacterial	Collapsing Visible capillary and arterial pulsation	3rd sound	Early diastolic LSB to apex (Austin Flint)	LV+
Tricuspid incompetence	Usually secondary to RV failure from mitral or pulmonary heart disease	May be atrial fibrillation Large V wave and sharp Y descent in jugular pulse	RV 3rd sound	Lower sternal diastolic	RV+

▲ Table 7.6

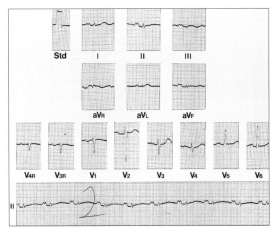

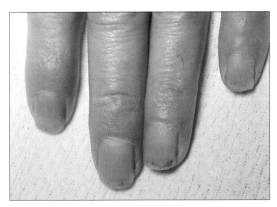

▲ **Figure 7.53 Bifid P waves, left atrial hypertrophy**. This ECG also shows a long P–R interval; and is the record from a patient with severe mitral stenosis. The long recording of lead II shows the bifid P waves particularly well

▲ **Figure 7.54 Polyarteritis nodosa**: splinter haemorrhages in the nails. These may also occur in cases of bacterial endocarditis

Mitral incompetence (Figures 7.31, 7.32)

Mitral incompetence often accompanies mitral stenosis; diagnosed by the presence of a mitral pansystolic murmur conducted to the axilla and enlargement of the left ventricle. The difficulties of diagnosis between mitral regurgitation due to disease of the valve cusps and to relative incompetence from papillary muscle–chordal dysfunction have been discussed under systolic murmurs. Unusual cases of rupture of the mitral cusps, chordae tendineae or papillary muscle may result in severe and sudden mitral incompetence, when the picture is dominated by the presence of pulmonary oedema of acute onset.

Aortic incompetence (Figures 7.19, 7.33, 7.38)

Aortic incompetence is characterized by an aortic diastolic murmur of classic distribution. The corroborative

signs in aortic regurgitation are of great value, especially the collapsing pulse, capillary pulsation and undue pulsation of the large arteries. The heart is enlarged, principally downwards and to the left. The enlargement is confirmed by a chest radiograph, in which the left ventricle is characteristically rounded. Electrocardiography may show left ventricular hypertrophy, phonocardiography the characteristic murmurs and echocardiography the dilated left ventricular cavity and perhaps the vibration of the anterior cusp of the mitral valve. The low-pitched diastolic murmur at the apex – the Austin Flint murmur – may make difficult the differentiation from a coincidental mitral stenosis, but the above-mentioned investigations should be decisive.

Aortic stenosis (Figures 7.13, 7.14, 7.37)

This was a less common lesion than the other valve diseases described until the declining incidence of rheumatic heart disease, but now increasingly recognized as non-rheumatic. A rough systolic murmur is often conducted into the neck. The characteristic anacrotic arterial pulse is usually present. Sometimes the murmur is transmitted to the apex (see page 155), and if there is a sufficiently severe degree of left ventricle hypertrophy, this ought to be recognized, often also with an audible and palpable fourth sound. Aortic regurgitation of some degree often accompanies stenosis. Special radiological and catheter studies, especially the pressure gradient across the aortic valve, may be necessary to establish the degree of obstruction, and its site. Echocardiography with Doppler estimation of valve gradient has revolutionized the evaluation of aortic stenosis and other valve lesions, and allows regular non-invasive assessment of valve gradients as well as visualization of the valve structure.

Bacterial endocarditis

This must receive special consideration if a valve lesion is found. It is suggested by the association of valve murmurs usually regurgitant with signs of septicaemia, including splenic enlargement, pyrexia, anaemia, embolic manifestations and the discovery of organisms in the bloodstream (blood culture). Characteristic signs in the fingers include clubbing, splinter haemorrhages in the nails (Figure 7.54) and tender red nodules in the finger pulp due to immune complex deposition (Osler's nodes). The condition may complicate congenital as well as acquired cardiac lesions.

CONGENITAL LESIONS

Congenital lesions (Table 7.7) have assumed a much more important role in diagnosis because of the possibility of surgical treatment. They are dealt with here in

CONGENITAL HEART DISEASE	
Without shunt	Aortic stenosis; bicuspid aortic valve Aortic coarctation Pulmonary stenosis; tricuspid stenosis Dextrocardia
With left-to-right shunt: no cyanosis	Atrial septal defect Ventricular septal defect Patent ductus arteriosus
With right-to-left shunt: cyanosis	Eisenmenger's syndrome Tetralogy of Fallot Pulmonary venous drainage to left atrium

◀ Table 7.7

a very brief fashion, but constitute a most important part of paediatric medicine.

History-taking is often unhelpful, but respiratory distress, cyanosis and signs of cardiac failure will have been noted. Failure to gain weight may be present, partly because of dyspnoea and distress during feeding.

Occasionally, the congenital abnormality is found by routine medical examination, but it should be remembered that auscultation is not easy in small children, and not all murmurs indicate serious underlying disease. Cardiac diagnosis in the seriously ill infant is a highly specialized practice, and depends to a very large extent upon a detailed knowledge of applied embryologic anatomy and the interpretation of echocardiograms and angiography.

As the child grows older, history-taking becomes less of a problem, signs correspond to those found in adults and problems of diagnosis which are non-urgent are dealt with in a way similar to the routine used in adults.

Atrial septal defect

Often asymptomatic until middle age, and found as an abnormality of the cardiac outline on routine chest radiograph, the signs depend upon the size of the left-to-right shunt at atrial level. The shunt itself is silent, but increased flow across the pulmonary valve produces a pulmonary systolic murmur. The prolongation of right ventricular systole, together with the usually present right bundle-branch block (Figure 7.49) causes wide fixed splitting of the second sound because of delay in pulmonary valve closure. The variation in the splitting of the second heart sound is reduced as the increased right atrial filling on inspiration contributes proportionately less because of the shunt from the left atrium. Increased flow to the right-sided chambers may occasionally produce a mid-diastolic murmur due to flow through the tricuspid valve. The large stroke volume from the right ventricle may produce an ejection sound from the pulmonary valve with an ejection systolic murmur in the pulmonary area.

On X-ray examination the right heart chambers are enlarged and the pulmonary artery and its branches are both enlarged and unduly pulsatile. Echocardiography and colour-flow Doppler clearly delineate atrial septal defect in the majority of cases and occasionally transoesophageal echocardiography is required. Cardiac catheterization will confirm the diagnosis by oxygen sampling and shunt calculation.

Ventricular septal defect (Figure 7.44)

Like atrial septal defect, ventricular septal defect may be found on routine examination of a symptomless patient, but here the loud pansystolic murmur audible in the left parasternal region, and often accompanied by a thrill, has long been recognized as typical. A very small defect may produce a lot of noise while a large defect, with equal pressures in the left and right ventricles and thus unaccompanied by left-to-right shunting, may be silent. There may be evidence of increased flow across the mitral valve shown by the presence of a diastolic murmur at the apex. The increased load placed on the left ventricle produces evidence of left ventricular hypertrophy, shown by ECG and radiology, while the increased blood flow through the lungs shows as an increase in size of the pulmonary artery and its branches, although this is rarely so marked as in atrial septal defect. Echocardiography with colour-flow Doppler again delineate the defect, though catheterization is required to calculate the shunt as with an ASD.

Patent ductus arteriosus (Figure 7.45)

The murmur is characteristically continuous in systole and diastole, as shunting from the aorta to the pulmonary artery is continuous also. If the shunt is sufficiently large, the load upon the left ventricle may cause left ventricular hypertrophy. There may be an audible 'flow' murmur across the mitral valve, the pulmonary artery and its branches enlarge and are pulsatile, while the pulse pressure widens in the systemic circulation because of the 'run off' from the aorta to the pulmonary artery during diastole.

Pulmonary stenosis (Figure 7.43)

When part of Fallot's tetralogy, it becomes one of the common causes of cyanotic congenital heart disease. As an isolated abnormality it is characterized by a midsystolic murmur, often sufficiently loud to be accompanied by a thrill, heard best in the second and third left intercostal spaces parasternally. Right ventricular hypertrophy is present, to a degree dependent on the severity of the stenosis (see Figure 7.67), and radiology will show poststenotic dilatation of the pulmonary artery, if the obstruction is at valve level. Echo-Doppler studies allow non-invasive evaluation of the gradient as with aortic stenosis.

Coarctation of the aorta

This is a common cause of cardiac failure in infancy. Often present with other congenital abnormalities, both cardiac and non-cardiac, it should not be missed if physical examination is properly performed with palpation of both femoral arteries. This should be an invariable routine in any patient presenting with systemic hypertension. The signs include absent or delayed femoral pulses, collateral vessels palpable around the shoulder girdle, and there may be a late systolic murmur present over these vessels and audible over the precordium also. The radiological finding of rib-notching is diagnostic.

Very complicated combinations of congenital malformations may occur, not only affecting the cardiovascular system but the other main systems also. In particular, the association of the skeletal deformities of Marfan's syndrome with septal and valve defects is well known.

DISORDERS OF HEART FUNCTION

The heart may be subject to disturbance of function with little or no anatomical change. This is seen in the *arrhythmias*, or abnormal rhythms, which, although commonly associated with pathological changes in the heart muscle, may occur quite independently. *Cardiac failure* is also a disturbance of function, but is almost invariably dependent upon structural defects. Apparent alteration of function is also observed in psychoneuroses and is referred to as effort syndrome.

ABNORMAL RHYTHMS

Many abnormal rhythms can be identified with reasonable certainty by skillful examination of the pulse, but some are very confusing and require not only examination of the pulse and heart, but graphic methods, for their elucidation. The more important disturbances of the heart rhythm and rate are:

Ectopic beats

These are extra contractions of the heart arising away from the normal pacemaker (sino-atrial node) and interrupting the normal, regular rhythm. They may be atrial or ventricular in origin and as they occur prematurely, before the ventricles have been properly filled, the beats are small. They are generally followed by a long pause until the next normal beat which may be obviously of bigger volume than normal, as the ventricle has had a longer filling time. These points are appreciated by feeling the pulse, but sometimes even if the beat is not sufficiently strong to produce a pulse wave, yet the heart sounds corresponding with it may be heard (Figures 7.55 and 7.56).

The most characteristic feature of ectopic beats is that they are not present all the time, though if very numerous they may appear to be, and may then imitate other irregularities, especially atrial fibrillation. They usually have no serious significance unless associated with known myocardial disease such as infarction, and tend to disappear when the heart-rate is increased by suitable exercise.

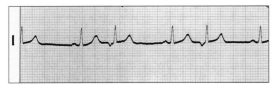

▲ **Figure 7.55 Atrial ectopics**. The P wave, arising from an ectopic focus, is inverted, but the following QRST complex is of normal form

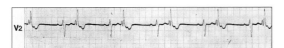

▲ **Figure 7.56 Ventricular ectopics**. These are 'coupled' to the preceding normal complex, but themselves are of abnormal form. The coupling interval, from normal to ectopic beat, is fixed, and the extra beats look like complexes with the form of a right bundle-branch block. This is because the ectopic focus from which they arise is part of, or close to, the left-sided conducting system (See Figure 7.12)

Atrial fibrillation

In this condition the atria cease to beat properly, individual areas of atrial muscle producing minute contractions or 'fibrillations' at a rate of 400–600 per minute which are conducted in an irregular pattern through the

AV node. In its turn this causes irregular action of the ventricles. The results are shown in a complete irregularity of the pulse and apex beat, manifested by a variation in the size of the beats and in the interval between them (Figures 7.57 and 7.58). Atrial fibrillation generally occurs with other serious heart disease, e.g. valve or myocardial disease, but may occur alone. It is most commonly associated with mitral stenosis, thyrotoxicosis and ischaemic heart disease.

The rate is generally rapid, and the force of some of the ventricular contractions may not be strong enough to open the aortic valves and allow transmission to the pulse. In such cases the ventricular rate will be greater than the pulse rate, and in fibrillation reliance should be placed on the heart rate rather than the pulse rate, both when making the diagnosis and in assessing the effect of treatment.

Atrial flutter

Comparable in many ways with atrial fibrillation, flutter may exist along with other forms of heart disease, or be an isolated phenomenon.

The atria beat at a great rate (200–400), but owing to refractory properties of the AV bundle, the ventricles usually respond to a smaller number of these contractions (2:1, 3:1, 4:1) depending upon the number of atrial impulses which 'penetrate' the AV node to cause ventricular action (Figure 7.59). Flutter may be suspected clinically when a high regular ventricular rate (120–200) persists for a long time (days to weeks). The usual ventricular rate is 160 or less. The tachycardia can sometimes be reduced temporarily by pressure over the carotid sinus (bifurcation of the common carotid artery below the angle of the jaw at the level of the upper border of the cricoid cartilage), causing vagal inhibition of conduction through the AV node.

Occasionally the rapid contractions of the atria communicate a pulsation to the jugular veins at a greater rate (usually twice) than that at which the ventricles are beating, and cannon waves appear when the atrium contracts on to a closed AV valve.

Sudden doubling or halving of the ventricular rate strongly suggests atrial flutter, with a varying degree of AV block.

Paroxysmal tachycardia

The heart beats regularly at a high rate (150–200, commonly over 160), and the condition may be mistaken for atrial flutter, but there is a 1:1 conduction and the ventricular rate is usually higher and the condition is of much shorter duration than flutter. Its duration is usually minutes to hours, and attacks may be stopped by simple measures such as a change of posture, or pressure over the carotid sinus. The pressure should be exerted firmly below the angle of the jaw on one side only for a period of about 1 minute, but ideally with ECG monitoring, and with resuscitation services at hand.

One of the most important signs is the characteristic sudden onset and offset, a sign which also applies in the case of flutter.

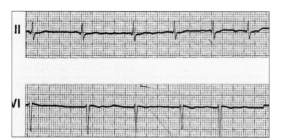

▲ **Figure 7.57 Atrial fibrillation (see Figure 7.13).** Leads II and V1 show complete irregularity of the QRST complexes, and absent P waves. This is the 'fine' type of atrial fibrillation

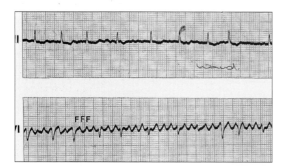

▲ **Figure 7.58 Atrial fibrillation, coarse (see Figure 7.57).** Leads II and V1 show total irregularity of the QRST complexes, with irregularly shaped and timed fibrillation, or 'f' waves

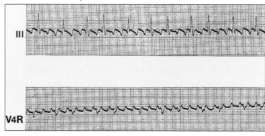

▲ **Figure 7.59 Atrial flutter** The flutter waves are regular in form and shape, representing atrial activity, with a rate of 300 per minute. There is a varying 2:1 and 3:1 atrioventricular block. The regular inverted 'P' waves in lead II give a characteristic 'sawtooth' pattern

When the patient is not seen during an attack, great attention should be paid to the story of the mode of onset and offset and the circumstances under which the attacks appear. Abnormal rhythms (paroxysmal tachycardia and flutter) are unexpected and unexplained, whereas simple tachycardia is often expected and provoked by emotion or exercise. Polyuria may occur after high heart rates, especially in paroxysmal tachycardia.

One of the most important developments in cardiac investigation has been the use of long-term monitoring of cardiac rhythm, using tape recordings over many hours. In this way, transient changes of rhythm, of great importance, may be successfully detected.

Simple tachycardia

It has already been observed that tachycardia may be produced in normal individuals by emotion, exercise, fevers, toxaemias – especially thyrotoxicosis – and other causes, and the pulse rate may be as high as is found in paroxysmal tachycardia or atrial flutter but rarely remains more than 140 when the patient is at rest.

In distinguishing simple tachycardia from abnormal rhythms, such as flutter or paroxysmal tachycardia, the student should note that exercise, emotion and other causes influencing a simple tachycardia do not alter the heart rate in abnormal rhythms.

Bradycardia

A slow heart rate – simple bradycardia – like tachycardia, may occur in perfect health, especially in athletes, and is common in old people. Rates of 60 are common, and may even be lower than 50.

Various non-cardiac conditions may be responsible for temporary bradycardia, notably the after-effects of febrile illnesses such as influenza and pneumonia; jaundice; increased intracranial pressure such as occurs in cerebral tumour; and hypothyroidism.

The most important cardiac condition in which bradycardia occurs is heart block, a condition in which the ventricles do not respond, in the normal way, to the impulses reaching the AV node. This may be the result of diminished conduction through the node itself, or through the more peripheral parts of the conducting system. When the ventricle fails to respond to the

impulses reaching the AV node, the condition is known as 'heart block'; 'partial' when the ventricles respond to some but not all the impulses, 'total' when all the impulses are without effect (Figures 7.60 and 7.61). The result is a higher atrial than ventricular rate, the latter usually varying between 30 and 50 according to the degree of block and to where the subsidiary pacemaking focus is situated. The intrinsic rate of the AV node itself is about 60 per minute and that of the peripheral parts of the conducting system is about 20, so that the more peripheral the subsidiary pacemaker the slower the ventricular rhythm, and this rhythm is not usually influenced by exercise or emotion.

In partial heart block irregular action may be present, and the rate may be suddenly increased (generally doubled) by exercise. The earliest stage of heart block may only be recognizable by electrocardiography, which shows prolongation of the P–R interval (Figure 7.60). At the other extreme, periods of ventricular standstill may occur in Stokes–Adams attacks (Figure 7.62).

From this description of cardiac arrhythmias the student will appreciate that in every case where the heart rate or rhythm appears abnormal it is essential to observe carefully:

1 The rate at the pulse and apex beat.
2 The variation of these with exercise and excitement.
3 The mode of onset and offset of the attacks, preferably by observation; if not, from the history.
4 The presence of any jugular pulsations and their rate.
5 The electrocardiogram without which the diagnosis of arrhythmias is not complete. It may be necessary to undertake long-term ECG monitoring.

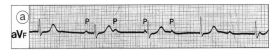

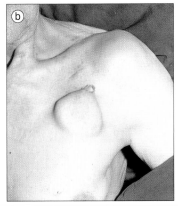

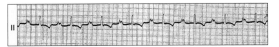

Figure 7.60 First degree heart block. P–R interval prolonged to 0.36 s. There is right and left atrial hypertrophy also

◀ **Figure 7.61 (a) Complete heart block**. The QRST complexes occur independently, at a rate of 47 per minute, from the P waves which are occurring at a rate of 88 per minute. The narrow QRS suggests this block is of congenital origin. (b) Cardiac pacemaker under the skin

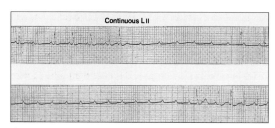

▲ **Figure 7.62 Ventricular standstill.** Normal atrial activity persists, but there is no ventricular activity for a period of 13 s. This is a continuous strip of electrocardiographic tracing, lead II

HEART FAILURE

The examination of the heart is not complete when a diagnosis of valve, myocardial, or other disease has been made. The most important question still remains to be answered, namely – What is the heart's capacity for work? This question has been partially discussed in describing the symptoms of heart disease, especially breathlessness, which, when it occurs without the customary degree of effort, is the earliest indication of cardiac failure. Later, objective signs appear which are usually of serious import. They result from failure of the ventricles to discharge their contents adequately into the systemic and pulmonary circulations. As a result the heart is unable to receive back from the systemic and pulmonary veins the optimum amount of blood.

In general the heart fails as a whole, i.e. both left and right ventricles, but in many cases the burden is laid on one ventricle more than the other, at least for a time. It is thus customary to speak of left and right heart failure.

LEFT VENTRICULAR FAILURE

This is liable to occur from the increased load which the ventricle must bear in hypertension or aortic valve disease. Similarly the damaged muscle in myocardial infarction and certain types of cardiomyopathy may be incapable of meeting the normal demands upon the heart. The left ventricle fails to discharge its contents successfully and the end diastolic pressure in the ventricle rises, causing a rise in the left atrial pressure, and hence in the pulmonary veins, resulting in pulmonary congestion and in more severe cases in pulmonary oedema.

The failure is often relatively sudden. Paroxysmal dyspnoea (page 131) and clinical signs of pulmonary congestion and oedema, cough, laboured breathing and crepitations at the base appear. There is little or no systemic venous congestion. Death may occur rapidly in severe cases due to ventricular fibrillation (Figure 7.63) or to the sudden onset of acute pulmonary oedema, with

flooding of the alveoli resulting in asphyxiation because no transfer of oxygen is possible. Copious frothy sputum accompanies the dyspnoea, the froth being pink with bloodstaining, and later may become more fluid, literally pouring from mouth and nose.

RIGHT VENTRICULAR FAILURE

This form of failure is usually produced more gradually and occurs especially in mitral stenosis and in respiratory diseases (e.g. chronic bronchitis and pulmonary fibrosis) because of pulmonary arterial hypertension which causes extra work for the right ventricle, which hypertrophies before it fails.

It is this form of failure which is chiefly responsible for the common *congestive heart failure*, which is a later feature of so many types of heart disease. Atrial fibrillation is often the precipitating factor of the actual failure, since ventricular function depends to a critical degree on atrial augmentation of filling.

Congestion is apparent in several ways. It is seen in the engorged external veins (Figure 7.21, page 143), in the enlarged and tender liver, in impairment of renal function shown by oliguria and concentrated urine; and in oedema.

These two types of failure, as previously mentioned, are commonly found together, but in varying degrees, and any attempt to separate them strictly would be artificial.

Both types of failure may disappear with treatment, leaving the causal state behind, but the failure may be repeated from time to time.

An acute form of right ventricular failure results from massive *pulmonary embolism* (Figure 7.64). There is usually a sudden onset of dyspnoea, retrosternal discomfort and faintness, accompanied by venous engorgement and peripheral circulatory failure with a right ventricular gallop rhythm produced by an early diastolic filling sound and accentuation of the pulmonary second

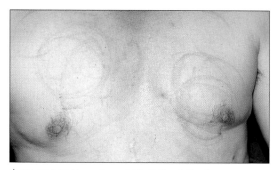

▲ **Figure 7.63 Burns from defibrillation following resuscitation from left ventricular failure caused by ventricular fibrillation**

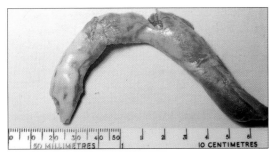

▲ **Figure 7.64 Pulmonary embolus successfully removed at operation from a 'saddle' position in the bifurcation of the pulmonary artery trunk**

sound. Multiple small emboli cause a more insidious form of congestive heart failure, consequent upon the development of pulmonary arterial hypertension.

Effort syndrome

This condition, historically called 'da Costa's syndrome', is an expression of a psychoneurosis, usually an anxiety state. Although there is no organic heart disease, the patient complains of apparent cardiac symptoms such as dyspnoea on slight exertion, palpitation or inframammary pain. There are often other symptoms arising from disturbance of the autonomic system, e.g. sweating, dizziness and syncope. It has no specific physical signs, the diagnosis being dependent on a properly taken history of the disorder, and the absence of any signs of organic cardiovascular disease.

SPECIAL INVESTIGATIONS

The special investigations include instrumental examination by means of the electrocardiograph, the phonocardiograph, the echocardiograph and also the radiograph. Cardiac catheterization is a more specialized procedure but necessary in certain heart conditions.

ELECTROCARDIOGRAPHY

The electrocardiogram (ECG) yields valuable data about electrical events occurring with cardiac muscle activity. Alteration of this activity results in departure from the normal pattern of the electrocardiogram and gives important information about the integrity of the heart muscle and the type of cardiac rhythm. For many years electrocardiograms were taken chiefly from what were known as the three standard leads. In lead I the patient is connected to the instrument by electrodes applied to

his right and left arms; in lead II the electrodes are from the right arm and left leg; in lead III from the left arm and left leg. Later it was found that further information could be obtained by the use of a precordial lead, in which one electrode was placed on the right arm or left leg and the other in various positions upon the chest (CR and CF leads). These leads were bipolar, and there was a considerable difference in voltage between them. In an attempt to establish a commonly accepted practice unipolar leads are now commonly used. In these, the three limbs are connected to a single terminal forming one electrode; the other electrode is in contact with the chest at various points from the right of the sternum to the axilla or back (V or voltage leads). Similarly, unipolar limb leads are derived from a single electrode joining the three limbs and a second electrode connected with one limb only (aVR, aVL, aVF). Fuller details of the relative value of these various methods of electrocardiography should be sought in specialized textbooks.

The excursion of the various waves is standardized by passing a current of known intensity through the instrument causing a deflection of 1 cm for 1 mV on the recording paper. Each record shows the method of time marking, vertical lines of 0.20 s (thick) and 0.04 s (thin) and horizontal lines of 1 mm with which the amplitude of the various waves and their distances apart can be measured.

THE INTERPRETATION OF THE ELECTROCARDIOGRAPH

The waves produced by the cardiac cycle are commonly named P, Q, R, S and T (Figure 7.65). The following description applies to these in the standard leads:

The P wave

P represents the spreading of electrical activity through the atria. It is absent in atrial fibrillation, when atrial activity is rapid, inco-ordinate and continuous. Abnormal P waves occur more frequently than the ventricular waves in atrial flutter with heart block, in which the atrial rate is greater than the ventricular. Normally the P wave is upright, but it is inverted in lead I in true dextrocardia and may invert in conditions in which the cardiac pacemaker is not in the sino-atrial node (e.g. paroxysmal atrial or nodal tachycardia and atrial flutter), but isolated inverted P waves may have no pathological significance.

P is followed by the ventricular events Q, R, S and T. The P–R interval is normally 0.14–0.18 s and represents the time taken by the excitatory process to pass from the atrium to the ventricle. It is measured from the beginning of the P to the beginning of the R waves. The P–R interval is increased (more than 0.22 s is generally considered

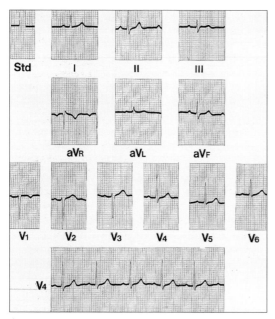

▲ **Figure 7.65 Normal electrocardiogram**. The continuous record at the bottom of the trace shows normal sinus rhythm, with normal sequence of PQRS and T

pathological) when the conduction through the atrioventricular bundle (of His) is decreased. This may merely indicate some temporary effect, e.g. digitalis poisoning, or may be a permanent condition in heart block, in which all grades of defective conductivity are found from slight prolongation of the P–R interval to complete atrioventricular dissociation. In the last case the atrial P waves bear no relationship to the ventricular events Q, R, S and T: the P waves occur at a normal rate of 72 (approximately) per minute; the QRST only at about 30 per minute, when the pacemaking focus is situated in the periphery of the conducting system.

The QRS complex

Q is the usually small initial downward deflection of the QRS complex, which corresponds with the initial part of ventricular septal activity. A deep or broad Q is abnormal and is often found over an area of cardiac infarction. R occurs next and is often the main deflection in the QRS complex. It is upright in all leads, and may be slightly notched even in health. S follows R and is normally a relatively small wave directed downwards. QRS together normally occupy no more than 0.12 s and QRS 'spread' – i.e. when the deflections occupy more than 0.12 s – indicates some impairment in conductivity through the branches of the atrioventricular bundle of His or their final arborization in the ventricular muscle. It is thus seen

in bundle-branch block, and in these cases the QRS is usually notched and bizarre in shape.

Ventricular extrasystoles produce a large QRS complex, with the final deflection in an opposite direction to the initial. Axis deviation of the heart, which can be physiological, varying with the body build and the phase of respiration, may be shown by alteration in the amplitude of the R and S waves in leads I and III. In right-axis deviation S is prominent in lead I and R in lead III. The signs are opposite in left-axis deviation. More pronounced changes of this kind, sometimes with T-wave inversion, are seen in left and right ventricular hypertrophy (Figures 7.66 and 7.67). Unipolar limb leads help in difficult cases, but care must be shown before pronouncing axis deviation as normal or abnormal.

The T wave

T represents the final electrical change coincident with ventricular contraction. It is upright and slightly rounded in lead I but frequently inverted (negative) in lead III in normal subjects as a part of left-axis deviation. Persistent negativity of the T wave in leads I and II is found in myocardial diseases, especially ischaemic, and may occur temporarily in toxaemias (e.g. digitalis poisoning and fevers).

Sometimes the S–T interval is modified. Instead of a flat portion, it may become curved, elevated or depressed. Such changes in the S–T interval occur with myocardial ischaemia.

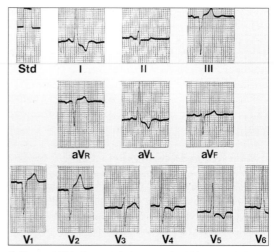

▲ **Figure 7.66 Left ventricle hypertrophy**. This record is from a patient with severe aortic stenosis. The leads V1–V5 are recorded at half sensitivity. There is left axis deviation, deep Q–S waves in leads V1 and V2, tall R waves in leads V5 and V6, and negative T waves in leads 1, aVL, V4, V5 and V6

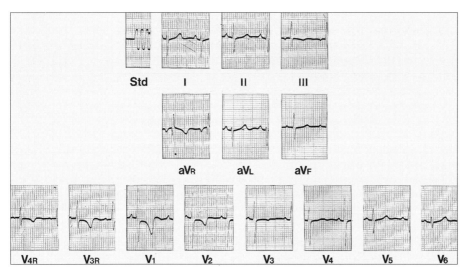

Std I II III

aVR aVL aVF

V4R V3R V1 V2 V3 V4 V5 V6

◄ **Figure 7.67 Right ventricle hypertrophy. This patient had severe pulmonary valve stenosis**. Leads V4R and V3R are recorded from right chest positions similar to V3 and V4 on the left. Right-axis deviation is present, with tall R waves in leads V4R, V3R (over the right ventricle), V1 and V2, with negative T waves in the same leads

PHONOCARDIOGRAPHY

This is used to record heart sounds and murmurs, and relate them to haemodynamic events, using a simultaneous tracing of carotid, jugular or apex pulse. It has been used far less since the advent of echocardiography and echo-Doppler for evaluation of structural cardiac lesions and murmurs.

Cardiac muscle activity is associated with low-frequency vibrations of considerable amplitude, much greater than that of heart sounds and murmurs, which have a frequency within the audible range. Since it is the latter that have to be recorded in phonocardiography, a filtering mechanism is used to remove high-amplitude, low-frequency vibrations and allow amplification of those in the higher-frequency, lower-amplitude range.

The terms, HF, MF and LF refer to the three frequency recordings found most satisfactory in clinical use – HF or high frequency being where most of the low frequency vibrations have been filtered out to allow amplification of low-intensity, high-frequency vibrations, e.g. the decrescendo diastolic murmurs of aortic incompetence. LF or low frequency corresponds to what is heard when using the bell end of a stethoscope, e.g. for the detection of a mitral diastolic murmur. MF is between HF and LF, and corresponds to what is heard with the diaphragm end of a stethoscope.

Phonocardiographs are obtained from crystal microphones applied to the chest wall and connected to a suitable recording apparatus through a series of amplifiers. The pattern commonly used is to record from the second and fourth right intercostal spaces by the sternal edge (2R and 4R), from the second, third and fourth left interspaces by the sternal edge (2L, 3L, 4L) from the position of the apex, both with the patient on his left side, and on his back, and from Erbs point – between the left sternal edge and the apex, corresponding to the V3 position in electrocardiography.

Together with the recording of heart sounds and murmurs, it is essential to record the lower-frequency events, i.e. the arterial pulse (usually carotid), the jugular venous pulse (JVP) and the movement of the apex beat (ACG). These recordings are needed for timing events in the cardiac cycle, but also have their own diagnostic value, e.g. in the recording of the arterial pulse in aortic stenosis (Figures 7.13 and 7.14). Several examples of normal and abnormal arterial and venous pulses have been illustrated in this chapter (Figures 7.12, 7.13 and 7.22). For recordings of apex cardiograms the reader is referred to more advanced books of cardiology, but the examples and descriptive legends included here give an indication of the usefulness of this technique.

ECHOCARDIOGRAPHY

Echocardiography is a non-invasive method of investigation used particularly for the demonstration of congenital cardiac abnormalities, the diagnosis of pericardial effusion and certain types of valve disease and the assessment of cardiac chamber size and function.

Echocardiography represents a development of naval sonar used for the location and detection of underwater objects and the mapping of the sea bed. In principle, it depends upon the emission and reflection of a beam of pulsed high-frequency sound, generated by a piezo-electric crystal, which acts as transmitter and receiver. The delay that occurs between the emission and return of the ultrasound is a measure of the depth of the reflecting surface, away from the energy source. Ultrasonic reflection occurs whenever there is a difference in the acoustic impedance of adjacent tissues. (Acoustic impedance is the product of the speed of sound in tissue and the density of the tissue.) Certain tissues are good reflectors, and send back narrow beams of high intensity – the heart valves are good examples, but when the valves become irregular and thicker, the beams reflected are wider and more diffuse. A change of impedance, say from fluid to denser tissue, as in a pericardial effusion, produces a reflecting layer which is clearly defined, and of great diagnostic value, but air-containing lung is a great absorber of ultrasound energy, and the interposition of lung between the heart and the transducer will make it very difficult to conduct this examination.

Display and recording of ultrasound has been developed into a method whereby the intensity of the reflected sound, shown as the brightness of a dot on an oscilloscope, at a calibrated distance from the ultrasound source, can be converted into a series of lines by sweeping the dots across the screen and recording the pattern produced. This is M-mode (or motion) echocardiography. The illustrations used here are mostly of M-mode echo traces.

A more recent extension of echocardiography is the 2-D (two-dimensional) echo, which is so arranged that a series of echo signals is produced and recorded in real time, so that in effect a moving picture of a cross-section of the heart can be obtained and recorded. Of great value in the diagnosis of congenital cardiac malformations, it is likely to be an area where considerable advances in technique will be made in the near future. Still frames, as in Figures 7.74 and 7.75 are not easy to produce and even less easy to interpret.

It is not possible here to illustrate many echocardiographic patterns, but the diagrams in Figures 7.68 and 7.69 show some of the normal and abnormal patterns of the mitral and aortic valves.

In Figure 7.68, number 1 shows the pattern of the mitral valve movement, in the normal heart, in sinus rhythm. At point D the anterior and posterior leaflets commence to separate. The larger excursion of the anterior leaflet can be measured and is the vertical distance between D and E. At the E point the two cusps are separated by their maximum amount, and the anterior cusp is almost in contact with the interventricular septum. Note that the posterior cusp is moving away from the anterior cusp.

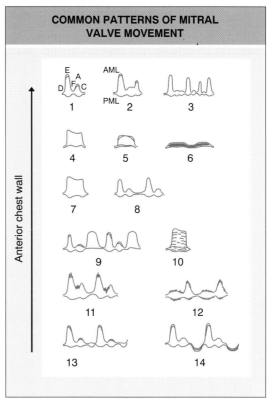

COMMON PATTERNS OF MITRAL VALVE MOVEMENT

▲ **Figure 7.68 Common patterns of mitral valve movement shown by M-mode echocardiography.** For explanations of numbers 1–14, see text

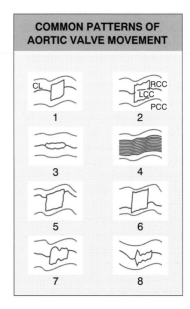

COMMON PATTERNS OF AORTIC VALVE MOVEMENT

◄ **Figure 7.69 Common patterns of aortic valve movement in M-mode echocardiography.** For explanations of numbers 1–8, see text

After point E, the mitral valve moves into a closed position as the ventricle fills, and the E to F slope represents the rate at which the closure movement occurs, the rate being markedly reduced in mitral stenosis. When atrial contraction occurs, the valve leaflets separate again to the A point, and the leaflets close at the point C when ventricular systole begins.

The excursion of the posterior leaflet is considerably less than the anterior and it should be emphasized that in the normal valve the movement in diastole is away from the anterior cusp, as the valve opens. The movement of the posterior cusp is less easy to record than the anterior, but is shown quite well in Figure 7.70.

Number 2 in Figure 7.68 is the normal valve in sinus rhythm, but with a slower rate, the extra separation of the cusps after F representing mid-diastolic flow into the LV.

Number 3 shows the result in atrial fibrillation, the valve movement being normal. The A point has disappeared, the excursion to E shows a varying amplitude, and if coarse atrial fibrillation is present, small separations of the cusps can be seen.

Number 4 shows the effects of mitral stenosis, in sinus rhythm, and with a mobile valve. The total excursion is limited only slightly, but the E to F slope is greatly reduced. A small A wave can be seen, but the posterior cusp moves anteriorly, in the same direction as the anterior cusps.

Number 5 shows more severe mitral stenosis, the A wave has disappeared and the cusps are thicker. Figure 7.36 (page 157) demonstrates this well, where the posterior cusp is also shown, moving anteriorly.

Number 6 shows a calcified immobile mitral valve, the echoes from the anterior and posterior cusps being very limited in amplitude and very dense in appearance. An example of this is shown in Figure 7.71.

Number 7 demonstrates the picture of a stiff left ventricle, as occurs in advanced systemic hypertension, or aortic stenosis. The amplitude of excursion may be slightly reduced, but of great importance is the fact that the posterior leaflet moves posteriorly, away from the anterior leaflet in diastole. This appearance closely mimics mitral stenosis, as in number 4, but the direction of movement of the posterior leaflet is the differentiating point.

Number 8 shows a normal valve, the chordae appearing as parallel lines best seen in diastole.

Number 9 is the appearance in hypertrophic obstructive cardiomyopathy (HOCM), where the valve movement is normal in diastole, but in systole the valve mechanism moves anteriorly, approaching the septum (systolic anterior motion, or SAM), producing obstruction in the left ventricular outflow tract.

Number 10 shows the characteristic appearance of a left atrial myxoma, when the echoes from the tumour fill the space behind the anterior cusps of the mitral valve as the mass descends into the valve opening. Differentiation from valve vegetations and left atrial thrombus may be difficult.

Numbers 11 and 12 show two varieties of mitral valve prolapse. Number 11 demonstrates late systolic prolapse of the posterior cusp, the start of the prolapse being simultaneous with the midsystolic click, followed by the systolic murmur, as in Figure 7.28. Number 12 is the echo picture of pansystolic prolapse of both leaflets, and is usually associated with symptomatic mitral regurgitation.

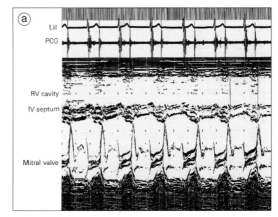

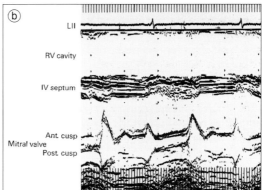

▲ **Figure 7.70 (a) Normal mitral valve movement**. This figure corresponds with pattern number 2 in Figure 7.68, but also shows a normal PCG, normal right ventricle, interventricular septum and normal left ventricle cavity size and movement. Note particularly the normal posterior cusp, moving away from the anterior cusp, during diastole. (b) Normal mitral valve movement. No PCG is shown here, and note the recording paper speed is faster than in (a). The normal E and F waves are shown, with the divergent movement of the posterior cusp of the mitral valve

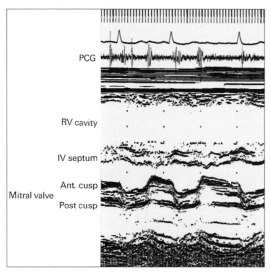

▲ **Figure 7.71 Mitral stenosis with regurgitation, pulmonary arterial hypertension**. The ECG shows the pattern of atrial fibrillation, the PCG is not helpful. From above downwards, the echogram shows a dilated right ventricle, normal thickness of the interventricular septum, a normal-sized left ventricle cavity, but the mitral valve is restricted in movement, the amplitude of which is low, the valves are slow to open and close, show dense echo shadowing, which represents calcification. The posterior cusp moves anteriorly, towards the anterior cusp, in diastole

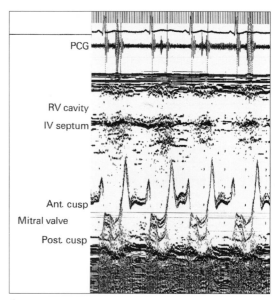

▲ **Figure 7.72 Mitral valve prolapse**. The PCG shows the midsystolic click and variable late systolic murmur present in this case. The echo from above downwards shows a normal right ventricle and IV septum. The mitral valve echo shows a sudden backwards prolapse of the posterior cusp, 1 ss of the anterior cusp, in late systole. The start of this sudden prolapse is coincident with the midsystolic click. Compare with number 12 in Figure 7.69

Numbers 13 and 14 show the mitral valve in aortic regurgitation. Number 13 diagrammatically is a reproduction of Figure 7.42, and represents a moderate grade of aortic regurgitation, with diastolic vibrations of a normally mobile anterior cusp of the mitral valve. The more severe grade of aortic regurgitation in number 14 shows fluttering of both cusps, with a reduced excursion of the valve opening.

In Figure 7.69 the common patterns of aortic valve movement are shown. Number 1 is normal. CL shows the closure line in diastole, central in position, ending with abrupt valve opening at the start of ejection, the cusps moving to the edge of the aortic wall. The right cusp (RCC) is anterior, the non-coronary, posterior cusp (PCC) being posterior. The resulting shape is a parallelogram, the cusps closing as abruptly as they open. Cusp opening corresponds to the position of the ejection click on the PCG; cusp closure corresponds to the position of the aortic component of the second sound.

Number 2 is also normal, but shows the rare appearance of the left coronary cusp. The fine vibrations are not abnormal.

Number 3 shows a relatively immobile aorta, and limited separation of otherwise normal valve cusps in a low cardiac output state.

Number 4 demonstrates the dense echoes appearing when the aortic valve is heavily calcified, where no discrete cusp movements can be seen, as in calcific aortic stenosis.

Numbers 5 and 6 show the eccentric closure line seen in a bicuspid aortic valve, where the cusps open normally, and are not yet stenosed. This pattern is suggestive, but not diagnostic, of a bicuspid valve.

Number 7 shows the aortic valve movement in HOCM (see Figure 7.68 for mitral valve movement). The aortic valve shows premature closure in mid-systole. The pattern, however, is not diagnostic, and may occur in other conditions.

Number 8 is the echo pattern of discrete subaortic stenosis, showing early systolic closure, particularly of the right coronary cusp. The premature closure is much earlier than in HOCM.

The tricuspid and pulmonary valves are difficult to demonstrate echocardiographically unless the right ventricle and pulmonary artery are dilated. Wall movement and ventricular function can be assessed by echocardiography. The internal measurements of the ventricle at end-systole and diastole can be measured, and stroke volume assessed.

Left atrial size can be shown quite accurately, as can a dilated aorta, for example in dissecting aneurysm. By gradual movement of the transducer so that the exploring beam of ultrasound passes from the apex of the ventricle upwards towards the aortic valve, it is possible to do an echo 'sweep' of the underlying structures, as in Figure 7.72. This technique can be used to visualize the left ventricle outflow tract, to show the presence of aortic–mitral continuity, aortic–septal continuity and, perhaps most important, in adult cardiology it helps to show the presence of a posterior pericardial effusion. The echo-free space of the effusion behind the ventricle disappears behind the left atrium where the pericardium

is reflected off the wall of that chamber. This is well shown in Figure 7.73.

Some final examples of echocardiography are given in Figures 7.74 and 7.75, with 'static' frames of 2-D echocardiography in Figures 7.76, 7.77 and 7.78.

Most modern echo machines, in addition to producing 2-D echocardiography, allow for measurements with continuous wave, pulsed wave and colour-flow Doppler. This allows the measurement of blood flow within the heart, and the calculation of gradients across the valves in the case of pulsed and continuous wave Doppler. Colour-flow Doppler visualizes colour coded-blood flow allowing the evaluation of regurgitation and intracardiac shunts.

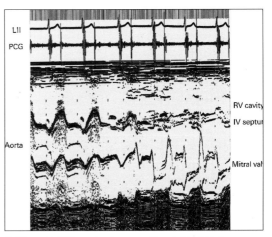

▲ **Figure 7.73 Normal aortic valve.** The diastolic closure line of the valve is very clearly seen. The 'box' or parallelogram of the opened valve is best seen in the fifth and sixth complete complexes in the figure. Note the closure line is central. The left atrial size is normal

▲ **Figure 7.74 Normal echo scan.** From left to right, the scan passes from aorta to the mitral valve, showing aortic continuity with the IV septum anteriorly, and with the anterior cusp of the mitral valve more posteriorly. The chamber sizes, valve movements and septal thickness are all normal

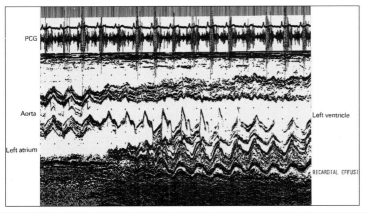

◄ **Figure 7.75 Echo scan, in a patient with uraemic pericarditis.** The PCG reveals the very loud pericardial friction noise. The right ventricle cavity size is normal, but the interventricular septum and the left ventricle posterior wall are thicker than normal. The aortic and mitral valves are normal. Where the echo of the mitral valve becomes apparent, moving from left to right (from aorta to left ventricle), an echo-free space widens as the pericardial effusion becomes apparent. The pericardium is reflected from visceral to parietal layers at this point, hence the effusion is behind the ventricle only, and not behind the atrium

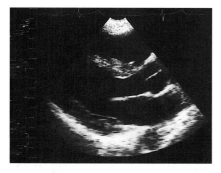

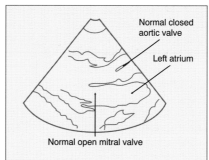

◀ **Figure 7.76 Two-dimensional (2-D) echo of a normal heart, long axis view**. The single line of aortic valve closure probably represents the central coaption of the valve cusps, but the widely open mitral valve is well seen

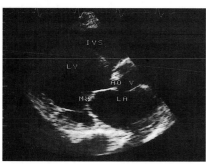

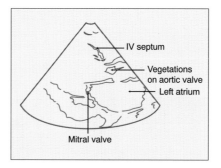

◀ **Figure 7.77 Two-dimensional (2-D) echo of vegetations on an aortic valve in a 72-year-old man with infective endocarditis**. The diagnosis was confirmed at surgery. The normal closed mitral valve is well seen

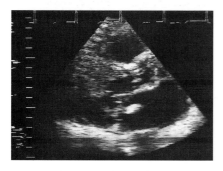

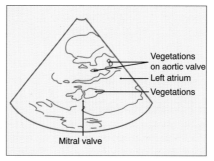

◀ **Figure 7.78 Two-dimensional (2-D) echo of vegetations on the aortic and mitral valves in a 76-year-old woman with infective endocarditis**. The vegetations on the mitral valve are particularly large

CARDIAC CATHETERIZATION

Catheterization of the right heart chambers is performed by the venous route, either through a femoral or an arm vein. The left heart chambers are approached retrogradely through the brachial or femoral artery, passing from aorta to left ventricle through the aortic valve. The left atrium is approached either through a patent foramen ovale, from right atrium to left, or by trans-atrial septal puncture, the catheter being introduced from the right atrium. All these manoeuvres, except in children, should be done using local anaesthesia only, since patient co-operation is needed for various movements and recordings.

Using a suitably designed cardiac catheter, it is possible with this method to:

1 Record intracardiac pressures and wave forms. With two or more catheters inserted, simultaneous pressure records from different sites can be recorded, e.g. left ventricle and aorta, in aortic stenosis (Figures 7.79 and 7.80).

2 Because of the ability to take blood samples from the catheter tip, arteriovenous oxygen differences can be determined in cardiac output studies, and blood sampling throughout the cardiac chambers will help to determine the site and severity of left-to-right shunting.

3 Injection of indicator solution and sampling downstream from the injection site, enables curves to be drawn of indicator dilution and these are of assistance in calculating cardiac output and in determin-

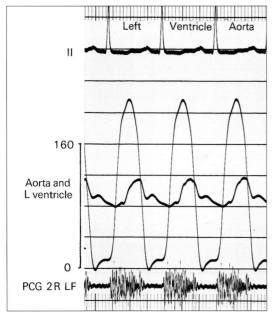

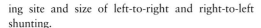

▲ **Figure 7.79 Cardiac catheter and PCG findings in aortic stenosis**. The PCG shows the systolic murmur, but the pressure tracings show a left ventricle pressure of 220 systolic, and an aortic pressure of about 115 systolic. The aortic pressure pulse is of small amplitude and is anacrotic. This patient had aortic valve stenosis of a severe degree

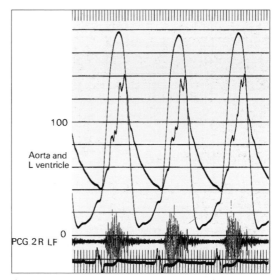

▲ **Figure 7.80 Cardiac catheter and PCG findings in aortic stenosis and regurgitatio**n. The PCG shows the systolic and diastolic murmurs, the pressure tracings a left ventricle systolic pressure of 180, with an aortic systolic pressure of 140. The aortic pressure pulse is of high amplitude, and although there is some delay in its upstroke, the diastolic fall to 40, almost equalling the ventricular end-diastolic pressure, is typical of severe aortic regurgitation

ing site and size of left-to-right and right-to-left shunting.

4 Injection of radiographic contrast material selectively into cardiac chambers or vessels is used, for example, in the quantification of mitral regurgitation, when contrast material is injected into the left ventricle and a film recording made of the subsequent cardiac cycles. Injection into the aorta helps to identify and quantify aortic regurgitation and injections into the left and right ventricles shows the interventricular septum and any defects therein. Coarctation of the aorta is readily shown by angiographic methods.

5 Left ventricular angiography, used to determine left ventricular function and morphology, is an important part of the now very common procedure of coronary arteriography. In this investigation, a special catheter is manipulated either by the femoral or brachial route to the left and right coronary orifice, and small volumes of contrast material are injected into the vessel, taking cine film in different views so as to build up a three-dimensional picture of the coronary arterial tree. This is a very important investigation, first to demonstrate the presence or absence of coronary arterial

pathology and secondly to show the precise anatomy of any obstructed lesions, a necessity if coronary artery bypass surgery is to be performed. Post-operatively, the integrity of the newly established bypass vessels can be confirmed.

6 Finally, it is possible, using a wide-bore catheter as a protective sheath, to insert biopsy forceps into left and right ventricles, and remove pieces of myocardium for histological examination.

PERIPHERAL VASCULAR DISEASES

Examination of the peripheral arteries and veins has already been described in relation to disorders of the heart (page 135). Diseases of these vessels themselves may, as in the case of the heart, be functional or structural in origin.

Functional disorders of the arteries consist of changes in vasomotor tone which may be diffuse or focal. A diffuse increase in arteriolar tone gives rise to hypertension which, though functional in origin, may have serious structural effects upon the arteries and left ventricle. Examples of focal disorders of arterial tone

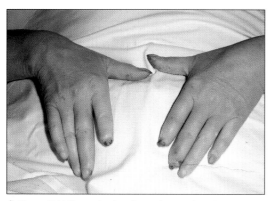

▲ **Figure 7.81 Case of scleroderma (systemic sclerosis) showing atrophy of terminal phalanges and early gangrene.** Similar appearances may be seen in other types of Raynaud's phenomena

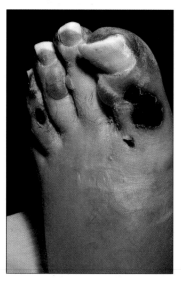

◀ **Figure 7.82 Cold injury to the feet: frostbite**

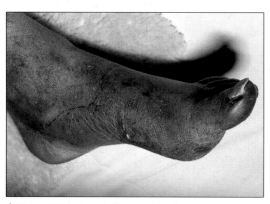

▲ **Figure 7.83 Ischaemic foot resulting from systemic embolus due to atrial fibrillation due to mitral stenosis**

are Raynaud's phenomenon (Figure 7.81), in which there is cold-induced spasm of the digital arteries, and migraine characterized by constriction followed by dilatation of the cranial arteries (see page 8). Erythrocyanosis frigidum (chilblains) also arises from an instability of vasomotor tone. Prolonged exposure to cold may induce gangrene from intense vasoconstriction (Figure 7.82).

Structural arterial disease is usually metabolic, degenerative or inflammatory in origin. The most important cause is *atheroma* in which arteries are damaged by the deposition of a lipoid material beneath the intima. This occurs most often in middle-aged men, especially those with disordered fat metabolism, as in diabetes and familial hyperlipidaemia. The degenerative process in the arteries is accelerated by hypertension and heavy smoking. Atheroma may be complicated by thrombosis, sometimes with embolism to more distal parts of the artery, and also by aneurysmal dilatation or rupture of the vessel. The aorta and its main branches and the coronary and cerebral arteries are most commonly affected.

Thrombosis and embolism may also lead to arterial occlusion in the absence of any primary disease of the artery. Thrombosis can occur in certain blood disorders (see Chapter 8), and emboli may arise from intracardiac thrombus, as in mitral disease, bacterial endocarditis or after myocardial infarction (Figure 7.83).

Inflammatory vascular disease or *vasculitis* is usually the result of an autoimmune process which may occur at any age and, unlike atheroma, favours the smaller peripheral vessels. The disease is often widespread and lesions in the kidneys, heart and lungs are of special importance. Infective forms of arteritis are now rare but two are worthy of mention:

1 Syphilitic aortitis causing dilatation of the proximal aorta leading to aneurysm and regurgitation.

2 Mycotic aneurysm due to infection of the arterial wall by an embolus from the aortic or mitral valve in patients with bacterial endocarditis.

The symptoms and signs of arterial disease are due either to narrowing of the lumen or to inflammation, distension or rupture of the wall. Luminal narrowing affects parts supplied by the diseased artery while changes in the vessel wall may also involve the structures surrounding it. The clinical features of some common arterial diseases will now be described.

OBLITERATIVE ARTERIAL DISEASE

The effects of coronary and cerebral arterial insufficiency are described elsewhere. The symptoms and signs of obstructed limb arteries depend upon the site and nature of the stenosis. The legs are much more commonly affected than the arms because the lower part of the aorta and its branches are more prone to atheroma. The ischaemic changes in the limb are sudden and profound when occlusion is by embolism. Narrowing by atheroma or thrombus is usually more gradual, allowing time for the development of a collateral circulation.

The commonest symptom of obliterative arterial disease is ischaemic muscle pain on effort ('intermittent claudication'). The level of the lesion determines the site of the pain which is most often in the calf but may occur in the buttock, thigh or sole of the foot. The pain resembles angina in that it is aching or cramping in character, regularly occurs after walking a certain distance, compels the patient to stop and disappears when he does so. Effort tolerance may progressively diminish until pain occurs even at rest and disturbs sleep. The patient may also complain that the foot on the affected side feels cold or numb and he may notice paraesthesiae or colour changes.

Inspection of the ischaemic limb may reveal cyanosis, pallor or trophic lesions in the skin, especially in the more peripheral parts. If the limbs are elevated and then quickly lowered to a dependent position, the veins re-fill and the colour returns more slowly on the side most severely affected. Trophic lesions include loss of hair, ulcers and gangrene (see Figure 3.39, page 42), seen first on the toes and later more proximally. The temperature of the skin will vary with the ambient temperature, but a difference between the two limbs, best detected with the dorsum or ulnar border of the hand, is significant. In patients complaining of effort pain, the dorsalis pedis and posterior tibial pulses are usually absent. The popliteal and femoral pulses may also be absent or diminished and a bruit may be audible over them.

SYSTEMIC HYPERTENSION

Although an abnormally high systemic blood pressure is rarely due to primary arterial disease, it is usually mediated by increased arteriolar tone. In most cases, a cause for this cannot be found though a family history is common, and to these the term 'essential' hypertension is applied. The majority of the remainder will be suffering from some form of chronic renal disease (see Chapter 5). Rarer causes include coarctation of the aorta and endocrine disorders such as phaeochromocytomas and Cushing's syndrome (see Chapter 12).

There is no evidence that hypertension of itself causes symptoms and indeed the majority of cases are discovered at a routine medical examination. Symptoms such as headache and dizziness are often due to the patient's anxiety about their blood pressure. Symptoms and signs

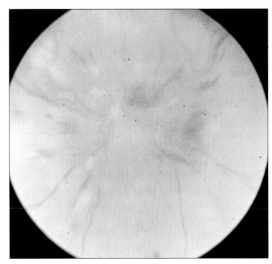

▲ **Figure 7.84 Malignant or accelerated hypertension: retinal haemorrhages, exudates and papilloedema**

are otherwise attributable either to the cause or to cardiac and arterial complications such as left ventricular failure and degenerative changes in the cerebral and coronary circulations.

The diagnosis is established by finding a persistent or recurrent elevation of the systemic blood pressure above 140 mmHg systolic and 90 mmHg diastolic even after a period of rest. An index of the severity of the hypertension is given by retinoscopy (Figure 7.84). The term 'accelerated (or malignant) hypertension' is applied to a severe rapidly progressive form of the disease associated with papilloedema and renal failure.

RAYNAUD PHENOMENON

This condition is characterized by intermittent spasm of digital arteries induced by cold and relieved by heat. Young women are most often affected and usually no underlying cause can be found (Raynaud's disease), but some cases are associated with occlusive arterial disease, arteritis, blood disorders, neurogenic lesions or repeated trauma to the hands.

The patient complains that, when exposed to cold, the fingers and less commonly the toes go numb and white, sometimes with patchy cyanosis. This is followed by redness, throbbing and tingling due to a reactive hyperaemia occurring either spontaneously or on re-warming. The hands may appear normal between attacks but trophic lesions develop in long-standing cases, especially those associated with organic disease. The fingers may then become thin and tapered with tight shiny skin ('scleroderma'), telangiectasia, deformed atrophic nails and infarcts causing painful ulcers at the fingertips (see Figure 7.81).

VASCULITIS ('CONNECTIVE TISSUE DISEASES')

It is appropriate here to consider a group of disorders characterized by inflammatory changes in connective tissues and in the walls of small peripheral vessels (necrotizing vasculitis). The cause is unknown but an autoimmune process, sometimes drug-induced, may be responsible in certain cases. These conditions are therefore distinguished by the clinical syndromes with which they present rather than by specific aetiological tests.

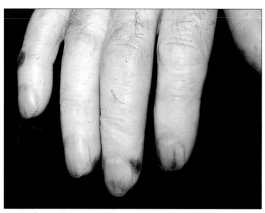

▲ **Figure 7.85 Digital infarcts in a patient with vasculitis**

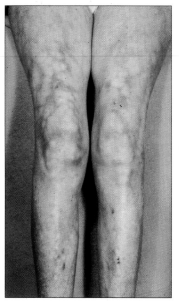

◀ **Figure 7.86 Livido reticularis**

1 Polyarteritis nodosa

The manifestations are so diverse that a purely clinical diagnosis may be impossible until several systems have been involved. The most characteristic features are renal failure, multiple organ infarction, asymmetrical peripheral neuropathy, intractable bronchial asthma and polymorph leucocytosis with eosinophilia. Splinter haemorrhages in the nails (see Figure 7.54) and small infarcts in the finger tips (Figure 7.85) may be seen in this and other vasculitic disorders.

2 Giant-cell arteritis

The inflammatory process mainly affects the cranial vessels of elderly subjects and tends towards spontaneous recovery. The temporal and occipital arteries may be tender, inflamed and pulseless. Sudden blindness can result from retinal artery occlusion (see Figure 1.1). The condition is often associated with painful stiffness of the proximal limb muscles (*polymyalgia rheumatica*).

3 Systemic sclerosis

This condition usually presents with a Raynaud phenomenon and the typical changes of scleroderma in the hands and face (see Figure 3.30 and Figure 7.81). Dysphagia and malabsorption from alimentary tract involvement, myocardial ischaemia and dyspnoea due to fibrosing alveolitis are other typical features of this disease.

4 Systemic lupus erythematosus

The name of this syndrome is derived from the red 'butterfly' rash which affects the nose, cheeks and other parts exposed to light (see Figure 3.11). Another cutaneous manifestation of connective tissue disease is livido reticularis (Figure 7.86), commonly associated with the anticardiolipsin antibody. Many organs may be involved including the joints, lung, heart, liver, kidneys, haemopoietic and nervous systems. As distinct from polyarteritis, systemic lupus is more common among women than men and is more often associated with leucopenia and thrombocytopenia than with leucocytosis.

5 Rheumatoid disease (see also Chapter 9)

A rheumatoid form of arthritis is a common feature of the vasculitic or connective tissue group of diseases and vasculitic lesions in the skin, eyes and elsewhere may be found in patients presenting with classic rheumatoid arthritis (see Figure 7.87).

An inflammatory cause for a peripheral vascular disorder should always be considered when the patient has fever or a raised ESR.

ANEURYSM

Congenital, inflammatory or degenerative changes in the arterial wall may lead to focal or diffuse dilatation and eventually rupture of the vessel (Figure 7.24). The cerebral arteries and the aorta are most commonly affected. Aneurysm of a cerebral artery, whether congenital ('berry' aneurysm), infective ('mycotic' aneurysm) or atheromatous, usually presents with subarachnoid or intracerebral haemorrhage (see Chapter 10). Aneurysm of the aorta may be of two kinds:

1 Saccular or fusiform.
2 Dissecting.

Saccular or fusiform aneurysms of the thoracic aorta are either syphilitic, degenerative (atherosclerotic) or posttraumatic in origin and usually manifest as mediastinal tumours with pressure effects upon surrounding structures (see Chapter 6). More common today is atheromatous aneurysm of the abdominal aorta. This causes a persistent aching or throbbing pain in the abdomen or back but may leak and simulate a perforated viscus with severe pain, circulatory collapse and abdominal rigidity. A tender fusiform pulsating mass may be palpable in the abdomen to the left of the midline and a bruit may be audible over it.

Dissecting aneurysm results from degenerative changes in the medial coat of the aorta. These changes are either congenital, as in Marfan's syndrome, or acquired when they may be associated with hypertension. Blood penetrates the intima, tracks through the media and may then either rupture the outer coat of the aorta or re-enter the lumen lower down. The process usually starts in the upper thoracic aorta giving rise to intense retrosternal pain simulating myocardial infarction or pulmonary embolism. Pain radiates to the back and, as the dissection proceeds, may descend towards the abdomen and the

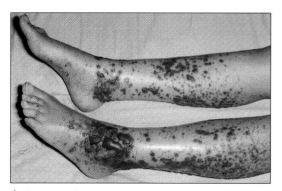

▲ **Figure 7.87 Cutaneous vasculitis in rheumatoid arthritis**

loins. The origins of the carotid and subclavian vessels may be affected to cause cerebral signs and absent radial pulses. Signs may also result from leakage of blood into the pericardial, pleural or peritoneal cavities.

VENOUS DISORDERS

The three most important abnormalities of veins are dilatation and tortuosity with incompetent valves (*varicose veins*), inflammation (*phlebitis*) and *thrombosis*. These three conditions may coexist or follow one upon the other. Each may both cause and result from impaired venous drainage and, because of gravity, the legs are affected more often than the arms. Predisposing causes include obesity, prolonged standing, pregnancy, pelvic tumours and chronic congestive cardiac failure. They also include conditions favouring thrombosis such as the postoperative state, immobilization, certain oral contraceptive agents and blood disorders (e.g. polycythaemia). Venous thrombosis may complicate malignant disease and give rise to the syndrome of *thrombophlebitis migrans* in which there are flitting episodes of inflammation in superficial veins as well as deep vein thrombosis.

The symptoms and signs of a venous disorder depend upon its duration and speed of onset. In cases of deep vein thrombosis (e.g. postoperative) the onset may be sudden with pain and discomfort in the leg. Physical signs include low grade fever, deep tenderness in the calf or thigh, increased girth of the affected limb and pitting oedema. Dorsiflexion of the foot may cause pain in the calf (Homans' sign). Symptoms and signs of pulmonary embolism (see page 172) may sometimes precede those of the venous thrombosis. Thrombophlebitis is recognized by the presence of a tender palpable cord in one or more segments of the superficial veins with reddening of the adjacent skin.

Venous stasis of long standing leads to secondary changes in the skin (Figure 7.88). There may be a network of superficial varices, eczema, pigmentation and ulceration. These changes are maximal in the lower part of the leg especially on the medial aspect above the ankle (see Figure 3.47, page 44). The subcutaneous veins will be tortuous and dilated but this may only be apparent when the patient is standing.

DISORDERS OF THE LYMPHATICS

There are few clinical signs peculiar to disorders of the lymph vessels. Amongst these are the red line around inflamed lymphatics draining an area of infection (Figure 7.89); yellow discoloration of the nails associated with congenital hypoplasia of lymphatics (Figure 6.42); nonpitting lymphoedema due to lymphatic obstruction by

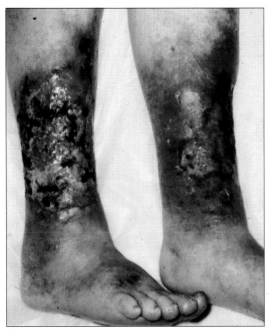

▲ **Figure 7.88 Venous stasis producing pigmentation, oedema and ulceration**

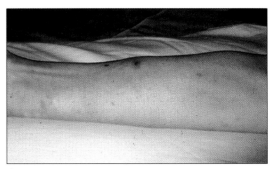

▲ **Figure 7.89 Lymphangitis secondary to an insect bite on the forearm**

malignant disease or radical surgical dissection, and the gross limb swelling of elephantiasis resulting from lymphatic obstruction by filarial parasites (see Figure 13.6). Obstruction of the thoracic duct may lead to a 'chylous' pleural effusion (see Chapter 6).

SPECIAL INVESTIGATIONS

Various radiographic and laboratory procedures are of value in the assessment of peripheral vascular disease. The arteries may be displayed by *retrograde aortography*, for which a catheter is passed into the aorta through the femoral artery. A radio-opaque material is then injected near to or within the origin of the relevant arteries. For *venography*, a radio-opaque material is injected into a vein near the ankle and will be carried upwards to display the veins of the leg and pelvis.

Non-invasive techniques are also available for the investigation of peripheral vascular disease. Doppler ultrasound can be used to assess both arterial and venous blood flow and ultrasound imaging has proved of value in the detection of aortic aneurysm and its differentiation from solid tumour. Plain radiographs of the abdomen or chest may be sufficient to demonstrate an aortic aneurysm, especially one which is calcified, and a radiograph of the thoracic inlet to exclude arterial compression associated with a cervical rib should always be taken in patients with upper limb ischaemia.

Relevant laboratory investigations include measurement of the serum lipoproteins and cholesterol in patients with atheroma; the ESR, tests for auto-antibodies (anti-nuclear and rheumatoid factors, etc.) and muscle or artery biopsy when a vasculitis is suspected; cryoglobulins and cold agglutinins in patients with a Raynaud phenomenon; and a Wassermann reaction to exclude syphilis as a cause of aortic aneurysm or regurgitation.

The investigation of a patient with hypertension consists mainly of excluding renal and endocrine causes (see Chapters 5 and 12).

The haemopoietic system

Under this heading are included the blood and those tissues concerned in its production or destruction: the bone-marrow, the lymph nodes, the spleen and the liver.

SYMPTOMS AND SIGNS OF HAEMATOLOGICAL DISEASE

The symptoms and signs of haematological disease include:

1 Symptoms and signs of anaemia.
2 Symptoms and signs of haemorrhage.
3 Enlargement of lymph nodes.
4 Enlargement of the spleen and liver.
5 Changes in the fundus oculi.
6 Changes in the mouth.
7 Changes in the skin.

These symptoms and signs are never sufficient for a diagnosis without examination of the blood and often of the bone-marrow. For this reason, this chapter is not restricted to a description of symptoms and physical signs.

ANAEMIA

This term means a deficiency in the haemoglobin content of the blood and usually a decrease in the number of red cells. The iron-containing pigment haemoglobin, which is responsible for the normal pink coloration of the mucous membranes and skin, carries the necessary oxygen to all the organs and tissues of the body.

The signs and symptoms which result from a deficiency of haemoglobin, are:

PALLOR OF THE SKIN AND MUCOUS MEMBRANES

Pallor of the skin without a corresponding loss of colour in the lips, tongue, buccal cavity and nail beds can frequently be disregarded, as many persons normally have a pallid complexion. In true anaemia, pallor occurs both in the skin and in the mucous membranes and varies in grade from a slight loss of colour, only appreciable to the experienced eye, to the extreme pallor of profound haemorrhagic anaemias or the lemon-yellow tint which is present occasionally in pernicious anaemia. In anaemias due to malignant disease an earthy pallor is often seen, and

in bacterial endocarditis the skin colour has been likened to café au lait. The degree of pallor of the mucous membranes is only a rough guide to the severity of the anaemia, which should always be corroborated by a haemoglobin estimation. It is important not to rely solely on the conjunctivae for evidence of anaemia in the mucous membranes, as infection of the former from other causes not uncommonly gives a false redness.

SYMPTOMS AND SIGNS OF OXYGEN DEFICIENCY

In the face of the reduced oxygen carrying capacity of the blood, both the respiratory and cardiovascular systems adapt in order to maintain tissue oxygenation. Dyspnoea may be as great as in certain forms of heart or lung disease, but the patient is only breathless at rest in very severe anaemia. With only a moderate anaemia the heart-rate is increased both at rest and on exertion. This compensatory mechanism is more marked in the elderly when both palpitations and angina are common symptoms. Sometimes right-sided heart failure may occur (see page 172). The deficient oxygenation of the blood also affects adversely most of the organs and tissues of the body. Dizziness, throbbing in the head and tinnitus are common and the patient complains of general lassitude and inability for physical or mental work. The function of the gastrointestinal tract may be affected, and loss of appetite, nausea, and constipation or diarrhoea may occur. Slight albuminuria is not unusual, and renal function may be impaired occasionally. A mild or moderate degree of fever is common when the anaemia is severe. It should be pointed out that the severity of the symptoms is not necessarily related to the degree of anaemia.

HAEMORRHAGE

Haemorrhage, especially in the form of melaena or occult bleeding from the gastrointestinal tract, is an important cause of anaemia (page 70). Spontaneous bleeding into the skin and from the mucosae–epistaxis, haemoptysis, haematuria, menorrhagia – is characteristic of certain forms of purpura (Figure 8.1 and see page 199). In haemophilia, haemorrhage is usually provoked by minor trauma and consists of haemarthroses and excessive bleeding from small breaches of the skin or mucosae.

ENLARGED LYMPH NODES

The common haematological diseases which present with lymph node enlargement are described on page 198.

Enlargement of the lymph nodes (Figure 8.2) is so common that a brief description of the characteristics of the nodes is necessary in differential diagnosis. The following points should be noted:

THE GROUP OR GROUPS OF NODES AFFECTED

The student should examine the area which the nodes drain. This is of particular importance when lymph node enlargement is due to local infection or malignant diseases. A more generalized enlargement may be found in infectious mononucleosis (glandular fever), the lymphomas and some blood diseases (page 198). In some parts of the world syphilis and plague are not uncommon causes of generalized enlargement which may also herald the onset of AIDS. The method for palpating axillary nodes is shown in Figure 8.3.

THE CONSISTENCY

A stony hardness, especially when accompanied by irregularity, suggests carcinoma. Nodes of moderate firmness are found in tuberculosis and other chronic infections and also in the infiltrations of leukaemia and the lymphomas. Sepsis and more rarely tuberculosis may cause abscess formation with characteristic 'fluctuation' on palpation (Figure 8.4).

THE ATTACHMENTS OF THE NODES

They tend to remain discrete in the lymphomas and leukaemias. Inflammatory changes often result in adherence of the nodes to the skin and subcutaneous tissues, which can no longer be moved freely over them. Carcinoma has a similar effect but with greater infiltration which anchors the nodes to the deeper structures.

THE PRESENCE OF TENDERNESS

Tenderness usually accompanies acute inflammatory changes in the nodes, especially those due to coccal

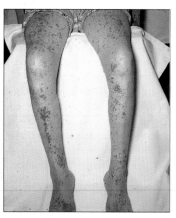

◀ **Figure 8.1 Purpura.** From a case of leukaemia in its terminal stages

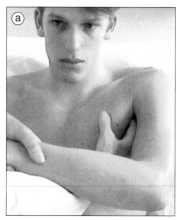

(a)

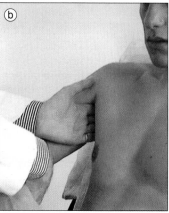

(b)

◀ **Figure 8.3 Palpating axillary nodes** (reproduced from *Clinical Examination of the Patient* by John Lumley and Pierre-Marc G. Bouloux, Butterworth–Heinemann, 1994)

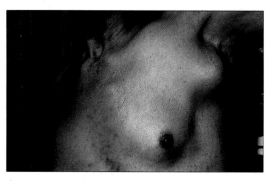

▲ **Figure 8.2 Enlarged axillary lymph nodes due to lymphoma**

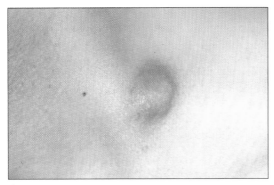

▲ **Figure 8.4 Tuberculous axillary node causing an abscess in an immunosuppressed AIDS patient**

infections. In these the superficial lymphatic vessels can frequently be seen as red streaks on the skin between the inflamed nodes and the original focus of infection (lymphangitis: see Figure 7.89, page 186).

A palpable lymph node, if soft, is not necessarily abnormal; a few lymph nodes can be felt in most healthy people, especially in the groins and axillae and in the necks of children.

ENLARGEMENT OF THE SPLEEN AND LIVER

The spleen may attain such huge dimensions that it causes a sense of weight and discomfort in the abdomen, of which the patient complains. More often the enlargement is moderate and only detected upon abdominal examination. Pain due to perisplenitis may also occasionally draw attention to splenic enlargement. It is experienced in the left hypochondrium and over the left lower ribs but is sometimes referred to the left shoulder (see Abdominal pain, page 51).

If the spleen is grossly enlarged, it may be seen on inspection occupying the left hypochondrium and, in extreme cases, extending across the middle line of the abdomen.

Palpation is the most useful method of determining splenic enlargement (Figure 8.5). The patient should be in a recumbent posture with the head on one pillow and the knees drawn up. Palpation should start well away from the spleen, below and to the right of the umbilicus, and the fingers of the right hand be gradually brought upwards until they encounter the sharp margin of the enlarged organ. At the same time the left hand is placed behind the lowermost ribs which are pressed forwards as the patient inspires deeply. A very large spleen

can be missed completely if the hand is pressed down on top of it. When the spleen is only slightly enlarged, it may be more easily felt with the patient lying half turned to his right side.

Two of the most distinctive features of an enlarged spleen are that it is sharp-edged and superficial, so that a light touch should be tried before resorting to deeper palpation. The edge should be defined and its medial border followed until the notch can be felt, although this is not always evident. The consistency of the organ should be noted, firmness being the usual characteristic in most haematological diseases. In infections the spleen is frequently soft and sometimes difficult to feel. Small degrees of splenic enlargement may not be detectable, as the organ must be moderately enlarged before it is palpable below the costal margin. When very large it may resemble the kidney in filling the left loin but can generally be distinguished by the sharp edges and the notch, if present. Moreover, it is impossible to get above the spleen on palpation. Rarely, in cases of perisplenitis, a friction rub may be heard.

Percussion may help to outline the borders of the spleen, especially when this is enlarged upwards. Dullness may be found between the ninth and eleventh ribs in the mid-axillary line, and as high as the eighth or seventh rib in cases of great splenic enlargement. Percussion is less satisfactory than palpation in determining enlargement of the spleen except when doubt exists as to the nature of a large tumour in the left hypochondrium which also fills the loin. In these circumstances the percussion note anteriorly is dull with a splenic tumour and resonant with renal enlargement.

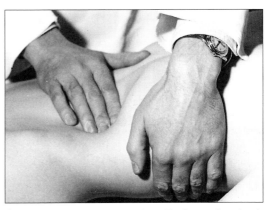

▲ **Figure 8.5 Palpation of the spleen.** The fingers of one hand are pressed gently into the abdomen and the patient is asked to take a deep breath. With the other hand the lowermost ribs are pressed forwards. This helps to bring an enlarged spleen in contact with the examining fingers

The main causes of enlargement of the spleen may be classified as follows:

Haematological disorders: Leukaemias, lymphomas, myelofibrosis, polycythaemia vera, haemolytic anaemias (except sickle cell anaemia), megaloblastic and iron-deficiency anaemias.

Vascular: Portal venous obstruction by cirrhosis of liver or thrombosis; disseminated lupus erythematosus (and other collagen disorders).

Infections: Septicaemias (bacterial endocarditis), infectious mononucleosis, brucellosis, enteric infections, miliary tuberculosis, tropical diseases (malaria, kala-azar).

Infiltrations: Amyloidosis, sarcoidosis, lipoidoses (e.g. Gaucher's disease).

The degree of splenomegaly can be of some diagnostic value. Extreme enlargement suggests chronic myeloid leukaemia, myelofibrosis, some forms of lymphoma, or, in certain tropical areas, chronic malaria or kala-azar. Conversely in acute infections, acute leukaemias and in the megaloblastic and iron-deficiency anaemias only the tip of the spleen may be felt.

Enlargement of the liver is a common accompaniment of splenomegaly in haematological diseases (see also Chapter 4, page 65).

CHANGES IN THE FUNDUS OCULI

These include retinal haemorrhages in thrombocytopenic purpura, leukaemia and severe anaemia. They may be punctate, splinter and flame-shaped, often with white centres. Flame-shaped haemorrhages around the optic disc are common in severe anaemia from any cause and do not necessarily signify an associated bleeding disorder. After sudden massive haemorrhage, particularly from the gastrointestinal tract, severe changes may occur with gross retinal haemorrhages and exudates, papilloedema and rarely permanent optic atrophy. Vitamin B_{12} deficiency may produce optic atrophy, which has occasionally been observed in the absence of anaemia. Leukaemia can cause retinal exudates and, when there is meningeal involvement, papilloedema also. Venous engorgement may occur in patients with polycythaemia.

CHANGES IN THE MOUTH

More can be learnt about blood disease by examination of the mouth than of any other part of the body. A smooth depapillated tongue (see Figure 8.11, page 195) is seen in cases of advanced iron deficiency, while the tongue in anaemia due to vitamin B_{12} or folic acid

deficiency tends also to be red and raw. Spontaneous bleeding from the gums is commonly observed in thrombocytopenic purpura and sponginess of the gums associated with pain is characteristic of acute leukaemia; sponginess and hypertrophy also occur in some patients with scurvy (see Figure 8.17, page 200). It should be remembered, however, that the commonest cause of spongy bleeding gums is chronic infection, i.e. gingivitis. Hypertrophy of the gums (Figure 8.6 and Figure 10.100, page 282) is sometimes seen in epileptic patients treated with phenytoin sodium (Epanutin) and this drug can also cause folic acid deficiency with megaloblastic anaemia; gum hypertrophy also occurs in myeloid leukaemia (see Figure 8.6) and almost always in the rare acute monocytic leukaemia. Lead poisoning may cause a blue discoloration of the gum margin.

Ulceration of the mouth occurs in a variety of haematological disorders, especially in acute leukaemia, but also in patients with folic acid or vitamin B_{12} deficiency and agranulocytosis.

Purpura in the mouth is seen in association with thrombocytopenia. The purpuric spots are usually similar to those observed in the skin but sometimes take the form of small blood blisters. Groups of petechiae on the soft palate are not uncommon in acute viral illnesses, particularly glandular fever, even in the absence of thrombocytopenia.

Infection of the mouth and throat, especially moniliasis (or 'thrush'), occurs with leukaemia or aplastic anaemia.

The lymphoid tissue in Waldeyer's ring should be examined in all patients with haematological disorders. It is commonly hypertrophied in patients with lymphosarcoma and chronic lymphatic leukaemia, and in these disorders the tonsils may be so large as to meet in the midline.

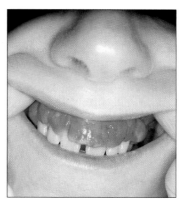

◀ **Figure 8.6**
Hypertrophy of the gums in a child with acute myeloid leukaemia

CHANGES IN THE SKIN

The various types of pallor observed in blood disorders have already been noted at the beginning of the chapter. Icterus is commonly found in patients with haemolytic anaemias. Purpura is characterized by haemorrhages into the skin, and the lesions can vary in size from a pin-head ('petechia') to a large bruise ('ecchymosis') (Figure 8.7).

The skin should be carefully examined for areas of infiltration in patients with leukaemia (Figure 8.8) and lymphomas, and for fungal and other infections in those with bone-marrow depression. Ulceration of the skin over the legs may accompany the hereditary haemolytic anaemias.

Polycythaemia vera causes cyanotic suffusion with injection of the superficial blood vessels over the face and upper half of the chest; the extremities tend to be warm and red and there are often scratch marks on the skin since pruritus is a common symptom. Pruritus with scratch marks may occur in any of the myeloproliferative disorders and also in Hodgkin's disease. Herpes infections may complicate leukaemia and lymphoma (see Figure 3.23).

A rare connective tissue disorder which may present with abnormal bleeding and bruising is the Ehlers–Danlos syndrome. A characteristic sign of this condition is the abnormal elasticity of the skin (Figure 8.9).

EXAMINATION OF THE BLOOD

Much information can be obtained from examination of the peripheral blood which is readily accessible and should be routinely examined. Venous blood is drawn with minimal stasis into a plastic tube containing the anticoagulant sequestrene.

CELL COUNTING AND ELECTRONIC COUNTERS

Automated blood cell analysers are now in widespread use. As a result of these technological advances the red cell indices dependent on these have become more valuable. These include the mean cell volume (MCV) and mean cell haemoglobin (MCH).

The most commonly used electronic counter measures red cell count, white cell count, haemoglobin concentration and MCV. With the aid of a small built-in calculator, it then derives the packed cell volume (PCV), mean corpuscular haemoglobin concentration (MCHC) and mean corpuscular haemoglobin (MCH), and prints the results out on a standard card.

The stained blood film

The films are spread on a glass slide and stained by one of the Romanowsky methods (Leishman, Giemsa). The

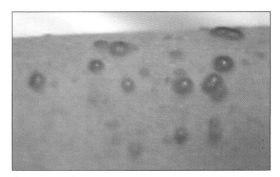

▲ **Figure 8.8 Chronic myeloid leukaemia: skin infiltration**

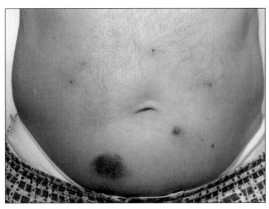

▲ **Figure 8.7 Petechiae and ecchymoses induced by subcutaneous heparin given to prevent venous thrombosis in a bed-bound patient with cardiac failure**

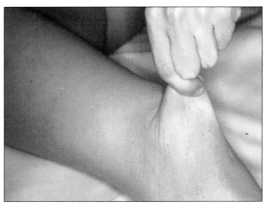

▲ **Figure 8.9 Abnormal elasticity of the skin in the Ehlers–Danlos syndrome**

size, shape and staining characteristics of the cells are observed. Small cells are known as microcytes and large cells as macrocytes. Microcytosis is produced by iron deficiency, and macrocytosis by an increase in reticulocytes (see below), deficiency of vitamin B_{12} and folic acid, excess alcohol intake and cirrhosis of the liver. When there is much variation in size, the phenomenon is known as anisocytosis.

Variation in shape is known as poikilocytosis, the cells appearing oval, pear-shaped, helmet-shaped or grossly irregular. Poikilocytosis is particularly striking in severe hypochromic and megaloblastic anaemias and in myelofibrosis. The presence of appreciable numbers of cells with spiny projections (burr cells) and red cell fragments (schistocytes) indicates severe damage to the cells and is found frequently in renal failure and sometimes in disseminated carcinomatosis. Spheroidal cells (spherocytes) appear on a stained film as small, round densely staining cells, and they are found in both hereditary spherocytosis and autoimmune haemolytic anaemias.

The pink coloration of the red cells is a criterion of their haemoglobin content. A decrease in haemoglobin is indicated by an exaggeration of their central pallor, and when the anaemia is severe, most of the red cells are colourless discs with a thin pink rim (hypochromic cells). Some of these hypochromic corpuscles may have a central stained area (target cells). In Britain hypochromic cells are almost always produced by iron deficiency. In many countries, particularly those in the Mediterranean region but also in immigrant areas of Britain, thalassaemia is a common cause.

The recognition of nucleated cells, which are the precursors of mature erythrocytes, is important. These cells are normally only present in the bone-marrow (see page 194). Red cell precursors, which are morphologically normal, are known as normoblasts or erythroblasts, and those with morphological abnormalities due to deficiency of vitamin B_{12} and folic acid are known as megaloblasts. Intermediate in position between mature erythrocytes and these nucleated cells are some large cells without a nucleus. These cells may be stained blue with the methylene blue of Leishman's stain, either uniformly (polychromasia) or with a fine blue stippling known as punctate basophilia. A reticulocyte contains a network or skein of basophilic material, which can only be demonstrated by vital dyes such as brilliant cresyl blue but is seen as a polychromatic cell on the routine smear.

The presence of erythroblasts in the peripheral blood is normal for the first month or so of life. It may occur after haemorrhage or haemolysis, and may also be produced by various disorders which act as irritants to the bone-marrow (e.g. infiltration of the bone-marrow with leukaemia or metastatic carcinoma). Megaloblasts are sometimes found in the peripheral blood in cases of severe anaemia due to deficiency of vitamin B_{12} and folic acid. Punctate basophilia is a characteristic feature of lead poisoning but occurs in many other types of anaemia. The phenomena of polychromasia and reticulocytosis usually indicate a physiological response by the bone-marrow to some specific stimulus such as haemorrhage, haemolysis or the administration of a specific haematinic (e.g. iron, vitamin B_{12}, folic acid) to a subject deficient in this substance.

In certain conditions clumps of red cells form on the blood film. These clumps may appear as agglutinated masses (auto-agglutination) or as intertwining columns (rouleaux). The former occur in severe types of autoimmune haemolytic anaemia, and the latter in diseases in which abnormal globulins are present in the serum, e.g. multiple myeloma.

THE WHITE CELLS (LEUCOCYTES)
The total leucocyte count
This is carried out by an electronic cell counter (see page 191). The total white cell count is more often of diagnostic value than a red cell count, and fortunately visual counting is less tedious to perform and an error is not so important as in a red cell count. For example, an error of 20 per cent between 8000 and 10,000 cells per mm^3 ($8 - 10 \times 10^9/l$) is not significant.

The normal leucocyte count in adults is from 4000 to 11,000 cells per mm^3 ($4–11 \times 10^9/l$). Slight fluctuations in the count occur during the day and also from day to day. In childhood and during pregnancy the count is usually increased by 2000–5000 cells per mm^3 ($2–5 \times 10^9/l$), and a more pronounced increase may occur after delivery and with strenuous exercise.

The stained blood film
The various types of white cell are identified and recorded as a differential count. One hundred white cells are counted and the number of each variety recorded. The cells are of two main types – granular and non-granular.

Granular cells
These cells, the granulocytes, include the neutrophil, eosinophil and basophil polymorphonuclear leucocytes which respectively contain fine pink granules, coarse red granules and coarse blue granules. They vary in size from 10 to 15 mm. In severe infections and other toxic conditions vacuoles and basophilic granules are sometimes found in the cytoplasm of the neutrophils; this is known as toxic granulation. The nuclei of the neutrophil polymorphs normally have two to five lobes, but less

than 10 per cent of the nuclei have five lobes. An increase in the number of cells containing multilobed nuclei is known as a 'shift to the right'; the converse is described as a 'shift to the left'. An increase in cells with more than four lobes in the nucleus is more probably due to disordered nuclear development than to increased age of the cells and is frequently the result of folic acid and vitamin B_{12} deficiency. A 'shift to the left' occurs in chronic myeloid and acute myeloblastic leukaemia, and in association with the leucocytosis found in various toxic conditions, e.g. burns and pyogenic infections.

Non-granular cells

These include the large and small lymphocytes (size 7–18 μm) and the monocytes (size 12–20 μm). The small lymphocyte has a darkly staining nucleus with a narrow rim of sky-blue cytoplasm. The large lymphocyte has a broader rim of cytoplasm which often stains less deeply. Usually granules are absent from the cytoplasm, but sometimes several bright red granules are found. Monocytes, often twice the size of a lymphocyte, have a lightly staining reticular and indented nucleus and a variable amount of greyish cytoplasm which is often filled with numerous reddish-blue granules.

The differential count of the white cells is represented by the following average normal figures:

Neutrophils	2.5–7.5 x 10^9/l
Lymphocytes	1.5–3.5 x 10^9/l
Monocytes	0.2–0.8 x 10^9/l
Eosinophils	0.04–0.44 x 10^9/l
Basophils	0–0.1 x 10^9/l

Immature white cells

In the examination of a stained blood film the presence of immature white cells, which are normally present only in the bone-marrow, is especially significant, and when these are abundant it generally indicates the presence of a leukaemia. Small numbers of immature white cells (myelocytes and metamyelocytes) may be found in various other disorders, e.g. myelofibrosis, disseminated carcinoma and megaloblastic and post-haemorrhagic anaemias. However, the most primitive form of white cell (blast cell) is usually found only in chronic myeloid (granulocytic) and acute leukaemias.

Abnormalities of the differential and total white cell counts

An increase in the total number of white cells is termed leucocytosis, and a decrease leucopenia. Both leucocytosis and a leucopenia are usually associated with a change in the differential count. For instance, in the leucocytosis which occurs in pneumococcal pneumonia there is an increase in the number of neutrophils, and in the leucopenia which occurs in hypoplastic anaemia there is a decrease in the polymorphonuclear leucocytes.

An increase in the number of neutrophils (neutrophilia) appears most frequently in sepsis (particularly coccal infections) if the body is capable of making a good defensive reaction. The count may rise to between 15,000 and 50,000 per mm³ (15–50 x 0^9/l). Neutrophilia of this grade is frequently seen in acute infections such as cellulitis, pneumonia and erysipelas, and where pus has actually been formed, e.g. in empyema, the count attains the higher levels. Neutrophilia may also be found following acute haemorrhage and myocardial infarction and in acute haemolytic anaemias, myelofibrosis, cachectic conditions such as carcinoma, and certain metabolic disturbances, e.g. gout, diabetic ketosis, or uraemia. In grave infections leucocytosis is often slight or absent owing to the profound toxaemia, which impairs the function of the bone-marrow. An eosinophilia occurs in parasitic infestations and allergic conditions, e.g. bronchial asthma, in some cases of polyarteritis nodosa, and in Hodgkin's disease. A lymphocytosis occurs in whooping-cough and during the convalescent stage of mumps and rubella. In infectious mononucleosis the blood picture is characterized by a lymphocytosis and monocytosis and by the presence of abnormal mononuclear cells.

The number of neutrophils may be diminished (neutropenia) in certain specific diseases, such as typhoid, influenza and measles, and in megaloblastic and hypoplastic anaemias. The syndrome called agranulocytosis, in which there is a complete disappearance of granulocytes usually presents with a sore throat or fever in a patient who is disproportionately ill. In susceptible persons certain drugs, e.g. sulphonamides and chloramphenicol, among many, may cause agranulocytosis by a direct toxic action on the granulocyte precursors in the bone-marrow. A decrease in the number of both granulocytes and lymphocytes occurs only rarely and is found in Felty's syndrome (rheumatoid arthritis and splenomegaly) and in disseminated lupus erythematosus. (For Leukaemias, see page 197.) A reduction in the lymphocyte count alone is a feature of AIDS.

THE BLOOD PLATELETS (THROMBOCYTES)

The platelets are small spherical, oval or rod-shaped bodies, and on staining they have a light blue cytoplasm packed with azure granules. They are concerned with the production of thrombi and the control of haemorrhage from the capillaries. In health they number 150,000–450,000 per mm³ (150–450 x 0^9/l). They are increased (thrombocytosis) as a reaction to carcinoma and chronic inflammatory states, in polycythaemia vera and sometimes in chronic myeloid leukaemia and after splenectomy or acute haemorrhage. A decrease in the number of platelets is termed thrombocytopenia, and the causes of this are discussed on page 199.

EXAMINATION OF THE BONE-MARROW

The marrow is obtained by inserting a special needle into the marrow cavity of the upper portion of the sternum, between the second and third ribs, under local anaesthesia. Alternative sites from which marrow may be obtained are the iliac crests, the spinous processes of the vertebrae and the ribs. A small quantity of material (about 0.2 ml) is aspirated into a 10 ml syringe, and stained films are made from it in the same manner as blood films.

In the cytological examination of the bone-marrow particular consideration should be given to the following:

1 The absolute numbers of the myeloid and erythroid series of cells and the ratio between these two groups of cells; this is known as the myeloid: erythroid ratio, and is usually in the region of from 2:1 to 6:1. These observations will determine whether there is a relative increase in activity of either the myeloid or erythroid series.
2 The morphological appearance of the erythroid series of cells in order to determine whether erythropoiesis is normoblastic or megaloblastic.
3 The morphological appearance of the myeloid series of cells, and in particular whether there is a predominance of primitive 'blast' cells.
4 The presence of cells which are normally either not found in the bone marrow or are only present in small numbers, such as lymphocytes, myeloma cells or tumour cells. A bone-marrow biopsy rather than an aspirate gives a more reliable guide to marrow infiltration and cellularity.
5 The quantity and morphology of the megakaryocytes, from which the blood platelets are produced.

THE DIAGNOSIS OF HAEMATOLOGICAL DISEASES

ANAEMIAS

There are three causes of anaemia:

1 Haemorrhage.
2 Defective erythropoiesis (red cell production).

3 Increased haemolysis (red cell destruction).

Of these the commonest is loss of blood.

Post-haemorrhagic anaemia

The most apparent cause for anaemia is acute haemorrhage, and where it is from obvious sources, e.g. wounds, haematemesis, haemoptysis or epistaxis. it should not escape notice. The loss of blood by profuse haemorrhage causes symptoms of shock, referable to the sudden decrease in blood volume (collapse, low blood pressure, tachycardia, thirst, etc.). These symptoms do not occur when the loss of blood is gradual and should not be confused with those of severe anaemia.

The possibility of concealed haemorrhage must not be overlooked as a cause of rapidly produced anaemia, and when symptoms of haemorrhage occur without obvious cause, such contingencies as melaena, haemorrhage into serous spaces or muscle or ruptured ectopic gestation should be considered. The blood picture in acute post-haemorrhagic anaemias shows an equal reduction in red cells and haemoglobin. The red cells are usually normochromic, and there are numerous polychromatic cells which are macrocytic.

Anaemias due to defective red cell production

Iron deficiency

This could have been considered in the previous section on post-haemorrhagic anaemias, as chronic blood loss is the most important cause. However, poor diet, impaired iron absorption and increased iron requirements (childhood, adolescence, pregnancy) are often important contributory factors and may be the chief causes of iron deficiency in the developing countries.

The blood picture is characterized by the low haemoglobin content of the red cells producing hypochromia and microcytosis. The MCH and MCV are reduced.

Iron-deficiency anaemia is most frequently found in women between 20 and 45 years, when the iron requirements are increased by menstrual haemorrhage and repeated pregnancies. When iron deficiency occurs in men, or in women who have passed the menopause, a particularly careful search should be made for sources of occult bleeding, especially from the gastrointestinal tract, e.g. peptic ulcer, hiatus hernia, gastric bleeding induced by aspirin and malignant disease of the stomach or large bowel.

The predominant symptoms are those of oxygen deficiency (page 187), but stomatitis and glossitis are common. Dysphagia (Plummer–Vinson syndrome) occurs rarely and the spleen may be palpable. Inflammatory and atrophic changes in the gastric mucosa, leading to impaired secretion of hydrochloric acid in the gastric juice, are frequently present. The nails may be spoon-shaped (koilonychia) (Figure 8.10), although this sign is comparatively rare. (See Chapter 3, page 41.)

Vitamin B₁₂ deficiency

Dietary deficiency of vitamin B_{12} commonly occurs in many developing countries. In the developed countries vitamin B_{12} deficiency is usually caused by impaired absorption, and dietary deficiency only occurs in those people who do not eat any food of animal origin (vegans). The conditions which cause impaired absorption of vitamin B_{12} are:

1　Deficiency of gastric intrinsic factor, which occurs in pernicious anaemia and following total gastrectomy and occasionally partial gastrectomy.
2　Diseases of the ileum (e.g. Crohn's disease) which is the site of vitamin B_{12} absorption.
3　The abnormal growth of bacteria in the small intestine, which assimilate vitamin B_{12} for their own metabolism. This may occur when there are strictures, fistulas and blind loops of bowel.
4　Infestation of the intestine with the fish tape-worm, *Diphyllobothrium latum*. This is confined to Scandinavia.

Vitamin B_{12} deficiency produces a macrocytic anaemia, and, when the anaemia is severe, marked anisocytosis and poikilocytosis. There is usually a decrease in the number of neutrophils and platelets in the blood. The bone-marrow picture is megaloblastic. It is advisable to confirm the presence of vitamin B_{12} deficiency by assaying the level of the vitamin in the serum before committing the patient to life-long treatment. This is usually done by a radio-assay method.

Pernicious anaemia is the most common of the diseases classified above. The disease is rare before the age of 40. Predominant symptoms, in addition to those of Hb deficiency, include sore tongue and loss of appetite and weight. Symptoms due to degenerative changes in the spinal cord and peripheral nerves are now rare (see page 271). Mental symptoms are not uncommon. The tongue is often smooth and red (glossitis; Figure 8.11), and the spleen may be palpable. Haemolysis results from the defective erythropoiesis and, when severe, gives rise to the characteristic lemon-yellow pallor. Petechiae may also occur. After giving histamine or pentagastrin, there is virtually always an absence of secretion of acid in the gastric juice.

Confirmation of the diagnosis of pernicious anaemia is obtained by demonstrating:

1　A macrocytic anaemia with megaloblastic marrow.
2　A low serum vitamin B_{12} level.
3　Impaired absorption of vitamin B_{12}, corrected by intrinsic factor, measured by radioactive isotope techniques.
4　Autoantibody estimation: anti-intrinsic factor and parietal cell.
5　Good response to vitamin B_{12} therapy.

Folic acid deficiency

The causes of folic acid deficiency are:

1　Dietary deficiency: This is widespread in many of the developing countries. In Western countries it occurs more commonly than was hitherto supposed in persons with impaired appetite, due in particular to psychiatric and gastric disorders.
2　Impaired absorption from the jejunum: extensive involvement of the jejunal mucosa is required before folic acid absorption is affected, and this occurs in

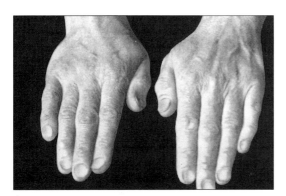

▲ **Figure 8.10 Koilonychia, from a case of iron-deficiency anaemia.** The nails show a spoon-shaped or salt-cellar defect

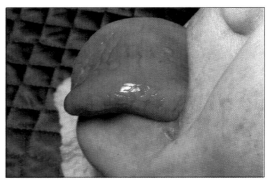

▲ **Figure 8.11 A smooth, red depapillated tongue with angular cheilosis.** These changes may be caused by deficiency of iron, folic acid or vitamin B_{12}

idiopathic steatorrhoea (coeliac disease) and in tropical sprue.

3 Increased requirements: megaloblastic anaemia due to increased folic acid requirements occurs frequently in pregnancy, unless prophylactic folic acid is given, and occasionally in certain other conditions: haemolytic anaemia, repeated haemorrhage, extensive dermatitis and widespread neoplastic disease, e.g. multiple myeloma, myelofibrosis and carcinomatosis.

4 Impaired utilization: certain drugs, notably phenytoin sodium (Epanutin), can antagonize the action of folic acid and thus cause megaloblastic anaemia.

The blood and bone-marrow pictures are indistinguishable from those due to vitamin B_{12} deficiency. Glossitis and icterus may be present, but neurological signs are most unusual. Free acid is frequently present in the gastric juice.

Folic acid deficiency is virtually always the main cause of megaloblastic anaemia of pregnancy. Otherwise it may be necessary to assay the serum levels of vitamin B_{12} and folic acid and to investigate the absorptive function of the gastrointestinal tract in order to distinguish anaemias arising from vitamin B_{12} and folic acid deficiency.

Other diseases

Other diseases in which red cell production is impaired are:

1 Lymphomas, see page 198
2 Diseases infiltrating the bone-marrow:
• Leukaemias, see page 198
• Myelofibrosis, see page 198
• Multiple myeloma (infiltration of bone-marrow; Bence Jones protein in urine; 'M' band in serum globulin on electrophoresis)
3 Infections, generally subacute or chronic lasting more than a month, e.g subacute bacterial endocarditis, chronic pyelonephritis
4 Renal and hepatic failure
5 Carcinomatosis
6 Hypoplastic anaemias due to toxic agents, e.g. irradiation, benzine derivatives, cytotoxic drugs, and in sensitive persons chloramphenicol, antithyroid drugs and other therapeutic agents
7 Endocrine disorders (hypofunction of the thyroid or adrenal cortex may produce a mild anaemia) Collagen diseases

Anaemias due to excessive red cell destruction

These can be classified into two main groups: hereditary and acquired.

Hereditary

In this group there is an abnormality of the red cells. The main examples are hereditary spherocytosis, the haemoglobinopathies, including the thalassaemias and sickle cell disease (Figure 8.12) and red cell enzyme deficiencies, e.g. drug-induced haemolysis and favism due to deficiency of glucose-6-phosphate dehydrogenase. The haemoglobinopathies occur mainly in the Negro race. Thalassaemia and glucose-6-phosphate dehydrogenase deficiency have a wide racial distribution in tropical, subtropical and Mediterranean countries, but occur very rarely in Northern Europeans.

Acquired

In this group the fundamental abnormality is outside the red cells. The main examples are acquired auto-immune haemolytic anaemia and erythroblastosis foetalis, in which there is a specific red cell antibody. Red cell destruction may also be produced by bacterial, metabolic, or chemical toxins, by burns and by protozoal parasites, e.g. septicaemia, uraemia, lead poisoning and malaria.

Clinical description

Haemolytic anaemia may be fulminating and acute or insidious and chronic, and the latter may be punctuated by episodes of more acute haemolysis. By and large the manifestations tend to be more severe in acquired auto-immune haemolytic anaemia than in hereditary spherocytosis, in which the mild cases have been described as 'more yellow than sick'.

During the acute episodes the symptoms often suggest an acute febrile illness with sudden weakness, headache, shivering, vomiting and aching pain in the limbs, back and abdomen. The abdominal pain may occasionally be so severe and be accompanied by such marked muscular rigidity as to simulate an acute surgical condition. Anuria or oliguria may develop, and the urine may be very dark due to haemosiderin or haemoglobin.

Pallor and jaundice of varying degree are found, more pronounced during the phases of acute haemolysis. Jaundice, however, is usually only slight unless the bile duct is obstructed by pigment gallstones. Splenomegaly, except in sickle cell anaemia, is common in acute and chronic haemolytic anaemias. The organ may be just palpable or it may be huge. Moderate enlargement of the liver may also occur. Chronic leg ulcers are common in sickle cell anaemia and may occur in hereditary spherocytosis.

Deformity of the skull with overgrowth of the maxillae occurs in certain congenital haemolytic anaemias. Patients with sickle cell anaemia tend to be tall and thin with long legs and often suffer from osteoarthrosis of the hip joints; rarely, cerebral infarction or haemorrhage may occur (Figure 8.12).

Haemolytic anaemia is usually associated with an increase in the number of reticulocytes in the peripheral blood and a slight to moderate rise in the levels of serum bilirubin and urine urobilinogen. However, these abnormalities are not only related to the degree of haemolysis but also to the capacity of the bone-marrow response and to liver function. Bile is only found in the urine when the patient develops obstructive jaundice due to the formation of pigment gallstones. When the haemolysis is severe, methaemalbumin can be detected in the plasma by Schumm's test (the spectroscopic detection of a haemochromogen band at 558 µm after the addition of concentrated ammonium sulphide to the serum or plasma), and haemoglobin and haemosiderin may occasionally be present in the urine.

The osmotic fragility of the red cells is always increased in hereditary spherocytosis. It is usually increased in acquired auto-immune haemolytic anaemia depending on the number of the spherocytes present, and it is decreased in thalassaemia. Acquired auto-immune haemolytic anaemia is diagnosed by the detection of an incomplete antibody coating the patient's red cells (direct Coombs' test), and quite frequently the incomplete antibody can also be detected in the serum (indirect Coombs' test). Occasionally when the evidence for increased haemolysis is equivocal or when splenectomy is being considered in auto-immune haemolytic anaemia, it is of value to determine the red cell survival and the principal sites of red cell destruction by methods using cells tagged with the radioactive isotope ^{51}Cr. For the laboratory diagnosis of the haemoglobinopathies, thalassaemia and red cell enzyme deficiencies the reader should consult a textbook of haematology.

LEUKAEMIAS

This is a group of conditions characterized by widespread proliferation of the leucocytes and their precursors in the tissues of the body. They are classified into acute and chronic forms, the distinction resting on the rapidity of the disease and on the stage of maturity of the predominant cells. Both the acute and chronic forms are further subdivided according to the dominant type of cell.

Acute myeloblastic leukaemia

This occurs particularly in adults and there is a slight predominance among males. The onset is sudden and the course short. Anaemia, fever and prostration rapidly develop. Often there are extensive haemorrhagic manifestations – petechiae, epistaxis, uterine bleeding – and necrotic lesions develop in the mouth and throat. There is usually slight or moderate splenomegaly. Enlargement of the lymph nodes is unusual except in the monocytic form when the cervical nodes may be considerably enlarged. There may be exquisite tenderness over the bones, the sternum and the tibiae especially. Moderate or severe anaemia is usually found, and the number of platelets is often below 100,000 per mm^3 (100 x 10^9/1). The total white cell count may be decreased or normal but is usually increased. Myeloblasts may form more than 60 per cent of the circulating white cells. In some cases they are completely absent with a neutropenia, but the bone-marrow is packed with them (aleukaemic leukaemia).

Acute lymphoblastic leukaemia

This variety occurs most frequently in childhood. The symptoms and signs are similar to those of the myeloblastic form but enlargement of the spleen and lymph nodes tends to be more pronounced. The blood and bone-marrow pictures can usually be distinguished from myeloblastic leukaemia by ordinary staining methods but special cytochemical stains and membrane marker studies are available to help.

Chronic myeloid leukaemia

This disease is rare before the age of 25 and most common between 30 and 65. The sex incidence is equal.

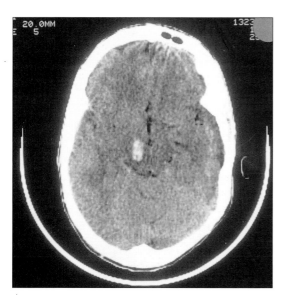

▲ **Figure 8.12 Intracranial haemorrhage in a 24-year-old patient with sickle cell disease**

The onset is insidious and early diagnosis is often accidental during the routine examination of a blood film. The symptoms may be classified into those resulting from anaemia, those caused by the gross enlargement of the spleen (abdominal discomfort or a visible mass) and those attributable to the increased metabolic rate (loss of weight, cachexia and excessive sweating). Dominant physical signs are the great enlargement of the spleen and to a lesser extent of the liver, and, later, anaemia. A well-marked leucocytosis is the rule with counts ranging from 100,000 to 750,000 per mm^3 (100–750 x 10^9/1). The increase is due to cells of the granulocyte series with neutrophils, metamyelocytes and myelocytes. There is only a small number of myeloblasts. The Philadelphia chromosome and a low leucocyte alkaline phosphatase score are usually present.

Myelofibrosis

This condition clinically may resemble chronic myeloid leukaemia as there is splenomegaly, leucocytosis and the presence of immature cells of the granular series. Myelofibrosis may be distinguished from myeloid leukaemia by the finding of marrow fibrosis in the former condition and by the presence in the latter of the Philadelphia chromosome (Ph$_1$) and decreased leucocyte alkaline phosphatase activity.

Chronic lymphatic leukaemia

In contrast to chronic myeloid leukaemia, this occurs mainly in elderly men. Enlargement of the lymph nodes is a salient feature, while splenomegaly is less marked than in myeloid leukaemia, and the total leucocyte count tends to be lower, the majority of the cells being mature lymphocytes.

LYMPHOMAS

This term is used to classify a group of neoplastic diseases that are characterized clinically by enlargement of the lymph nodes and spleen. The principal members of this group are Hodgkin's disease and the non-Hodgkin's lymphomas. In most cases it is impossible to distinguish these disorders from one another, either clinically or from examination of the blood and bone-marrow, and lymph node biopsy is necessary to confirm the diagnosis.

Hodgkin's disease

This condition may occur at any age but is observed chiefly between the age of 20 and 40 years. Males are affected more often than females. The course of the disease may be variable but the prognosis has improved dramatically with modern treatment. Enlargement of the

superficial groups of lymph nodes is usually the presenting symptom, and constitutional symptoms, also known as 'B' symptoms (night sweats, recurrent fever, loss of weight), if present, are signs of poor prognosis. The enlarged lymph nodes are usually painless. They remain discrete, have an elastic character on palpation, and do not become adherent to the skin. The fever sometimes exhibits periodicity (the Pel–Ebstein phenomenon). Palpable enlargement of the spleen and liver and involvement of abdominal and thoracic lymph nodes indicate a later state of the disease. The presence of cold agglutinins may cause digital infarction (Figure 8.13).

Anaemia is common and is rarely associated with haemolysis. There may be either a neutrophilia, an eosinophilia or a lymphopenia. The histological appearance of the lymph nodes is characterized by the wide variety of proliferating cells; these include neutrophils, eosinophils, lymphocytes, plasma cells and multi-nucleated giant cells (Reed Sternberg cells).

Other forms of lymphoma

These non-Hodgkin's lymphomas can be divided into a low grade group in which the cause is indolent, and a higher histological grade with a more aggressive clinical course and for which more intensive treatment is necessary. The age incidence of these diseases tends to be higher than in Hodgkin's disease and the disease is more often clinically disseminated at diagnosis (Figure 8.14)

HAEMORRHAGIC DISEASES

After injury to a vessel, the process of normal haemostasis takes place in three phases:

1 Vessel wall contraction.
2 Platelet aggregation and plugging of the injured area.
3 The formation of an insoluble fibrin clot from soluble fibrinogen due to the activation of the intrinsic

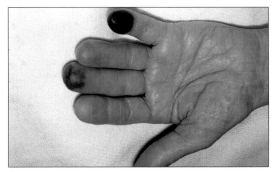

▲ **Figure 8.13 Digital infarction due to intravascular thrombosis caused by cold agglutinins in Hodgkin's disease**

and extrinsic blood clotting system; this third step takes a few minutes to get under way.

There is, in addition, a fibrinolytic system which actively removes the clot. Thus the haemorrhagic diseases can result from abnormalities of blood vessels, platelets or the intrinsic or extrinsic clotting systems. Diseases affecting the smaller blood vessels or platelets produce the clinical picture of purpura. Disorders of the clotting systems may be congenital (e.g. haemophilia) or acquired (deficiency of prothrombin or fibrinogen).

Purpura

This is characterized by extravasation of blood into the skin, causing purple spots varying in size from a pinhead (petechiae) to large bruises (ecchymoses). Sometimes haemorrhage also occurs from the mucosae, for example, in the nose, gastrointestinal tract and uterus. Purpura is due to increased capillary permeability and this may result from a deficiency in the number (thrombocytopenia) or function (thrombasthenia) of platelets, or from damage to the capillary walls by antibodies (allergic purpura), vitamin C deficiency (Figure 8.15), drugs and bacterial and metabolic toxins, e.g. bacterial endocarditis and uraemia.

In elderly persons purpura frequently occurs on the back of the forearms and hands. This is called senile pur-

pura and results from rupture of small vessels due to increased mobility of the inelastic skin. Similar lesions are caused by prolonged corticosteroid therapy (Figure 8.16).

Thrombocytopenic purpura may be primary (idiopathic thrombocytopenic purpura) due to the development of platelet antibodies, or secondary due to suppression of the bone-marrow as in hypoplastic anaemia, pernicious anaemia, acute and chronic leukaemias (see Figure 8.1, page 188), secondary carcinoma and certain forms of drug therapy. The spleen is rarely enlarged in idiopathic thrombocytopenic purpura, and then it is only just palpable.

One type of allergic purpura is referred to as the Henoch–Schönlein syndrome and is characterized by haemorrhage from the gastrointestinal tract and kidneys, serous effusions into the joints and purpuric and urticarial skin rashes. It is frequently related to infection with the haemolytic streptococcus.

The closure of capillaries which occurs after injury depends on normal platelet numbers and function, and therefore the bleeding time is prolonged in cases of thrombocytopenic purpura. In other types of purpura the bleeding time may be prolonged, but sometimes it is normal. The measurement of bleeding time has been made more accurate by modifying the Ivy technique by the use of a template device which allows a standardized incision to be made on the skin of the forearm. The bleeding time using a template is normally between 2.5 and 8 minutes.

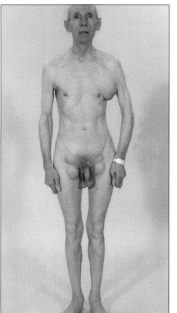

◀ **Figure 8.14 Lymphoma: enlargement of axillary and inguinal lymph nodes**

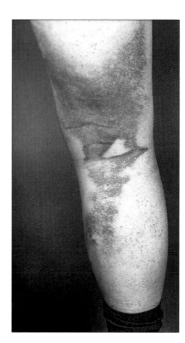

◀ **Figure 8.15 Scurvy: bruising of the thigh**

Scurvy

Scurvy, both in adult and infantile forms, is due to a deficiency of vitamin C in the diet. There may be extensive ecchymoses on the legs (Figure 8.15), and petechiae occur characteristically around the hair follicles. Haemorrhages from any mucous membrane may take place but are most commonly seen in the mouth (Figure 8.17), where the spongy bleeding gums (if the patient has teeth) are always a suggestive feature in a patient who has been undernourished or incorrectly fed.

Congenital clotting disorders

Haemophilia

This is a sex-linked hereditary deficiency of clotting factor, either factor VIII (haemophilia A) or factor IX (haemophilia B or Christmas disease), and each is almost entirely confined to males. The female cases are either carriers who typically have very mild symptoms, or women who acquire antibodies to clotting factors (usually factor VIII) in whom the haemophilia is often untreatable. A male haemophiliac transmits the carrier state to all his daughters, and they in turn transmit the haemophilic state to 50 per cent of their sons. A careful family history must therefore be taken in bleeding disorders.

The diagnosis of haemophilia should be considered when profuse haemorrhage occurs from such minor causes as cuts and tooth extraction, and when there are episodes of spontaneous haemorrhage into the muscles and joints, peritoneal cavity and the renal and gastrointestinal tracts. Recurrent haemarthroses may lead to ankylosis of the affected joints, especially the knees, with disuse atrophy of adjacent muscles. The initial bleeding time is normal as this depends on capillary contractility and not on the coagulability of the blood. There is a tendency, however, for the bleeding to recommence after an interval of several minutes. The clotting time of the blood is prolonged, but to confirm the diagnosis it is necessary to demonstrate a low or absent factor VIII or factor IX.

von Willebrand's disease

More common than haemophilia, this condition affects the sexes equally and is due to a lack of the factor VIII-carrying protein (known as von Willebrand's factor). Patients present with bleeding more typical of platelet deficit since von Willebrand's factor is essential for platelet aggregation.

Acquired clotting disorders

Haemorrhage due to vitamin K dependent coagulation factor deficiency may occur in severe liver disease (see Chapter 4) or as a result of anticoagulant therapy.

Hypofibrinogenaemia can also result from destruction of the liver but is more commonly produced by release from the tissues into the circulation of thromboplastin, which consumes fibrinogen by bringing about intravascular clotting and secondary activation fibrinolysis. The condition usually occurs as a result of:

1 Obstetrical complications – abruptio placentae and intra-uterine retention of a dead fetus.
2 Extensive physical trauma.
3 Pulmonary surgery.

It is termed 'disseminated intravascular coagulation'.

The clinical picture may present with the sudden appearance of severe bleeding from mucous membranes and extensive ecchymoses, or in some cases the bleeding may be only slight. The clotting time of the blood is greatly prolonged. The failure of the blood to clot rapidly after the addition of thrombin distinguishes hypofibrinogenaemia from other disorders of coagulation.

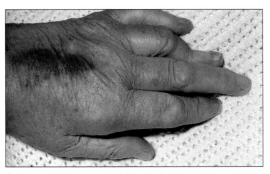

▲ **Figure 8.16 Purpura on the back of the hand of a patient receiving corticosteroid therapy for rheumatoid arthritis.**
Note the deformities of the interphalangeal joints

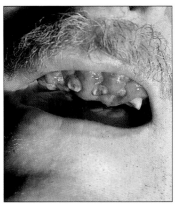

◀ **Figure 8.17 Scurvy showing the condition of the gums**

The skeletal system

The skeletal system provides not only the strength to support the body and to protect vital organs, but also the flexibility to permit a wide range of movement at the joints of the axial skeleton and the limbs. The following description of the symptoms and signs arising in the skeleton especially refers to those generalized disorders affecting bones and joints. The student must be aware, however, of the orthopaedic and traumatic lesions of this system.

SYMPTOMS

The chief symptoms arising in the skeletal system are pain, deformity, impaired movement and cracking and creaking.

PAIN

Pain may originate from bone and periosteum, the capsule and synovia of joints, the ligaments, tendons and muscles. Bone pain is usually continuous, aching and disturbs sleep, whilst that arising in the joints and their adnexae is more often sharp, related to posture or to movement and accompanied by a feeling of stiffness. Pain in the limb joints is usually well localized with the exception of the hip, when discomfort may be referred to the knee. In the vertebral column, however, degenerative osteoarthritis in the cervical or lumbar spine often produces referred as well as local pain. The former is produced by pressure on nerve roots and may indicate the segmental level of the lesion giving rise to brachial neuritis and sciatica (see page 266). Sneezing, coughing and straining at stool may aggravate the discomfort by raising the intraspinal pressure.

DEFORMITY

The patient or relatives may notice painless alteration in the appearance of the skull and face (Paget's disease, Figure 9.1, or acromegaly), hands (Heberden's nodes), legs (Paget's disease or rickets), joints (Charcot's neuropathy), or the gradual loss of height and spinal curvature in osteoporosis of the vertebrae.

IMPAIRED MOVEMENT

When movement is limited by pain and stiffness the skeletal system is usually at fault but diminished movement without these symptoms suggests a neurological lesion. In rheumatoid arthritis stiffness is noted especially on first awakening in the morning and symptoms may improve as the day progresses. However, in osteoarthritis, movement is restricted after using the joints at the end of the day or on first using the joints after a period of immobility.

CRACKING AND CREAKING

Minor clicks in the finger joints produced by passive hyperextension are of no significance nor are clicks arising in the shoulder joint or scapula, sometimes heard during auscultation of the chest. Snowball crunching in the knee during active or passive movement is heard when the articular cartilage is badly damaged as a result of osteoarthritis.

CONSTITUTIONAL SYMPTOMS

Fever and sweating with joint involvement accompany septic arthritis and rheumatic fever, and the latter may be associated with a skin eruption - erythema marginatum. Rashes can be diagnostic in psoriatic arthropathy, Reiter's disease and systemic lupus erythematosus. Breathlessness and pleuritic chest pain may precede or accompany the arthritis in rheumatoid disease and other connective tissue disorders. Eye symptoms such as conjunctivitis in Reiter's disease, dry eyes in Sjögren's syndrome, or a painful iritis in ankylosing spondylitis may give useful clues. Blue sclerae may be noted in children

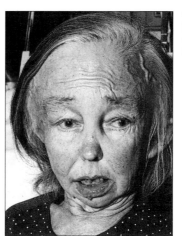
◀ Figure 9.1 Paget's disease: enlargement of the head

with multiple fractures due to osteogenesis imperfecta (Figure 9.2). Raynaud's phenomenon may herald rheumatoid arthritis, systemic sclerosis or systemic lupus erythematosus (Figure 9.3) and genital symptoms such as urethritis in Reiter's disease or penile and vaginal ulceration in Behçet's syndrome should merit specific inquiry. Alteration in bowel habit may accompany ankylosing spondylitis, Reiter's disease or systemic sclerosis and bulky stools indicating malabsorption may be associated with osteomalacia. Painful recurrent mouth ulcers suggest Behçet's syndrome and in Paget's disease blindness and deafness may be disabling complications.

SIGNS

Physical examination should first consist of a general inspection of the patient with special attention to stance, gait, posture, height, skeletal proportion and the performance of simple tasks such as dressing, bending or rising from a chair.

The observer should note the appearance of the face and then examine the skull, jaw, rib cage, spinal column and pelvis, and each limb in turn, comparing one side with the other and noting any abnormality in structure or function of the joints and adjacent tissues: the bones, cartilage, synoviae, bursae, ligaments, tendons, fascia, muscles, subcutaneous tissue and overlying skin.

INSPECTION

Inspection will reveal any gross deformity, displacement or enlargement of bone such as occurs in tumours (primary or secondary), Paget's disease (Figure 9.1) and osteomalacia.

On inspection of the joints, the examiner will look for swelling, discoloration and deformities, including ulnar deviation of the fingers, spinal scoliosis (Figure 9.4), flexion of the knee and clawing of the toes. He will then observe the range of active movement and the patient's ability to use the joints for everyday purposes such as gripping, putting on shoes, eating and combing the hair. Nodular lesions, swelling of tendon sheaths and muscle wasting around the joint (see Figure 9.16) are also noted, remembering that muscle wasting can give a false impression of joint enlargement. Particular attention is paid to the distribution of joint changes through-

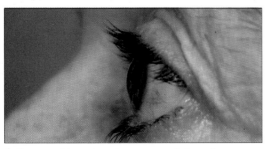

▲ Figure 9.2 Blue sclerae in osteogenesis imperfecta

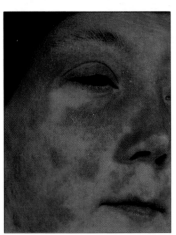

◀ Figure 9.3 Butterfly rash in systemic lupus erythematosus

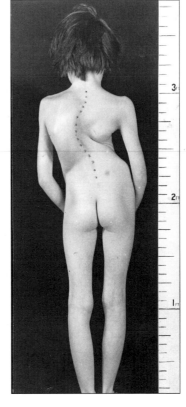

◀ Figure 9.4 Thoracic scoliosis: idiopathic or adolescent type

out the body since this may be of prime importance in the differential diagnosis of arthritis (Table 9.1).

PALPATION

Palpation must be gentle and sudden sharp movements avoided. The patient's face should be watched for signs of distress when the joints are moved or tender parts are explored. Palpation is used to detect a raised temperature over a bone or joint. For this purpose the back of the fingers may be more sensitive than the palmar surface. An increased temperature indicates a high blood flow (e.g. Paget's disease) or inflammation (e.g. septic arthritis, rheumatoid arthritis or rheumatic fever). Palpation is also used to elicit tenderness over bones or ligaments; to determine the anatomical origin and consistency of any swellings (fluid, synovial, bony, cartilaginous, tendinous, sub-cutaneous); to measure the range and power of movement at each joint and, at the same time, to note crepitus or abnormal mobility. Examples of unusual mobility are observed in Charcot's knee joints and the Ehlers–Danlos syndrome in which lax ligaments permit hyperextensibility (Figure 9.5). Fluid accumulations within the joint or adjacent bursae can be recognized by the presence of fluctuation. This is most easily detected in a knee joint, when a brisk depression of the patella causes displacement of the fluid and a slight knock of the patella against the underlying bone (patella tap).

MOVEMENT

To assess the range and power of a joint is an important part of the clinical examination. Active movements test the function not only of the joint under consideration but also the tendons, muscles and nerves, whereas passive movements test the state of the joint itself and are therefore more useful. When movement is limited by pain or fixation an attempt should be made to determine the cause. If the bone, cartilage or synovial membrane is diseased, movement is limited in all directions and tenderness is generalized. If the capsule or ligament is damaged, movement towards the affected structure relieves the pain. Tenderness will be detected locally and an effusion may be present. If an intra-articular structure is present, such as a detached semilunar cartilage in the knee, movement is restricted by pain when the joint is compressed towards the detached fragment and relieved by movement away from it.

Complete lack of joint movement because of pain is due to recent trauma or acute inflammation, but if painless, is due to ankylosis or arthrodesis.

The direction and degree of passive movements to be found in the joints of a healthy subject are shown in Table 9.2 and these should be recorded in all patients presenting with an arthropathy. Joint movement is measured by the goniometer, a protractor with long hinged arms, preferably transparent (Figure 9.6). Movement is recorded by the neutral zero method whereby all joints are considered to be neutral when the subject is standing upright to attention with the hands flat against the thighs.

A rough measure of temporomandibular movement is given by the distance between the incisor teeth when

ARTHRITIS: DISTRIBUTION OF JOINT CHANGES	
Disease	**Joints most commonly affected**
Rheumatic fever	Large ('flitting')
Rheumatoid arthritis	Small peripheral (MP and proximal IP)
Ankylosing spondylitis	Central (sacro-iliac, spine, hip)
Infective arthritis	Large (usually one only)
Osteo-arthritis	Weight bearing. Terminal IP (Heberden's nodes)
Gout	Small peripheral (1st metatarsophalangeal especially)
MP = metacarpophalangeal/metatarsophalangeal; IP = interphalangeal	

▲ Table 9.1

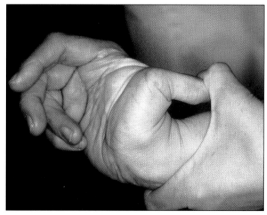

▲ **Figure 9.5 Hyperextensibility of the right thumb joint in Ehlers–Danlos syndrome.**

JOINT MOVEMENTS: SYSTEM OF EXAMINATION	
Joint	**Movements**
Jaw	Open and shut Protrusion and retraction Side to side
Spine (cervical and thoracolumbar)	Flexion and extension Lateral flexion (R & L) Rotation (R & L)
Shoulder	Flexion (180) and extension (60 Abduction (180) and adduction (45) Internal (80) and external (60) rotation
Elbow	Flexion (150)
Wrist (and forearm)	Flexion and extension (70) Ulnar (30) and radial (20) deviation Pronation (80) and supination (80)
Fingers: MP joints IP joints	Flexion (90) and extension (45) Flexion (90)
Hip	Flexion (120) and extension (30) Abduction (45) and adduction (30) Internal (80) and external (60) rotation
Knee	Flexion (135)
Ankle and foot	Plantar (50) and dorsal (20) flexion Eversion (5) and inversion (5)
Toes: MP joints IP joints	Flexion (40) and extension (40) extension (40) Eversion (15) and inversion (5) Flexion (90)

The figures in parentheses indicate range of movement in degrees. MP = metacarpophalangeal/metatarsophalangeal; IP = interphalangeal

▲ Table 9.2

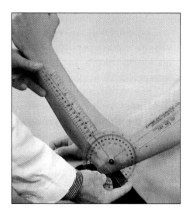

◀ Figure 9.6 The goniometer (reproduced from *Clinical Examination of the Patient* by John Lumley and Pierre-Marc G. Bouloux, Butterworth–Heinemann, 1994)

second mark 10 cm higher with the spine extended. On full flexion of the spine, the distance between these two points should increase by 4–6 cm in the healthy adult (Figure 9.7). The sacroiliac joints are virtually immobile but can be examined by local palpation and by lateral compression or 'springing' of the pelvis. These manoeuvres may induce pain or discomfort, a useful early sign of ankylosing spondylitis. Examination of the knee joint should include an assessment of the stability of the joint with particular reference to any undue 'play' in the lateral or anteroposterior plane. The range of knee joint movement is illustrated in Figure 9.8.

Active movements are used to measure the power of joint action which may be impaired not only if the bones or joints are deformed but if tendons are disrupted or muscles wasted, as in rheumatoid arthritis. Power should be recorded on a simple scale, such as one recommended by the British Medical Research Council:

0 No movement
1 Flicker of movement
2 Movement with gravity eliminated
3 Movement possible against gravity
4 Movement possible against gravity and resistance
5 Normal power

ILLUSTRATIVE DISEASES: DISEASES OF BONE

OSTEOMALACIA

Osteomalacia, or softening of the bones, results most commonly from deficiency of vitamin D, a vitamin concerned with the absorption and metabolism of calcium and phosphate and with the normal mineralization of osteoid tissue. The plasma levels of calcium and

the mouth is fully opened. Shoulder movements may be scapulo-thoracic in origin; mobility of the gleno-humeral joint itself can only be measured after fixation of the scapula. For examination of forearm pronation and supination, the arm is adducted at the shoulder and the elbow held in the flexed position. An index of the range of lumbar spine flexion can be obtained by making a mark at the lumbosacral junction and a

phosphate are usually reduced and the alkaline phosphatase raised. At one time, the commonest form of osteomalacia was rickets, a condition due to deficient dietary intake of vitamin D from the small intestine (see Malabsorption syndrome, page 74). The chief manifestation of osteomalacia is bone pain, which is usually generalized and persistent but may become acute and localized when 'pseudo-fractures' (Figure 9.9) occur. Muscle weakness, skeletal deformities and tetany due to hypocalcaemia are features of severe cases. Other signs of malabsorption may also be found (see page 74). The clinical features of childhood rickets are sim-

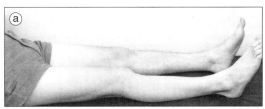

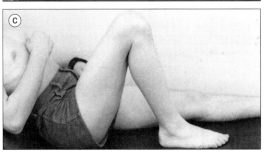

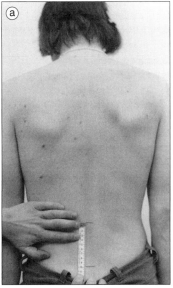

◀ **Figure 9.7 Evaluation of lumbar spine mobility.** With the patient standing upright 10 cm is measured upwards from the lumbosacral junction. The patient is then asked to bend forwards and the 10 cm should extend to 15 cm in an individual of average build. This affords a reproducible and readily repeated test of the lumbar spine mobility

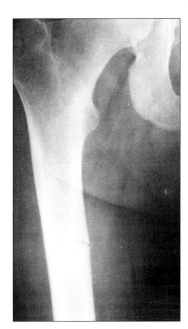

▲ **Figure 9.8 Examination of the knee.** This is conventionally recorded as three figures, e.g. 0–30–130. (a) 0 in this instance shows that, when extended, the knee is straight. (b) 30 indicates a 30° extension lag on straight-leg raising and reflects impairment of quadriceps function. (c) 130 demonstrates that flexion is possible to 130°

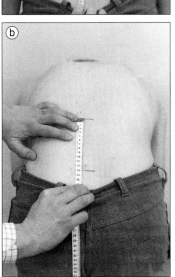

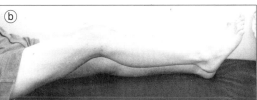

◀ **Figure 9.9 Osteomalacia.** Pseudo-fractures are seen in the cortex of the femoral shaft and in the pubic ramus

ilar to those of adult osteomalacia with the addition of tender swellings at the ends of long bones due to increased epiphyseal activity (Figure 9.10) and characteristic deformities of the skull, chest and legs.

OSTEOPOROSIS

Osteoporosis is a condition in which there is a decrease of bone mass due to loss of the glycoprotein matrix. Plasma levels of calcium, phosphate and alkaline phosphatase are usually normal. Osteoporosis occurs most commonly in elderly women (senile or postmenopausal osteoporosis), but bone resorption may also result from prolonged inactivity, deficient intake or absorption of calcium and from certain endocrine disorders, e.g. hyperthyroidism, Cushing's syndrome and corticosteroid therapy (Figure 9.11).

Episodic backache is a characteristic symptom of osteoporosis, the principal signs of which are attributable to compression and collapse of the vertebrae resulting in kyphosis and loss of height. In severe cases the lower ribs may override the pelvis and characteristic horizontal skin folds then appear over the lower chest and abdomen. In the senile group especially there is an increased susceptibility to fracture of the femoral neck and the lower end of the radius.

PAGET'S DISEASE (OSTEITIS DEFORMANS)

This is a chronic progressive bone disease of unknown cause, the incidence of which increases with age. It is characterized by rapid bone formation and resorption which at first is localized but later may extend to involve much of the skeleton. The skull and the weight-bearing bones of the spine, pelvis and leg are most commonly affected.

The clinical features include enlargement of the skull (see Figure 9.1), kyphosis and thickening and bowing of the long bones of the leg (Figure 9.12). The disease may be symptomless but bone pains are common, and there is an increased skin temperature over areas of active disease due to the high blood flow through the bone; this increased blood flow may lead to dyspnoea from high output cardiac failure. The excessive bone growth can encroach upon neural structures adjacent to skull or spine and cause such symptoms as nerve deafness and paraplegia. Osteogenic sarcoma is a rare complication. The plasma level of alkaline phosphatase is raised and the urinary excretion of hydroxyproline increased.

DISSEMINATED NEOPLASIA OF BONE

Perhaps the most common serious disorder of bone in medical practice is metastatic carcinoma secondary to a primary lesion in the breast, prostate, lung, kidney or thyroid. Bone metastases usually present with pain, a 'pathological' fracture or a bony swelling at the site of a malignant deposit. The plasma alkaline phosphatase (and, in the case of prostatic carcinoma, the acid phosphatase also) is raised with osteosclerotic metastases (e.g. breast and prostate). There may be evidence of primary or secondary tumours in other organs.

Diffuse neoplastic bone disease can also be secondary to malignant change within the bone-marrow

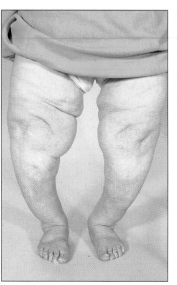

◀ **Figure 9.10 Epiphyseal enlargement.** Marked enlargement of the epiphyses of the ankles in a case of rickets. Note also bow-legs

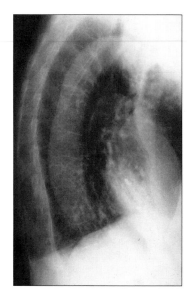

◀ **Figure 9.11 Lateral chest radiograph showing osteoporotic vertebral bodies less dense than the aorta and other intrathoracic contents**

itself, as in the case of certain lymphomas (e.g. Hodgkin's disease) and leukaemias (see page 197). A special example of this is multiple myeloma, a neoplasm of the plasma cells in which there is widespread destruction of the skeleton associated with anaemia, hypercalcaemia, impaired renal function and an increased susceptibility to infections.

HYPERPARATHYROIDISM
See page 312.

DISEASES OF JOINTS

INFLAMMATORY
Rheumatic fever
This disease is the result of a reaction to infection with β-haemolytic streptococci and therefore generally

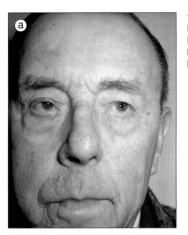
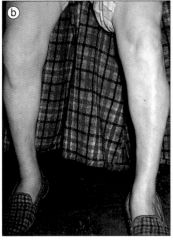

◀ **Figure 9.12 Paget's disease.** Note (a) the large head and (b) the bowing of the legs

appears 2–3 weeks after a sore throat. It now occurs mainly in those areas where overcrowding and poor economic conditions still prevail. The relative rarity of rheumatic fever today is also due to the effective antibiotic treatment of streptococcal infections.

Rheumatic fever usually presents in the school-age child or sometimes during pregnancy. The onset is generally sudden with high fever and profuse sweating. The large joints are most often attacked, but the active signs of inflammation usually manifest themselves in one joint at a time and remain 24 hours on average, before they appear in another joint. The arthritis, however, does not pass away completely from the joint first affected but remains in a subacute form. Thus it is common for one joint to show acute inflammation signs while several others are affected to a lesser extent. Each affected joint is hot, swollen and exquisitely tender. The skin over it may be reddened.

The illness may be accompanied by other rheumatic manifestations, including skin rashes (e.g. erythema marginatum), subcutaneous nodules, choreiform movements and evidence of cardiac involvement, such as a pericardial rub, systolic murmur or tachycardia disproportionate to fever. Chronic disease of the mitral and aortic valves are important complications (see Chapter 7, page 166) which may present in adults whose original rheumatic illness was too slight to be recalled.

Rheumatoid disease
Rheumatoid disease is an inflammatory condition in which immunological mechanisms play an important role. Arthritis is its principal manifestation, but the disease can affect the lungs (fibrosing alveolitis), eyes (episcleritis and kerato-conjunctivitis (Figure 9.13), pericardium and peripheral nerves. Splenomegaly and lymphadenopathy also occur. Rheumatoid nodules may be found in the subcutaneous tissues, especially over the elbow, forearm and hand, but also in the lungs and other organs (Figure 9.14). Anaemia is common and amyloi-

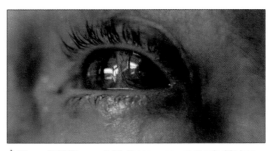

▲ **Figure 9.13 Rheumatoid disease: recurrent scleritis has led to gross scleral thinning and secondary glaucoma**

dosis a rare complication. A rheumatoid form of polyarthritis may accompany systemic disorders such as systemic lupus erythematosus and polyarteritis nodosa (Figure 9.15).

Rheumatoid arthritis is more common in women than in men and most often presents in the fourth and fifth decades. The onset may be acute or insidious and the course remittent or progressive. Although the disease process may eventually become inactive, some degree of permanent dysfunction and deformity is the rule, and in many cases disability is severe and lasting.

Although any joint in the body may be involved, the inflammation typically affects the small joints of the hands and feet in a symmetrical manner, notably the proximal interphalangeal and the second and third metacarpophalangeal joints. The terminal interpha-

langeal joints are usually spared (in contrast with gout and the psoriatic form of arthritis). Other joints commonly involved include the wrists, elbows, knees, ankles, joints of the feet, cervical spine and, occasionally, the temporomandibular joints.

The chief symptom of rheumatoid arthritis is painful joint stiffness, especially on first wakening in the morning, but constitutional symptoms such as fatigue, anorexia and weight loss also occur. In acute disease the affected joints are swollen and warm, tender to touch and painful on motion. In advanced cases there will be diminished range of joint movement due to synovial thickening, weakening of the joint capsule, muscle wasting, tendon dislocation and rupture and destruction of articular surfaces. These pathological processes lead to the characteristic deformities including spindle shaped swelling of the proximal interphalangeal joints sometimes with a buttonhole protrusion (Boutonniere deformity), hyperextension of the same joint with flexion of the distal joints (Swan neck deformity), ulnar deviation of the metocarpophalangeal joints, and a Z deformity of the thumb with hyperextension of its interphalangeal joint and flexion deformities of the wrist, fingers and knees (Figure 9.16).

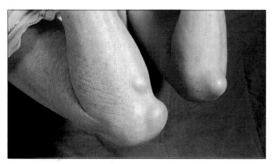

▲ **Figure 9.14 Rheumatoid nodules over the elbows and forearms**

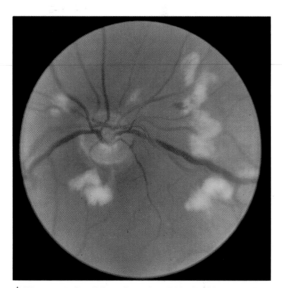

▲ **Figure 9.15 Fundal exudates (cytoid bodies) in systemic lupus erythematosus**

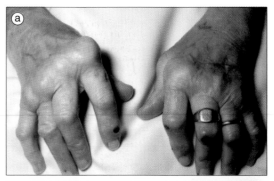

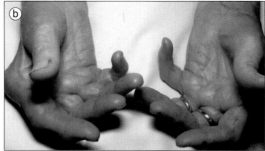

▲ **Figure 9.16 Rheumatoid arthritis showing muscle wasting, flexion deformities, joint swelling and vasculitic lesions**

Ankylosing spondylitis

Like rheumatoid arthritis, ankylosing spondylitis is an inflammatory condition of uncertain cause which may be associated with systemic lesions, notably iritis, aortic regurgitation and apical pulmonary fibrosis. Ankylosing spondylitis differs from rheumatoid arthritis in that it occurs most often in young men and chiefly involves the proximal or 'central' joints of the body: the sacro-iliac, intervertebral, costovertebral, hip and, occasionally, the shoulder joints.

The patient complains of back pain especially in the early stages when there may be tenderness over the sacro-iliac joints. Later, examination will show abnormal rigidity of the spine, reduced chest expansion and fixation of the hip joints. In untreated cases, a flexion deformity of the spine may develop with forward displacement of the head (Figures 9.17 and 9.18).

Reiter's syndrome

This disorder is largely confined to young men and is characterized by conjunctivitis, non-bacterial urethritis or enterocolitis, various mucosal and skin lesions and a polyarthritis. It is usually venereal but not gonococcal in origin. The arthritis particularly affects the lower limb and consists of an acute inflammatory reaction which can be followed by permanent joint damage.

Infective arthritis

Bacterial infection, which usually involves only one or two of the larger joints, has become infrequent as a cause of arthritis since the development of effective antibiotics. Gonorrhoea, tuberculosis, typhoid, dysentery and pneumococcal and staphylococcal infection are among the commoner causes. Pyogenic infection may also occur in a rheumatoid joint, especially after intra-articular corticosteroid injections.

Other forms of inflammatory arthritis

Varying patterns of inflammatory joint disease occur in association with psoriasis, ulcerative colitis, Crohn's disease, brucellosis, erythema nodosum and many other conditions. Some of these may resemble rheumatoid arthritis. In psoriatic arthritis several patterns of joint involvement are described. Typically the distal interphalangeal joints are deformed whereas in rheumatoid arthritis these are often spared. A single joint such as the wrist may be the only manifestation and a symmetrical polyarthritis resembling rheumatoid arthritis is recognized. Pain in the lower back in psoriasis suggests a spondyloarthropathy and the rare arthritis mutilans consists of deformity, destruction and disability often in a finger (opera glass finger) (Figure 9.19). Psoriatic nails show thimble pitting, thickening, crumbling and dis-

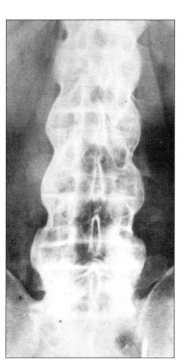

◀ Figure 9.17 Ankylosing spondylitis: radiograph of the lumbo-sacral spine showing bony bridging between the vertebral bodies. Note also obliteration of the sacro-iliac joints

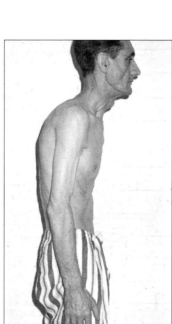

◀ Figure 9.18 Characteristic posture in ankylosing spondylitis. Due to the dorsal kyphosis, the neck is hyperextended to maintain horizontal gaze

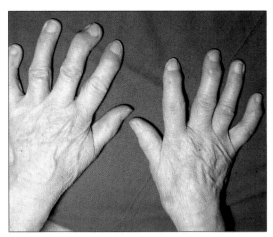

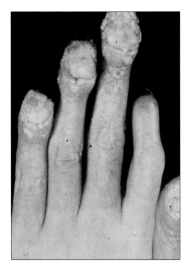

▲ Figure 9.19 Psoriatic arthritis involving the terminal interphalangeal joints and nails

coloration of the nail plate indistinguishable from fungal changes and separation of the nail from the nail plate produces onycholysis (Figure 9.20).

DEGENERATIVE
Osteo-arthritis

This degenerative non-inflammatory condition of the joints increases in frequency with age. It is by far the commonest cause of arthropathy in the elderly but may come on at an earlier age as a result of repeated trauma from postural and mechanical defects, occupational stresses or obesity. It follows that the weight-bearing joints – the spine, hip and knee especially – are chiefly involved. In contrast to rheumatoid arthritis, the distal interphalangeal joints are commonly affected to produce the characteristic Heberden nodes, especially in women (Figure 9.21). Joints with a large range of mobility such as the neck, shoulders and base of the thumb are also specially prone to osteo-arthritis.

The patient most often complains of aching pain and stiffness on using the joints especially after a period of immobility. Those patients having vertebral arthritis may also suffer from root pains due to neural compression from osteophytes or disc protrusions. Examination may show enlargement of the affected joint due to bony hypertrophy, and there may be transient effusions, particularly in the knee. Passive motion of the joint may be accompanied by pain and palpable crepitus but, except in the hip, the range of movement is often unrestricted.

Neuropathic joint disease

In certain neurological disorders, loss of pain and proprioceptive sensations deprive the joint of its normal protective reactions. The resulting impairment of joint posture and stability leads to degenerative changes resembling those of osteoarthritis. The final state is a grossly enlarged and disorganized joint with an excessive range of painless mobility ('Charcot joint') (Figure 9.22). The hip and knee are most commonly affected in tabes, the foot in diabetic neuropathy and the shoulder and elbow in syringomyelia.

METABOLIC DISORDERS
Gout

This is a syndrome characterized by an excess of uric acid in the blood. Often there is an inherited factor, with either increased synthesis of uric acid or its decreased excretion by the kidney, or both. Gout may also be sec-

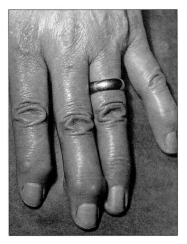

◀ Figure 9.21
Heberden's nodes

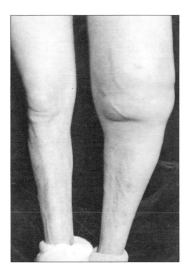

◀ **Figure 9.22**
Charcot's joint.
The left knee joint is
disorganized but
painless

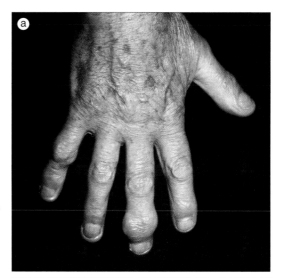

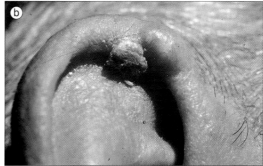

▲ **Figure 9.23 Gouty tophi.** (a) Around interphalangeal joints.
(b) In the ear (one has ulcerated)

ondary to increased cellular breakdown (as in polycythaemia and chronic myeloid leukaemia) or to the use
of certain drugs (e.g. thiazide diuretics) which impair the
renal excretion of urates. Sodium urate is deposited in
the joints, cartilage (e.g. of the ear) and kidneys to produce the three principal features of the disease: arthritis, tophi and renal failure.

Gout usually presents in middle life and is uncommon in women. A family history can often be obtained.
The classic attack consists of a rapidly developing
painful swelling of one joint, usually the first metatarsophalangeal, which is extremely tender with shiny hot
redness of the overlying skin and oedema of the surrounding parts. The temperature may be raised and the
illness can be mistaken for a bacterial infection such as
cellulitis. The attack usually subsides within a week and
may be followed by a complete remission. However, in
some cases, the deposition of urates in the joints and
periarticular tissues may gradually cause a crippling
form of polyarthritis with gross deformity. The feet,
ankles, knees, fingers, hands, wrists and elbows are the
joints most frequently affected.

When gout is suspected as a cause of arthritis, the
clinical examination should include a careful search for
tophi and for evidence of renal damage (albuminuria,
hypertension etc.). Tophi may be seen under the skin,
especially in the helix of the ear (see Figure 9.23(b)) and
around the joints (Figure 9.23(a)); they consist of pale
yellow deposits of sodium urate, sometimes forming
large masses that ulcerate and discharge a pasty material through the skin. However, tophi are found in only
a small proportion of cases, and the clinical diagnosis is
usually made from the history alone.

SPECIAL INVESTIGATIONS

Radiology plays an important part in the investigation
of bone and joint disease. Radiographs of bone reveal
fractures and pseudo-fractures, deformity and areas of
resorbtion or thickening. CAT scans show bone structure in greater detail and radioactive bone scanning
reveals increased activity in Paget's disease and bony
metastases not visualized on conventional radiographs.
In disease of the limb joints it is advisable to compare
one side with the other. It should be noted that radiology is usually unhelpful in diagnosing early gout since
punched out areas in the bone do not appear until there
are clinical tophi. In osteoarthritis, the involved bone
margins show sclerotic thickening with loss of joint
space and outgrowth of bony spurs – osteophytes. In
the early stages of rheumatoid arthritis, soft tissue
swelling over the affected joint may be visualized but

later typical erosions appear at the margin of the articular surfaces which eventually are destroyed and subluxation can occur (Figure 9.24). The sacro-iliac joints in ankylosing spondylitis show subtle marginal sclerosis in the early stages but later there may be fusion of vertebral bodies and calcification of ligaments spreading upwards from the sacrum producing the characteristic bamboo spine (see Figure 9.17).

Investigations of value in the differential diagnosis of bone disorders include the plasma and urinary levels of calcium and phosphorus, the plasma alkaline and acid phosphatases and the urinary total hydroxyproline excretion.

The erythrocyte sedimentation rate (ESR) is raised in the presence of inflammation and may thus help to differentiate active inflammatory from degenerative forms of arthropathy. The finding of a raised antistreptolysin titre (evidence of recent streptococcal infection) would support a diagnosis of rheumatic fever while the presence of rheumatoid factor (positive Latex flocculation test) suggests rheumatoid arthritis. Detection of LE cells or anti-nuclear antibodies in the blood may indicate systemic lupus erythematosus and ankylosing spondylitis occurs almost exclusively in those who have the HLA B27 antigen. In septic arthritis, the causative organism may be recovered from cultures of the synovial fluid, and a positive complement fixation test may be found in those cases due to gonorrhoea. In gout, the serum uric acid is raised, monosodium urate crystals are present in the synovial fluid of the affected joints and tests of renal function may be abnormal. Tabes can be identified as the cause of a neuropathic arthrosis by the Wasserman reaction and fluorescent treponema antibody test, and diabetes by the finding of impaired glucose tolerance.

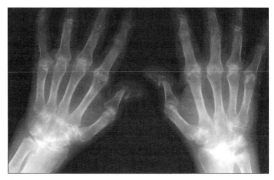

▲ **Figure 9.24 Advanced rheumatoid arthritis: radiograph showing subluxation of MP joints, ulnar deviation, erosions and cystic changes in metacarpals and phalanges**

The nervous system

The diagnosis of neurological conditions is one of the most satisfying skills in clinical medicine. It depends on taking a careful history which often suggests the likely pathological process (see page 277) and eliciting physical signs which indicate the site of the lesion based on an understanding of neuroanatomy and physiology.

The physical signs include changes in motor power and sensation, alteration in reflexes and disturbances in the function of the brain, cranial nerves and spinal cord. Some of the signs are due to loss of function in the damaged areas which are likely to be lasting as are the 'release phenomena' due to loss of control of one part of the nervous system over another. Other physical signs are transient such as epilepsy or spinal shock, but nonetheless valuable evidence of the anatomical site of the lesion.

MENTAL FUNCTION AND CONSCIOUSNESS

The brain is concerned with the maintenance of consciousness and mental function in addition to its role controlling motor power, sensation and the control of vital functions such as respiration and cardiac action.

MENTAL FUNCTION

The general *intelligence* of different individuals varies enormously, but the patient's relatives are often able to assist in determining whether his mental activity has changed of late. *Memory* and *orientation* in space and time should be tested by asking the patient to state the names of his nearest relatives, the address of his home, the date of his birth, the place where he is at the present time and the day of the week. His ability to obey simple commands should also be noted.

Loss of memory for recent events is more common than loss of long-term memory. It can be tested by asking the patient to recall something he has just read or to repeat something he has just been told. Episodes of unconsciousness due, for example, to trauma or epilepsy may be followed by a period of memory loss which can precede the onset of the coma (*retrograde amnesia*). In Korsakov's psychosis an attempt is made to disguise the memory defect by the elaborate invention of recent happenings (*confabulation*).

Mental symptoms such as hallucinations, delusions and abnormalities of conduct may result from organic brain disease as in cerebral arteriosclerosis and neoplasm.

DISTURBANCES OF CONSCIOUSNESS

Mental function naturally depends upon full consciousness. This may be lost partially, *stupor*, or completely, *coma*, apart from the physiological cyclical loss of consciousness which we know as sleep. The partial unconsciousness which is accompanied by restlessness of the body and mind is called *delirium*. All phases of this state are seen, from tossing and turning in bed with periodic chattering, to the wilder types in which the patient throws himself about and struggles violently, frequently shouting at the top of his voice. These changes in consciousness are often found in severe cerebral lesions such as trauma, vascular insults and tumours but may be caused by fever and toxaemias, which exert an indirect effect upon the brain. Consciousness may also be lost as a result of global cerebral damage or the switching off of reticular activity.

Coma

Coma may be divided into six stages:

1 Alert.
2 Drowsy but response to verbal stimulation.
3 Unconsciousness, no response to verbal commands but withdrawal response to pain.
4 Unconsciousness with flexion of upper and lower limbs to pain (decorticate).
5 Unconscious with hyperextension of upper and lower limbs to pain (decerebrate).
6 Unconsciousness with no response.

The Glasgow Coma Scale (Table 10.1) is used to grade the conscious level numerically to assess whether there is deterioration or improvement.

THE GLASGOW COMA SCALE		
Eye opening	**Best verbal response**	**Best motor response**
Spontaneous 4	Orientated 5	Obeying 6
To speech 3	Confused 4	Localizing 5
To pain 2	Inappropriate 3	Withdrawing 4
None 1	Incomprehensible 2	Flexing 3
	None 1	Extending 2
		None 1
Best total 15, worst 3		

▲ **Table 10.1**

SPEECH DEFECTS

Speech is one of the highest functions of the human brain. It is not surprising, therefore, that it is disordered in many gross diseases of the brain which affect other mental functions. For speech to be carried out normally not only must the higher centres be intact, but the motor mechanism which controls the muscles of articulation must be perfect. Disorders of speech can thus be divided at once into two groups:

1 Those affecting the higher centres in the brain – *dysphasia* or *aphasia*, a disturbance of speech as an intellectual function.
2 Those interfering with the motor execution of speech – *dysarthria* or *anarthria* (see The 12th cranial nerve, page 233, and Bulbar paralysis, page 257).

DYSPHONIA

Dysphonia may result from paresis, inflammation or neoplasm of the vocal cords and may occasionally be hysterical.

Other forms of language impairment to be differentiated from aphasia are stuttering (defined as repetition of part of a word, usually the initial consonants), poverty of speech when there is intellectual impairment and language abnormalities such as the neologisms of schizophrenia.

APHASIA

Aphasia is a defect of language production due to brain damage. It usually affects all modules of language such as speech production and comprehension, reading and writing.

Localizing Value of Aphasia

More than 90 per cent of right-handed people have language function represented in the left cerebral hemisphere. However, the reverse does not apply, and the left hemisphere is dominant in 70 per cent of normal left handers. Left handers appear to have a diffuse representation of language function for their recovery from aphasia may be better than would be expected in right handers.

The most important areas for language production in the left hemisphere are (see Figure 10.1):

1 Broca's area located in the posterior part of the inferior frontal gyrus.
2 Wernicke's area in the posterior part of the superior temporal gyrus.
3 The inferior parietal lobule.
4 Frontoparietal operculum.

Speech may also be impaired by lesions in other parts of the left hemisphere, especially sub-cortical areas.

Examination of the Aphasic Patient

A full history is taken from the patient in so far as the aphasia allows, and if necessary from a relative or close friend. Previous speech abnormalities such as stuttering and reading or writing difficulties should be recorded and whether there is any history of deafness. Language skills and usage need to be noted as well as the patient's natural language. Hand preference is important including ambidexterity as well as any family history of left-handedness. Speech should be assessed for fluency, and the patient should be asked to repeat words or phrases and to name common objects. In addition to the patient's spoken speech, comprehension of spoken language and reading and writing should be ascertained.

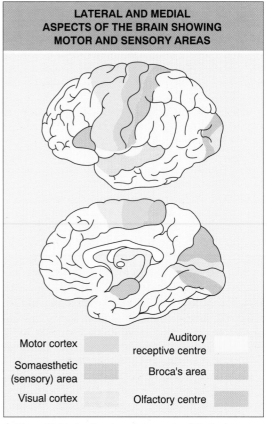

LATERAL AND MEDIAL ASPECTS OF THE BRAIN SHOWING MOTOR AND SENSORY AREAS

Motor cortex	Auditory receptive centre
Somaesthetic (sensory) area	Broca's area
Visual cortex	Olfactory centre

▲ **Figure 10.1 Lateral and medial aspects of the brain showing motor and sensory areas (key on the left) and respective association areas (key on the right)**. These figures should be compared with Figure 10.39, page 235

Spontaneous Speech

This may be fluent or non-fluent. At its most severe, *non-fluent aphasia* consists of a complete loss of speech and phonation. It is usually found in the immediate aftermath of left-sided hemisphere damage. Following some recovery, simple utterances such as 'yes' or 'no' may be produced indiscriminately without any meaning or sense. In emotional speech some propositional speech may break through, and some patients may only speak automatically such as swearing.

When the aphasia is less severe a grammatic, telegraphic speech with a high information content is produced, but lacks the enrichment of auxiliary and relational words. In contrast to non-fluent aphasia where the word output is reduced, *fluent aphasia* is near or above normal in terms of output which may be incomprehensible because it contains non-existent words – neologisms, wrong words, paraphasias which themselves may be whole word substitutions and semantic errors such as dog instead of cat, or syllabic errors such as tip for top.

Non-fluent speech is associated with anterior hemisphere lesions and fluent speech with posterior hemisphere lesions.

Other abnormalities include circumlocutions because the correct word cannot be found, *echolalia* with repetition of words without understanding, *palilalia* with repetitions of increasing frequency. These are usually manifestations of diffuse brain disease such as Alzheimer's or encephalitis and may also be found in psychoses. Abnormalities of speech may be particularly obvious when the patient is asked to discuss constrained topics as quite severe aphasia may be missed if concentration is restricted to 'small talk'.

A naming defect is common to many speech defects and *nominal dysphasia* should be tested for by asking the patient to name common objects and the parts of the body. It is important to mix the subject material rather than to restrict this test to a single area such as bodily parts.

Reading assessment must take account of the patient's educational prowess and after he has been asked to read aloud his comprehension should be tested.

In motor aphasia the ability to write is usually lost – *agraphia*, but in testing for its loss the possibility of weakness in the arm and hand must first be excluded. The patient's writing ability should be tested first by single words then sentences at first to dictation and then spontaneously. Sometimes the writing will be confined to one half of the page, suggesting unilateral neglect. Associated neurological signs may be helpful. A contralateral hemiparesis is usually present in Broca's aphasia and less often in Wernicke's. A visual defect however is commonly present in Wernicke's and rarely Broca's. It must be remembered that when discussions are held at the bedside that many patients with aphasia retain some understanding of the spoken word.

Acquired aphasia usually develops after middle life since the commonest cause is a vascular lesion, usually cerebral thrombosis or embolism. In younger life, aphasia may result from cerebral tumour or abscess and is an occasional feature of migraine.

DYSARTHRIA

Speech is often altered in character without being lost. Some types of abnormal speech may be recognized spontaneously, but others are made apparent when the patient attempts to repeat certain difficult phrases. In lesions of the basal ganglia speech is unusually slow and monotonous; in cerebellar ataxia (e.g. disseminated sclerosis) it has an interrupted character described as *staccato* or *scanning* (sometimes with an explosive element). The speech in cases of palatal paralysis has a nasal quality as air escapes through the nose. Lesions of the recurrent laryngeal nerve cause whispered speech due to paralysis of the vocal cord (aphonia) and this is usually accompanied by a bovine cough. In bulbar paralysis, whether of nuclear or supranuclear origin, all stages between difficult speech and complete absence (*anarthria*) may be present, and the patient frequently mumbles indistinguishable sounds although fully aware of what he wishes to say.

THE CRANIAL NERVES

A systematic examination of the cranial nerves is essential in every neurological case. Not only may primary lesions of the nerves, their nuclei or their cerebral controlling centres be found, but the secondary involvement of these by diseases of the brain or its meninges frequently gives most important localizing data.

If there are signs of paralysis of muscles supplied by a cranial nerve, it is necessary to consider whether the lesion is situated in the upper or lower motor neuron, just as in the case of paralysis of the limbs. The cranial nerve lesion may then be described as either *supranuclear* or *infranuclear*.

When the lesion has been localized, its pathology must be determined. The common pathological processes responsible for cranial nerve paralysis are similar to those mentioned for the nervous system as a whole.

THE 1ST OR OLFACTORY NERVE

The olfactory nerves are not often of great clinical importance. Their anatomical position renders them liable to damage by tumours, especially subfrontal meningioma, or by head injuries, especially when a fracture involves the anterior fossa. The result will be loss of the sense of smell, *anosmia*, which is particularly significant if unilateral. The patient often confuses this with loss of the sense of taste, as flavours depend upon the sense of smell, not the sense of taste. In total olfactory lesions, only the primary sensations of taste (sweet, bitter, sour and salt) remain.

The perception of smell appears to be situated in the uncus and pyriform cortex, lesions of which may be associated with perversions of smell. Similar perversion may occur as an aura in epilepsy, and in mental disorders.

Examination

The olfactory nerves must be tested by substances which do not stimulate the sensory endings of the 5th nerve. Ammonia and acetic acid, therefore, must not be used. Peppermint, turpentine and oil of cloves are suitable and should be applied to each nostril in turn.

THE 2ND OR OPTIC NERVE

This is the most important of the cranial nerves. Not only does it serve the most highly organized special sense, that of sight, but it spreads out into the retina, the examination of which so often reveals signs of disease in other parts of the body.

A few important anatomical facts must be recalled. The impressions of light from the whole of each retina are taken in the optic nerve to the optic chiasma. Here the fibres from the left half of each retina pass into the left optic tract, those from the right half to the right optic tract. Most of the fibres of each optic tract pass on to the lateral geniculate body; some to the pretectal area which presides over the reflex action of the pupils and movements of the orbital muscles. From the lateral geniculate body the fibres make their way, via the optic radiation on each side, to the occipital cortex. Through the medial part of each optic tract communication is established between this optical system and the oculomotor nuclei. The pupillary reflexes are also controlled through special fibres in the optic nerve which leave the optic tract to reach the pretectal area, which in its turn communicates with the 3rd nerve nucleus.

The various parts of these optical paths may now be considered in relationship to surrounding structures. The nerve itself may be involved as it enters the orbit, or by lesions in the anterior fossa of the skull or of the frontal lobes. The chiasma lies in close contact with the pituitary gland and the internal carotid arteries and may be damaged by lesions of these structures such as pituitary tumour or carotid aneurysm (Figure 10.2); also by meningeal changes such as arachnoiditis following skull injury. Each optic tract, as it diverges from its fellow in front of the

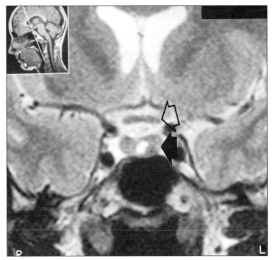

▲ Figure 10.2 MRI pituitary macroadenoma (closed arrow) touching optic chiasma (open arrow)

interpeduncular space, winds round the corresponding crus in close association with the posterior cerebral artery which supplies it. The tract may be affected by disease, either of the artery or of the crus. Finally, each optic radiation passes through the posterior limb of the internal capsule and sweeps round the posterior horn of the lateral ventricle to the visual cortex (area 17), the lower fibres having first descended through the temporal lobe.

The effects of lesions in the different parts of these visual pathways will be seen in Figure 10.3.

EXAMINATION OF THE OPTIC NERVE AND ITS CONNECTIONS

The patient must first be asked whether he has noted any visual changes. His visual acuity may then be tested, and an ophthalmoscopic examination of the retina and optic discs made. Finally the visual fields may be tested.

VISUAL ACUITY

Acuity of vision is tested by means of special charts (Snellen types) with lines of print varying in size (Figure 10.4). Each eye is tested separately. Central visual acuity is conventionally recorded as a fraction. For example, if the patient standing at 6 metres' distance can read only the largest type, which he should be able to read at 60 m, his visual acuity is said to be 6/60. Similarly, if he can read no further down the type than that line which should be read at 18 m, his visual acuity is stated to be 6/18, and ability to read the penultimate line (line 7 in the diagram) is expressed as 6/6, i.e. normal vision. Colour vision is tested using Ishihara charts (Figure 10.5).

COURSE OF VISUAL FIBRES

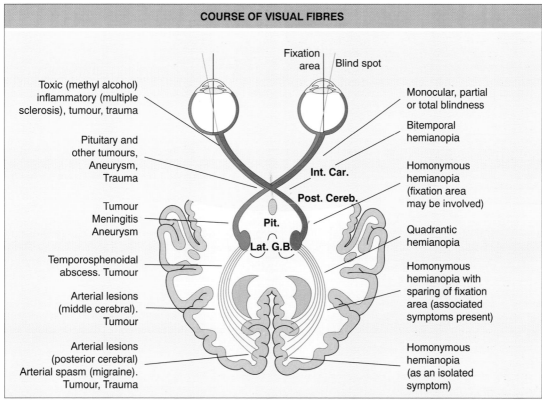

Fixation area

Blind spot

Toxic (methyl alcohol) inflammatory (multiple sclerosis), tumour, trauma

Monocular, partial or total blindness

Pituitary and other tumours, Aneurysm, Trauma

Bitemporal hemianopia

Int. Car.

Homonymous hemianopia (fixation area may be involved)

Post. Cereb.

Tumour Meningitis Aneurysm

Pit.

Lat. G.B.

Quadrantic hemianopia

Temporosphenoidal abscess. Tumour

Arterial lesions (middle cerebral). Tumour

Homonymous hemianopia with sparing of fixation area (associated symptoms present)

Arterial lesions (posterior cerebral) Arterial spasm (migraine). Tumour, Trauma

Homonymous hemianopia (as an isolated symptom)

▲ **Figure 10.3 Course of visual fibres.** On the left side are shown the common lesions in the various parts of the course of the fibres, on the right the results of the lesion. Int. Car. = internal carotid artery; Pit = pituitary gland; Post. Cereb. = posterior cerebral artery; Lat. G.B. = lateral geniculate bodies. (based on a drawing by Mr A. McKie Reid)

TESTING COLOUR VISION

60

F

36

H P

24

N F U

18

T A Z X

12

A H X N T

Z U P T A D

6

X D F P N H Z

5

D X U N Z T F H

◀ **Figure 10.4 Snellen's test types**. Reduced in size from standard chart seen at 6 m. (By courtesy of Messrs Hamblin)

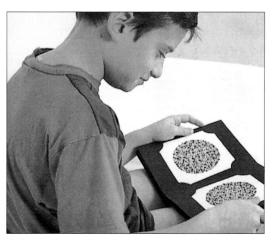

▲ **Figure 10.5 Testing colour vision.** (Reproduced from *Clinical Examination of the Patient* by John Lumley and Pierre-Marc G. Bouloux, Butterworth–Heinemann, 1994)

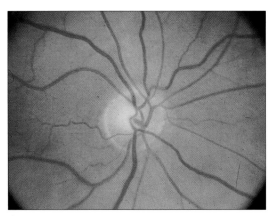

▲ **Figure 10.6 Normal retina and optic disc.** Note the well-defined margin and paler shade of the disc. The vessels radiate from the centre of the disc, the veins being broader and deeper in colour than the arteries.

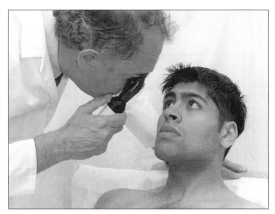

▲ **Figure 10.7 Method of using the ophthalmoscope**

OPHTHALMOSCOPIC EXAMINATION

The retinae and optic discs (Figure 10.6) can be examined with an ophthalmoscope (Figure 10.7) even by the inexperienced, and it cannot be overemphasized that the student should use every opportunity of becoming familiar with the physiological variations in the fundus and the commoner types of pathological changes. These include changes in the optic disc, such as pallor, swelling (papilloedema and optic neuritis), cupping and atrophy; and various forms of retinitis and retinopathy, either primary or associated with systemic disease, such as hypertension, blood dyscrasias, renal disease and diabetes.

The Optic Disc

The optic disc is as individually characteristic as a fingerprint. Its pattern is probably only repeated in identical twins.

Inspection of the disc calls for a definite plan. Colour – pink or paler; margin – clear-cut, blurred or absent; contour – elevated, flat or cupped; crescents – at the temporal margin as in myopia; the distribution of the vessels; lamina cribrosa – the floor of the disc – whether abnormally obvious as in glaucoma or not visible as in oedema; and finally, abnormalities such as neuroglia, pigment deposition, haemorrhages and opaque nerve fibres.

Papilloedema

Papilloedema or choked disc (Figure 10.8) is a non-inflammatory swelling of the optic disc or nerve head usually associated with increased intracranial pressure such as results from space-occupying lesions in the cra-

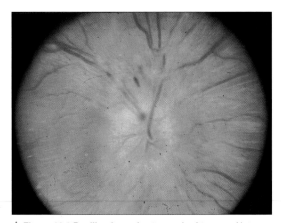

▲ **Figure 10.8 Papilloedema due to cerebral tumour.** Note blurring of the disc margin and of the lamina cribrosa. Most of the vessels disappear near to the margin of the disc (cf normal retina, Figure 10.6). Note also the exudates that radiate from the disc and the two small haemorrhages immediately above the disc

nium, malignant hypertension and chronic carbon-dioxide retention. Papilloedema may also arise from occlusion of the retinal veins or cavernous sinus by thrombosis or other causes. Unilateral papilloedema with contralateral optic atrophy (Foster Kennedy sign) occurs when a tumour presses upon the optic nerve and blocks the posterior opening of the optic canal, while increased intracranial pressure causes papilloedema in the other eye.

Pathogenesis of Papilloedema (Figure 10.9)

The subarachnoid space of the optic nerve sheath is in direct communication with the cerebral subarachnoid space. The retinal artery, vein and lymphatics run in the nerve, and cross the subarachnoid space of the nerve sheath about 1 cm behind the eyeball. Increased pressure in the cerebral subarachnoid space is transmitted into the nerve sheath. The relatively thin walls of the vein and lymphatics, with the low pressure of their fluid contents, permit them to be compressed more than the artery. The inflow of blood to the retina is practically unchecked, while the outflow of venous blood and lymph is obstructed. This results in increased transudation of lymph into and oedema of the optic disc.

Other features to be noted are the engorgement of the veins, blurring of the disc margin, and apparent disappearance of the blood vessels as they 'mount' the elevated disc.

Optic Neuritis

Inflammation or demyelination may affect the optic nerve at any point. When the anterior part of the nerve, the optic disc, is involved the disc is oedematous, but the swelling is not as great as in papilloedema; the disc colour is usually more red, and the disc appears cloudy due to inflammatory exudates not only in the disc but in the overlying vitreous. The differential diagnosis between papilloedema and optic neuritis is, however, not always easy using an ophthalmoscope but in optic neuritis there is invariably a central scotoma. In neurological practice multiple sclerosis is the only common cause.

Retrobulbar neuritis is the condition in which the nerve lesion lies behind the lamina cribrosa. There is little if any disturbance of the disc, but there is often a central scotoma.

This state of affairs has been described as one in which 'neither the ophthalmologist nor the patient sees anything'. The most common cause of retrobulbar neuritis is multiple sclerosis. Other causes are meningitis and avitaminosis. Optic atrophy may follow as well.

Optic Atrophy (Figure 10.10)

The common feature of all varieties of optic atrophy, whatever their aetiology or pathogenesis, is pallor of the optic disc and loss of visual acuity. When the optic atrophy follows severe optic neuritis or a vascular occlusion the visual failure will be rapid but in other conditions it may be slow and progressive. Optic atrophy may result from many lesions and pathological processes, but the old terms of the past such as primary, secondary and consecutive optic atrophy are no longer used. The causes of optic atrophy are:

1 Optic neuritis.
2 Papilloedema.
3 Optic nerve damage due to trauma.
4 Glaucoma.
5 Ischaemia.
6 Familial, e.g. retinitis pigmentosa, Friedreich's ataxia, Leber's disease.

The Retinopathies

The most important retinopathies are:

1 Hypertensive.
2 Diabetic.

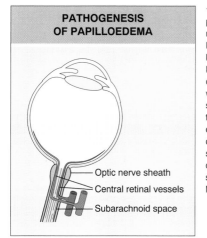

PATHOGENESIS OF PAPILLOEDEMA

Optic nerve sheath
Central retinal vessels
Subarachnoid space

◀ **Figure 10.9 Pathogenesis of papilloedema.** The swelling may be measured by the ophthalmoscope. Both eyes of the examiner should be kept open and unaccommodated as if looking at a distance. A vessel near the centre of the disc is brought into focus with the highest possible plus lens. The same vessel is followed until it leaves the disc and is focused again. The difference, e.g. between +6.0 and +3.0 dioptres, is the measure of the swelling. In this case it would be 3 dioptres (3 dioptres = 1 mm of swelling). (based on a drawing by Mr A. McKie Reid)

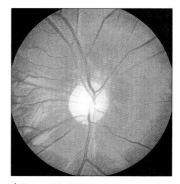

▲ **Figure 10.10 Primary optic atrophy.** The disc is pale and stands out vividly against the red fundus; the margin is sharply defined. The vessels are attenuated

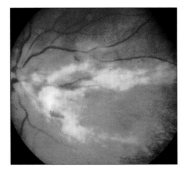

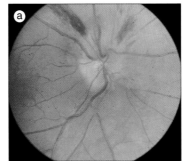

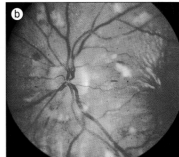

▲ **Figure 10.11 CMV retinopathy in AIDS resembling 'pizza pie'**

▲ **Figure 10.12 Hypertensive retinopathy.** (a) Papilloedema, flame-shaped haemorrhages, and arterial narrowing. Contrast with (b) which shows a few haemorrhages and many exudates, some of which appear as a star-shaped figure near the macula

Viral infections such as toxoplasmosis and cytomegalovirus may cause a retinopathy especially in immunosuppressed AIDS patients (see Figure 10.11).

Hypertensive retinopathy

Hypertensive retinopathy has been classified into four stages according to the appearances and life prognosis (Figure 10.12).

Grade I: narrowing of the vessels.

Grade II: marked variation in the calibre of the vessels with pressure by the artery on the vein at arteriovenous crossings, so that the vein is kinked and its peripheral calibre is engorged while the part central to the crossing is attenuated.

Grade III: the addition of flame-shaped or round retinal haemorrhages and cotton wool patches of exudate.

Grade IV: the addition of papilloedema and increased haemorrhages and exudates.

The first two grades are an age-related phenomenon seen in normal individuals; they have a low specificity. Variation in the calibre of the retinal arterioles is perhaps the best early sign of grade II hypertensive retinopathy.

Diabetic Retinopathy (Figure 10.13)

The retina is spattered sparsely or thickly with minute red dots which are micro-aneurysms. Larger blot and dot haemorrhages appear next; then waxy-looking exudates with harder edges than the cotton-wool patches in hypertensive retinopathy. Larger haemorrhages appear with irregular veins, and, later, new-formed vascular plexuses, venous loops and coils which may protrude into the vitreous. Vitreous haemorrhages and detachment of the retina may follow with blindness as a result.

FIELDS OF VISION

Whenever the visual field is found to be abnormal by rough tests, accurate charts should be prepared by

perimetry. As a rough test, the examiner may compare the patient's visual fields with his own. The examiner and the patient sit facing each other, with opposite eyes closed and each fixes his gaze upon the other's nose. The examiner then holds out his arm to its full extent equidistant between himself and the patient and asks the patient to say when he sees any movement of the examiner's finger. If no movement is detected, the hand is brought in, kept still and the finger moved again. The examiner compares his own first sighting of the movement with the patient's. When a perimeter is used, a record must be made of the visual field for

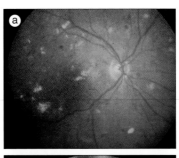

◀ **Figure 10.13 (a) Diabetic retinopathy, showing** microaneurysms, 'blot and dot' haemorrhages and waxy-looking exudates. (b) Laser photocoagulation scars in periphery of retina in a diabetic

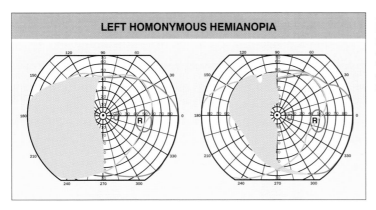

▲ **Figure 10.14 Left homonymous hemianopia**. Tumour right parietal lobe; male, aged 50. Visual acuity: right and left eyes 6/6. Fixation area spared. Perimetry with white object 5 mm in diameter – daylight. (based on a drawing by Mr A. McKie Reid)

each colour separately (white, red, green and blue). The colour fields are the first to be restricted in most cases. Lastly, it is essential not to overlook central scotomas, i.e. patches of impairment in the central area of the field of vision.

Blindness in the whole of the visual field occurs from lesions of the retina or optic nerve, less commonly from occipital lobe lesions. Blindness in one-half of each visual field is known as *hemianopia*. If it affects the same – that is right or left – half of each field, it is called right or left *homonymous hemianopia* (Figure 10.14). This occurs, for example, in lesions of the optic tract and also of the optic radiation. If the right side of one field and the left side of the other are affected, the condition is known as *crossed* or *heteronymous hemianopia*. There are two types of this, *bitemporal hemianopia* (Figure 10.15) when the outer

half of each visual field is affected, and *binasal hemianopia* when the inner halves are involved. Bitemporal hemianopia not infrequently results from tumours of, or adjacent to, the pituitary gland (Figure 10.16) and binasal hemianopia may be caused by calcification and expansion of both internal carotid arteries. A field defect affecting one eye only indicates a lesion anterior to the chiasma, either of the optic nerve or of the retina itself.

Quadrantic defects ('quadrantic hemianopia') (Figure 10.17) occur from lesions involving the optic radiations or, less commonly, the occipital lobe. The restriction of the visual field is less than one-half, usually about one-quarter. It is to be observed that most forms of hemianopia are irregular, and in their early stages may appear quadrantic. This is particularly so when the temporal loop of the optic radiation is affected.

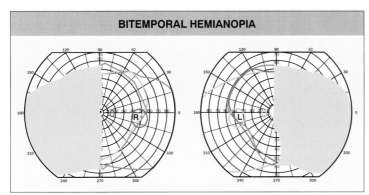

▲ **Figure 10.15 Bitemporal hemianopia.** Pituitary tumour, 6 years' history. Visual acuity: right eye 6/9, left eye 6/24. Sparing of fixation area. Perimetry with 5-mm white object – daylight. (based on a drawing by Mr A. McKie Reid)

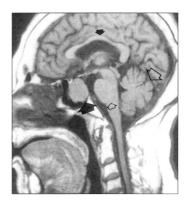

▲ **Figure 10.16 MRI sagittal scan showing pituitary tumour (closed large arrow), normal pons (open small arrow), normal vermis (open large arrow) and normal corpus callosum (closed small arrow)**

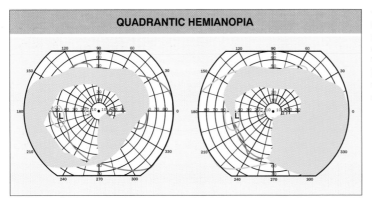

QUADRANTIC HEMIANOPIA

◀ **Figure 10.17 Quadrantic hemianopia.** Subcortical haemorrhage left parietal lobe; male, aged 58. Accompanied by weakness of right arm and leg and blurring of speech. Visual acuity: right eye 6/12 left eye 6/9. Perimetry 4 months after onset with 2-mm white object – daylight. (based on a drawing by Mr A. McKie Reid)

OCULOMOTOR AND PUPILLARY INNERVATION (THE 3RD, 4TH, 6TH AND SYMPATHETIC NERVES) (see Figure 10.18)

Anatomical considerations

The muscles which move the eyeball and those which are responsible for the pupillary reactions are all innervated by the 3rd, 4th, 6th and sympathetic nerves, and these nerves are tested together. The 3rd and 4th nerves have their nuclei in the midbrain and the 6th nerve nucleus is in the floor of the fourth ventricle in the pons.

The 3rd nerve emerges at the upper border of the pons, passes through the cavernous sinus and superior orbital fissure and supplies all the orbital muscles except the superior oblique and lateral (external) rectus. It also sends fibres to the levator palpebrae superioris, and, through the ciliary ganglion, controls the muscles of accommodation (the sphincter of the pupil and ciliary muscle).

The 4th nerve and its fellow decussate before emerging lateral to the frenulum veli and each winds round the crus and enters the orbit through the superior orbital fissure to supply the superior oblique.

The 6th nerve appears between the pons and medulla and also passes through the cavernous sinus and superior orbital fissure to enter the orbit. It supplies the lateral (external) rectus.

The *sympathetic* fibres concerned with the oculomotor mechanism arise in medullary centres and run in the spinal medulla to the 1st and 2nd thoracic nerves, through which they emerge to pass upwards in the cervical sympathetic trunk to the superior cervical ganglion where they synapse. Postganglionic fibres pass upwards from the ganglion in company with the internal carotid artery to be distributed by way of the nasociliary branch of the ophthalmic division of the trigeminal nerve and the long ciliary nerves to the dilator pupillae, and by way of the upper branch of the oculomotor nerve to the involuntary fibres in the levator palpebrae superioris.

The oculomotor muscles work in unison so as to secure conjugate movements of the eyes in a vertical or lateral plane, during which the visual axes remain parallel and in convergence. This simultaneous action of the oculomotor muscles is obtained by special centres in the brainstem, in close association with the nuclei of the 3rd,

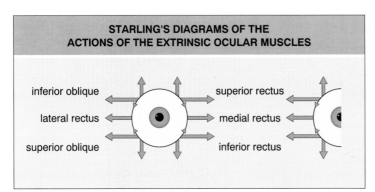

STARLING'S DIAGRAMS OF THE
ACTIONS OF THE EXTRINSIC OCULAR MUSCLES

inferior oblique

lateral rectus

superior oblique

superior rectus

medial rectus

inferior rectus

◀ **Figure 10.18 Starling's diagram of the actions of the extrinsic ocular muscles**

4th and 6th nerves. These centres probably control the reflex movements of the eyes, while similar conjugate movements of voluntary origin are under control of the higher cortical centres.

Examination

The patient should be asked if he sees double (*diplopia*), and note should be taken of squint (*strabismus*), drooping of the eyelid (*ptosis*) or oscillation of the eyeballs (*nystagmus*).

The condition of the *pupils* should be observed, whether they are equal in size and regular in outline, whether abnormally dilated or contracted, and whether they react normally to light and accommodation.

In testing the reaction to light the patient should focus on a distant point and the ambient light should not be too bright. A strong light is then shone into each eye in turn, ensuring that the light does not fall on the other eye and the pupil contracts. If the afferent path of the reflex arc is interrupted by an optic nerve lesion, the direct response to light will be lost. Sometimes the pupil size slowly waxes and wanes as the light source remains constant. This is known as hippus and implies an intact Edinger–Westphal nucleus (3rd nerve).

A *consensual* reflex may be obtained by shining a light into one eye and noting the contraction of the pupil in the other. The value of this reflex is in the recognition of retrobulbar neuritis, one of the earliest signs of disseminated sclerosis. If the afferent path of the reflex arc for pupillary reactions is interrupted by retrobulbar neuritis, the direct response to light will be lost. But the efferent limbs of the reflex arc (from the 3rd-nerve nuclei) are intact, so when a light is shone into the normal eye, the other pupil will contract, though it may show no response to direct light.

In testing the reaction to accommodation the patient is told to look at the far wall of the room. The observer's

finger is then suddenly held vertically about 15 cm in front of the patient's nose, and the patient is told to look at it. As the eyes converge, the pupils should contract equally as the patient accommodates for the finger, and dilate as the finger is moved away.

To test the *ocular movements* (Figure 10.19) the patient's head must be fixed, and he must be asked to move the eyes in turn to the right, to the left, upwards and downwards as far as possible in each direction. Any limitation of movement is noted (see Figures 10.20–10.22).

Common Lesions

These are usually lower motor neuron lesions, i.e. affecting the nuclei or nerves. The causes include trauma, meningeal infection or haemorrhage, multiple sclerosis, peripheral neuropathy and local lesions within or behind the orbit (e.g. tumour, aneurysm). Upper motor neuron lesions, e.g. cerebral haemorrhage, or thrombosis affecting the cortical or midbrain centres, are often transient and produce paralysis of conjugate movements rather than of individual nerves or muscles (see page 226). In myasthenia gravis, ocular pareses, especially ptosis, tend to be bilateral, to vary from time to time and to increase with fatigue.

Third-nerve paralysis

If this is complete, the eye is immobile except in the direction it is moved by the lateral (external) rectus (Figures 10.20–10.22). It cannot be moved upwards, downwards or inwards. There is usually external strabismus owing to the unopposed action of the 6th nerve. Diplopia results in most cases, the type varying with the muscles principally involved, but it may be masked

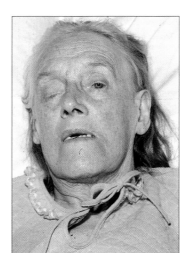

◀ **Figure 10.20 Right 3rd-nerve paralysis.** Complete ptosis obscures the other physical signs

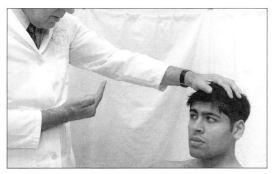

▲ **Figure 10.19 Testing the ocular movements**. The patient's head must be fixed by the examiner's hand

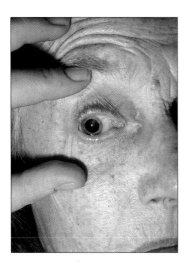

◀ **Figure 10.21 Same patient as Figure 10.20.** Note the large pupil and that the eye looks downwards and outwards due to the unopposed action of the 4th and 6th cranial nerves

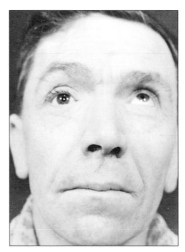

◀ **Figure 10.22 Another case with residual 3rd-nerve paralysis of the right side following meningitis.** Shows failure of the superior rectus when the patient attempts to look upwards

by ptosis. Ptosis gives a narrow palpebral fissure (Figures 10.20, 10.23; see Figure 10.27), owing to paresis of the levator palpebrae superioris, and there is compensatory wrinkling of the forehead on the same side. This wrinkling, due to overaction of the frontalis muscle, may raise the eyelid and mask the narrowing of the palpebral fissure, especially if the ptosis is slight. If the fingers are pressed firmly on the eyebrow against the bone, however, so as to prevent the eyelid from being raised by the frontalis, the ptosis at once becomes apparent. The pupil is fixed and dilated owing to unopposed action of the sympathetic on the dilator pupillae. In 3rd and 6th nerve paralyses secondary deviation may also be observed, i.e. the non-paralysed muscles force the eye farther to the lateral angle than normal and this in its turn results in erroneous projection, so that the patient points farther to one side than the object really is.

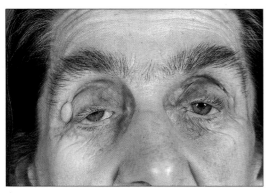

▲ **Figure 10.23 Bilateral partial ptosis due to carcinomatous neuromyopathy**

Sometimes only portions of the nucleus of the 3rd nerve are affected, and the result is paresis of individual orbital muscles such as the superior or inferior rectus or the inferior oblique. This happens especially with central lesions involving the 3rd nucleus, while peripheral lesions of the nerve give complete paralysis. Paralysis of the superior rectus becomes apparent in abduction or in attempting to look upwards, which also reveals the paralysis of the inferior oblique. Adduction shows up the paralysis of the medial (internal) rectus. A lesion affecting the anterior part of the third nerve, as in some forms of neuropathy, will spare the fibres to the pupil (Figure 10.24(a) and (b)).

Fourth-nerve paralysis
Superior oblique paralysis is difficult to determine objectively, but on looking downwards the patient complains of diplopia, particularly when the eye is adducted, i.e. turned towards the nose. Isolated lesions of the 4th nerve are extremely rare.

Sixth-nerve paralysis
The patient is unable to move the eyeball outwards (Figure 10.19). Unopposed contraction of the medial rectus eventually leads to internal strabismus with corresponding diplopia.

If the 6th nucleus is paralysed abduction is limited, i.e. the patient is unable to look towards the side of the lesion with the affected eye, but the unaffected eye moves normally (Figure 10.24(c) and (d)).

Diplopia
Double vision has been referred to under paralysis of the oculomotor muscles. The patient may complain spon-

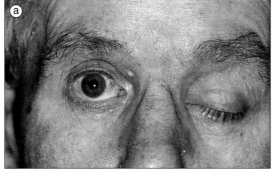

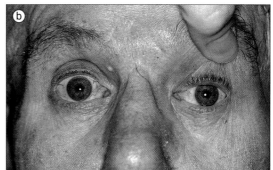

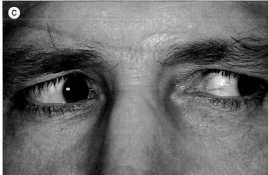

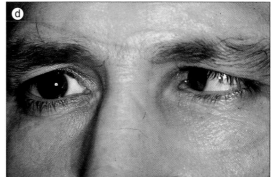

▲ **Figure 10.24 (a) Complete left ptosis due to 3rd nerve palsy.** (b) Same case – note the normal pupil size in the left eye which is looking down and out. (c) Paralysis of right 6th nerve.

Normal movement of both eyes to left. (d) Same patient. Paralysis of lateral movement of right eye due to right lateral rectus palsy

taneously or only after questioning that he sees double. The diplopia may be present in all positions of the eye but increases when an attempt is made to move the eye in that direction towards which the paralysed muscle would normally move it.

The symptom results from strabismus because the images from the two eyes do not fall on corresponding parts of the retina and two images are seen instead of the one, which is the normal result of binocular vision (Figure 10.25). The visual axis is a line drawn from the point of fixation through the nodal point of the eye so as to reach the retina at the macular lutea. If an image falls on the retina to the temporal side of the macula, it is projected to the nasal side of space (in front of the observer), and vice versa. In paralysis of the internal rectus it may be impossible to direct the eye so that the image of the fixation point falls on the macula. The image falls on the retina to the temporal side of the macula, and the object is falsely projected to the nasal side of the fixation spot. True fixation and projection take place in the unaffected eye, and hence crossed diplopia occurs. When the squint is of long standing the patient may learn to disregard the false image, and diplopia no longer occurs.

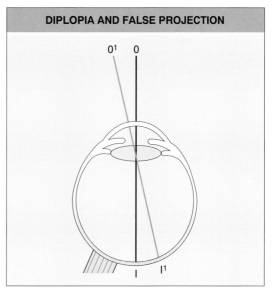

DIPLOPIA AND FALSE PROJECTION

▲ **Figure 10.25 Diplopia and false projection (see text).** O = fixation spot; O1 = fixation spot or object falsely projected to nasal side of space; I = image at macula; I1 = image on temporal side of macula. . (based on a drawing by Mr A. McKie Reid)

The position of the images as seen by the patient is often useful in determining the nature of the ocular paresis. The false (more peripheral) image is the one seen by the paralysed eye, the true one by the normal eye.

Strabismus (squint)

This sign has been mentioned as occurring in oculomotor paralysis (Figure 10.26). Concomitant strabismus is due to an imbalance in the action of opposing muscles. Many cases of squint are non-paralytic and are called 'concomitant'. The main differences between paralytic and concomitant squint may be summarized as follows:

Paralytic strabismus

1. Known cause and sudden onset
2. Diplopia present
3. Limitation in ocular movements
4. Deviation of visual axis varies as the gaze is turned in different directions
5. No amblyopia (blindness)
6. False projection
7. Vertigo may occur

Concomitant strabismus

1. Gradual onset in early childhood
2. No diplopia
3. No limitation of movement
4. Deviation of visual axis does not vary
5. Eye may be amblyopic
6. No false projection
7. No vertigo

The descriptions which have been given of an oculomotor paralysis apply only to lower motor neuron lesions. If the lesion is supranuclear, individual orbital muscles are not affected, therefore squint and diplopia do not occur. Instead, muscles controlling a particular movement are paralysed. In most cases this results in *conjugate deviation*, in which the eyes are persistently turned towards the side of the lesion, as the centres enabling the patient to gaze to the side opposite from the lesion are paralysed. In irritative processes there may be conjugate deviation towards the side opposite the lesion due to overaction of the affected muscles.

Cervical sympathetic paralysis (Figures 10.27, 10.28)

The sympathetic may be involved by diseases in the cervical cord such as syringomyelia, or by lesions in the neck, such as trauma, surgical resection (Figure 10.27)

or malignant lymph nodes. The pupil is contracted owing to unopposed action of the 3rd nerve. Slight ptosis occurs from paresis of the involuntary muscle fibres in the upper eyelid giving the impression of recession of the eyeball (enophthalmos), and sweating may be absent on the affected side of the head and neck. This combination of meiosis, ptosis, and anhidrosis is known as Horner's syndrome.

Pupillary abnormalities

Make sure first that no mydriatics have been used recently.

The pupils may be abnormally dilated (*mydriasis*) in conditions of sympathetic overactivity, e.g. hyperthyroidism and anxiety, or from the adhesions of iritis. They are contracted (*meiosis*) in neurosyphilis, especially tabes, and in morphine poisoning.

Inequality in the size of the pupils in lesions of the 3rd nerve or sympathetic affecting one side only, and in diseases such as syphilis or iritis which may produce more advanced changes on one side.

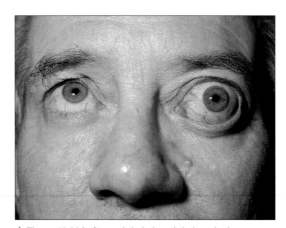

▲ **Figure 10.26 Left exophthalmic ophthalmoplegia**

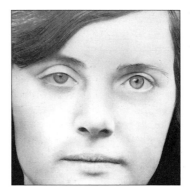

◀ **Figure 10.27 Right sympathetic nerve paralysis.** The right eye shows ptosis, causing narrowing of the palpebral fissure, and meiosis from unopposed action of the 3rd nerve

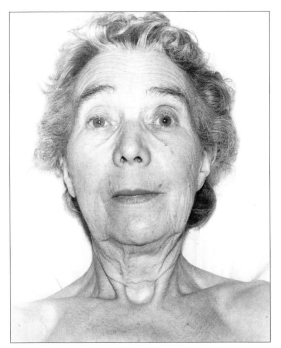

▲ Figure 10.28 Right Horner's syndrome in same patient as in Figure 10.36. Lesion in base of brain

Irregularity may result from the synechiae of iritis, but syphilis and encephalitis are sometimes responsible.

Argyll Robertson pupil: Argyll Robertson described the pupil in neurosyphilis as small, constant in size and unaltered by light or shade; contracts fully on convergence and dilates when effort to converge is relaxed. The pupils are also unequal, irregular in outline and eccentric, and the central part of the iris may be depigmented. The site of the lesion causing these changes in the pupil is probably in the pre-tectum of the midbrain behind the optic tract and 3rd-nerve nucleus. Diabetes is now a more common cause than tabes for pupillary changes of this kind ('diabetic pseudotabes').

The myotonic pupil is a rather rare condition which may erroneously suggest tabes, especially as the knee jerks or ankle jerks are sometimes absent. The abnormality is, however, usually unilateral, and the affected pupil is of normal size or dilated. The reaction to light is lost or very slow and that to accommodation sluggish. The condition is generally found in young women and is unexplained, but it is not associated with clinical or spinal-fluid signs of syphilis. It is also known as the Adie–Holmes syndrome.

The pupil in cerebral injury: Changes in the pupils provide important diagnostic and prognostic information after head injuries or cardiac arrest. Inequality of the pupils may indicate rising intracranial pressure due,

for example, to an expanding haematoma. Dilated pupils unreactive to light for several minutes suggest that brain damage is irreversible and that further attempts to resuscitate the patient are unlikely to succeed.

THE 5TH OR TRIGEMINAL NERVE
Anatomical considerations

This nerve has motor and sensory roots. Both have their nuclei in the pons. The sensory nucleus also makes connections with the medulla and spinal cord through the substantia gelatinosa. The motor and sensory roots emerge from different parts of the brain but come closer together as they approach the trigeminal ganglion on the petrous portion of the temporal bone. Into this ganglion the sensory root enters, but the motor portion lies beneath the ganglion and later joins the mandibular division of the 5th nerve.

From the trigeminal ganglion the three divisions of the 5th nerve emerge:

1 Ophthalmic.
2 Maxillary.
3 Mandibular.

These divisions are responsible for reception of sensation from the greater part of the face, forehead, parietal and temporal regions, nasal and buccal mucosae and conjunctivae.

The mandibular division makes connections through the lingual and facial nerves with the chorda tympani, which is responsible for the sensation of taste in the anterior two-thirds of the tongue. Motor fibres innervate the muscles of mastication, of which the most important are the temporals, masseters and pterygoids.

Examination

The sensory and motor functions of the nerve must be tested.

Sensation

Sensation may be tested as elsewhere in the body by the use of cotton wool and a pin over each area of the face and buccal mucosa supplied by the three divisions of the 5th nerve. A light wisp of cotton wool touching the cornea normally produces closure of the eye, but if there is anaesthesia of the cornea the reflex will be abolished. Loss of the corneal reflex may precede other signs of a trigeminal nerve lesion. If the 5th nerve has been paralysed for some time, serious effects may appear, especially ulceration of the cornea and dryness of the nasal and buccal mucous membrane, with anosmia and difficulty in chewing.

Motor power

The position of the teeth should be noted to see if there is any deviation of the jaw. The temporal and masseter muscles should then be palpated while the patient clenches his teeth; any difference in the strength of contraction on the two sides is noted. The side-to-side movements (pterygoids) may be tested by asking the patient to move the jaws in a ruminating manner against the resistance of the observer's fingers. If the lesion is in the upper neuron the paresis is rarely marked owing to bilateral cortical innervation. The jaw jerk, scarcely detectable in health, is brisk when there is a bilateral upper neuron lesion above the level of the trigeminal motor nucleus. Wasting of the muscles of mastication will be present in lower neuron lesions of considerable standing, giving the face and temple on the affected side a hollowed-out appearance.

Lesions

Pontine lesions which involve the 5th nucleus often produce pyramidal tract and other characteristic signs. Outside the pons the nerve may be involved by tumours at the base of the brain, especially in the cerebello-pontine angle, and more rarely the trigeminal ganglion or individual branches may be affected by tumours or neuropathies. Lesions of the upper cervical cord, such as syringomyelia, may involve the spinal prolongation of the trigeminal sensory nucleus to cause loss of facial pain and temperature sensation, especially over the forehead.

Trigeminal neuralgia

This affection of the 5th nerve needs special consideration in view of its frequency. It is commoner in old age, especially in women. Any or all of the three sensory branches may be involved, and the patient complains of sudden severe lancinating pain over the distribution of the affected divisions. The attacks are often provoked by touch, cold or the movements of the face in eating or talking. The second and third divisions are usually primarily affected, but the first may follow. Localized tenderness is usually present over the same area, but there is never any sensory loss. Trigeminal neuralgia comes in attacks, at first short, but later of long duration. Long periods of freedom are common. The cause is usually compression of the sensory root by a dilated artery and rarely it may be an early symptom of multiple sclerosis. It must be distinguished from other types of facial pain, e.g. those associated with dental and sinus disease, in which the classic paroxysms do not occur. A good history is imperative.

Ophthalmic herpes (Figure 10.29)

Herpes zoster commonly affects the first division of the trigeminal nerve and may result in severe and intractable pain, especially in older patients. Sensory loss and corneal ulceration may occur.

THE 7TH OR FACIAL NERVE
Anatomical considerations

The facial nerve arises from its nucleus in the pons, where its fibres course around the nucleus of the 6th nerve. The nerve emerges in the cerebello-pontine angle in company with the 8th nerve. Both enter the internal (auditory) acoustic meatus, but later the 7th nerve leaves the 8th and runs in the facial canal to its point of exit at the stylomastoid foramen. Thereafter the nerve is distributed to the facial muscles, all of which it supplies except the levator palpebrae superioris (3rd nerve). In its course through the aqueduct the facial nerve gives off two branches which have localizing value:

1 The nerve to the stapedius.
2 The chorda tympani.

In cases of facial paralysis it is often possible, if these anatomical data are borne in mind, to determine fairly accurately the part of its course in which the nerve has been damaged. Simultaneous involvement of the 6th nerve is suggestive of a pontine lesion; concurrent affection of the 7th and 8th nerves is common in lesions at the cerebello-pontine angle; excessive response to sounds in one ear ('hyperacusis') indicates that the lesion has also

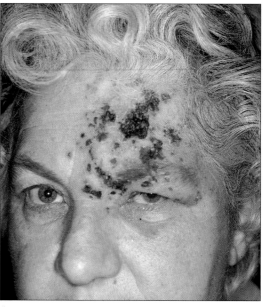

▲ **Figure 10.29 Left ophthalmic herpes**

affected the nerve to the stapedius in the facial canal; and loss of taste over the anterior two-thirds of the tongue implies that the 7th nerve has been damaged in the facial canal before the origin of the chorda tympani. In the commonest type of facial lesion, Bell's palsy, these collateral signs are not commonly present, as the nerve is affected either at or after it has left the stylomastoid foramen, or sometimes in its course through the temporal bone.

Examination

The examination of the facial nerve is primarily designed to test the movements of the facial muscles. The patient should be asked in turn to show the teeth, puff out the cheeks, wrinkle the forehead by looking upwards and close the eyes (see Figure 10.31).

Taste on each half of the anterior two-thirds of the tongue should be tested as described on page 232, but the loss of taste is often more easily determined by questioning. Finally, note should be taken of any abnormal acuity of hearing on the affected side.

Lesions

Facial paralysis results quite commonly from both upper and lower neuron lesions.

Upper neuron paralysis

This only affects the muscles of the lower part of the face, as the occipito-frontalis and orbicularis oculi muscles are bilaterally innervated from the cortex (Figure 10.30). Vascular lesions of the brain are commonly responsible, the paralysis occurring on the opposite side to the lesion (see also page 255). The angle of the mouth droops, the paralysed cheek is puffed out loosely with each expiration. On the other hand, the forehead can be wrinkled normally and the eye closed (cf. lower neuron lesions).

Lower neuron paralysis

If the paralysis is complete the whole side of the face is smooth and free from wrinkles (Figures 10.31). The lower eyelid droops and the angle of the mouth sags. Saliva may dribble away from the mouth and tears flow over the lower lid. In attempting to look upwards or frown, the wrinkling on the normal side contrasts with the smoothness of the affected side. The patient is unable to close the eye which also rolls upwards in the attempt. The mouth cannot be moved so as to expose the teeth, and when the cheeks are puffed out the paralysed side balloons more than normal. Attention should be paid to complaint of alterations in taste or hearing in view of the anatomical connections of the 7th nerve.

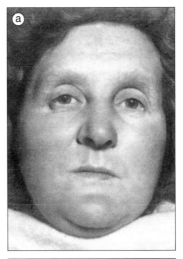

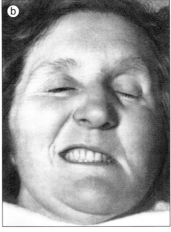

◀ **Figure 10.30 Upper neuron facial paralysis (left).** (a) Face at rest. (b) Showing the teeth. Note normal eye closure

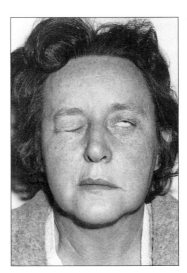

◀ **Figure 10.31 Lower motor neuron facial paralysis showing inability to close the left eyelid with upward rolling of the eye.** Note also the drooping of the left angle of the mouth and loss of the nasolabial fold

If the paralysis does not improve quickly, conjunctival infections may result from inability to close the eye.

Although the cause is often unknown, it is usually probably due to inflammation and compression of the nerve within the facial canal. Other causes include tumours of the pons or cerebello-pontine angle (Figure 10.32), trauma, osteomyelitis of the petrous temporal bone due to chronic middle ear infection, parotid tumours and herpes zoster affecting the geniculate ganglion. This last condition may be associated with a herpetic eruption on the pinna of the ear (Ramsay–Hunt syndrome, Figure 10.33).

THE 8TH OR VESTIBULO-COCHLEAR NERVE

It is convenient under this heading to consider the functions and disturbances of the inner ear which contains three different organs:

1 The cochlea, the true organ of hearing.
2 The three semicircular canals, constituting the organ of dynamic equilibrium.
3 The two otolith organs, utricle and saccule, constituting the organ of static equilibrium.

The cochlear nerve carries impulses from the spiral ganglion in the modiolus of the cochlea via cochlear nuclei in the pons and thence, via the lateral lemniscus and medial geniculate body, to the superior temporal gyrus of the opposite cerebral hemisphere.

The vestibular nerve conveys impulses from the organs of equilibrium and terminates in nuclei within the medulla which then communicate with the cerebellum and midbrain and, by way of the vestibulo-spinal tract, with the spinal cord.

The two nerves run as a common trunk in close association with the 5th and 7th in the cerebello-pontine angle and are usually involved in pathological conditions affecting the region, e.g. cysts, acoustic neuromas and cerebellar abscesses.

Disturbances of the cochlear system

These manifest themselves essentially with deafness and tinnitus.

Deafness

The existence of significant hearing loss can easily be established by testing the patient's ability to hear a watch or a soft whisper. Each ear is tested separately, the other being firmly occluded by the finger. The tests should be carried out in a room free of distracting noise, and the examiner should know beforehand the distance at which a normal ear can hear his watch or his voice. A soft whisper should normally be audible at about three feet.

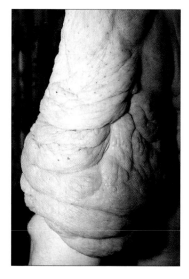

◀ **Figure 10.32 Plexiform neurofibroma of the upper arm.** This patient also has a cerebello-pontine neurofibroma of the 8th cranial nerve

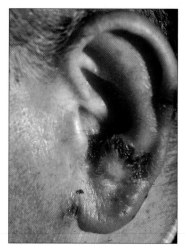

◀ **Figure 10.33 The Ramsay–Hunt syndrome. Geniculate herpes**

Tinnitus

This symptom is variously described by the patient as 'ringing', 'buzzing', 'hissing', 'singing' or other form of noise in the ear. It may precede deafness as a symptom of 8th-nerve disease. It is also common in ischaemia of the auditory apparatus due to anaemia, atheroma or postural hypotension and after high dosage of salicylates and quinine. It is most commonly present when the inner ear is actively deteriorating but can also occur in the course of middle ear disease. In some cases, fortunately rare, distressing tinnitus can be caused by disease in the central nervous system, and cases have been recorded in which even section of the 8th nerve has failed to suppress the sensation.

Tuning-fork tests: Tuning-forks emit pure tones and enable more accurate information to be obtained by comparison of AC (air-conducted) hearing with BC (bone-conducted) hearing.

Principles of tuning-fork tests: For tuning-fork tests, the vibration frequency should be 256, twice that used for testing vibration sensation in the skin. In AC hearing the sound traverses the outer and middle ears to reach the cochlea where it stimulates the organ of Corti. In BC hearing the sound traverses the skull bones to reach the organ of Corti.

Thus pathological conditions in the outer and middle ear will reduce AC hearing but will have no effect on BC hearing, i.e. conductive deafness. Pathological conditions in the inner ear or central pathways will reduce both AC and BC hearing, i.e. perceptive deafness.

In other words, if BC is normal, the inner ear must be normal, but if BC is reduced, the inner ear or central pathways are at fault.

Schwabach's test is the simplest of all. The examiner, assumed for simplicity to have normal hearing, strikes the fork and places it on the subject's mastoid asking him to indicate when the sound becomes inaudible. The examiner then places the fork on his own mastoid. If he can still hear it, the patient's BC is reduced and the diagnosis is perceptive deafness.

Rinne's test: In a case of conductive deafness, bone conduction (BC) is normal and found to be greater than air conduction (AC): thus, when AC is no longer heard at the external auditory meatus the tuning-fork can still be heard when placed on the mastoid process.

In perceptive deafness AC and BC will be impaired by both routes. If such a hearing loss is confined to one ear, comparison with the normal ear will reveal increased perception for both AC and BC.

Weber's test: If a tuning-fork is placed in the midline of the skull, the sound reaches both inner ears by bone conduction (i.e. not by the normal route through the middle ears). Thus so long as the inner ear is normal (as in middle ear deafness) the sound aroused by such a fork is unaffected. If, however, the inner ear is impaired the sound evoked is also impaired (Figure 10.34). Now consider a patient with unilateral deafness. If the lesion is in the inner ear, the sensation is quieter on that side than on the normal side, i.e. the patient lateralizes to the healthy ear. But in unilateral conductive deafness the sensation from the deaf ear is just as great as from the normal ear and therefore the sound does not lateralize. Indeed, the sound may actually lateralize to the deaf ear because the conduction defect has excluded background noise. The student should test this observation for himself by occluding one external meatus and applying the

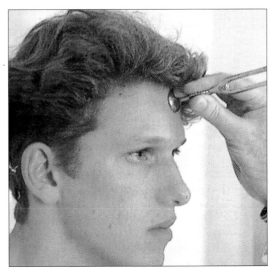

▲ **Figure 10.34 Weber's test.** (Reproduced from *Clinical Examination of the Patient* by John Lumley and Pierre-Marc G. Bouloux, Butterworth–Heinemann, 1994)

tuning-fork to the centre of his forehead. The sound will be louder on the side of the occlusion.

Limitation of tuning-fork test: The above tests often give valuable qualitative information but are unable to give quantitative estimates of auditory acuity. For the latter purpose the otologist now depends on the audiometer. A more serious weakness of tuning-fork tests is that bone-conducted vibrations reach all parts of the skull irrespective of where the fork is placed. Thus the examiner ostensibly testing BC on the right ear may obtain misleading answers because the patient will also be hearing with his left ear. In audiometry this error is obviated by masking the opposite ear, i.e. temporarily obtunding it with a special noise which blocks out the testing tone. For a full account of audiometry the student is referred to specialist textbooks on otology.

Disturbances of the vestibular system

These include vertigo and nystagmus.

Vertigo

Many conditions, including some of psychological origin, are associated with vague sensations of dizziness or light-headedness. True labyrinthine vertigo involves a sense of movement, usually rotation, in relation to the environment. In its most severe form, vertigo is accompanied by vomiting, pallor, sweating and an inability to remain upright. The spinning sensation is made worse by movement, and the patient usually lies motionless with the eyes tightly closed.

Positional vertigo is a transient feeling of dizziness when the head is placed in certain positions, especially dorsiflexion. This can be due to disorder of the otolith mechanism. If a patient complains of positional vertigo, the effect of posture should be determined. The head is lowered to beyond the horizontal offering support if required. The development of nystagmus recorded either immediately or after an interval indicates positional nystagmus. The patient should be warned that vertigo may develop and asked if the symptoms resemble those of the presenting complaint.

Ménière's syndrome is caused by pathological changes within the inner ear. Usually all three end-organs are affected to a greater or lesser degree. Thus:

1 The semicircular canals set up sensations of movement of varying severity as described above.
2 The cochlear disturbance reveals itself with tinnitus and deafness.

In a typical attack the patient complains of intense rotational dizziness, sweats, nausea and vomiting and may show nystagmus. The episode lasts for some hours and slowly subsides although some unsteadiness, deafness and tinnitus may persist for weeks and, in severe cases, may become permanent. Remissions last for months if not years.

Nystagmus
Nystagmus, i.e. uncontrollable pendular movement of the eyes, can arise from:

1 Disturbance of visual function.
2 Disturbance of labyrinthine function.
3 Disturbance of the central nervous system with involvement of the visual pathways.

In congenital blindness the eyes, lacking a focal point, oscillate aimlessly. Miner's nystagmus is not fully explained, but may have some connection with poor illumination. Optokinetic nystagmus is characteristically seen in railway passengers gazing at the passing scenery. The eyes fix on a certain point (e.g. a telegraph pole) and follow it until further fixation becomes impossible. They then rapidly jerk back to a new focal point and so the process continues.

Labyrinthine nystagmus is due to disturbance of the semicircular canals. As there are three sets of canals, in three planes in space, nystagmus can occur in three directions, i.e. horizontal, vertical and rotary. Characteristically, there is a slow component and a quick component.

Nystagmus of central origin occurs in lesions which involve the cerebellum and vestibular apparatus, or the pathways in the pons and medulla between these. The commoner neurological disorders include disseminated sclerosis, tumours and other lesions of the cerebellum, and more rarely tumours and syringomyelia affecting the pons or medulla, and Friedreich's ataxia.

Irrigation of the ear, with either hot or cold water, sets up convection currents in the endolymph of the semicircular canals and so produces nystagmus. A similar effect can be produced by rotating the patient in a special rotating chair. By evaluating the nystagmus under such controlled conditions of stimulation, useful information can be obtained, not only about the labyrinth but also about the vestibular tract in general. The absence of nystagmus when the ear is irrigated with cold water is one of the criteria used in the diagnosis of brain death (see Chapter 16).

For details of caloric and rotary tests otological textbooks should be consulted.

THE 9TH OR GLOSSOPHARYNGEAL AND 10TH OR VAGUS NERVES
Anatomical considerations
The glossopharyngeal and vagus nerves are usually considered and examined together owing to their close association. They arise in medullary nuclei and leave the base of the skull through the jugular foramina.

The 9th nerve carries taste fibres from the posterior third of the tongue and innervates certain of the muscles concerned in swallowing, but in its motor function the nerve overlaps with the vagus.

The 10th nerve has a wide distribution and constitutes an important part of the autonomic nervous system, carrying parasympathetic fibres to the heart, lungs and gastrointestinal tract. Special physiological tests are needed to examine the visceral functions of the vagus nerve, although some of its autonomic effects may be evident in such signs as bradycardia (vagal overaction) or diarrhoea (vagal suppression). Direct clinical examination of the vagus depends chiefly upon testing the function of the branches to the voluntary muscles of the pharynx, soft palate and larynx.

Examination
1 The sensation of taste is tested in suspected lesions of the 7th and 9th nerves. The anterior two-thirds of the tongue may show loss of taste sensation in 7th-nerve lesions, and the posterior third when the glossopharyngeal nerve is affected.
Substances that are sweet, salt, sour and bitter (sugar, salt, vinegar and quinine) should be used in turn by placing a little on one-half of the anterior two-thirds of the tongue. The patient should not speak, but write down what he tastes. A weak

galvanic current is recognized as a metallic taste and is particularly useful in testing the posterior third (glossopharyngeal nerve).

2 Test the pharyngeal reflex by tickling each side of the pharynx with a wooden spatula (Figure 10.35). Unilateral abolition of the reflex only results from organic lesions. In these cases the pharynx will move like a curtain towards the normal side. Bilateral abolition of the palatal reflex is sometimes found in hysterical subjects.

3 Ask the patient to say 'Ah'. Normally the uvula moves backwards in the median plane, but in vagal paralysis it is deflected to the normal side.

4 Note any difficulty in deglutition or speaking. In vagal paralysis regurgitation of food through the nose and a nasal voice sometimes occur.

5 Hoarseness or aphonia calls for a laryngoscopic examination. The left recurrent laryngeal branch of the vagus may be damaged by mediastinal tumours, causing abductor paralysis.

The effects of a supranuclear lesion of the vagus are discussed under Pseudobulbar paralysis (page 256).

THE 11TH OR SPINAL ACCESSORY NERVE

The spinal accessory nerve supplies the sternomastoid and trapezius muscles. It emerges from the skull through the jugular foramen, and has relations centrally with the 9th and 10th nerves.

Examination

The patient should be asked to shrug his shoulders, when the trapezii come into action, and then to rotate the head against resistance, in which the sternomastoid of the opposite side is employed (Figure 10.36).

Sometimes in 11th-nerve paralysis the vertebral border of the scapula stands out, rather like the 'winged scapula' of serratus anterior paralysis.

THE 12TH OR HYPOGLOSSAL NERVE

The hypoglossal nucleus is in the medulla, the upper portion of which is in the floor of the 4th ventricle near the midline. The nerve fibres pass through the medulla to emerge between the olive and the pyramid from where they pass across the posterior fossa. The nerve leaves the skull through the hypoglossal canal and having passed downwards and forwards towards the hyoid bone turns medially and then downwards over the carotid arteries from where it reaches the tongue.

Examination

The patient should be asked to protrude the tongue. In lower neuron paralysis the affected side is wasted, wrinkled and may display fasciculation (Figure 10.37).

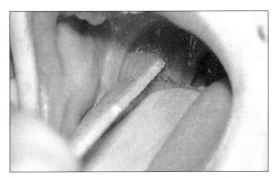

▲ **Figure 10.35 Gag reflex.** The anterior fauces on each side are gently touched with a wooden spatula. (Reproduced from *Clinical Examination of the Patient* by John Lumley and Pierre-Marc G. Bouloux, Butterworth–Heinemann, 1994)

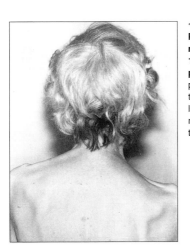

◄ **Figure 10.36 Paresis of the right trapezius in 11th-nerve paralysis.** The patient is shrugging the shoulders: the left moves upwards normally, but not the right

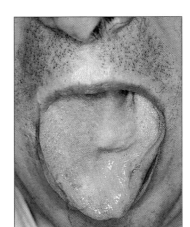

◄ **Figure 10.37 Left hypoglossal palsy showing atrophy of the tongue**

The tongue deviates to the affected side as in cases of facial paralysis, but in the latter the deviation can be rectified by straightening the corner of the mouth with the fingers. Dysarthria is often present. More commonly, as in motor neuron disease, there is bilateral involvement of the tongue. Abnormality can then be detected by noting crenation of the edges of the tongue and generalized fasciculation; the latter should be looked for when the tongue is at rest within the mouth. In supranuclear lesions of the 12th nerve the tongue may be small and immobile, resulting in dysphagia and dysarthria (see also page 256).

THE MOTOR SYSTEM: ANATOMICAL AND PHYSIOLOGICAL CONSIDERATIONS

The neurons responsible for voluntary motor action run in two relays. The first extends from the cortical cells in the motor area, which is found in the precentral gyrus, and is distributed to cranial nerve nuclei and to different parts of the spinal cord, there to terminate with internuncial neurons in the grey matter of the ventral horns. These in turn synapse with the anterior horn cells which give rise to the motor nerve root supplying voluntary muscles. To the first relay the name *upper motor neuron* is given; to the second *lower motor neuron* (Figure 10.38).

THE UPPER MOTOR NEURON

The upper motor neuron starts in the precentral gyrus (area 4) in groups of cells which control movements rather than individual muscles. These cells are arranged in a fashion which has been proved experimentally and is shown on the accompanying diagram (Figure 10.39). It will be observed that the motor area covers a considerable region of the cortex, and it follows that a small lesion may affect only a small part of the motor area, e.g. that governing movements of the hand, and lead to a strictly limited paralysis.

From these cortical cells, projection fibres known as the *corticospinal (pyramidal) tract* pass through the substance of the brain in the *corona radiata*, converging towards the *internal capsule*, where they are densely packed. The result of quite a small lesion in this region may be an extensive paralysis – usually the face, arm and leg on the contralateral side. The position of the fibres in the anterior two-thirds of the posterior limb and in the genu of the internal capsule is shown in Figure 10.40. The relative position of the motor fibres for different parts of the body is not the same as in the motor cortex. (Cf. Figure 10.39.)

Sensory fibres and visual paths in the capsule may be involved simultaneously with the motor fibres but lie more posteriorly.

From the internal capsule the fibres pass through the *midbrain* and *pons* to the *medulla (oblongata)*, where the bulk of them decussate and travel down the lateral columns of the *spinal cord* as the crossed corticospinal tract. The few fibres which do not decussate, but form the uncrossed corticospinal tract, have little clinical importance (Figure 10.38).

In the brainstem some of the fibres terminate in relationship with the nuclei of the cranial nerves. They form the upper neurons of these nerves, the lower neurons starting from each cranial nerve nucleus.

As in the internal capsule, the dense aggregation of corticospinal tract fibres in the midbrain, pons and

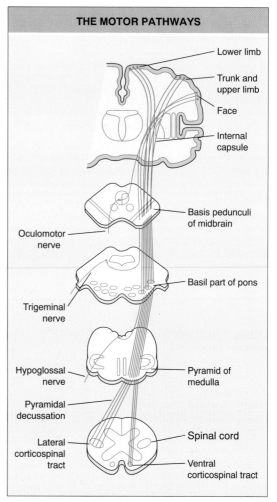

THE MOTOR PATHWAYS

- Lower limb
- Trunk and upper limb
- Face
- Internal capsule
- Basis pedunculi of midbrain
- Oculomotor nerve
- Basil part of pons
- Trigeminal nerve
- Hypoglossal nerve
- Pyramid of medulla
- Pyramidal decussation
- Lateral corticospinal tract
- Spinal cord
- Ventral corticospinal tract

▲ **Figure 10.38 The motor pathways**

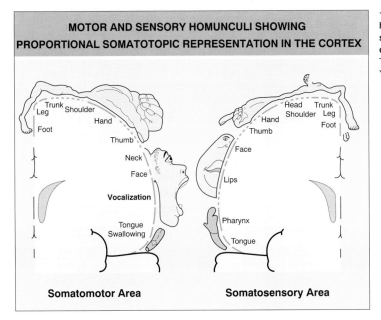

MOTOR AND SENSORY HOMUNCULI SHOWING PROPORTIONAL SOMATOTOPIC REPRESENTATION IN THE CORTEX

Somatomotor Area

Somatosensory Area

◀ **Figure 10.39 Motor and sensory homunculi showing proportional somatotopic representation in the cortex**. (After Penfield W. and Rasmussen T. (1950) The Cerebral Cortex of Man, New York, Macmillan)

medulla renders a lesion in these parts unusually disastrous in its results. Paralysis is often extensive and bilateral, and other brainstem structures (sensory fibres, cranial nerve nuclei, etc.) may be damaged.

The fibres of the corticospinal tracts pass along the spinal cord for a varying distance, some ending in the upper and some in the lower segments of the cord in close proximity to the anterior horn cells. Between the terminations of the corticospinal fibres and the anterior horn cells there appear to be short internuncial neurons.

The results of corticospinal tract destruction will vary with the level at which the tract is interrupted: for example, if in the cervical regions, both arms and legs will be paralysed; if in the lower thoracic regions, only the legs. Certain movements, notably of the upper part of the face, the jaw and the larynx, are bilaterally represented in the cortex and are therefore little affected by unilateral lesions of the corticospinal system. Bilateral lesions may cause dysarthria and dysphagia (see page 256).

Motor apraxia

This is defined as an inability to perform a purposeful movement. An intention begins in the auditory association cortex of the dominant hemisphere, passes to the parietal cortex and enters the premotor cortex and finally the motor cortex. Interruption to this pathway at any point may result in an ideomotor apraxia. It should be noted that whole body movements are relatively well pre-

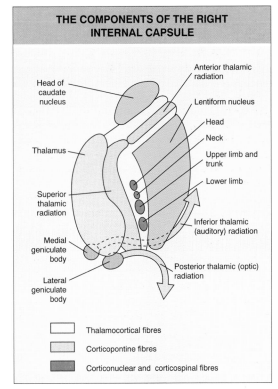

THE COMPONENTS OF THE RIGHT INTERNAL CAPSULE

Head of caudate nucleus

Thalamus

Superior thalamic radiation

Medial geniculate body

Lateral geniculate body

Anterior thalamic radiation

Lentiform nucleus

Head

Neck

Upper limb and trunk

Lower limb

Inferior thalamic (auditory) radiation

Posterior thalamic (optic) radiation

Thalamocortical fibres

Corticopontine fibres

Corticonuclear and corticospinal fibres

▲ **Figure 10.40 The components of the right internal capsule: horizontal section**. (After Carpenter M. B. and Sutin J. (1983) Human Neuroanatomy. Baltimore, Williams and Wilkins)

served even when ideomotor apraxia is substantial. This may be tested for by giving the patient with apparently normal function of his limbs and no paralysis of the hands a box of matches instructing him to strike one. He is unable to take a match out of the box and strike it.

THE LOWER MOTOR NEURON

From the anterior horn cells, fibres pass out as the anterior nerve roots to become eventually the peripheral nerves, in many of which sensory fibres are present. The motor fibres end in the voluntary muscles. This lower neuron may be interrupted by lesions in the anterior horn cells, in the nerve roots, in the peripheral nerves, or at the termination in the muscle (motor end-plate). The results will differ in the distribution of the paralysis, and the effects of a lesion of the anterior horn cells or nerve roots will be entirely motor; in peripheral nerve damage sensory changes often occur as well.

The lower motor neuron is influenced by the upper neuron and also by the extrapyramidal system, and mod-

ifications of muscle tone and reflexes result when the correct balance between these neurons is lost (see Table 10.2). The trophic changes often found in diseases chiefly affecting the lower neuron are due mainly to associated damage to the sensory and autonomic systems.

Anterior horn cells: muscle weakness and fasciculation.
Nerve roots: muscle weakness.
Peripheral nerve: muscle weakness and sensory loss.
Motor end plate: myasthenia gravis syndrome.

THE EXTRAPYRAMIDAL SYSTEM

The basal ganglia are located in the fore- and midbrain and include the putamen, globus pallidus, caudate nucleus, substantia nigra and red nucleus. The basal ganglia receive impulses from the cerebral cortex, thalamus and reticular formation and connect with the anterior horn cells via the striospinal fibres, vestibulospinal, rubrospinal, tectospinal and reticulospinal tracts.

◀ Table 10.2

CLINICAL DISTINCTION BETWEEN UPPER AND LOWER MOTOR NEURON LESIONS	
Upper neuron	**Lower neuron**
Paralysis affects movements rather than muscles	Individual muscles or groups of muscles affected
Wasting only from disuse, therefore slight. Occasionally marked in chronic severe lesions	Wasting pronounced
Spasticity of 'clasp-knife' type. Muscles hypertonic	Flaccidity. Muscles hypotonic
Cyanosis and oedema may result from disuse; no gross trophic changes (except in infantile hemiplegia)	Skin often cold, blue and shiny. Ulceration may result
Tendon reflexes increased (see page 246). Clonus often present	Tendon reflexes diminished or absent
Superficial reflexes diminished or modified (see page 250). Note especially absent abdominal reflexes. Babinski and Hoffmann signs, and increased jaw jerk	Superficial reflexes often unaltered unless sensation is also lost or when appropriate LMN is interrupted
Associated movements sometimes present	No associated movements. Fasciculations and myotatic irritability often present

In summary, these ganglia and tracts bring the anterior horn cells of the spinal cord under the influence of the subcortical nuclei which therefore modify the programme of muscular action. The basal ganglia integrate components of skilled motor tasks such as writing and walking.

Lesions of the extrapyramidal system do not result in paralysis but interfere with the delicate precision characterized in perfect movement. For example, lesions of the globus pallidus lead to increased duration of movement in the contralateral limbs whilst loss of inhibition caused by lesions of the red nucleus may lead to involuntary movement of the contralateral limbs.

THE CEREBELLUM

This part of the brain lies closely packed below the tentorium in intimate contact with the pons and medulla and the cranial nerves (5–12) which take origin in the neighbourhood. It is not surprising, therefore, that lesions of the cerebellum are frequently accompanied by signs of involvement of these neighbouring structures.

The cerebellum has elaborate connections with other parts of the nervous system, notably with the vestibular organs, the cerebral cortex and pons, and the spinal cord. These connections make the explanation of cerebellar symptoms complex, but, in general, muscular co-ordination depends upon the connections of the cerebellum with the higher parts of brain, while tone and equilibrium are more particularly associated with its connections with the lower parts. Modern work tends to assign disturbances of equilibrium to the flocculo-nodular lobe, while hypotonia and disorders of movement appear to be related to the neocerebellum.

SYMPTOMS OF DISEASE OF THE MOTOR SYSTEM

The chief symptoms of motor system disease are weakness, stiffness, unsteadiness and tremor.

WEAKNESS

The patient may complain merely of weakness in a limb or other part of the body. To this the name paresis is given. When the part is immovable or nearly so the term paralysis is applied. A paralysis affecting one side of the body is known as hemiplegia; if it is confined to one limb, monoplegia; if it affects both legs, paraplegia; or both arms and both legs, either tetraplegia or quadriplegia. Paralysis is as obvious to the patient as to the doctor; paresis may only be discovered on examination.

In upper neuron lesions paralysis is, to some extent, selective. The limbs are affected more than the trunk, and smaller and more precise movements of the hands are usually interfered with more than the grosser movements, e.g. of the shoulders (Figure 10.41). In the lower limb dorsiflexion of the ankle is usually affected and also flexion at the knee and hip, while extension at the knee, hip and toes is little affected.

Paralysis arising from the lower neuron lesions affects individual muscles or groups of muscles controlled by particular segments of the cord. Knowledge of the segmental control is of localizing value, e.g. in spinal cord compression, and the table indicates the motor distribution of the main spinal segments (Table 10.3).

STIFFNESS

Stiffness in one or more limbs may be due to spasticity from interruption of the corticospinal tract. The rigidity of extrapyramidal disease is more generalized and

PRINCIPAL SEGMENTAL REPRESENTATION OF MUSCLES	
C4	Scaleni, trapezius, levator scapulae, diaphragm
C5	Levator scapulae, scaleni, supraspinatus, rhomboids, infraspinatus, teres minor, biceps, brachioradialis, deltoid, supinator longus, serratus anterior, pectoralis major (clavicular part)
C6	Subscapularis, pronators, teres major, latissimus dorsi, serratus anterior, pectoralis major
C7	Triceps, extensors and flexors of wrist and digits
C8	Small hand muscles
Th1	Interossei and small hand muscles
Th1 to 10	Intercostals
Th5 to 11	Abdominal muscles
L1	Quadratus lumborum
L3	Sartorius, adductors of hip, iliopsoas
L4	Quadriceps femoris, abductors of hip
L5	Flexors of knee
S1	Calf muscles
S2	Small foot muscles
S3, 4	Pelvic muscles

▲ Table 10.3

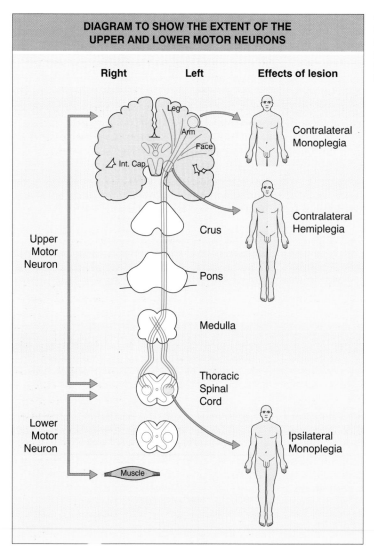

◄ Figure 10.41 Diagram to show the extent of the upper and lower motor neurons and the effects of a lesion in different parts of the motor system. Only the common positions for a lesion have been illustrated

may lead to stiffness of the neck and trunk muscles as well as the limbs. Dysphagia and dysarthria may also occur in extrapyramidal or bilateral pyramidal lesions.

UNSTEADINESS

Patients with cerebellar dysfunction will complain of loss of balance with a tendency to fall towards the side of the lesion. They may feel unable to control the movements of their hands for everyday purposes such as writing, shaving and eating. They may also notice inco-ordination of speech.

TREMOR (see also page 240)

A persistent rhythmic tremor at rest can be one of the most disabling symptoms of extrapyramidal disease; the patient may find that the tremor is influenced by emotion. The action or intention tremor of cerebellar origin occurs mainly when a movement is attempted so that the patient's purpose is frustrated. The clonic tremor of pyramidal disease usually affects the lower limb and tends to occur when the foot is held in dorsiflexion because of stretching of the Achilles tendon.

PHYSICAL SIGNS OF DISEASE OF THE MOTOR SYSTEM

The prime function of the motor system is to permit precise and well-ordered voluntary contractions of the muscles. The examination of the motor system is firstly concerned, therefore, with testing this movement. Many incidental observations are made, however, which have a direct or indirect bearing on the integrity of the motor neurons. Briefly these fall under the following headings: trophic changes, atrophy or hypertrophy of muscles; fasciculations and myotatic irritability; contractions and contractures; involuntary movements; abnormal postures and gaits. Inspection is the chief method by which these physical signs are elicited, and they are often noted before muscular power and tone are tested. In the interpretation of these abnormal signs, the integrity of the sensory system and reflex arcs must be taken into account (see below), but the signs are more conveniently described in the present section.

TROPHIC CHANGES

The colour, temperature and texture of the skin should be recorded and any oedema or ulceration noted.

Such changes may result from neurological disease which causes sensory loss, e.g. peripheral neuropathy and syringomyelia, from disturbances of the autonomic nervous system and sometimes from disuse.

ATROPHY AND HYPERTROPHY

The contour and size of the muscles should be noted.

Atrophy is a characteristic of lower motor neuron lesions (Figure 10.42), but also occurs in the myopathies (page 259) and to a lesser extent from disuse, especially in rheumatoid arthritis.

For accuracy the circumference should be measured and compared with the normal side. Each limb must be measured at the same level. In the case of the legs, for

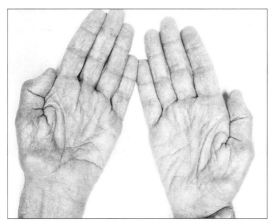

▲ **Figure 10.42 Wasting of the small muscles of the hand. From a case of progressive muscular atrophy.** Note especially the flattened thenar eminences

example, the measurement may be made 15 cm below the lower border of the patella with the limbs extended. The distribution of the atrophy helps in diagnosis, tending to be distal in neuronal disease and proximal in certain myopathies.

Hypertrophy is more difficult to recognize. Slight grades may result from increased occupational use of certain groups of muscles, or occasionally as a developmental defect. Without such cause, the presence of apparent muscular hypertrophy usually suggests muscular dystrophies. In the pseudohypertrophic form of muscular paralysis the relatively great calves and buttocks stand out in marked contrast with the atrophic flexor muscles of the thighs.

FASCICULATIONS AND MUSCULAR IRRITABILITY

Fasciculations are not uncommonly seen in chronic degenerative lesions of the anterior horn cells, particularly progressive muscular atrophy and amyotrophic lateral sclerosis. They may be provoked by tapping. The muscle fibres produce a quivering of the skin by their irregular contractions. Fasciculation can be an important early sign of motor neuron disease and can occur in muscles which are not grossly wasted. Fasciculations may occur even in health and should not be regarded as pathological unless the patient is warm and relaxed, for shivering from any cause may give rise to similar movements. Nor should they be confused with myokymia, a familiar and harmless phenomenon in which there is twitching of the orbicularis oculi or less commonly other muscles ('live flesh'). Wasting muscles as in lower neuron lesions are often irritable and contractions can be produced easily by a light tap.

CONTRACTIONS AND CONTRACTURES

When a group of muscles is paralysed the action of unopposed groups causes the limb to assume an abnormal position. This happens by virtue of *muscular contraction*. In time fibrotic changes take place in the paralysed muscles and their tendons, resulting in true contractures, which are of a permanent and progressive nature. The effects of contraction (see Muscle tone – rigidity, page 244) can be overcome by passive movement, but this is not possible with contractures unless considerable force is used.

In upper neuron lesions affecting the corticospinal tracts alone, e.g. cerebral hemiplegia and spinal paraplegia, the limbs are in an extended position; but if the lesion also involves the extrapyramidal tracts below the vestibular nucleus, an attitude of flexion in the limbs results. *Paraplegia in flexion* is thus indicative of a more severe lesion of the spinal cord than *paraplegia in extension*.

The attitude resulting from these types of paralysis may become permanent if contractures are allowed to ensue.

INVOLUNTARY MOVEMENTS

If movements of the limbs, face or trunk are observed, their exact distribution and type must be recorded. Factors aggravating or diminishing the movements should also be noted, especially the effect of voluntary movement, sleep and emotion.

Choreiform movements

Choreiform movements are irregular and spontaneous. They are quick and apparently purposeless and may occur anywhere in the body but may be predominant on one side (hemichorea). Emotion and voluntary effort usually increase them, but during sleep they disappear.

They are seen in *rheumatic chorea* (Sydenham's chorea), popularly but incorrectly called 'St Vitus's dance', a disease which has now become uncommon. Children are most frequently affected, and the involuntary movements cause the child to drop things and to 'pull faces'. Weakness of the affected side is common, and may be so extreme as to be called 'paralytic chorea'. Particular signs such as the jack-in-the-box tongue, a rapid protrusion and withdrawal of the tongue, depend upon the inability to sustain posture. The syndrome of chorea is in all probability attributable to lesions in the extrapyramidal system though possibly cortical.

In *Huntington's chorea* similar involuntary movements are seen, but as this disease is familial and occurs in the fourth and fifth decades and is associated with progressive dementia, no difficulty is found in distinguishing it from rheumatic chorea. Moreover the movements are slower. Unlike the movements of rheumatic chorea they are probably a release symptom due to a lesion of the basal ganglia.

Athetosis

In cases of hemiplegia of long duration, especially infantile hemiplegia, peculiar slow 'snake-charming' movements may be seen, known as 'athetosis'. They chiefly affect the hands and consist of alternate flexion and extension at the wrists and fingers, with spreading of the latter.

Athetosis is only seen when some degree of voluntary movement is retained by the paralysed limb. Occasionally the movements occur in the feet (hyperextension of the big toe), and great facial contortion may result if the affection is bilateral. The phenomenon is thought to arise from a lesion in the extrapyramidal system and its cortical connections and is sometimes found without upper neuron signs. It is in the nature of a release symptom.

Hemiballismus

Hemiballismus is a swinging movement of violent nature of an arm and leg. The movements are of greatest ampli-

tude at the shoulder and hip, but the affected limbs are usually flaccid. A vascular lesion is the usual cause when it affects the contralateral subthalamic nuclei.

Habit-spasms and tics

It is sometimes difficult to distinguish choreiform movements from the more purposive movements seen in habit-spasms and tics. These are of many different types. Some are very simple, such as shrugging the shoulders or blinking the eyes; others are highly complex, affecting many groups of muscles and perhaps associated with verbal abnormalities such as the frequent uncontrollable repetition of the same word or sentence. A more common and special form is a stammer.

The most important point of distinction from chorea is the repetition of the same movements, though a new movement may replace an old one. The movements may go on for much longer than chorea, e.g. months, without much variation in intensity. Disease of the eyelids may, for example, cause blepharospasm, which normally passes away when the local cause is cured. There will be no other abnormal physical signs.

Tremors

Tremors are shaking movements, fine or coarse, which are usually most evident in the hands but may affect the head ('titubation') or other parts of the body.

Tremors of *metabolic* origin may be fine, as in hyperthyroidism (see Chapter 12), or irregularly coarse or flapping as in hepatic, renal and respiratory failure (see Chapters 4, 5 and 6). Fine or coarse tremors may also be seen in certain *toxic* states such as alcoholism. If the patient is asked to extend the arms, fine tremors can be felt by touching the fingers lightly or seen by using the technique shown in Figure 10.43. Coarse flapping tremors are brought out by full extension of the wrists when the arms are outstretched.

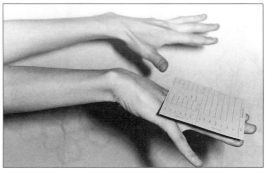

▲ **Figure 10.43 A method of demonstrating fine tremors by laying a thin piece of cardboard on the outstretched hand**

Tremors of *neurological* origin are of two kinds: static and action.

Static tremors are those which are relatively independent of movement or posture. The classic example is the rhythmic 3–5 per second coarse tremor of Parkinsonism which often first affects the index finger and thumb of one hand ('pill-rolling'). This is followed later by flexion–extension movements of the wrist and pronation–supination movements of the forearm. In its early stages, the tremor is inhibited for a few seconds by skilled activity but later may spread to involve the whole body.

Action tremors are usually evident on voluntary movement or during the active maintenance of a posture; they are common in adults and tend to increase with age. They are aggravated by emotional tension and quite often suppressed by alcohol. The tremors are fine affecting the hands, head and voice. The tremor best demonstrated by voluntary movement is that characteristic of cerebellar dysfunction (intention tremor). An intention tremor is illustrated by asking the patient to touch the tip of the nose accurately with the tip of his index finger when the excursion of the involuntary movement will increase as the finger approaches the nose (see Figure 10.64).

Another form of action tremor is the clonic tremor of a pyramidal tract lesion. Although this may occur spontaneously, it is usually provoked by dorsiflexion of the foot when the patient puts his toes on the ground.

CONVULSIVE MOVEMENTS

These are described on page 279.

A rare type is *myoclonus* which consists of a sudden shocklike contraction producing recurring muscle jerks. The movements may be generalized or confined to one part of the body. When the palate is involved the patient may have noticed an inability to sustain an even pitch when speaking or singing. This usually follows damage to the brainstem from cerebrovascular disease, but myoclonus may be an expression of a familial tendency with or without epilepsy and of encephalopathies such as Creutzfeld–Jacob disease or subacute sclerosing encephalitis.

ABNORMAL POSTURES

The posture of the patient, both erect and recumbent, must be observed when possible. Abnormal postures may be observed when the proper control of muscular tone and movement is affected. Lesions of the motor neurons – upper, lower and extrapyramidal – and of those tracts such as the posterior columns and cerebellar tracts which convey proprioceptive sensations may each result in altered posture.

Upper Neuron Lesions

In hemiplegia the paralysed arm is adducted, flexed at the elbow, fingers and wrist, and the forearm pronated. The hip also is adducted, the knee extended and the foot often inverted and plantar flexed. (See Figure 10.46.)

Lower Neuron Lesions

These include lesions of the anterior horn cells, nerve roots and peripheral nerves. They cause different types of posture dependent upon the groups of muscles paralysed. The posture will result at first chiefly from unopposed action of antagonistic groups of muscles, but later the contractures in the paralysed muscles may overcome this and cause a more permanent abnormal attitude of the limb.

Thus a lesion which picks out the extensor muscles of the wrist will result in the familiar 'wrist drop', seen in certain cases of peripheral neuropathy or lesions of the radial nerve. (See also Erb–Duchenne paralysis, page 257.) Other examples include the posture of the hand in ulnar and median nerve paralysis and in progressive muscular atrophy (Figure 10.44) and the result of paralysis of the long thoracic nerve (winged scapula, Figure 10.45).

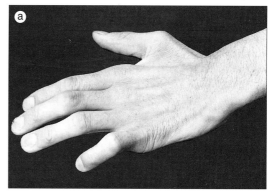

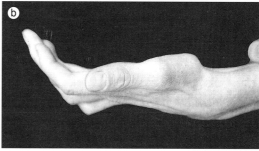

▲ **Figure 10.44 (a) Claw hand (main-en-griffe) from a case of** progressive muscular atrophy. Showing the wasting of the interosseous muscles. (b) Another view of the same hand

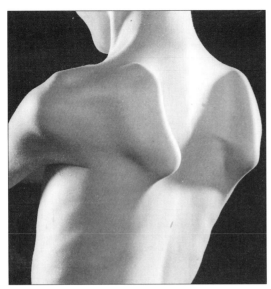

▲ **Figure 10.45 Winging of the scapulae from weakness of both serrati anterior in muscular dystrophy**

Extrapyramidal system

Lesions may result in Parkinsonism and cause an increase of tone in the flexor muscles in particular, and the result is an attitude of flexion. The patient stands with the knees slightly bent, the shoulders drooping and the chin sunk into the chest. The arms are partially flexed at the elbows and the hands at the metacarpophalangeal joints; but extension occurs at the wrists and interphalangeal joints. The lack of movement of the facial muscles is responsible for the vacant expression (Figure 10.77).

Lesions of Sensory and Cerebellar Systems

An example of the former is *tabes dorsalis* (affecting the posterior columns, see page 269) which leads to loss of tone in the muscles and sometimes modifies the posture. In tabes the hypotonus may result in abnormal extension at the knee joints – genu recurvatum. To preserve balance the patient stands with the feet well apart. Cerebellar lesions have a similar effect.

Abnormal Postures at Rest

Even when the patient is confined to bed, suggestive postures may be discovered. The retraction of the head and arching of the back (opisthotonos) are valuable signs of meningeal irritation; deviation of the head and eyes to one side is often seen in cerebral haemorrhage.

In *dystonia*, abnormal postures result from the contraction of antagonistic muscles and may be generalized or localized to one area, e.g. torticollis. The acute onset of dystonia is most often seen as a side effect of drug therapy such as Phenothiazines, Levodopa and Metoclopramide.

GAITS (Table 10.4)

The study of the gait is complementary to that of the posture in a neurological case.

The patient should be asked to walk across the floor with the legs uncovered and unhampered by clothes.

Spastic gaits are probably the commonest abnormal type. They result from upper motor neuron lesions such as hemiplegia and paraplegia.

In *hemiplegia* the affected limb is stiff and extended with the foot plantar-flexed. To avoid catching the toe against the ground at each step, the limb is sometimes circumducted in the arc of a circle (Figure 10.46).

The 'scissors' gait of *diplegia* results from contractures in the adductors of the thighs and is seen in the cerebral diplegia of children (Little's disease). The legs may cross in the act of walking (Figure 10.47).

Various types of *paraplegia* resulting from spinal cord compression, disseminated sclerosis, etc. cause bilateral stiffness of the legs and plantar flexion of the feet so that the patient walks on the toes.

Lesions involving the posterior columns and cerebellum cause *ataxia*, i.e. an unsteady, uncontrolled gait.

A somewhat similar gait results from other posterior column lesions, as in subacute combined degeneration and occasionally multiple sclerosis, though in these two diseases the spasticity resulting from corticospinal tract involvement may mask the ataxia. In Friedreich's ataxia the disorder of gait is due to involvement of the cerebellar tracts and posterior columns.

The ataxia of *cerebellar disease* (tumours, vascular lesions, etc.) is shown by a characteristic reeling or 'drunken man's' gait with a special tendency to fall to one side, usually to the side of the lesion owing to the loss of muscle tone on that side.

The gait in *extrapyramidal lesions* (Parkinsonism) is stiff, and the short steps taken by the patient give a quick shuffling appearance, a phenomenon known as *festination*. In classic cases, if pushed gently forwards, the patient appears 'to hurry after his centre of gravity' (*propulsion*). If pushed backwards he continues in the same direction until he falls or is stopped (*retropulsion*). Lateropulsion is a similar movement sideways, more rarely seen. On walking, the arms do not swing freely.

Another characteristic of the gait in Parkinsonism is that, on being asked to walk away and then turn round, the patient carries out a 'military' turn in three or four steps instead of swinging around on the ball of the foot.

◀ Table 10.4

ABNORMAL GAITS		
Descriptive term	**Explanation**	**Site of lesion**
Spastic (arm still)	Increased tone Circumduction	Upper motor neurone
Scissors	Bilateral adduction and contractures	Bilateral upper motor neurone
Wide based ataxia	Loss of balance	Posterior columns
Drunken ataxia	Hypotonia and inco-ordination	Cerebellum and connections
Festinating (arm still)	Hypertonicity Bradykinesia	Extrapyramidal
High stepping	Foot drop	Peripheral neuropathy Poliomyelitils Progressive muscular atrophy
Waddling	Hip muscle weakness Hip damage	Muscular dystrophy
Limping	Short or painful leg	Leg or foot
Astasia-abasia	Cannot stand or walk	Hysteria

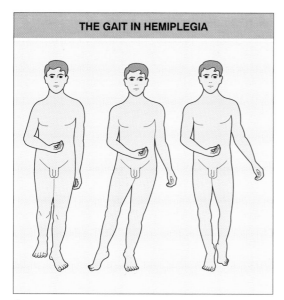

THE GAIT IN HEMIPLEGIA

▲ Figure 10.46 The gait in hemiplegia

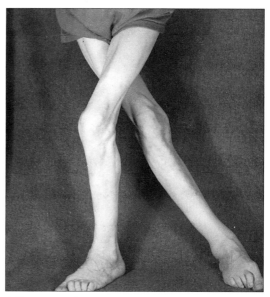

▲ Figure 10.47 Congenital cerebral diplegia. Cross-legged progression. 'Scissors' gait

Peripheral neuropathy commonly leads to foot-drop as a result of peroneal muscle weakness. The patient adopts a characteristic *high steppage* gait to avoid dragging the toes along the ground.

When pain is produced by weight-bearing the patient puts the foot down carefully and takes a short step to remove the weight off the painful limb as soon as possible. A *limping gait* may also be associated with a short leg or a deformed foot.

Other special types of gait, less frequently observed, are the *waddling gait* of muscular dystrophies caused by weakness of the glutei, also seen in congenital dislocation of the hips, and the contorted gait of Huntington's chorea.

Hysteria may also produce many peculiarities of gait. One special, though uncommon form, generally seen in children, is known as *astasia-abasia*, an inability to stand or walk.

Lastly it is necessary in suspected *myopathies* to watch the way in which the patient rises from the recumbent to the erect posture (Figure 10.48). In the Duchenne type of muscular dystrophy this is highly characteristic. The patient rolls over, gets on to his hands and knees and takes the weight of the body with the hands while he extends the knees. He then levels the trunk upright with the hands placed on the thighs. Occasionally paralysis of the extensor muscles of the thighs – e.g. from anterior poliomyelitis – has a similar result.

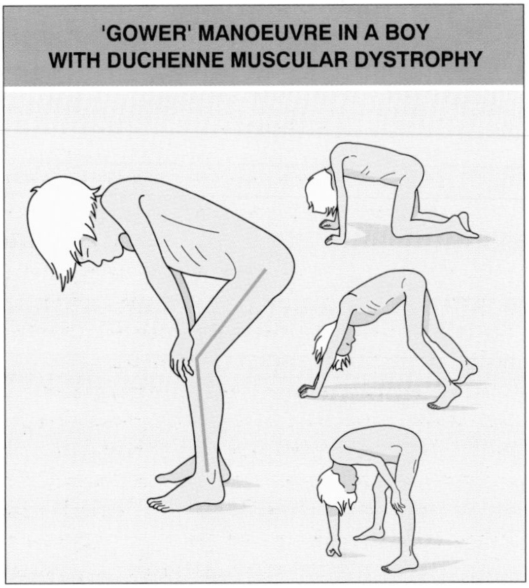

'GOWER' MANOEUVRE IN A BOY WITH DUCHENNE MUSCULAR DYSTROPHY

▲ Figure 10.48 'Gower' manoeuvre in a boy with Duchenne muscular dystrophy

MUSCLE TONE

Muscle tone is maintained by the continuous activation of alpha motor neurons by muscle spindles acting as stretch receptors. Inhibition of this tone is exerted by corticospinal, corticoreticulospinal and corticorubrospinal tracts and this is an example of a release phenomenon. Vestibular nuclei are independent of cortical control and facilitate anti-gravity extensor muscle action, whereas corticospinal and rubrospinal fibres activate flexor muscles. The vestibulospinal and reticulospinal tracts are important in equilibration, locomotion and maintenance of an upright posture. Reticulospinal fibres innervate axial and proximal limb muscle but corticospinal tracts innervate distal limb muscles. Thus section of the brainstem below the vestibular nuclei produces decerebrate rigidity and following a stroke above the vestibular nuclei there is spasticity of limbs especially affecting the extensor muscles.

In order to test muscle tone it is essential that the patient should be warm and relaxed. Not all joints need to be assessed and flexion and extension of the elbows and knees and pronation and supination of the forearm are suitable for screening purposes. The posture of the limb may indicate a discrepancy between the flexors and extensors as in decerebrate or decorticate states (see page 213).

Any pain in the joint or limb should be noted since this might cause voluntary resistance to movement. The limb is held on either side of the joint to be tested and passively moved through the full range of mobility, and this is repeated using the range of speeds from slow to fast.

Hypertonia

Hypertonia occurs in lesions of the upper motor neuron and extrapyramidal system.

Spasticity is typical of an upper motor neuron lesion. When the limb is moved the maximum resistance is noticed almost at once, but it gives way suddenly after some effort on the part of the examiner and allows the limb to be moved with comparative ease ('clasp-knife' effect). Spasticity is usually maximal in the flexors of the arms and the extensors of the legs.

Rigidity is a feature of Parkinsonism and may be of two kinds: 'cog-wheel' rigidity, in which the resistance to movement diminishes in jerky steps; this is probably due to a combination of tremor and rigidity. In cases without tremor, rigidity is of the 'lead pipe' variety. Extrapyramidal rigidity is often greater in the head, neck and shoulder than in the limbs. Rigidity may be activated by contraction of muscles in an unaffected limb. If there is doubt about an increase in tone the patient is asked to clench their teeth or grip the contralateral hand or swing the contralateral arm when the rigidity in the limb under examination will become more apparent.

Hypotonia

Hypotonia occurs in lower motor neuron and cerebellar lesions or when there is a loss of muscle afferents as in tabes dorsalis. Passive movement is unduly free, often through a greater range than normal.

MOTOR POWER

Muscle weakness may be suggested by lack of spontaneous movement in the affected part (limb or face) observed when the patient walks into the room or during the consultation.

After this preliminary inspection the examiner proceeds to test the muscular strength of the limbs and trunk using the MRC grading classification of muscle power rather than using inexact terms such as weakness (see Table 10.5).

At each important joint the action of the extensors and flexors, abductors and adductors, pronators and supinators, etc. must be tested without any load and then against the resistance of the physician's hand and compared with the same muscles in the opposite limb. Movements of head and trunk (flexion, extension and rotation) must be similarly tested. The hand grip is important but allowance must be made for the normal variation in power according to handedness. Attention must also be given to the patient's ability to perform more complex but everyday movements such as buttoning a coat or combing the hair. Loss of skilled movements may be an important early sign of an upper motor neuron lesion. *Bradykinesia,* a slowness in initiating and maintaining movement, is seen in Parkinsonism.

The importance of the distribution of muscular weakness has already received attention. When confined to one limb it is known as a monoplegia, if involving one half of the body hemiplegia. If both legs are affected the muscular weakness is known as a paraplegia and if there is weakness of all four limbs the terms quadriplegia or tetraplegia are used.

Weakness predominates in the extensors of the arms and flexors of the legs, but with cortical lesions affecting, for example, the hand global loss of motor function predominates.

It is common for the degree of muscle weakness to fluctuate during the examination but the fatigability should be formally tested by abducting the shoulder to 90°. The patient is asked to maintain this position for about a minute and is then re-tested. In myasthenia gravis and myopathies the abducted arm position cannot be sustained as the muscle tires. In the legs elevation of the hip to 45° provides comparable information.

Muscle relaxation may be prolonged following voluntary contraction in *myotonia.* The patient is asked to clench the fist tightly and release suddenly. In myotonia there is significant delay before the fingers may be straightened – a sign that may also be noted by the alert examiner when shaking hands with the patient, who may have complained of difficulty in letting go of items held in the hand such as a banister rail or bus handle. To demonstrate myotonia the thenar eminence is tapped with a patella hammer or the tongue with a spatula when the affected muscle stays dimpled for several seconds (Tinel test).

REFLEXES

Reflex action is an immediate motor or secretory response to an afferent sensory impulse. For clinical purposes such reflex action is spoken of as a 'reflex', of which several types are differentiated:

1 Deep or tendon reflexes.
2 Superficial or skin reflexes.
3 Organic or visceral reflexes.

In health these should be present, and, in the case of deep and superficial reflexes, equal on the two sides of the body. It must be recognized, however, that past disease, or some present disability not necessarily of neurological significance, may modify them. Thus the abdominal reflexes may be absent owing to laxity of the abdominal wall after repeated pregnancies.

The clinical importance of reflexes depends partly on their localizing value (Table 10.6), and partly on the information they give as to the integrity of the neurons, sensory and motor, which form the reflex arc. If the tendon reflexes of the arm are altered, this will place the lesion higher than if those of the legs only are modified. Again, exaggeration of the deep reflexes is an important sign of an upper motor neuron lesion, while their loss is commonly found in lesions of the lower motor neuron or afferent sensory path.

MRC CLASSIFICATION OF MUSCLE POWER	
0	Total paralysis
1	Flicker of contraction
2	Movement with gravity eliminated
3	Movement against gravity
4	Movement against resistance but incomplete
5	Normal power

▲ Table 10.5

SEGMENTAL LEVELS OF SOME OF THE COMMONER REFLEXES*	
Deep reflexes	**Superficial reflexes**
Ankle jerk S1, 2	Plantar reflex S1, 2
Knee jerk L3, 4	Abdominal reflexes T7–11
Biceps jerk C5, 6	Cremasteric reflex L1
Triceps jerk C7, 8	
Radial jerk C6	
Jaw jerk pons	
* Variations of these levels are given by different authors.	

▲ **Table 10.6**

TENDON REFLEXES

These reflexes are elicited by striking a tendon and so stretching it. This forms the sensory impulse which passes up afferent nerve fibres to the spinal cord. Internuncial fibres convey the impulse to the anterior horn cells, which discharge a motor impulse to the muscles supplied from that segment (Figure 10.49).

Diminution or absence will result if the reflex arc is interrupted by injury or disease. It may be interrupted in the motor limb, in the sensory limb or in the spinal cord itself. Peripheral neuropathy and root lesions are the commonest causes for absent tendon reflexes. Tendon reflexes are also abolished by spinal cord shock, e.g. severe injury to the cord. Lesions of the muscles themselves (dystrophies, involvement in scar tissue) will, of course, prevent the muscular contraction which is the visible evidence of the reflex. Loss of tendon reflexes is bilateral in states of coma. Lastly it must be borne in mind that in some persons the deep reflexes are sluggish and occasionally absent without pathological cause, especially the ankle jerks in the elderly. Abolition of a reflex by a segmental lesion of the cord is particularly valuable in localization (see Table 10.6).

Exaggeration of the deep reflexes is an important sign of an upper motor neuron lesion, especially if unilateral or accompanied by other signs. The reason for this exaggeration (a 'release phenomenon') is not fully understood, but it appears that the higher centres in the pyramidal (corticospinal) and extrapyramidal sys-

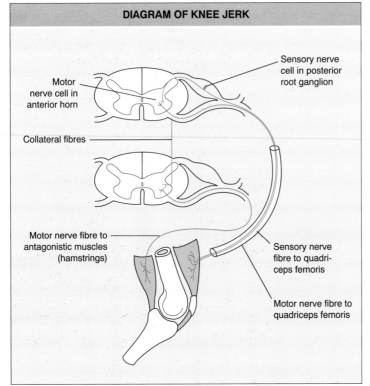

DIAGRAM OF KNEE JERK

Motor nerve cell in anterior horn

Sensory nerve cell in posterior root ganglion

Collateral fibres

Motor nerve fibre to antagonistic muscles (hamstrings)

Sensory nerve fibre to quadriceps femoris

Motor nerve fibre to quadriceps femoris

◀ **Figure 10.49 Diagram of knee jerk**

tems restrain the overactivity of the stretch reflexes, and when the restraint is lost these reflexes are more easily excited.

Moderate exaggeration of the tendon reflexes without other signs may occur in nervous persons and in conditions of hyperexcitability of the nervous system, e.g. tetanus.

The more important deep reflexes follow, and the methods by which they are elicited. Each reflex is graded according to the strength of the response which should be observed as a muscle contraction as well as a movement of the distal limb. The gradings are:

0	Absent even with reinforcement.
+/–	Present only with reinforcement.
+	Just present.
++	Normal.
+++	Exaggerated.

KNEE JERK

If the patient is able to sit, he should cross one leg over the other and allow the upper leg to hang loosely. A more mobile patient should be asked to sit with both legs hanging loosely over the edge of the couch or bed (see Figure 10.51). This position permits a more rapid comparison of the two knee jerks. The tendon hammer is held lightly between index finger and thumb, raised by extension of the wrist and then allowed to fall and strike the tendon by virtue of its own weight (Figures 10.50 and 10.51). A sharp tap on the patellar tendon then produces a contraction of the quadriceps extensor of the knee. The leg is momentarily shot forward if the contraction is sufficiently great, owing to the extension of the knee joint. If the legs are fat, the quadriceps tendon should be located by palpation to ensure that the tendon hammer strikes it properly.

Alternatively the patient may be recumbent, and his legs should be supported behind the knee with one hand and the patellar tendon tapped (Figure 10.50).

When the knee jerks are apparently absent they may be reinforced. The patient is asked to lock his hands and try to pull them apart while the physician strikes the patellar tendon (Figure 10.51). This is one method of producing a slight general increase of tone.

Apart from diminution or exaggeration of the knee jerks, certain special responses may be observed occasionally. In chorea they may be sustained, that is, after the contraction of the quadriceps has occurred, the leg seems to hover momentarily before falling to the resting position. Somewhat similar is the pendular knee jerk of acute cerebellar disease, present on the same side as the lesion. In myasthenia gravis the knee jerks

and other reflexes tire rapidly in common with voluntary muscular action. The reflexes in hypothyroidism show a normal immediate response but with a delayed return to the resting position, the biceps and ankle jerks especially (Figure 10.52).

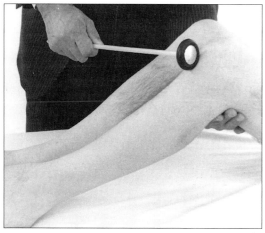

▲ **Figure 10.50 Knee jerk.** The knees are supported and a brisk tap made on each side to compare the response

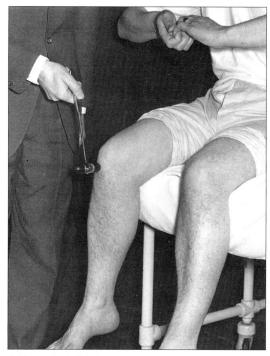

▲ **Figure 10.51 Reinforcement of knee jerks.** The patient pulls upon one hand with the other while the observer strikes the patellar tendon

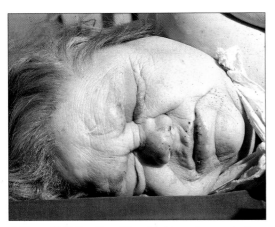

▲ **Figure 10.52 Hypothyroidism.** The biceps, knee and ankle jerks all showed delayed relaxation.

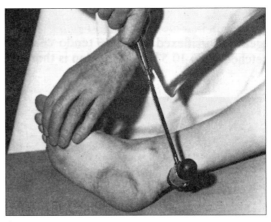

▲ **Figure 10.53 Ankle jerk.** When the patient is unfit to kneel this test can be carried out in bed

ANKLE JERK

If the patient is in bed the knee should be flexed, the hip externally rotated and the foot gently dorsiflexed until the tendo calcaneus (Achilles) is tensed but not overstretched (Figure 10.53). The tendon is then struck with a percussion hammer, each side being tested in quick succession for clear comparison of the responses. The ambulant patient may kneel (as shown in Figure 10.54). The result is a brisk plantar flexion of the foot.

TRICEPS JERK

The arm is supported at the wrist and flexed to a right-angle. The triceps tendon is struck just proximal to the point of the elbow (Figure 10.55), and the resulting contraction of the triceps causes extension at the elbow.

BICEPS JERK

The elbow is flexed to a right-angle and the forearm slightly pronated. The thumb is then placed over the biceps tendon and struck with a percussion hammer (Figure 10.56). The result is a contraction of the biceps, which causes flexion and slight supination of the forearm.

RADIAL JERK (SUPINATOR JERK)

The elbow is flexed to a right-angle and the forearm placed midway between pronation and supination. The styloid process of the radius is tapped with a percussion hammer (Figure 10.57). The result is a contraction of the brachioradialis causing flexion at the elbow and partial supination of the forearm.

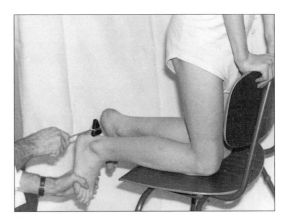

▲ **Figure 10.54 Ankle jerk.** A tap on the tendo calcaneus (Achilles) causes contraction of the gastrocnemius.

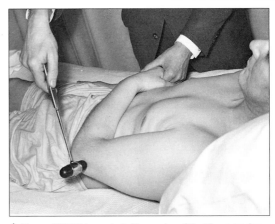

▲ **Figure 10.55 Triceps jerk.** Percussion of the triceps tendon causes contraction of the muscle with extension at the elbow

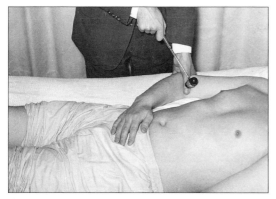

▲ **Figure 10.56 Biceps jerk**. A tap on the biceps tendon causes contraction of the biceps and flexion of the forearm

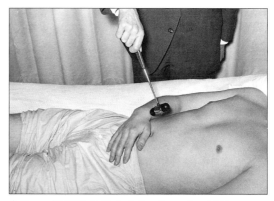

▲ **Figure 10.57 Radial jerk**. A sharp tap on the styloid process of the radius causes flexion at the elbow and partial supination of the forearm

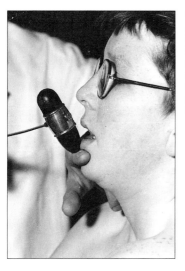

◄ **Figure 10.58 Jaw jerk. The finger lies on the lower jaw and is struck with the hammer.** A contraction of the masseters may result

HOFFMANN'S SIGN

This indicates increased tendon reflex activity in the finger flexors. The distal phalanx of the middle finger is first flexed and then abruptly released. If the sign is positive the thumb and index finger will then flex with a flicking motion.

JAW JERK

The jaw is allowed to relax and the mouth to hang open loosely. The finger is placed on the lower jaw and is struck with the hammer. A brisk response suggests a lesion of both corticopontine (pyramidal) tracts (Figure 10.58).

CLONUS

Closely allied to the tendon reflexes is clonus, a series of involuntary contractions of certain muscles initiated by stretching their tendons. Clonus is usually found when the tendon reflexes are grossly exaggerated and is therefore commoner in organic (upper neuron) than functional nervous disorders. It is of more significance when it is increased by continuing and increasing the stimulus (stretching the tendon) than if it is abolished. The former type is called 'true' or 'inexhaustible' clonus, the latter 'spurious' or 'exhaustible'. In many cases, however, the spurious clonus may become true as the malady progresses. Clonus occurs in two main types in clinical practice: ankle clonus and patellar clonus.

Ankle clonus

Ankle clonus is elicited by sharply pressing up the foot into the dorsiflexed position (Figure 10.59). This results in contractions of the calf muscle leading to plantar flexion of the foot, and in upper motor neuron disease the contractions usually continue as long as pressure is made.

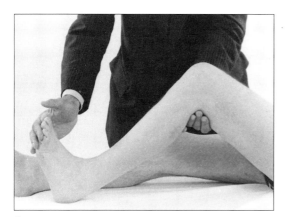

▲ **Figure 10.59 Ankle clonus**. The foot is sharply dorsiflexed. If clonus is present the calf muscles give series of jerky contractions

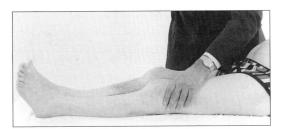

▲ **Figure 10.60 Patellar clonus**. The patella is pressed firmly and sharply downwards. If clonus is present a series of jerky contractions of the quadriceps takes place, continuing while pressure is exerted

Patellar Clonus

With the leg extended at the knee, the patella is fitted into the angle between the thumb and first finger (Figure 10.60). A sharp downward movement of the hand will induce contractions of the quadriceps which pull the patella upwards and continue so long as pressure is exerted.

SUPERFICIAL (CUTANEOUS) REFLEXES

These include the plantar responses, abdominal reflexes, cremasteric reflex, ciliospinal reflex and corneal reflex. All consist of a contraction of certain muscles when a particular area is stimulated by stroking or pinching.

PLANTAR REFLEX

If the sole of the foot is stroked firmly with a moderately sharp object such as a key, the great toe becomes plantar flexed. The stimulus should be applied to the outer half of the sole from the heel to the base of the small toes. This is the normal response which occurs in adults (Figure 10.61(a)). It may be absent without organic disease, especially when the feet are cold or damp, or if there is anaesthesia of the skin or paresis of the relevant muscles.

In infants, the response consists of extension of the great toe and occasionally spreading of the small toes in a fan-like manner. In adults such a response is always pathological, and is known as *Babinski's sign* (Figure 10.61(b)). Occasionally a Babinski response may result from stimulation over a wider area, e.g. the leg. If an excessive stimulus is applied, dorsiflexion of the toe may occur as part of a general withdrawal of the foot even in normal people. For this reason, the effect of a gentle stimulus with the thumb alone should always be tried before any form of implement is used. When the great toe is fixed due to osteoarthritis, flexion seen in the hip and knee may be an important sign.

Babinski's sign indicates that the corticospinal tracts are out of commission. This may be temporary, as in some types of coma and after epileptic fits, but as a permanent phenomenon it is found in such lesions of the upper motor neuron as cerebral vascular disease, multiple sclerosis and subacute combined degeneration. Occasionally in cases of paraplegia in extension a crossed response is obtained, namely, a Babinski sign on the stimulated side, and a plantar flexion of the opposite foot.

ABDOMINAL REFLEXES

To elicit these reflexes a sharp object, e.g. a metal pencil or key, is drawn firmly but lightly across the abdominal wall, on each side in turn (Figure 10.62). The four quadrants of the abdomen are examined in this way. In a healthy young adult the natural response is a contraction of the underlying abdominal muscles and a deviation of the linea alba to the same side. The response is generally brisker in the upper part of the abdomen (*epigastric reflex*).

In infants the abdominal reflexes are not present, and in adults obesity or laxity of the abdominal wall may abolish them. The abdominal reflexes often fatigue easily and may disappear after repeated stimuli. Acute abdominal lesions and sensory loss may also abolish these reflexes, but the most important cause of *absence* or *diminution* is a lesion of the corticospinal system. It is of greater significance, too, if the reflex is lost on one side only (e.g. in hemiplegia).

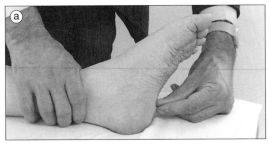

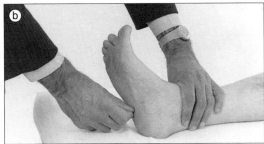

▲ **Figure 10.61 Plantar reflex**. (a) Normal response. (b) Babinski's sign

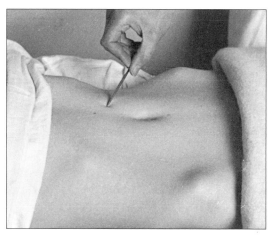

▲ **Figure 10.62 Abdominal reflex**. The skin of the abdomen is lightly stroked with a pencil. Brisk contraction of the underlying abdominal muscles normally occurs

One of the commonest nervous diseases in which the abdominal reflexes are bilaterally lost is multiple sclerosis.

CREMASTERIC REFLEX

This reflex consists in a retraction of the testicle by the cremaster muscle when the inner side of the thigh is stimulated by stroking the skin or pressure over the sub-sartorial canal. It is often difficult to elicit in older men, though easy in children. Loss occurs in corticospinal lesions, but is rarely of importance unless unilateral. It is not to be confused with the *dartos reflex* in which the scrotum contracts under the influence of cold.

CILIOSPINAL REFLEX

If the skin of the neck is pinched, the pupil normally dilates. The sympathetic trunk and pathway in the spinal cord must be intact for this reflex to occur, and its abolition therefore suggests a lesion of one of these. Loss of the ciliospinal reflex is used as a measure of the depth of coma and also as one of the criteria for the diagnosis of 'brain death'.

CORNEAL REFLEX

Light touch with cotton wool on the corneal surface of the eye normally produces blinking in both eyes. This reflex may be bilaterally abolished in coma of any type. Abolition may be confined to one side only. The loss then indicates a lesion either of the efferent limb (7th nerve) or of the afferent sensory limb (5th nerve ophthalmic division) on the same side. This reflex is important in the early diagnosis of 5th-nerve lesions, testing as it does for anaesthesia of the cornea.

PHARYNGEAL REFLEX

Irritation of the pharynx with a spatula produces contraction of the pharyngeal muscles. This may be absent in hysteria and in 9th and 10th cranial nerve lesions.

GRASP REFLEX

When the examiner's finger is drawn across the patient's palm, it may be grasped firmly if there is a lesion of the opposite frontal lobe.

ORGANIC OR VISCERAL REFLEXES

There are many reflexes governing the function of motile viscera such as the heart, lungs, bladder and gastrointestinal tract. These reflexes are mediated by the autonomic nervous system and may be abnormal in cases of autonomic neuropathy. An important example is the cardiovascular response to changes in posture. An abnormality in this reflex is suggested by a fall in systolic blood pressure on changing from the supine to the upright posture. In neurological practice, however, disturbances in the function of bladder and bowel are of prime importance.

MICTURITION

The activity of the bladder is under voluntary as well as reflex control. The detrusor muscle of the bladder is unstriated with a mainly parasympathetic cholinergic innervation via the S2–4 roots and pelvic nerve (Figure 10.63). The urethra on the other hand is encircled by striated muscle fibres which enable voluntary closure of the external sphincter; these fibres are supplied by the sacral somatic nervous system via the pudendal nerve. The reflex responses to bladder distension are co-ordinated in the brainstem reticular formation with a higher centre for voluntary control in the superior frontal gyrus.

In neurological disorders, the relative involvement of inhibitory and facilitatory pathways determines whether hesitancy and retention or precipitancy and incontinence are predominant. An acute spinal lesion causes retention of urine but, after a few weeks, reflex bladder evacuations occur in response to bladder distension. Lesions of the cauda equina usually result in persistent incontinence.

The reflex responses of the bladder may be studied by measuring pressure changes during distension with fluid. Frequent detrusor muscle contractions during filling are suggestive of an upper motor neuron lesion. When only a few weak contractions are induced by a large volume of fluid, a lower motor neuron lesion is likely.

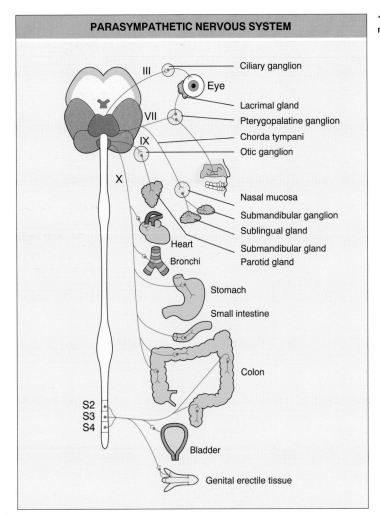

PARASYMPATHETIC NERVOUS SYSTEM

- Ciliary ganglion
- III
- Eye
- VII
- Lacrimal gland
- Pterygopalatine ganglion
- Chorda tympani
- IX
- Otic ganglion
- X
- Nasal mucosa
- Submandibular ganglion
- Sublingual gland
- Heart
- Submandibular gland
- Bronchi
- Parotid gland
- Stomach
- Small intestine
- Colon
- S2
- S3
- S4
- Bladder
- Genital erectile tissue

◀ **Figure 10.63 Parasympathetic nervous system**

DEFAECATION

Constipation or faecal incontinence may accompany the corresponding disorders of micturition in neurological diseases.

SEXUAL REFLEXES

The reflexes governing penile erection and seminal ejaculation are mediated by similar pathways to those of micturition so that impotence is a common accompaniment of neurological disturbances of the bladder.

MASS REFLEX

The mass reflex occurs in severe spinal cord lesions. After a period of flaccid paralysis with retention of urine and constipation, there occurs with paraplegia in flex-ion a periodic involuntary evacuation of the bladder and rectum. On the application of a stimulus (pin-prick or stroking the sole of the foot) to any point below the level of the lesion, especially in the midline of the body, the legs are vigorously drawn up, Babinski's sign occurs, the skin sweats below the lesion and the bladder and some-times the bowel are evacuated.

CO-ORDINATION

The co-ordination of movement depends among other factors upon the integrity of the sensory paths in the posterior columns and the cerebellum and its connections. Lack of proper co-ordination is known as *ataxia*.

In the *arms* the co-ordination of movement may be tested by asking the patient to touch the tip of the nose with the index finger of each hand in turn (Figure 10.64). Tests for co-ordination should be carried out with the eyes open, then closed, to distinguish sensory from motor ataxia (see below). The patient should be able to do this accurately both slowly and rapidly. Ataxia of the arms is seen in disseminated sclerosis and other cerebellar lesions.

In the legs ataxia is best observed by watching the patient's attempt to walk (see Gaits, page 242 and Table 10.4). In bed the 'heel-to-knee' test (Figure 10.65) may be made. The patient is instructed to touch each knee in turn with the opposite heel and then run it down his shin. The degree of ataxia in the affected limb may be roughly gauged by the clumsiness of the attempt. Ataxia in the legs is well seen in tabes and other lesions (Friedreich's ataxia, subacute combined degeneration) where the posterior columns are diseased. It also results from cerebellar lesions and some forms of peripheral neuropathy.

It is important to note that in the posterior column (sensory) type of ataxia the inco-ordination can be partially corrected by ocular impressions. The ataxia is therefore made worse by closing the eyes. In cerebellar (motor) ataxia the degree of ataxia may be little influenced by ocular impressions. These facts are the basis of *Romberg's sign*. The patient first stands with the eyes open and brings the heels as closely together as possible without losing his balance. The eyes are then closed, and normally the patient sways slightly. In posterior column lesions, he often sways to the extent of falling if unsupported. In sensory ataxia (posterior-column lesions) an error of projection is often present, e.g. when the patient attempts to touch the nose with the finger he fails to do so. This differs from the jerky movements of the arm in intention tremor (page 241), which is essentially a manifestation of cerebellar (motor) ataxia. Romberg's sign may be positive in cases of labyrinthine or cerebellar disease in which ocular impressions may partially compensate for the disorder of balance.

Other features of cerebellar ataxia (dysmetria and dysdiadochokinesia) are considered on page 262.

It must be remembered that the sensory impulses upon which co-ordinated movement depends may be interrupted in the brain itself – for example, in the thalamus or post-central gyrus. Cerebral lesions which injure these parts may therefore result in ataxia. Examples are seen in thalamic tumours or vascular lesions, internal capsular haemorrhage, and tumours of the post-central gyrus.

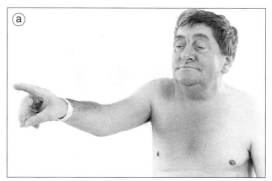

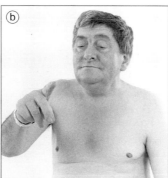

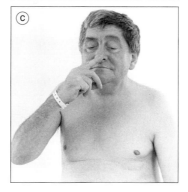

◀ **Figure 10.64 Method of testing for ataxia in the arms**. This method also demonstrates the presence of any 'intention' tremor

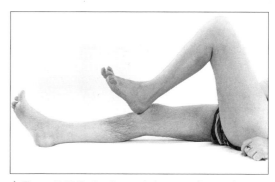

▲ **Figure 10.65 Testing for ataxia in a recumbent patient**. The 'heel-to-knee' test

LESIONS OF THE UPPER MOTOR NEURON

HEMIPLEGIA (see also Cerebral haemorrhage, page 274)

Vascular lesions are by far the commonest causes of hemiplegia, especially thrombosis of the middle cerebral artery or its branches causing infarction in small (cortical) or larger (internal capsular) areas of the brain. The extent of the paralysis varies with the number of motor fibres affected. In complete hemiplegia the face, arm and leg are paralysed, but the trunk and some cranial muscles escape, at least partially, because they are bilaterally represented in the cortex.

These signs may persist for less than 24 hours in which case the episode is known as a *transient ischaemic attack*. If they persist for longer than 24 hours and are not progressive the episode is known as a completed stroke. There may be an initial period of cerebral shock during which there is deep unconsciousness, loss of reflexes and conjugate deviation of the eyes away from the side of the lesion. At first the limbs may be flaccid but they become spastic when the signs of an upper motor neuron lesion develop. These are:

1 Muscle weakness.
2 Increased tone often with clonus.
3 Increased tendon reflexes.
4 Loss of abdominal reflexes.
5 Extensor plantar response.

These signs are in the limbs opposite to the side of the intracerebral lesion because of the decussation of the pyramidal tract in the medulla. If the patient partially recovers, contractures of muscles may occur in the elbow, wrist, knee and ankle and the characteristic posture and gait may develop as described (Figures 10.46 and 10.66).

Whatever the position of the lesion these signs of hemiplegia are the same provided all the corticospinal tract fibres are affected. From the short account of the anatomy of the motor tract given on page 258 it follows, however, that a complete hemiplegia more frequently results from a small lesion situated in a region where the fibres are closely crowded together, e.g. the internal capsule, crus, pons, or medulla. In the cortex a small lesion results in a more limited paralysis.

Even where the hemiplegia is complete one limb may be more affected than the other. Thus in internal-capsular thrombosis it is common for slight movement to remain in the leg though the arm is devoid of any. That the fibres to the leg are not so completely destroyed is shown by the quicker recovery of this limb. The facial paralysis is only partial and does not include the forehead or eye (cf. Bell's palsy, page 229) because the occipito-frontalis and orbicularis oculi muscles are supplied by a part of the 7th nerve nucleus which is governed by corticobulbar fibres from both sides of the brain.

Localization of the lesion

Certain special features help to localize the lesion causing the hemiplegia.

In the cortex, monoplegia, or paralysis of an even smaller group of muscles, is common. Aphasia is a frequent accompaniment if the left side of the brain is affected. Jacksonian fits may occur if the lesion is in or near the cortex.

In the internal capsule the hemiplegia is generally complete, and if the lesion extends into the posterior limb sensory changes and sometimes homonymous hemianopia on the same side as the paralysis may result (Figure 10.38). In the midbrain an ipsilateral third nerve paralysis may accompany a contralateral hemiplegia (Weber's syndrome) (Figure 10.67). When the red nucleus is involved unilateral tremor is found on the same side as the third nerve palsy (Claude's syndrome).

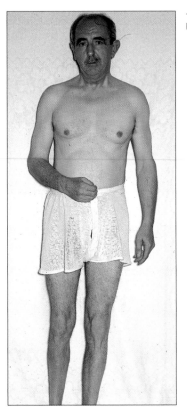

◀ **Figure 10.66**
Right hemiplegia

Tumours in the interpeduncular space may have a similar effect by pressure on the midbrain, but polydipsia and polyuria of hypothalamic origin may also be present.

In the pons other types of crossed lesion may occur when a contralateral hemiplegia is associated with an ipsilateral 6th and 7th nerve palsy (Millard–Gubler syndrome) or with a 7th nerve palsy alone (Foville syndrome). Strictly unilateral lesions of the pons are not common, and hemiplegic signs may therefore be present on both sides in variable degrees. Pinpoint pupils and hyperpyrexia are occasionally seen in cases of pontine haemorrhage. If the medial lemniscus is involved, ataxia and loss of deep sensibility may be present on the opposite side.

Crural and pontine lesions are not common and are generally vascular or neoplastic (Figure 10.68). In hemiplegia arising from lesions below the pons (7th nucleus) the face is spared.

In the medulla crossed paralyses also occur – hemiplegia on one side and paralysis of the 9th, 10th, 11th or 12th nerves on the other. As in pontine lesions the damage is rarely confined to one side, and frequently extends into the sensory tracts.

A lesion below the decussation of the corticospinal tracts in the lower medulla causes a hemiplegia on the same side. A lesion below the cervical region of the spinal cord will affect the leg alone (see Brown-Séquard's syndrome, page 268).

CAUSES OF HEMIPLEGIA

Vascular lesions are by far the commonest cause of hemiplegia (stroke) including cerebral embolism, haemorrhage and thrombosis. Disease of the extracerebral as well as intracerebral arteries will determine the extent of brain damage (page 273).

In a completed stroke abnormal physical signs develop within 24 hours and persist thereafter before any recovery occurs. A more gradual onset of hemiplegia is typically seen in primary and secondary malignancy, brain abscess and subdural haematoma.

Tumours and other space occupying lesions in the brainstem such as tuberculoma may present rapidly but degenerations such as a multiple sclerosis, Friedreich's ataxia and motor neuron disease may have a longer history.

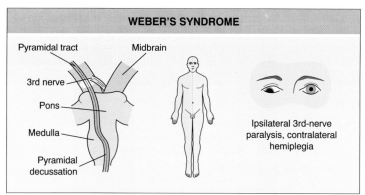

WEBER'S SYNDROME

Pyramidal tract · Midbrain · 3rd nerve · Pons · Medulla · Pyramidal decussation

Ipsilateral 3rd-nerve paralysis, contralateral hemiplegia

◄ **Figure 10.67 Weber's syndrome.** A lesion in the midbrain interrupting the pyramidal (corticospinal) tract fibres and simultaneously involving the 3rd nerve. Result: Contralateral paralysis of face, arm and leg (upper neuron type), with ipsilateral 3rd-nerve palsy (lower neuron type). Note the dilated pupil and the eye fixed in the downward and outward position

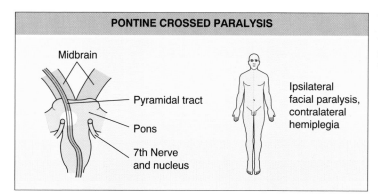

PONTINE CROSSED PARALYSIS

Midbrain · Pyramidal tract · Pons · 7th Nerve and nucleus

Ipsilateral facial paralysis, contralateral hemiplegia

◄ **Figure 10.68 Pontine crossed paralysis.** A lesion in the pons involving the nucleus of the 7th nerve, causing facial paralysis on the same side, and paralysis of the opposite arm and leg

PARAPLEGIA

This means paralysis of both lower limbs, but if the lesion is in the cervical region the arms may also be affected (quadriplegia). The signs are similar to those of hemiplegia, but bilateral (Figure 10.69). The paralysis is generally spastic, though severe lesions of the cord may cause an initial flaccid paralysis from spinal cord shock (see also Paraplegia in flexion and extension, page 239); the tendon reflexes are increased; the abdominal reflexes are lost if the lesion is above this reflex arc; Babinski's sign and clonus are present. Another important sign is loss of sphincter control, not generally present if the corticospinal tract is damaged on one side only.

Many diseases of the spinal cord are characterized by a combination of spastic paraplegia with sensory changes – for example, compression paraplegia and subacute combined degeneration. They will be described in the discussion of the sensory system.

UPPER MOTOR NEURON BULBAR PARALYSIS (PSEUDO-BULBAR PARALYSIS)

This term is applied to cases of difficulty in articulation and swallowing, sometimes with facial rigidity, due to *bilateral* involvement of the corticospinal fibres to the cranial nerve nuclei. It is usually due to bilateral cerebral thrombosis affecting the internal capsular region. Mild bilateral hemiplegic signs are present together with the

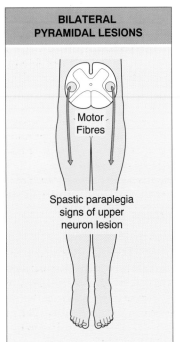

BILATERAL
PYRAMIDAL LESIONS

Motor
Fibres

Spastic paraplegia
signs of upper
neuron lesion

◀ **Figure 10.69**
Bilateral pyramidal lesions, e.g. multiple sclerosis. For signs of upper neuron lesion see page 254

bulbar symptoms and generally some emotional instability. The jaw jerk is increased, a sign which helps to differentiate this syndrome from Parkinsonism.

The history is one of hemiplegia, often slight on one side, followed after an interval (sometimes months or years) by similar affection of the opposite side. The first 'stroke' does not interfere with bulbar activities as the cortical control of these is bilateral. Pseudo-bulbar paralysis also results from motor neuron disease.

LESIONS OF THE LOWER MOTOR NEURON

The lower neuron may be injured or diseased in the cranial nerve nuclei or spinal anterior horn cells, in the anterior nerve roots, or in the nerves themselves.

The commonest acute lesion of the anterior horn cells is poliomyelitis (infantile paralysis). A chronic degeneration of the anterior horn cells also occurs as a part of motor neuron disease (progressive muscular atrophy).

The anterior nerve roots may be damaged by trauma, especially that associated with cervical spondylosis, and more rarely vascular, inflammatory and neoplastic lesions. The effects are similar to and frequently indistinguishable from disease of the anterior horn cells.

Lesions of the peripheral nerves are generally due to trauma, inflammation and various toxic or metabolic disorders (neuropathies). The results depend upon the distribution of the nerve and the position in which it is affected. When the nerve is purely motor (e.g. the long thoracic nerve to the serratus anterior) paralysis of the muscles supplied results; but as the majority of nerves are 'mixed', i.e. contain both motor and sensory fibres, muscular paralysis is frequently accompanied by sensory changes.

Some examples of lower neuron lesions may now be considered in more detail.

LESIONS OF THE ANTERIOR HORN CELLS AND OF THE BULBAR NUCLEI
Acute poliomyelitis (Infantile paralysis)

This disease is commonest in children and young adults, but has become less frequent since the introduction of preventive inoculation. It is infectious (virus) in origin, and the onset is therefore like other febrile illnesses, with which it is not uncommonly confused unless or until paralytic symptoms appear.

Pain in the back and tenderness of the limbs are suggestive early symptoms. Fever is often accompanied by signs of meningeal irritation (see page 271). In a few days a *flaccid paralysis* occurs and establishes the diagnosis. It is generally maximal at the onset, but occasionally extends with a new bout of fever. The extent is variable. Sometimes only a few muscles are affected; sometimes the greater part of all the limbs and trunk may be involved. The distribution of paralysis corresponds with the affected segments of the spinal cord (see Table 10.3, page 237). Involvement at the cervical and thoracic levels may lead to respiratory failure due to phrenic and intercostal nerve paralysis. The muscles most commonly singled out are those of the lower limbs, especially the extensors of the thigh, tibialis anterior, and peronei and of the feet and toes.

The signs of a lower neuron lesion are present: rapid wasting of the paralysed muscles (Figure 10.70), loss of tendon reflexes, flaccidity and trophic changes in the skin. Although acute poliomyelitis is now rare in the developed countries, it remains the commonest cause in adult life of a wasted and shortened limb.

Motor neuron disease

This is a progressive degenerative condition of middle or later life which may affect both upper and lower motor neurons, i.e. the corticospinal tracts, anterior horn cells and motor nuclei of the brainstem. Lower motor neuron signs are usually found mainly in the arms and consist of weakness, wasting and fasciculation especially in the small muscles of the hand (see Figure 10.42, page 239), where there may be a 'claw' deformity (see Figure 10.44, page 241). The tendon reflexes in the arms may be either diminished or increased according to whether the lower or upper neuron lesion predominates. In the legs, the tendon reflexes are usually exaggerated and the plantar responses extensor. Involvement of medullary nuclei may

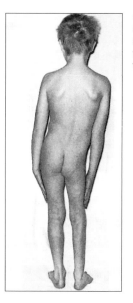

◀ **Figure 10.70 Poliomyelitis, showing wasting and shortening of the right leg with compensatory tilting of the pelvis**

lead to bulbar paralysis (see below) while bilateral corticospinal tract disease above the medulla will result in pseudo-bulbar paralysis. The absence of sensory symptoms and signs helps to distinguish this condition from syringomyelia and cord compression.

Bulbar paralysis

Reference has been made to this as a manifestation of motor neuron disease.

The principal symptoms are increasing difficulty in articulation due to paresis of the tongue (12th nucleus), difficulty in swallowing from paresis of the soft palate and pharynx, regurgitation of fluids through the nose and nasal voice (10th and 9th nuclei). The tongue wastes, shows fasciculation, and its movement is more and more limited. The larynx may also be involved. (See also Cranial nerves, page 233.) The process is essentially a chronic one, and death usually results from an inhalation pneumonia consequent upon the swallowing defect.

More rarely, bulbar paralysis of this type may be an acute process due to acute poliomyelitis, encephalitis or to vascular lesions. It may also be imitated by a peripheral neuropathy affecting the 9th, 10th and 12th cranial nerves. In myasthenia gravis bulbar symptoms are present but improve after a rest, only to recur after use of the affected muscles.

LESIONS OF THE ANTERIOR NERVE ROOTS

The anterior nerve roots contain autonomic preganglionic fibres and motor fibres which are distributed to the muscles in a segmental fashion so closely resembling that of the anterior horn cells as to make a diagnosis between a lesion of one or the other impossible unless other signs of spinal cord disease (e.g. corticospinal tract signs) are present.

The commonest lesions of the anterior nerve roots are traumatic, e.g. brachial plexus injuries, and the student's knowledge of anatomy has a direct practical application in such cases. It is not possible here to deal with the many varieties of traumatic lesions of the anterior nerve roots or the peripheral nerves. One example of a lesion of the anterior nerve roots may, however, serve as an illustration: the obstetrical palsy of Erb–Duchenne type.

Erb–Duchenne paralysis

In this condition the 5th cervical anterior nerve root is torn at birth. The result is a paralysis of the muscles governed by this segment – the deltoid, brachioradialis and biceps. From action of the unopposed muscles the hand and arm are held in the characteristic position. The arm is adducted and extended at the elbow, and the forearm pronated, giving the 'waiter's hand' position.

No lesion of an individual nerve could produce such a combination of muscular paralyses, and the cause can be narrowed down to a lesion of the anterior horn cells or the corresponding nerve root of the 5th cervical segment. The characteristics of a lower neuron lesion will be present, and the absence of sensory changes will further exclude a peripheral nerve lesion.

LESIONS OF THE PERIPHERAL NERVES
Traumatic lesions
Here again the student must be prepared to work out on anatomical grounds the nerve or nerves affected. The problem is made easier by the combination of muscular paralysis and anaesthesia corresponding with the distribution of an individual nerve. The paralysis, again, is of the lower neuron type, and in the area supplied by the sensory fibres of the nerve all types of sensation are lost.

As an example of a peripheral nerve lesion paralysis of the radial nerve may be taken.

Radial nerve paralysis
This is of particular interest to the physician, as not only is the radial the nerve most commonly injured, but it is sometimes affected in neuropathies.

The nerve, including its posterior interosseous branch, has a large motor distribution, comprising the triceps, brachioradialis, extensor carpi radialis longus and brevis and extensor digitorum. When it is injured high up (for example, in 'crutch paralysis' or 'Saturday night paralysis' due to pressure on some hard object during alcoholic stupor) these muscles are paralysed in varying degrees. The main result is wrist-drop, i.e. an inability to use the extensors of the wrist, and weakness of the extensors of the digits.

The sensory changes are limited owing to overlap with other nerves. Generally the anaesthesia is confined to a small area on the back of the thumb and the skin between this and the index finger.

Entrapment syndromes
Constriction or entrapment of a peripheral nerve may give rise to pain and paraesthesiae as well as objective motor and sensory changes in the distribution of the nerve. The three nerves most prone to such constriction are the median nerve in the carpal tunnel at the wrist, the ulnar nerve between the two heads of the flexor carpi ulnaris at the elbow and the lateral cutaneous nerve of the thigh as it passes behind the inguinal ligament.

The *carpal tunnel syndrome* occurs especially in middle-aged women doing ordinary housework or heavy manual work. It may also complicate pregnancy, rheumatoid arthritis and hypothyroidism. The typical story is of severe pain and paraesthesiae, which may involve the whole arm as well as the hand, waking the patient from sleep. In the morning, the hand feels stiff and swollen and paraesthesiae may recur throughout the day. There may be few objective signs of a median nerve lesion although abductor pollicis brevis may be weakened in chronic cases. *Ulnar nerve constriction* is less common but occurs more often in men. There is a slowly progressive ulnar nerve palsy, sensory symptoms preceding motor effects. *Meralgia paraesthetica* is the name given to the burning pain, paraesthesiae and sensory loss over the lateral aspect of the thigh which results from entrapment of the lateral cutaneous nerve, usually in obese men.

Peripheral neuritis and neuropathies
Many cases formerly regarded as neuritis do not justify the term as they are not inflammatory in origin. For those which do not fall under this heading the term *neuropathy* is preferable.

Neuritis
Examples of this are:

1   Lesions of the main nerve trunks as in leprosy (Figure 10.71). There is an actual inflammatory change in the nerves and sensory manifestations, notably anaesthesia, are present. Similar changes may occur locally when nerves are involved in a septic area.
2   Acute polyneuritis (Guillain–Barré syndrome). This commonly follows a virus infection and is due to a non-infective inflammatory reaction in the peripheral nerves. The onset is usually sudden with a symmetrical paresis which starts in the legs but may rapidly ascend to affect the arms, the respiratory musculature and the cranial nerves. Paraesthesiae occur, but objective sensory changes are usually minimal. There is a lower motor neuron type of paresis with flaccidity and absent tendon reflexes. Unless the patient succumbs to respiratory failure, recovery is usually complete within a few months.
3   A type of shoulder-girdle neuritis (neuralgia amyotrophy) may occur after inoculation. It causes pain in the distribution of the 5th and 6th cervical nerve roots and there is usually weakness and wasting of the muscles. This is thought to be inflammatory but may be imitated in older people by a neuropathy due to cervical spondylosis.

Polyneuropathies
Many diseases can result in peripheral nerve changes. They include infections such as diphtheria in which the organism remains localized to the throat, but the toxins affect the nerves. Poisons have a similar effect,

e.g. arsenic, lead and carbon tetrachloride used in industry, isoniazid and nitrofurantoin used in treatment. Among important metabolic causes may be mentioned diabetes (Figure 10.72), uraemia, amyloid disease and porphyria. Deficiency diseases which are responsible include beriberi, pellagra and chronic alcoholism which leads to vitamin deficiency. Deficiency of vitamin B_{12} can cause a peripheral neuropathy as well as degeneration of the cord. The condition is not uncommon in malignant diseases, but the mechanism is more obscure.

Most varieties of neuritis and neuropathy show the signs of lower neuron involvement with loss of reflexes

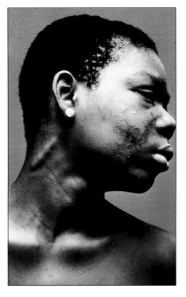

◀ **Figure 10.71 Great auricular nerve showing thickening due to leprosy**

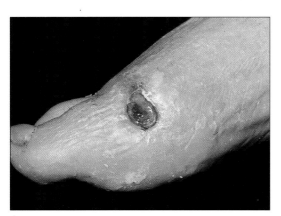

▲ **Figure 10.72 Painless trophic ulcer in a diabetic with polyneuritis**

together with sensory changes, but in some the motor signs predominate (e.g. lead poisoning) and in others there may be sensory loss alone (e.g. certain malignant neuropathies). The degree and distribution of the signs vary much in the individual case and help in deciding the aetiology. The causal agency may also be suspected by associated non-neurological signs, e.g. alcoholism, exposure to poisons, diabetes and diphtheria.

LESIONS OF THE MUSCLES: THE MYOPATHIES

A few diseases apparently have their pathological seat in the muscles themselves, the motor neurons, both upper and lower, remaining intact. These diseases are often characterized by muscular weakness, and their diagnosis is therefore made during the examination of the motor system. The same applies to certain diseases in which there is some disorder of transmission of impulses at the myoneural junctions, viz. myasthenia gravis, and also to the phenomenon of myotonia which consists of difficulty in relaxing muscles.

MUSCULAR DYSTROPHIES

Muscular atrophy due to primary changes in the muscles, as distinct from neural muscular atrophy, occurs in certain families. This familial nature of the dystrophies is all-important in diagnosis. They usually appear in childhood or, in some forms, in adolescence. In many cases, alongside of the wasting of certain groups of muscles, there is apparent hypertrophy of others, really due to overgrowth of fat and connective tissue.

Various types of dystrophy are described, according to the groups of muscles affected, the age of onset and the mode of inheritance.

Duchenne type

This is inherited by boys as a sex-linked recessive characteristic. It presents in early childhood and is usually fatal in adolescence. The *atrophy* is seen especially in the latissimus dorsi and lower halves of the pectorals, but the biceps, peronei and hamstrings are also affected. Winging of the scapulae results from wasting of the serratus anterior. Lordosis is common owing to wasting of the flexors of the thighs. By contrast with these wasted muscles, those of the calves and buttocks and the deltoids and spinati are enlarged owing to pseudohypertrophy. The gait is waddling and the classic method of rising from the supine to the erect posture is described on page 244. In this and other forms of muscular dystrophies, the serum creatine kinase (a muscle enzyme) is characteristically raised.

Facio-scapulo-humeral type

This starts at about the same age as, or somewhat older than the Duchenne type. The distribution of muscles affected is indicated by the name. The facial weakness causes a characteristic myopathic facies with drooping of the lower lip and wasting of the facial muscles (Figure 10.73(a)). The shoulder-girdle muscles (especially trapezius and serratus anterior) and the muscles of the upper arm (biceps, triceps and pectorals) are involved, causing drooping of the shoulders and winging of the scapulae (Figure 10.73(b)).

Limb girdle type

This manifests later than the other kinds, usually in adolescence. It is inherited as an autosomal recessive and therefore affects both sexes. The biceps, triceps, brachioradialis, and to a lesser extent the quadriceps and glutei, are the paretic muscles.

Dystrophia myotonica

This condition is transmitted by dominant inheritance and usually presents in adult life. There is diffuse muscle weakness and wasting but involvement of the facial muscles with ptosis is a characteristic feature (Figure 10.74) Myotonia consists of a failure of muscle relaxation after voluntary contraction. When the patient grips the examiner's hand, he is unable to release it.

MYASTHENIA GRAVIS

This is a disease in which there is muscle weakness, usually without wasting, due to a failure of normal neuromuscular transmission. The muscles tire easily, especially towards the end of the day. Any muscle group can be involved but those supplied by the cranial nerves are commonly affected first so that the patient complains of ptosis, diplopia, dysarthria, dysphagia or difficulty in chewing or holding up the head. Simple tests for muscle fatigue will demonstrate the patient's inability to sustain activities such as opening and shutting the eyes or mouth, clenching and unclenching the fist or raising the head from the pillow. The diagnosis can be established by intravenous injection of edrophonium chloride (Tensilon) which results in a rapid, dramatic but transient improvement in muscle power (see Figure 10.75).

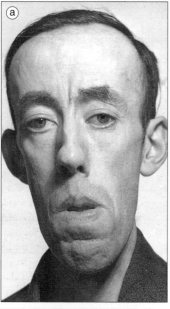

(a)

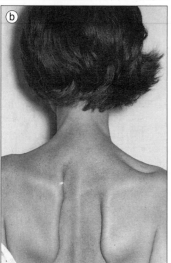

(b)

◀ **Figure 10.73 (a) Myopathic facies.** The loose parting of the lips is due to weakness of the orbicularis oris. (b) Muscular dystrophy. Shoulder girdle distribution. Note winging of scapula

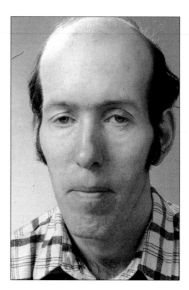

◀ **Figure 10.74 Dystrophia myotonica**

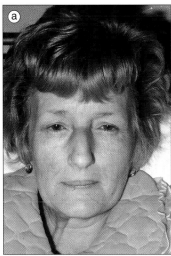

◀ **Figure 10.75 (a) Myasthenia gravis.** (b) Same patient after injection of edrophonium chloride

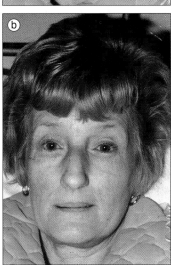

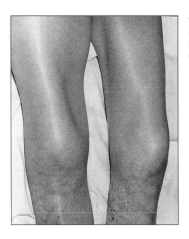

◀ **Figure 10.76 Diabetic myopathy:** wasting of quadriceps

ACQUIRED MYOPATHIES

In this group, the weakness and wasting mainly affect proximal limb muscles. The commoner causes are carcinoma, connective tissue disorders such as dermatomyositis and polymyositis, vitamin D deficiency, especially due to malabsorbtion and endocrine conditions including diabetes mellitus (Figure 10.76), thyrotoxicosis and corticosteroid therapy. The myopathy associated with thyrotoxicosis and carcinoma especially of the bronchus may be accompanied by a myasthenic-like syndrome in which symptoms worsen toward the end of the day and muscle testing reveals increased fatigability. However there is no response to the intravenous injection of edrophonium chloride and this is known as the Eaton–Lambert syndrome.

LESIONS OF THE EXTRAPYRAMIDAL SYSTEM

PARKINSONISM

This disease is a good example of a degenerative process affecting the basal ganglia (corpus striatum). It appears insidiously in elderly persons who at first may complain only of a vague tiredness or stiffness of the limbs with difficulty in the performance of fine movements. Relatives may notice that the patient has been slowing up and the whole illness is often attributed by patient and doctor alike to 'rheumatism' or 'old age'. Like hypothyroidism, Parkinsonism is usually not recognized until some years after its onset. Early diagnosis depends more upon general inspection of the patient's posture, gait and facies than on a detailed neurological examination. Parkinsonism is characterized by three principal signs, which depend on disordered function in the extrapyramidal system. These are:

1 Poverty of movement (akinesia).
2 Muscular rigidity.
3 Tremors.

The chief disability arises from a complex disturbance in which voluntary movements are slowed (bradykinesia) or absent altogether (akinesia). This, combined with muscular rigidity, causes difficulty in carrying out everyday activities such as washing, dressing and writing. The gait is shuffling, and the patient appears to hurry in the direction he is going (festination), or if gently pushed backwards may continue in this direction (retropulsion), gathering speed and tending to fall unless stopped. The patient does not swing his arms when walking, and in turning round does so 'by numbers'. The attitude is one of flexion, the head depressed on the chest, the shoulders bowed, the knees and elbows slightly bent. The rigidity of the facial muscles gives a characteristic immobility to the face which is known as the 'Parkinsonian facies' (Figure 10.77). The expression is fixed and staring; blinking is infrequent, the patient smiles little or not at all; the mouth is often slightly open and saliva dribbles away. The voice is monotonous and later dysarthria and dysphagia may result from rigidity of the bulbar muscles.

The tremor is not always present, but in many cases is the first sign observed. It is described as 'pill-rolling' owing to the characteristic movement of the thumb and index finger. Later the tremor extends to the whole hand, to the leg on the same side and finally to other parts of the body. Both rigidity and tremor may for a long time be unilateral. It may be momentarily controlled by an effort of will, or by muscular movement, only to return when these cease. The combination of tremor and increased muscle tone give rise to the typical 'cog-wheel' rigidity; this can best be elicited by passive flexion and extension of the elbow.

Encephalitis lethargica was a common cause of Parkinsonism, but is no longer so. Some cases are of unknown aetiology, though bearing some resemblance to the postencephalitic syndrome. Others can be associated with cerebral arteriosclerosis, with manganese poisoning or with disturbance of copper metabolism in Wilson's disease. Parkinsonism is observed as a reversible side-effect of phenothiazine tranquillizers and as a result of head injury in the 'punch drunk' syndrome of professional boxers.

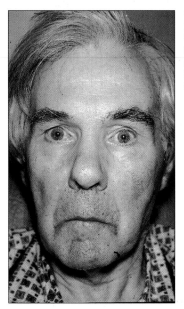

◀ **Figure 10.77 Parkinsonian facies. Note fixed stare and dribbling which has caused angular stomatitis**

LESIONS OF THE CEREBELLUM

Cerebellar lesions may involve the vermis as in medulloblastoma or ependymoma in children. The early sign is loss of balance but as the tumour spreads other features due to involvement of adjacent structures become apparent.

More commonly, the lesion involves the lateral lobe, as in otitic abscess, and produces a variety of signs which are due mainly to abnormalities of tone and postural fixation; not only are the muscles in action affected but also those passively maintaining the background of correct posture. It is important to note that the signs of unilateral cerebellar disease are on the same side of the body as the lesion. The signs are as follows:

LOSS OF MUSCLE TONE (HYPOTONIA)
Hypotonia is conspicuous only in acute cerebellar lesions. The limbs are unduly flaccid and can be moved through unusually large ranges of movement. The hypotonia is generally accompanied by slight weakness, because perfect muscular action is impossible with atonic muscles. Hypotonia also explains the swinging or 'pendular' response when the knee jerk is elicited with the legs hanging freely (see Figure 10.51, page 247).

MUSCULAR INCO-ORDINATION
This is seen in the ataxic (drunken) gait so often present. The patient tends to fall to the affected side. Ataxia in the arms may be demonstrated by asking the patient to make a fist and then to pronate and supinate the forearms rapidly. On the affected side this cannot be properly accomplished *(dysdiadochokinesia)*. Intention tremor is another example. When the patient attempts to touch the nose with the finger, the arm and hand become increasingly shaky until the nose is reached (see Figure 10.64, page 253). The precision of movement which depends upon the appreciation of the force and rate of muscular contraction is also lost. This is known as *dysmetria*.

OCULAR DISTURBANCES
The commonest is *nystagmus* (oscillations of the eyeball – see page 232), usually lateral, but sometimes rotary. Nystagmus is again a defect of postural fixation and can be regarded as an intention tremor of the orbital muscles. Occasionally *skew deviation* is observed, one eye being turned upwards and outwards, the other downwards and inwards.

ALTERED POSTURES
The position of the head is sometimes altered. It is retracted, with the face turned upwards towards the

lesion. When the middle lobe is affected a position may be assumed similar to that of meningeal disease - the head retracted, the back arched, and the legs extended. The natural tendency of the patient to lean towards the side of the lesion may be over corrected, producing an abnormal attitude.

These signs of cerebellar disease are present chiefly on the side of the lesion. Signs may be present on the opposite side due to involvement of surrounding structures. This is particularly so in tumour. The 6th nerve, owing to its propinquity, frequently suffers in cerebellar tumours, with consequent paralysis of the lateral (external) rectus (see also Cranial nerves, page 224).

SPEECH DEFECTS

These generally take the form of 'staccato' speech, in which each syllable is pronounced as though it was a word. Here the muscles of articulation are affected by the defect of postural fixation.

In tumours of the cerebellum the general signs of increased intracranial pressure come on earlier than in supratentorial lesions.

THE SENSORY SYSTEM: ANATOMICAL AND PHYSIOLOGICAL CONSIDERATIONS

From the sensory nerve endings in the epidermis the fibres conveying sensation run in the peripheral nerves and enter the spinal cord through the posterior nerve roots. In the cord they dissociate to run in different tracts, some ending in the cord itself, some in the gracile and cuneate nuclei of the medulla, some proceeding to the thalamus, and some passing directly to the cerebellum, their impulses thus not reaching consciousness, but supplying proprioceptive information to this region of the brain. From the thalamus a last relay conveys the sensory impulses to the post-central area of the cerebral cortex.

The path taken by the different types of sensation is of great importance in clinical neurology.

PATH IN THE PERIPHERAL NERVES

All types of sensation are conveyed by the peripheral nerves, but they arise from special end-organs in the skin, muscles and tendons. The modes of sensibility include cutaneous sensations, i.e. light touch, cold, warmth and pain, and deep impressions (proprioception) such as painful and painless pressure, postural sensibility and vibration sense. There are no nerves that are specially for discrimination and localization, though the end-organs may afford some localizing facilities (Figure 10.78).

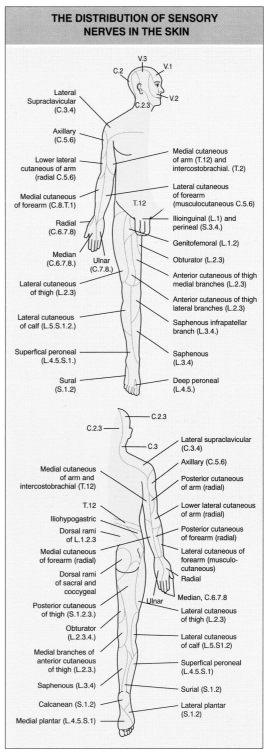

THE DISTRIBUTION OF SENSORY NERVES IN THE SKIN

▲ Figure 10.78 The distribution of sensory nerves in the skin

PATH IN THE POSTERIOR NERVE ROOTS

From the peripheral nerves the various types of sensation enter the cord through the posterior nerve roots, in which the fibres are arranged in segmental fashion similar to the motor fibres in the anterior nerve roots (Figure 10.79). Lesions in the posterior roots are not common but must be considered when segmental anaesthesia is present.

PATH IN THE SPINAL CORD

In this part of their course the fibres of sensation are grouped entirely differently from the arrangement in the peripheral nerves.

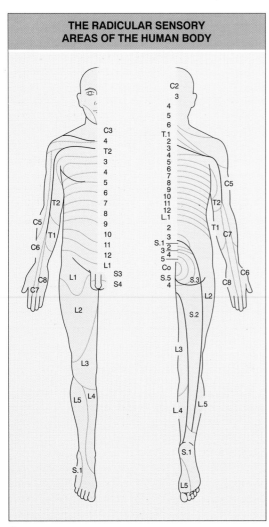

THE RADICULAR SENSORY AREAS OF THE HUMAN BODY

▲ **Figure 10.79 The radicular sensory areas of the human body**

Touch fibres cross to the opposite side soon after their entry and run in the anterior spinothalamic tracts. Some also pass up the posterior columns crossing to enter the anterior spinothalamic tract at successive levels up to the gracile and cuneate nuclei in the medulla. A lesion in the lateral column will thus result in partial loss of tactile sensation (and loss of pain and temperature) on the opposite side below the level of the lesion, together, of course, with motor paralysis on the same side of the type already discussed.

Pain and temperature sensibility is conveyed by fibres which cross after traversing a few segments of the cord above their point of entrance. In crossing they pass closely in front of the central canal and ascend the opposite lateral spinothalamic tract to the thalamus. A lesion near the central canal (e.g. syringomyelia or intramedullary tumour) will involve these fibres and cause a limited loss of pain and temperature sense corresponding to the affected segments. Touch is affected to a much smaller extent, initially at least, because of the double pathway in the cord ('dissociated sensory loss').

Deep sensibility fibres pass up the posterior columns to the gracile and cuneate nuclei before crossing to the opposite side. Lesions of the posterior columns therefore result in loss of the proprioceptive sensations (deep pressure; muscle joint and tendon position; vibration sense) on the same side as the lesion and considerable loss of touch also occurs.

PATHS IN THE MEDULLA AND BRAIN

Leaving the spinal cord the sensory paths are continued in the following manner. *Touch* fibres pass through the medulla, pons and crus in the formatio reticularis, ending in the thalamus. *Pain and temperature* fibres run to the outer side of the medulla separate from the tactile fibres, but in the pons and crus the touch, pain, and temperature paths approximate and pass upwards to the thalamus. *Proprioceptive* sensations differ from pain, temperature and part of touch, the fibres of which have already crossed in the cord, by continuing uncrossed until they reach the medial lemniscus, where the superior sensory decussation takes place (Figure 10.80).

From these anatomical and physiological data will be seen that *dissociated anaesthesia*, i.e. loss of some types of sensation, with preservation of others, is most likely to occur in cord lesions, less commonly in midbrain lesions, but very rarely in lesions of the peripheral nerves.

THE THALAMUS

Each thalamus is an ovoid mass of grey matter lying in the floor of the third ventricle and one of the largest of

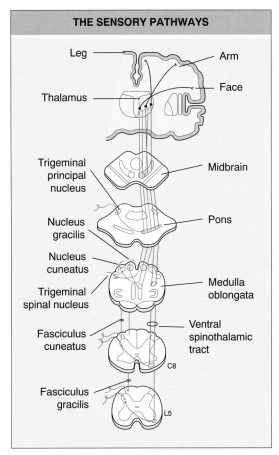

THE SENSORY PATHWAYS

Leg

Arm

Face

Thalamus

Trigeminal
principal
nucleus

Midbrain

Nucleus
gracilis

Pons

Nucleus
cuneatus

Trigeminal
spinal nucleus

Medulla
oblongata

Fasciculus
cuneatus

Ventral
spinothalamic
tract

C8

Fasciculus
gracilis

L5

▲ **Figure 10.80 The sensory pathways**

the basal ganglia. The nuclei of the thalamus have several functions:

1 All forms of somatic sensory fibre relays are projected from the thalamus to the primary sensory area in the post central gyrus.
2 Motor impulses from the corpus striatum, substantia nigra and cerebellum exert their influence on corticospinal and corticobulbar motor pathways via the thalamus.
3 Awareness of nocioceptive stimuli occurs in the thalamus so that these may be excessive, unpleasant and prolonged in thalamic disorders.
4 Sensory input is recognized as agreeable or disagreeable in the thalamus and connections with the pre-frontal cortex influence mood and personality.
5 The anterior nucleus of the thalamus is part of the limbic system which influences memory and instinctive behaviour.

6 The thalamus is concerned with activation and arousal and its intralaminar nuclei generate much of the low voltage cortical activity seen in the EEG of alert individuals.

Thus the results of a thalamic lesion are:

Hemianaesthesia, excessive sensibility to painful stimuli, spontaneous pains, and misinterpretation of other stimuli (e.g. light touch or tickling may give an unpleasant sensation), possibly ataxia and choreiform movements from concurrent involvement of the corpus striatum. These signs are present on the side opposite to the lesion.

Lesions of the thalamus are commonly vascular or neoplastic. If vascular, they are rarely confined to the thalamus but involve the internal capsule, so that hemiparesis is also present.

THE PARIETAL LOBES

Sensory fibres pass from the thalamus via the internal capsule to the sensory cortex behind the central sulcus in the parietal lobe (see Figure 10.39). Complex forms of sensation are appreciated in the parietal lobes and lesions may give rise to spatial disorientation and astereognosis (see page 267). *Apraxia* may also occur, i.e. the inability to perform a particular movement although the patient is aware of what he wishes to do and has no paralysis preventing him from doing it. This can be tested by asking the patient to use a key or pencil.

The parietal lobes, together with the frontal lobes, are also concerned with higher intellectual functions.

SENSORY SYMPTOMS IN NERVOUS DISEASES

The subjective sensations commonly experienced in disease of the nervous system fall into two groups:

1 *Paraesthesiae.*
2 *Pain.*

Certain phenomena are described under the objective examination, though they may well be appreciated by the patient, i.e. anaesthesia or ataxia.

PARAESTHESIAE

These consist of such sensations as 'pins and needles', pricking, numbness and band-like sensations around the trunk. They are common as transient phenomena when the peripheral nerves are stretched or subjected to pressure. A familiar example is the paraesthesia produced by compression of the lateral popliteal nerve after sitting too long with the legs crossed. Equally they may herald serious disease of the nervous system (e.g. spinal tumour, subacute combined degeneration, multiple sclerosis). The distribution of the paraesthesiae has localizing value.

PAIN

Impulses interpreted as pain in the consciousness are carried by the nervous system whatever their origin may be, but the description of pain as a symptom of visceral disease is considered under the various systems and on pages 5–8. Special types of pain associated with lesions of the nervous system need mention here.

Peripheral nerve pain

This may occur in various forms of injury, neuritis and neuropathy. Sensory loss accompanied by pain follows the distribution of the nerve and may be associated with motor changes.

Sometimes pain occurs alone, i.e. without motor or sensory changes. In time, however, objective changes indicating involvement of the nerves may appear. For example, sciatica is neuralgic pain referred to the muscles supplied by the sciatic nerve, but sooner or later it is usual for some objective signs to appear such as pain on stretching the nerve or tenderness over its course. There may also be loss of the ankle jerk on the affected side. Disc lesions are held to be responsible for many cases, but pelvic examination is necessary to exclude the presence of neoplasms. Another example is the neuralgia preceding, or more commonly following, herpes zoster. (See also Trigeminal neuralgia, page 228.)

Root pains

These are often of a neuralgic type but are characteristically increased by coughing and sneezing. They follow the distribution of the particular root or roots affected, and may at first be unaccompanied by objective evidence of root irritation. It is therefore of great importance to ascertain the exact distribution of pains in the trunk. Examples may be seen in the girdle pains of tabes and the half-girdle pains of herpes zoster, a virus infection of the posterior-root ganglia associated with a vesicular rash followed by scarring and sensory loss in the same area as the pain (Figure 10.81). Cervical and lumbar root pains are distributed to the appropriate limb and are most often due to spondylosis with disc protrusions. Tumours arising from the meninges of the cord produce pain of a root type, at first confined to one side, later spreading to the other. The 'lightning pains' of tabes are an example of a root pain in the limbs.

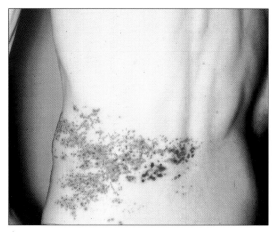

▲ **Figure 10.81 Herpes zoster (shingles) at T12, L1.** The vesicles in this case are haemorrhagic

Causalgia

This is an unusual type of burning pain, generally occurring after limb injuries in cases where the nerve damage is comparatively slight.

Visceral pains

Excluding pains due to visceral disease, pains of a visceral type may occur in the well-known visceral crises of tabes. The commonest of these is the gastric crisis, in which epigastric pain and vomiting may erroneously suggest a diagnosis of gastric ulcer.

Headache and thalamic pain are considered elsewhere (pages 5–9).

PHYSICAL SIGNS: EXAMINATION OF THE SENSORY SYSTEM

In all neurological cases a thorough investigation of the perceptions of sensations is valuable, and in many diagnosis depends chiefly upon this.

The examination must test *tactile sensation and discrimination, deep sensibility, perception of pain and temperature, joint and vibration sense, co-ordination of movement and stereognosis.*

When the exact localization of the lesion is of direct therapeutic importance, the areas of disturbed sensibility should be carefully charted (simple line drawings of the body are readily obtainable) (cf. Figures 10.78 and 10.79). This is the more important as it enables the observer to appreciate changes in the distribution of anaesthesiae, etc., which may take place from time to time. The recognition of a sensory 'level' is of particular relevance to the diagnosis and localization of spinal cord compression. The appropriate stimulus (touch, prick, vibration, etc.) is applied at about one-inch intervals down each side of the trunk in turn, both front and back. The spinous processes of the vertebrae may be used for testing vibration sense. Particular attention is paid to the 'saddle' area of the buttocks and perineum where sensory loss may be the only sign of a cauda equina lesion. Sensory levels and areas of sensory loss may be lightly marked with a skin pencil prior to recording on a chart.

TACTILE SENSATION

This is best tested by gently touching the skin with a wisp of cotton wool; the patient's eyes should be covered. If an area of *anaesthesia* is found, it should be carefully compared with the corresponding area on the opposite limb or part of the body. The anaesthesia may be graded as slight (*hypoaesthesia*) when sensation is merely dulled, or complete when it is entirely absent. If the touch is more acutely felt than normal, *hyperaesthesia* is said to be present. If it is felt as a perverted sensation, e.g. tingling or pain, the term *paraesthesia* or *dysaesthesia* describes it.

TACTILE DISCRIMINATION

This is tested by determining at what distance apart two points of a compass can be distinguished as separate entities. This varies greatly in different parts of the body. It corresponds with the richness of touch spots which are numerous on the tongue and nose so that the points of the compass can be distinguished a few millimetres apart, whereas on the lower part of the back they may need to be separated by several inches.

Tactile discrimination is less sensitive in cortical lesions.

DEEP SENSIBILITY (PRESSURE PAIN)

This may be tested by firm pressure with a blunt object such as a pencil, or by pinching the muscles, tendons, etc. Testicular pain on squeezing is another form of pressure pain, often absent in tabes.

This type of sensation is often retained when cutaneous sensibility is lost.

PAIN

Pain sensibility may be tested by pricking with a pin; heavy pressure must be avoided, otherwise pressure pain may be induced.

The patient's expression should be noted and compared with his statement about the sensation and the time relationship between the stimulus and the response noted. The term *analgesia* signifies absence of the sense of pain, and in dissociated 'anaesthesia' the part may be analgesic without being anaesthetic.

TEMPERATURE DISCRIMINATION

Two test tubes of water, cold and warm (not hot), may be conveniently used. They should be interchanged frequently so that the patient cannot guess which is being used.

SENSATIONS OF JOINT MOVEMENT AND POSTURE

The joint must be moved passively, making sure that the muscles to it are completely relaxed. In the case of the great toe, for example, the patient should know when it is extended or flexed without moving it himself (Figure 10.82). When the limb (especially the upper) is put in a certain position it should be possible for the patient to put the opposite limb in a similar position.

VIBRATION SENSE

This is tested by placing a tuning-fork of low pitch over the superficial bones, e.g. tibia or phalanges. The patient is normally conscious of a vibratory tremor, not merely the touch of the fork.

STEREOGNOSIS

This requires not only an appreciation of the form of the object but of its weight and texture. It may be tested by asking the patient to identify familiar objects such as a key, a coin or a pencil. Impairment of such appreciation results from lesions in the higher parts of the sensory system, e.g. in the parietal lobes.

With certain lesions *sensory suppression* is found. This means that when touch or pin-prick is tested on either side of the body independently, sensation is normal, but when the two sides are tested simultaneously the sensation is appreciated on the normal side only.

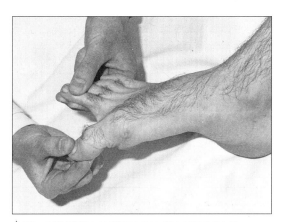

▲ **Figure 10.82 Toe position sense.** The patient should recognize that the toe is in the flexed position. To prevent him from obtaining this information by the sense of touch, the other toes are kept well away from the toe which is moved

ILLUSTRATIVE LESIONS OF THE SENSORY NEURONS

A few diseases affect chiefly the sensory neurons but many involve concurrently the motor neurons. As lesions of the motor neurons have already received attention, it will be convenient to use as illustrations some diseases in which sensory and motor lesions are combined, but in which the sensory changes are more notable.

Lesions of the sensory neurons have a similar causation to those of the motor system.

LOCALIZATION

The localization of a lesion of the sensory neurons depends partly on the distribution of the disturbance of sensation and partly on its type. This has been partially discussed in the sections on anatomy and physiology, and may be recapitulated here.

From an anatomical point of view lesions of the peripheral nerves result in anaesthesia corresponding to the distribution of the sensory fibres (see Figure 10.78); segmental anaesthesia results from root lesions (see Figure 10.79). Complete transverse lesions of the spinal cord cause anaesthesia in the limbs and trunk below the level of the lesion. Unilateral lesions result in the dissociation of anaesthesia found in the Brown-Séquard syndrome (opposite). Lesions of the brainstem may also result in dissociation, some types of sensation being lost on the same side of the body, some on the opposite side. Lesions of the thalamus, internal capsule or cortex result in hemi-anaesthesia affecting the face, arm and leg on the opposite side of the body.

As regards the type of anaesthesia, all varieties of sensation may be lost in peripheral nerve lesions and complete transverse lesions of the spinal cord although, in the former case, some sensations may be affected more than others. *Dissociated anaesthesia*, e.g. abolition of pain and temperature sense with preservation of touch sensibility, may result from a lesion of the lateral spinothalamic tract or of the grey matter of the cord near the central canal. Such a lesion may occur in syringomyelia and intramedullary tumours which interrupt the pain and temperature fibres as they cross over from one side to the other.

Dissociated anaesthesia also results from brainstem lesions (particularly the medulla), as in syringomyelia of these parts, or thrombosis of the posterior inferior cerebellar artery.

The loss of proprioceptive sensations (joint movement, vibration sense, etc.), with little or no loss of tactile, thermal or pain sensibility, is characteristic of lesions of the posterior columns (tabes, subacute combined degeneration) or of their continuation fibres to the medulla.

When anaesthesia is central in origin (thalamus, internal capsule and cortex) it is rarely so complete as in peripheral lesions, and it affects the distal parts of the limbs more than the proximal. It is further characteristic of thalamic lesions that the response to sensory stimulation is exaggerated and frequently perverted (touch may produce an unpleasant sensation almost amounting to pain). Spontaneous pain may also occur. Such symptoms may be thought to be hysterical. In lesions of the sensory cortex the higher types of sensation are impaired (asterognosis) (see also page 267).

BROWN-SÉQUARD SYNDROME (Figure 10.83)

Although not common, this phenomenon is an excellent illustration of one type of dissociated anaesthesia. The lesion consists of a hemisection of the cord and is usually traumatic (e.g. stab wound), though tumours and other conditions such as multiple sclerosis may produce the same effect.

On the side of the lesion the sensations from tendons, muscles, and joints, vibration sense and tactile discrimination are lost. On the opposite side pain and temperature sense are abolished and to a lesser extent touch. In

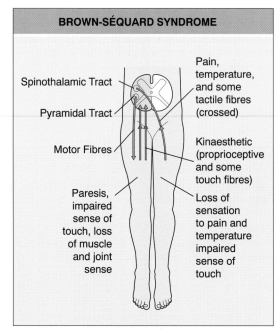

BROWN-SÉQUARD SYNDROME

Spinothalamic Tract

Pyramidal Tract

Motor Fibres

Paresis, impaired sense of touch, loss of muscle and joint sense

Pain, temperature, and some tactile fibres (crossed)

Kinaesthetic (proprioceptive and some touch fibres)

Loss of sensation to pain and temperature impaired sense of touch

▲ **Figure 10.83 Brown-Séquard syndrome. Hemisection of the cord.** As touch has a double pathway, it may be impaired on each side, as shown in the diagram, or may be preserved on both sides

addition, motor and vasomotor signs are added: on the side of the lesion there is paralysis of the upper neuron type, and signs of vasomotor paresis. A limited lower neuron paralysis may also be present, corresponding with the segments of the cord affected.

SYRINGOMYELIA

This condition results from obstruction to the flow of cerebrospinal fluid between the spinal subarachnoid space and the cisterna magna or through the foramina in the roof of the fourth ventricle. The commonest cause of obstruction is the Chiari malformation in which a tongue of cerebellum projects down through the foramen magnum, but arachnoid adhesions following meningitis may be responsible in some cases. The resulting distension of the central canal or perivascular spaces in the spinal cord interrupts the pain and temperature fibres crossing here but only affects part of the touch fibres, those in the posterior columns remaining intact. Pain and temperature sense are therefore lost while common touch and postural sensibility are preserved. When the spinothalamic tract is interrupted there is loss of sensation below the level of the lesion. When segmental fibres only are involved, there is a lower as well as an upper limit to the area of anaesthesia; this is referred to as suspended anaesthesia. Injuries due to the non-appreciation of pain and heat may first call attention to the disease (Figure 10.84). Charcot's joints (see page 210) may occur in the upper limbs in chronic cases.

Motor signs are also generally present. If the lesion extends into the anterior horn cells there will be a lower neuron type of paralysis corresponding with the spinal segments affected. As these are usually the lower cervical and upper dorsal segments, the paralysis affects the small muscles of the hand, as in motor neuron disease.

Involvement of the lateral columns often gives upper neuron signs on one or both sides, but the degree of paralysis is rarely great. Less often, the posterior columns are damaged, with corresponding loss of deep sensibility, etc. Signs of involvement of these long tracts are found only below the level of the lesion and are thus evident in the legs rather than the arms. A rare type of syringomyelia affects the brainstem – syringobulbia. Here the bulbar nuclei are affected, and dissociated anaesthesia may be present in the face.

TABES DORSALIS (Figure 10.85)

This is now a rare disease resulting from syphilis and characterized pathologically by degeneration of the posterior nerve roots of the spinal cord and of some cranial nerves. The symptoms and signs are mainly sensory.

Pain is an early symptom. It may be described as 'lightning' or hot and sharp, striking limbs at right angles and band-like sensations ('girdle pains') may be felt around the chest. Sensory loss may produce symptoms of 'walking on air' or 'cotton wool' due to anaesthesia of the soles of the feet. Visceral crises involving the larynx, stomach, kidney and heart are analogous to lightning pains and may be accompanied by vomiting simulating an abdominal or cardiac catastrophe. Difficulty in commencing micturition or defaecation and painless urinary retention may reflect tabetic involvement of the lumbo-sacral roots.

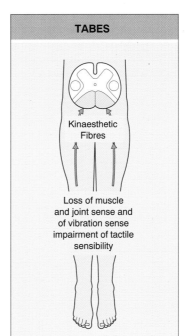

◄ Figure 10.85 Tabes. Lesion of the posterior columns. The lumbar and sacral segments are generally affected

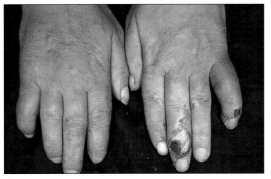

▲ Figure 10.84 Syringomyelia. showing burns and whitlows. Note also the resorption of the terminal phalanges (especially the right hand) and the puffy appearance of the hands (the 'succulent' hand)

Unsteadiness and ataxia of the legs especially in the dark will result from loss of proprioception.

The physical signs include loss of the ankle and less commonly the knee jerk due to interruption of the sensory limb of the reflex arc. There may be scattered areas of anaesthesia and analgesia in the limbs and trunk and on the lips and nose. Deep pain sensation is lost when the tendo Achilles is squeezed. Romberg's sign is present due to joint positional loss. Painless injury to joints of the leg may result in Charcot deformity which may also be accompanied by perforating painless foot ulcers. Cranial nerve signs include Argyll-Robertson pupils, optic atrophy and ptosis which is responsible for the 'tabetic facies'.

COMPRESSION OF THE SPINAL CORD (see also CAUDA EQUINA LESIONS)

Compression of the cord illustrates a combination of motor and sensory phenomena varying in type and degree according to the nature and site of the compressive lesion. A number of causes may be responsible, e.g. fractured spine, cervical spondylosis, Paget's disease, extramedullary tumours and primary and secondary malignant disease. As in many diseases the symptoms vary with the rapidity with which the compression occurs. In sudden catastrophes, such as fracture of the spine, immediate paralysis and loss of sensation below the level of the lesion results. When the compression is more slowly produced as by tumour, there are often pains in the limbs or around the trunk due to root irritation. These are increased by sneezing, coughing and movements of the spine and often precede other signs. Later the general symptoms consist of progressive paraplegia with characteristic upper motor neuron signs together with sensory loss, sphincter paralysis and impotence. The level of the spinal compression can be located by finding paralysis, sensory loss and altered reflexes at or below the affected segment of the cord. As previously described, the finding of a level below which power or sensation is impaired is of great importance in determining the site of a spinal lesion. It must be remembered, however, that spinal nerves supply the skin and muscles ('dermatomes and 'myotomes') of the trunk at a level two or three vertebrae lower than the vertebral level at which they arise (Figure 10.86). Certain infective and metastatic lesions can be located by finding tenderness on pressure over the affected vertebra.

Useful evidence of compression is also obtained by examination of the cerebrospinal fluid. The protein is greatly increased without any cellular increase and occasionally is so great that spontaneous coagulation occurs, and the fluid may assume a yellow colour, *xanthochromia*. The fluid removed from above the level of

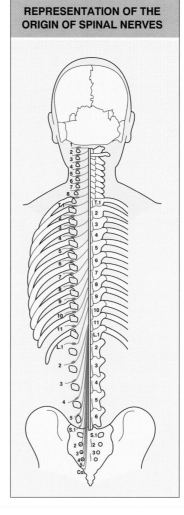

REPRESENTATION OF THE ORIGIN OF SPINAL NERVES

◀ **Figure 10.86** Diagrammatic representation of the origin of the spinal nerves, showing the position of their roots and ganglia respectively in relation to the vertebral column. The nerves are shown as thick black lines on the left side. (From Cunningham's Textbook of Anatomy, Oxford Medical Publications)

the obstruction, e.g. by cisternal puncture, remains normal. Queckenstedt's test, i.e. pressure on the jugular veins, fails to cause the normal rise of pressure noted at lumbar puncture.

Certain types of intramedullary tumour do not produce these compression symptoms but tend to imitate other centrally situated lesions of the spinal cord such as syringomyelia.

CAUDA EQUINA LESIONS

These result in combined motor and sensory symptoms varying considerably in distribution according to the particular nerve roots affected.

Their characteristic features are a saddle-shaped area of anaesthesia over the genitalia, perineum and buttocks, with disturbances of micturition and defaecation

– especially retention of urine – and motor paralysis of the lower neuron type affecting all or several groups of muscles in the lower limbs. Both the anaesthesia and muscular paralysis have a root distribution; so also has pain if present.

SUBACUTE COMBINED DEGENERATION

The degeneration of the spinal cord which occurs in cases of vitamin B_{12} deficiency is another example of combined motor and sensory lesions of the cord, but in this instance there is usually a peripheral neuropathy as well and sometimes an organic psychosis due to cerebral cortical degeneration. Anaemia may be absent but sternal puncture may reveal a megaloblastic marrow, and the diagnosis is supported by the finding of a reduced serum level of vitamin B_{12}. (See also page 192.)

Symptoms of a peripheral neuropathy usually occur first (numbness or tingling in the hands and feet), followed later by unsteadiness of gait, ultimately resulting in gross ataxia due to degeneration of the posterior columns. Vibration sense is also lost. Simultaneously the pyramidal tracts are affected with a consequent spastic paraplegia and other signs of upper motor neuron disease. In severe cases, and in the terminal stages, the increased tendon reflexes may become diminished or lost and the paralysis flaccid. Disturbances of micturition and defaecation and trophic changes in the skin, may occur, as in other spinal cord diseases.

FRIEDREICH'S ATAXIA

This disease also illustrates the effects of a simultaneous involvement of motor and sensory tracts. It is familial, being transmitted by recessive autosomal inheritance, and usually becomes manifest in childhood.

The posterior columns and cerebellar tracts are affected, causing ataxia both of the arms and legs. Other cerebellar signs include nystagmus, head tremor and scanning speech. Affection of the corticospinal tracts gives signs of an upper motor neuron lesion, especially Babinski's sign and spasticity. The tendon reflexes are, however, lost owing to an interruption of the sensory limb of the reflex arc in the posterior nerve root. There are often congenital skeletal deformities, especially pes cavus and scoliosis.

Other types of familial ataxia are described bearing a close resemblance to Friedreich's disease.

MENINGES

The meninges form a continuous membrane over the whole brain and extend down to cover the spinal cord.

The pia and arachnoid are in close contact in most places, and between them circulates the cerebrospinal fluid, which is more plentiful in the 'cisterns', where the pia and arachnoid separate from one another to accommodate it. The pia-arachnoid follows the convolutions of the brain closely and carries the blood vessels in its substance.

These facts explain the necessity for considering the meninges, both cerebral and spinal, as a whole, and of remembering that some of the symptoms and signs in meningeal disease may be due to spread of the disease process from or into the brain itself and to involvement of the cranial nerves which are partly or completely ensheathed by the meninges.

Whatever the cause of meningeal irritation, the symptoms and signs are similar. They will be modified by the part of the membranes which is most affected, e.g. cerebral or spinal; by the actual pathology, e.g. inflammation or haemorrhage; and by the rapidity with which the membranes are affected. They may be conveniently grouped as follows.

1 SYMPTOMS AND SIGNS OF INCREASED INTRACRANIAL PRESSURE (see page 281)

Headache, vomiting and sometimes papilloedema may result from the increased tension on the meninges by the accumulating cerebrospinal fluid between the pia and arachnoid, and also from hydrocephalus if adhesions or exudate have obstructed the free circulation of the fluid. The headache is frequently referred to the nape of the neck and may be very severe. Vomiting may be explosive and not preceded by nausea.

2 SIGNS OF MENINGEAL IRRITATION

The characteristic phenomenon of neck rigidity occurs early and later changes to definite head retraction (Figure 10.87). To test neck rigidity the observer attempts passively to flex the head on the chest and with

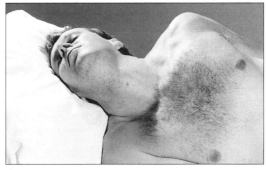

▲ **Figure 10.87 Head retraction**. A sign of meningeal irritation

his other hand notes the tautness of the neck muscles. When the spinal meninges are much affected, particularly in infants, the phenomenon of opisthotonos may be seen. The body is then arched backwards and held rigidly. This sign is but one example of the muscular rigidity which occurs in meningeal irritation.

Two special signs depend upon traction of the inflamed meninges and spinal nerves.

Kernig's sign: The hip is flexed to about 90° and any attempt then to straighten the knee results in pain and spasm in the hamstrings (Figure 10.88).

Brudzinski's sign: The head is flexed on the chest, which causes the lower limbs to be drawn up. The sign is valuable if it is suspected that the head retraction (which relieves tension on the spinal nerves) is partly voluntary.

3 SIGNS OF BRAIN INVOLVEMENT

Some spread of the disease process may take place to the brain itself or the meningeal infection may have arisen in the brain. As examples of the resulting signs may be mentioned motor phenomena such as fits and paresis, mental disturbances and so forth (Figure 10.89).

4 SIGNS OF CRANIAL NERVE INVOLVEMENT

These are found in chronic forms of basal meningitis but only rarely in acute disease unless treatment has been delayed or ineffective. The oculomotor, 7th and 8th nerves are most commonly affected.

5 CHANGES IN THE CEREBROSPINAL FLUID

Early lumbar puncture is necessary so that the cerebrospinal fluid can be examined and an accurate diagnosis made.

MENINGITIS

This may be caused by the meningococcus, by the pneumococcus and other cocci, by *mycobacterium tuberculosis* and by virus infections. *Haemophilus influenzae* is an important cause in children while in diabetic, leukaemic, HIV positive and other immunosuppressed patients, a variety of other organisms including fungi can produce meningitis. Whichever organism is responsible, the results are similar, though special clinical signs may help in distinguishing one type from another. Tuberculous meningitis is often suggested by a long prodromal period and by the discovery of other tuberculous lesions. Cerebrospinal fever (meningococcal meningitis) is rapid in onset, often found in epidemics and sometimes accompanied by a petechial or roseolar rash, which has given it the name 'spotted fever'. Pneumococcal meningitis is a likely diagnosis if signs of pneumonia are found, or in cases of pneumococcal otitis

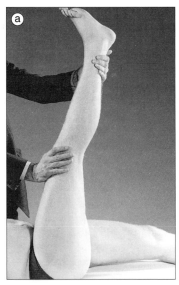

Figure 10.88 Kernig's sign. (a) Negative response. The leg can be well extended. (b) Positive response. The leg cannot be extended to more than a right-angle when the thigh is well flexed on the abdomen

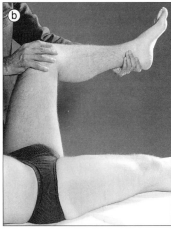

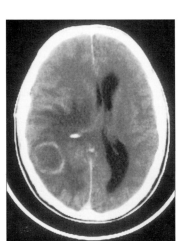

Figure 10.89 Toxoplasmoma in AIDS – CT scan showing enhancing ring lesion

media. It may also be a primary infection. Direct extension of sepsis from the skull bones, e.g. osteomyelitis resulting from chronic sinus infection or mastoiditis, and trauma, account for some cases. *Viral meningitis* is accompanied by changes in the cerebrospinal fluid similar to those of polio-encephalitis. The term *meningism* is given to a condition of meningeal irritability due to toxaemia without any actual inflammation of the meninges. It occurs especially in pneumonia and is most common in children. The headache is said to cease when delirium begins, whereas in meningitis it continues.

The diagnosis not only of the type of meningitis, but of the disease itself, is not complete without examination of the cerebrospinal fluid.

Meningitis is an inflammatory disease and fever is a symptom. It is variable in degree, and the pulse rate may be proportionately increased at first, but later tends to become slower owing to the increase in intracranial pressure.

THE CEREBRAL VESSELS (Figure 10.90)

Atheroma may affect the cerebral arteries or the extracranial arteries which feed them. Thus the supply of blood to the brain may be interrupted both within and without the skull. This is of importance because of the difficulty it causes in topographical diagnosis which may be essential from the point of view of treatment.

The flow of blood may be greatly reduced by conditions which cause a fall of blood pressure, as in shock or haemorrhage. Similar effects are caused by external pressure upon the neck arteries, e.g. vertebral artery compression in cases of cervical spondylosis.

The amount of damage resulting from brain infarction after vascular occlusion depends upon the site of the occlusion and the adequacy of collateral circulation through the circle of Willis. Infarction is especially likely to follow the occlusion of small end arteries, such as the perforating vessels supplying the internal capsule. Atheroma is particularly common in the middle cerebral artery, but changes in the carotid, basilar and vertebral arteries are certainly important contributory causes. Similarly, haemorrhages may arise from an atheromatous cerebral artery, and emboli may occur in mitral disease, atrial fibrillation, bacterial endocarditis and cardiac infarction. Atheromatous plaques may be responsible for microemboli from extracranial arteries.

It is therefore necessary in a case of 'stroke' that the condition of the arteries arising from the arch of the aorta and those in the circle of Willis and in the cerebral vessels proper should be considered as a whole.

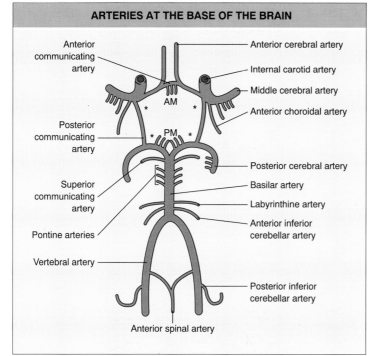

ARTERIES AT THE BASE OF THE BRAIN

Anterior communicating artery — Anterior cerebral artery — Internal carotid artery — Middle cerebral artery — Anterior choroidal artery — AM — Posterior communicating artery — PM — Posterior cerebral artery — Superior communicating artery — Basilar artery — Labyrinthine artery — Pontine arteries — Anterior inferior cerebellar artery — Vertebral artery — Posterior inferior cerebellar artery — Anterior spinal artery

◀ **Figure 10.90 The arteries at the base of the brain showing the circulus arteriosus (circle of Willis).** The groups of the central branches are anteromedial (AM) and posteromedial (PM)

Information about the arteries in the neck may be obtained by careful palpation of the carotid vessels, by auscultation to search for any murmurs by Doppler studies and, if necessary, by the use of arteriography.

Subject to the conception that any change in the flow of blood through the extracranial vessels will modify the results of changes in the cerebral vessels themselves, the following comments may be made.

The middle cerebral artery

The middle cerebral artery supplies the lateral aspects of the anterior two-thirds of the brain, including the internal capsule. This is the commonest site for cerebral thrombosis and usually results in hemiplegia and hemianaesthesia (cortical type), on the opposite side, particularly in the face, tongue and upper limb. Aphasia of various types is also common and may occur alone. Hemianopia due to involvement of the optic radiation in the internal capsule may also occur.

The anterior cerebral artery

The anterior cerebral artery supplies the medial aspects of the anterior two-thirds of the brain. Motor and sensory impairment are more marked in the lower limb than in the arm and may be accompanied by mental deterioration.

Posterior cerebral artery

The posterior cerebral artery mainly supplies the occipital pole of the brain, and occlusion results in contralateral hemianopia (Figure 10.91).

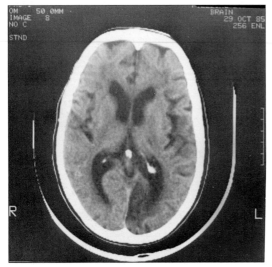

▲ **Figure 10.91 Left occipital infarction producing right homonymous hemianopia**

Carotid artery

This may be the site of stenosis which interferes with the blood supply to the intracranial vessels. Any insufficiency of this kind may make lesions, for example, in the middle cerebral, of much more serious significance. The suspicion of a carotid artery stenosis should lead to careful examination of the neck for the pulsation (inequality or absence) of the carotid vessels or presence of a systolic murmur over the bifurcation of the carotid. Fleeting episodes of ischaemia due either to microemboli or diminished perfusion may affect the territory supplied by the carotid. The most characteristic of these is *amaurosis fugax*, or transient blindness, due to impaired circulation through the retinal artery.

Vertebrobasilar system

Partial occlusion may occur without symptoms if the circulation in the carotid artery and the circle of Willis is adequate. Transient ischaemic attacks from vertebrobasilar insufficiency are common and may consist of vertigo, migraine-like visual disturbances, facial paraesthesiae, dysphasia, hemiparesis, hemianaesthesia or 'drop' attacks in which the patient suddenly falls without loss of consciousness. These may be provoked by vertebral artery compression on extending or turning the head, especially when there is cervical spondylosis. Another less common cause is stenosis of the subclavian artery proximal to the origin of the vertebral artery producing reversal of flow in the latter when the arm is in use ('*subclavian steal*').

Infarction of brain within the territory supplied by the vertebrobasilar system (brainstem, cerebellum and occipital pole) can produce a variety of syndromes in which the most constant features are vertigo, ipsilateral cerebellar and cranial nerve signs (5th–10th) with contralateral spinothalamic and pyramidal tract signs.

INTRACRANIAL HAEMORRHAGE (see Table 10.7)

The site and therefore the clinical features of intracranial haemorrhage depend to some extent upon the cause. Intracerebral haemorrhage is usually due to atheroma and (or) hypertension, subarachnoid haemorrhage to aneurysm and subdural or extradural haemorrhage to trauma.

Intracerebral haemorrhage

Generally involves the internal capsule (middle cerebral) and usually causes abrupt loss of consciousness with hemiplegia, but these may be preceded by intense headache and vomiting. The subjects commonly have hypertension as well as cerebral arteriosclerosis. Blood may appear in the

COMMON FEATURES OF CEREBROVASCULAR DISORDERS PRODUCING STROKE					
	Onset	**Course**	**Loss of consciousness**	**Associated findings**	**CSF**
Intracerebral haemorrhage	During activity Headache	Minutes to hemiplegia	Rapid coma	Hypertensive retinopathy and cardiomegaly Bleeding diathesis	Bloody
Cerebral thrombosis	At rest Variable onset	Minutes to hours to hemiplegia	Unusual	Atherosclerosis and cardiovascular disease	Clear
Cerebral embolism	Instantaneous	Rapid recovery	Possible	Cardiac arrhythmia Mitral stenosis Myocardial infarction Carotid murmur	Clear
Subarachnoid haemorrhage	Sudden headache	May relapse early	Common	Hypertension Neck stiffness Subhyaloid haemorrhage	Bloody
Subdural haemorrhage	Gradual Preceding trauma	Days Weeks Months	Eventually	Headache, vomiting Confusion Papilloedema Bradycardia	Xantho-chromia

▲ Table 10.7

cerebrospinal fluid and cause neck rigidity (Figure 10.92). Thrombosis also occurs within the same vascular territory but is less likely to be associated with coma, has a better recovery prospect and often a more limited paralysis, because branches of the middle cerebral rather than the main stem may be picked out. Cerebral embolism may occur in the young (mitral stenosis with atrial fibrillation or subacute bacterial endocarditis) or older persons with myocardial infarction. Hemiparesis occurs, rarely associated with unconsciousness, and usually suddenly on the dislodgement of the embolus.

Subarachnoid haemorrhage

The usual cause is the leakage or rupture of a congenital aneurysm on the cerebral arterial circle of Willis or less commonly an angioma (Figure 10.93). Sometimes in older persons a degenerate artery bursts, or trauma may be responsible. Hypertension is a common precipitating cause. The clinical manifestations vary. Meningeal symptoms – slowly or suddenly produced – include head retraction, neck rigidity, Kernig's sign, pyrexia and other signs which may lead to a wrong diagnosis of meningitis. A systolic murmur arising from an aneurysm or angioma may be heard on auscultation over the skull or the closed eye.

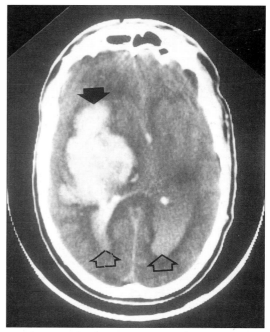

▲ **Figure 10.92 Massive intracerebral haemorrhage from right middle cerebral artery (closed arrow).** Note spill of blood into posterior horns of lateral ventricles (open arrows)

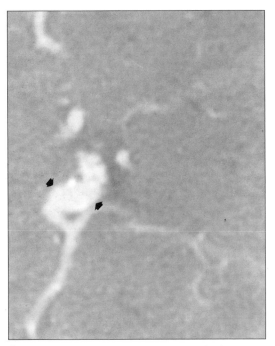

▲ **Figure 10.93 Aneurysm of anterior communicating artery in suspected subarachnoid haemorrhage.** CT scan with intravenous enhancement

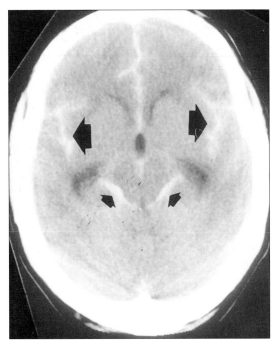

▲ **Figure 10.94 Acute subarachnoid haemorrhage with high density blood (white) throughout subarachnoid space notably in Sylvian fissures (large arrows) and ambient wing cisterns (small arrows)**

The truth is established on lumbar puncture when pure blood or heavily bloodstained fluid is withdrawn. CT scanning is an alternative method of diagnosis when blood may be seen throughout the subarachnoid space (Figure 10.94). After settling, the supernatant fluid remains straw coloured, thus distinguishing the blood from that due to imperfect lumbar puncture. The blood is evenly mixed throughout the fluid, whereas in the case of a 'traumatic tap' the first sample obtained is usually more heavily stained than subsequent samples.

In a patient who survives the first haemorrhage the aneurysm becomes lined with clot. This tends to be removed after a few days so that a second bleed commonly occurs about 10 days after the first. This fact is relevant to surgical treatment of the aneurysm which should be attempted within 10 days of the original haemorrhage.

Subdural haemorrhage

Sometimes a comparatively minor injury to the skull may result in a gradual leakage from the cortical veins into the subdural space, and a haematoma is formed causing pressure symptoms as it slowly increases in size; it may therefore be confused with cerebral tumour unless the history of trauma is elicited (Figure 10.95). The symp-

toms manifest themselves in a few days, weeks or months after the injury, and concussion may not have occurred. Headache, vomiting, drowsiness, mental confusion and bradycardia are common, but subject to remarkable fluctuation, seldom seen to the same extent in tumour. Papilloedema of moderate degree may develop. Variable changes in the pupillary, tendon and superficial reflexes result, hemiplegia may develop, and drowsiness changes to stupor or, later, coma and death, if unrelieved.

THE DIAGNOSIS OF DISEASES OF THE NERVOUS SYSTEM

THE ANATOMICAL DIAGNOSIS

Diagnosis may often be achieved with more precision in diseases of the nervous system than in other parts of the body.

The reason for this is that disturbances of function are closely related to the anatomical site of the lesion. This is well illustrated in the examples already given of affections of the motor and sensory tracts in the spinal cord, of the localizing value of the abolition of tendon reflexes and the modification of reflexes, as in the case

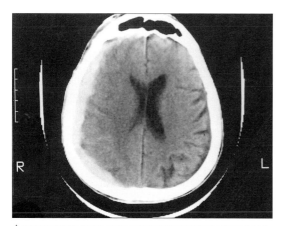

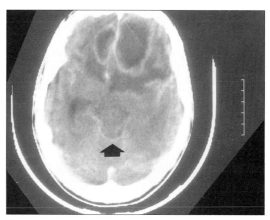

▲ **Figure 10.95 Acute right subdural haematoma from head injury.** Crescentic high density lesion on brain surface with midline shift and effacement of sulci and compression of ipsilateral ventricle

▲ **Figure 10.96 Frontal lobe abscesses which developed over four days**. Note compression of quadrigeminal cisterns (arrow) indicating incipient tentorial coning

of Babinski's sign. It has been seen how a combination of signs may lead to a topographical diagnosis of such diseases as motor neuron disease, subacute combined degeneration, neuropathies and myopathies.

Similarly, damage to the motor system in the brain may result in characteristic patterns as in the complete hemiplegia of an internal capsular lesion. Special functions of other parts of the brain may be lost or altered and cause impairment of intellect, memory and personality when the frontal lobes are affected.

Involvement of cranial nerves may have great localizing value if associated with other neurological signs, but not if the nerve alone is involved because of the long course of certain cranial nerves.

By contrast with examination of other systems, e.g. the heart, the nervous system stands almost alone in enabling the patient to co-operate fully in the diagnosis and displaying the higher faculties of the brain in speech, thought, memory and reasoning. A routine for recording examination of the nervous system is given in Table 10.8.

THE AETIOLOGICAL DIAGNOSIS

This has a close bearing on the anatomical diagnosis, for it is known that certain types of pathological process repeatedly occur in the same site.

The virus of poliomyelitis has a selective affinity for the anterior horn cells, the virus of herpes zoster favours the posterior nerve root, and deficiency of vitamin B_{12} leads to degenerative changes in the peripheral nerves, posterior column and pyramidal tracts – to give but a few examples.

It sometimes happens, therefore, that the anatomical picture of the lesion suggests its pathology.

The medulloblastoma of childhood is an example. This tumour brings headache, vomiting, papilloedema and other signs associated with an expanding lesion within the skull, but cranial nerve lesions, especially oculomotor pareses, are common, and there is some inco-ordination of movement of a cerebellar type. Such features in a young child indicating an involvement of the brainstem, cerebellum and cervical cord are rarely caused by anything other than medulloblastoma, though tubercular meningitis has certain symptoms and signs in common.

Time relationships are also closely bound up with aetiology. Trauma often causes instantaneous effects, as does haemorrhage into the brain or spinal cord.

Inflammatory lesions develop in a matter of days (Figure 10.96), while neoplastic conditions may take weeks or months, and degenerative processes may require months to years before revealing a diagnosable clinical picture.

The aetiology in neurological disease does not differ in principle from the causes at work in other parts of the body, but emphasis can be placed upon certain causes which are common.

ILLUSTRATIVE DISEASES

In conclusion, three common diseases of the nervous system will be described to illustrate some important principles in neurological diagnosis. *Epilepsy* is a paroxysmal disorder of cerebral function, and the patient may be in perfect health at other times. Diagnosis depends upon an accurate account of the attack and a careful physical examination to exclude the early signs of a

A ROUTINE FOR RECORDING EXAMINATION OF THE NERVOUS SYSTEM	
Cerebral dominance	Left- or right-handed
Mental state	Orientation, memory, intelligence, grasp of information, behaviour, mood, talk, delusions, hallucinations, insight
Speech	Dysarthria, dysphasia, stuttering
Stance and gait	Romberg's test
Skull and spine	Congenital or acquired deformities. Bruits. Symmetry of development

Cranial nerves	1 Recognize test odours with either nostril
	2 Visual acuity: near and distance vision
	  Visual fields; scotomas
	  Optic disc and retinae
	3,4,6 Enophthalmos or exophthalmos. Ptosis
	  Pupils equal, central, circular and regular
	  Pupils react to light, direct and consensual and to convergence
	  External ocular movements. Nystagmus
	5 Corneal reflexes. Facial sensation
	  Jaw opens centrally; normal power
	  Jaw jerk
	7 Facial asymmetry or weakness (upper and lower divisions)
	8 Hears whispered voice at 3 ft, either AC>BC; Weber's test not lateralized
	9, 10 Palate elevation; gag reflex; cough and voice
	11 Sternomastoids and trapezius: weakness, wasting or fasciculation
	12 Tongue: wasting, fasciculation, protrusion (central or elevated)

Motor system	Posture
	Muscle bulk
	Fasciculation
	Tone
	Voluntary movements – power
	       fine movements
	       akinesia
	       bradykinesia
	Co-ordination
	Involuntary movements – tremor
	       chorea
	       athetosis
	Tendon reflexes
	Superficial reflexes
	Plantar responses (Babinski sign)

Sensory system	Light touch (cotton wool) Pain (sharp pin) Temperature (hot and cold tubes) Joint position sense Vibration sense (128 Hz) 2-point discrimination (compasses)
Peripheral nerves	Palpation Response to percussion
Autonomic system	Sweating on peripheries Blood pressure control – postural hypotension Heart-rate control – Valsalva manoeuvre

▲ Table 10.8

focal cause. A *space-occupying lesion* such as tumour exemplifies an organic and progressive focal process which may sometimes be precisely localized by clinical examination based on a knowledge of the functional anatomy of the nervous system. *Multiple sclerosis* is characterized by episodes of neurological disturbance which may be scattered over a long period of time and accompanied by multifocal signs. Special investigations are of little value, and diagnosis may sometimes rest upon the history alone.

EPILEPSY

Epilepsy consists of a recurrent transient disturbance of cerebral function usually accompanied by an abnormal and excessive discharge from cerebral neurons. Epilepsy is classified as 'idiopathic' or 'symptomatic' according to whether a specific cause can be found. The causes include high fever in children, cerebrovascular disease in the elderly, trauma, tumour, metabolic disorders such as uraemia and the withdrawal of alcohol or sedative drugs. A familial incidence is common especially in the idiopathic form.

Epilepsy may manifest itself as generalized convulsions (*grand mal*), minor momentary attacks (*petit mal*, myoclonic, etc.) and focal epilepsy (psychomotor, Jacksonian).

GENERALIZED CONVULSIONS (GRAND MAL)
The fits of epilepsy follow, in classic cases, such a definite sequence of events as to make their recognition easy. The events are:

1 The aura.
2 The cry.
3 The tonic stage.
4 The clonic stage.
5 Postepileptic phenomena.

Usually there is no apparent precipitating cause, but occasionally the attack seems to result from some specific sensory stimulus or emotion, such as music or flickering light.

1 The aura
This is a warning occurring a short time before the fit. It usually takes the form of a peculiar subjective phenomenon, e.g. tingling in one hand, queer sensations in the epigastrium, sense of constriction around the leg, visual or auditory sensations. The aura is generally constant for the same individual. It is important, though dif-

ficult, to distinguish an aura of motor character (trivial twitchings followed by other phenomena) from true Jacksonian or focal epilepsy.

2 The cry
As the patient falls to the ground the respiratory muscles are in a state of tonic spasm and a grunting cry is emitted. The patient is unaware of this as he falls unconscious.

3 The tonic stage
The muscles of the whole body are in tonic contraction. The body is therefore rigid, the hands and jaws clenched. The cessation of respiratory movements causes cyanosis and engorgement of veins in the neck. Occasionally the muscular involvement is unequal, twisting the body to one side. This stage lasts about half a minute and passes into –

4 The clonic stage
Clonic movements affect the whole body almost instantaneously. The limbs are alternately flexed and extended, and the movements rapidly increase in excursion and then diminish in intensity and frequency. The convulsions last about three minutes. During them the patient may injure himself by the champing movements of the jaw (laceration of the tongue, injury to the teeth, frothy and often blood-stained saliva on the lips) or by contact with surrounding hard or dangerous objects. During the clonic stage incontinence of urine and more rarely of faeces also occurs.

5 Postepileptic phenomena
Following the clonic stage, coma of short duration occurs during which the tendon reflexes are abolished and the plantar responses are extensor. The pupils are dilated and the corneal reflexes absent. There may be a slight rise in temperature, more pronounced if a succession of fits occurs – status epilepticus. Usually the patient passes from coma into a natural sleep which lasts for several hours and from which he awakes with a headache. More rarely *postepileptic automatism* results: the patient may perform acts (e.g. undressing or walking) of which he afterwards has no recollection. In some cases 'psychic equivalents' of epilepsy may be found – e.g. complete change in personality and habit and liability to criminal acts of which the patient later has no knowledge.

MINOR MOMENTARY ATTACKS
Petit mal
This is a term used to describe transient 'absence' attacks in children, accompanied by a diagnostic 3 per second 'spike and dome' pattern in the electroencephalograph

(see Figure 10.104). There is a sudden interruption of activity lasting only a few seconds with blankness of expression, perhaps a momentary twitching of the face or limbs, but the child rarely falls, objects held are seldom dropped and incontinence is unusual. A family history is common and most cases are 'idiopathic'.

Myoclonic seizures

These consist of violent jerking movements usually of one or both arms. Other transient motor forms of epilepsy in children include sudden bowing of the head (*Salaam attacks*) and *akinetic seizures*, in which the child suddenly falls to the ground without loss of consciousness.

FOCAL EPILEPSY
Psychomotor epilepsy

This is the commonest form of seizure in which the symptoms arise from one particular focus in the brain, in this case the temporal lobe. This focus may be an identifiable structural lesion, especially in adults, but many cases are idiopathic. Sensory hallucinations, especially of taste and smell, are accompanied by mental and emotional phenomena including 'dreamy' states, which may be pleasant or otherwise, and a sensation known as *déjà vu*, in which surroundings or events seem strangely familiar. The motor features of temporal lobe epilepsy consist of purposive but inappropriate movements which include smacking the lips, chewing, muttering or more complex activities such as undressing. The patient may also display anger, laughter and other motor manifestations of the emotional disturbance. These attacks may be distinguished from *petit mal* and other forms of minor epilepsy by the fact that movements are co-ordinated rather than clonic and last for minutes rather than seconds.

Jacksonian epilepsy

This was first described by the pioneer neurologist Hughlings Jackson. It generally consists of a localized fit without loss of consciousness. The convulsive movements usually start in the same group of muscles and extend in a 'march'. Thus twitchings may be observed in the right hand followed by movements of the arm and shoulder-girdle, and then of the whole of the right side, sometimes spreading to the left. Occasionally the attack ends in generalized convulsions, in which case consciousness may be lost. Such a history suggests an irritative lesion of the brain such as tumour or trauma, though the story in these two examples will be quite different.

The physical examination in cases of Jacksonian epilepsy is more likely to yield signs than in the case of the idiopathic variety, though not always so. The com-

monest sign is a hemiparesis (Todd's paralysis), which may last for several hours after an attack. The attacks are not always motor in character but may be sensory with visual, auditory or other sensory phenomena.

The electroencephalogram (EEG) has proved the clear vision of Hughlings Jackson when he defined epilepsy as an excessive, sudden and unruly discharge of neuronal cells. For during the attacks distinctive waves appear, indicating that there is a dysrhythmia of the electrical potentials of the brain, due in its turn to physicochemical changes (see Figure 10.104). These may be congenital, but it is not surprising that one or more of the several factors causing symptomatic epilepsy may modify the physicochemical state of the brain.

OBSERVATION AND CAUSATION OF EPILEPTIC FITS

It is useful to provide the nursing staff or relatives with a questionnaire to cover the points described in the various forms of epilepsy. Often the patient has no knowledge of the attack unless there has been injury or incontinence. This particularly applies to nocturnal attacks. Sometimes he feels ill afterwards or behaves strangely and knows that something has happened, but generally one must depend upon information provided by an intelligent observer.

True *petit mal* is usually idiopathic and Jacksonian fits are usually symptomatic, but in every case of epilepsy a careful search must be made for an organic cause by thorough general and neurological examination and by appropriate investigations (see page 285). Hypertrophy of the gums (Figure 10.97) and megaloblastic anaemia may be found in epileptic patients who are taking phenytoin sodium.

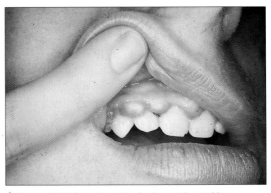

▲ **Figure 10.97 Gum hypertrophy in a patient taking phenytoin sodium for epilepsy**. The patient, a female, also had megaloblastic anaemia due to folic acid deficiency. (See also page 190)

HYSTERICAL FITS

These can usually be distinguished from epilepsy, though *petit mal* may cause difficulties. They are commoner in women. Hysterical 'convulsions' are so violent as to be obvious purposeful struggling. Incontinence and injury do not occur for they are too unpleasant, but manifestations such as shutting the eyes against resistance and persistent general rigidity or movements all increase if the patient feels that she is attracting attention. It is important to note that hysterical fits may be a result of organic brain disease and are not uncommon in epileptic subjects.

NARCOLEPSY AND CATAPLEXY

These rare conditions, which usually occur together, resemble epilepsy in that they each consist of a paroxysmal but transient disturbance of cerebral function. The cause is unknown and is not associated with structural disease of the brain. Narcolepsy is characterized by bouts of uncontrollable sleep from which the patient can easily be roused. In cataplexy, there are abrupt but momentary episodes of muscular weakness usually precipitated by emotion such as laughter. Other features of this syndrome are hypnagogic hallucinations (vivid dreams on first falling to sleep) and sleep paralysis (inability to move on first waking).

SPACE-OCCUPYING LESIONS

The recognition and localization of an intracranial space-occupying lesion is of the greatest importance, because the condition can often be relieved and sometimes cured by surgical treatment. Examples of such lesions include tumour, abscess, cyst, haematoma and aneurysm (Figure 10.98). The two principal manifestations are increased intracranial pressure and focal signs.

SYMPTOMS AND SIGNS OF INCREASED INTRACRANIAL PRESSURE

Whatever the cause of a rise of intracranial pressure, certain common symptoms and signs result. The most important of these are headache, vomiting, papilloedema, disturbances of cerebration, fits, bradycardia and respiratory arrhythmias.

Headache

This symptom is considered on pages 8–9 as it results from many conditions not primarily affecting the nervous system. As a feature of increased intracranial pressure it may occur in paroxysms of great severity, often with periods of freedom, be mild or even absent. The headache is usually maximal in the early morning, sometimes waking the patient, and then improves after he gets up from bed. It is sometimes over the site of a tumour, but more often it is generalized (Figure 10.99).

Vomiting

Typical cerebral vomiting is not preceded by nausea and is sometimes projectile in character. This is often seen in meningitis. In children especially, the gastric contents may be ejected quite forcibly through the mouth. Vomiting due to increased intracranial pressure is, however, not commonly of this cerebral type. It may resemble other forms of sickness preceded by nausea. Vomiting is a late sign of raised intracranial pressure and is usually associated with severe headache.

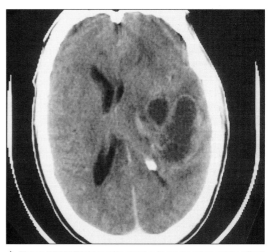

▲ **Figure 10.98 Right cystic astrocytoma causing mass effect displacing midline structures**. Patient presented with headache and contralateral hemiparesis

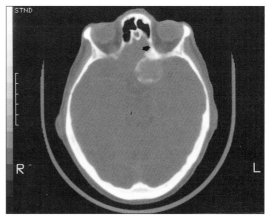

▲ **Figure 10.99 Left frontal hemangioma**. Patient presented with left frontal headache

Papilloedema (choked disc) (Figure 10.100)

This is the sign of greatest importance in the diagnosis of increased intracranial pressure, though it does not correlate well with the level of the pressure and may take several days to develop. The patient may complain of impaired vision, which is confirmed by the discovery of enlargement of the blind spot and contraction of the periphery of the visual field. In many cases no subjective visual changes are present, emphasizing the necessity of examining the retina in all neurological cases. The objective sign consists in swelling of the optic nerve head to an extent of several dioptres. (See also the 2nd cranial nerve, page 216 *et seq.*)

Mental changes

Mental confusion and apathy are common but late signs in most cases of increased intracranial pressure (see Cerebration and consciousness, above) and stupor or coma follow in severe unrelieved cases.

Fits (see also page 279)

It is important to remember that generalized convulsions resembling idiopathic epilepsy are a commoner manifestation of increased intracranial pressure than localized fits. Fits occurring first in middle life should emphasize the necessity of excluding organic cerebral disease.

Bradycardia

The general rise of intracranial pressure in time causes slowing of the heart rate owing to its effect on the vagal centres in the medulla; a grave sign of most value when the normal heart rate for the individual is known.

Respiratory arrhythmias

Increasing intracranial pressure impairs the cerebral circulation including that of the medulla with involvement of the activities of the respiratory centre. This may result in abnormalities of the rate or rhythm of respiration such as Cheyne–Stokes breathing (see page 111).

FOCAL SIGNS (Table 10.9)

It is important to localize a space-occupying lesion as accurately as possible, because upon this will depend the success of any operative treatment. The earlier the anatomical diagnosis can be made, the more likely is the treatment to be successful, not only because the encroachment of even a simple tumour upon the brain substance is attended by grave results, which increase the longer the tumour remains, but also because the slight localizing signs of the early stages are often masked by increasing intracranial pressure. Moreover, the disturbances of consciousness which have been mentioned (impairment of intellect and increasing stupor) soon render the patient unable to help in the diagnosis of the condition by his accurate history.

This preamble emphasizes the necessity for paying due attention to the slightest focal signs in the early stages of intracranial disease. These signs depend upon the abolition or alteration in function of the various parts of the brain and the cranial nerves which proceed from it. Some areas – for example, the motor area – have well-defined functions, the loss or alteration of which will almost certainly occur when a lesion affects them.

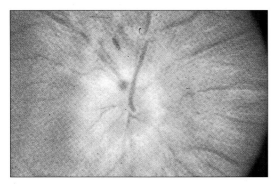

▲ Figure 10.100 Papilloedema

LOCALIZING FOCAL SIGNS IN THE CEREBRUM	
Site	**Symptoms and signs**
Frontal lobe	Personality change, facetiousness Anosmia Optic atrophy and papilloedema
Precentral gyrus	Focal convulsions and hemiparesis

Parietal lobe	Spatial disorientation,
	  astereognosis, alexia,
	  homonymous hemianopia

Temporal lobe	Psychomotor convulsions Memory and emotional disturbances Sensory aphasia Homonymous hemianopia
Occipital lobe	Homonymous hemianopia Papilloedema
Cerebellum	Disturbances of equilibrium and tone Papilloedema
Pituitary	Bitemporal hemianopia

▲ Table 10.9

Others – for instance, the frontal lobes – may be the seat of gross changes without symptoms or signs of real localizing value. In this connection it is well to note that supratentorial tumours are relatively silent, while below the tentorium lesions generally produce early focal signs.

Those focal signs which appear earliest are of greatest value, for they are more likely to be due to the original lesion. The same signs appearing later may merely result from secondary changes in the neighbourhood of the lesion, e.g. meningitis or thrombosis, or from displacement of intracranial structures by rising pressure.

Local signs are of even greater value than general ones in the diagnosis of cerebral lesions, for whereas such signs as headache, vomiting and retinopathies may be caused by hypertension, blood diseases and other conditions, local signs such as paresis or disturbances of sensation indicate a local lesion. Sometimes a combination of signs is known to be associated with a particular type of tumour. For example, a medulloblastoma is the commonest cerebral tumour of childhood and causes a combination of signs, indicating both the position of the tumour in the vermis and surrounding structures and its pathology. Local signs may now be discussed in more detail and grouped according to the various parts of the brain affected.

Mental disorder should draw attention to the frontal, parietal or temporal lobes. Frontal tumours may reach a considerable size and produce no focal signs other than personality changes, sometimes with loss of inhibitions and urinary incontinence. Temporal lobe lesions cause impairment of memory and emotional disorders (see also under Epilepsy, page 279), while parietal lesions are characteristically associated with spatial disorientation (see also page 265). It should be noted that any tumour interfering with the circulation of the CSF (especially in the posterior fossa) may cause intellectual impairment secondary to hydrocephalus.

Motor phenomena such as Jacksonian fits and paresis point to lesions in the precentral gyrus and the neighbouring subcortical regions. Paralysis with involvement of the cranial nerves suggests lesions in the midbrain – crura, pons or medulla. They are more fully described under the motor system, page 254 *et seq.*

Cortical sensory disturbances, i.e. astereognosis, loss of point discrimination and of the perception of small variations in temperature, suggest a lesion of the parietal lobe.

Aphasia may suggest temporal lobe involvement if of the auditory type, a lesion of areas 18 or 19 when visual, or an affection of Broca's centre (area 44) in the inferior frontal gyrus, when essentially motor (see Figure 10.1). Aphasia is a sign which must be used with caution for localizing purposes, owing to the difficulty in analysing different types.

Perversions of smell, when local nasal causes have been excluded, may throw suspicion on the uncus.

Hemianopia, especially homonymous and quadrantic types, is found in lesions of the optic radiation and area 17 of the occipital cortex (see Figure 10.1). Bitemporal hemianopia suggests a tumour in the region of the pituitary.

Cranial-nerve palsies are sometimes of localizing value and are particularly found when the tumour is situated at the base of the brain, though when not accompanied by other neurological signs they may be due to lesions involving only the nucleus or its nerve.

Disturbances of equilibrium and muscle tone are the most important symptoms suggestive of cerebellar tumours.

It must not be forgotten that the functions of several adjacent areas may be affected successively as the tumour grows, so that new signs continue to appear. An important example is the acoustic neuroma which usually presents with unilateral nerve deafness followed in succession by signs of vestibular nerve damage (absent caloric reaction), signs of trigeminal involvement (absent corneal reflex), facial paresis, cerebellar ataxia and contralateral pyramidal tract signs from medullary compression. This tumour may be associated with generalized neurofibromatosis (Figure 10.101). The possibility of tumour should be considered when any localizing signs are present, especially when these appear gradually over a period of some months. If signs of increased intracranial pressure (see page 271) occur concurrently, the diagnosis becomes more certain. The reverse, however, is commonly the case, namely, the signs of increased intracranial pressure occur early and the localizing signs only later. In such

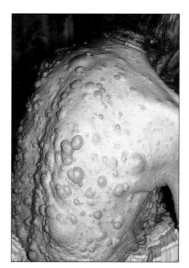

◄ **Figure 10.101 Neurofibromatosis (von Recklinghausen's disease)**. This condition is sometimes associated with an acoustic nerve tumour

cases the careful exclusion of other diseases causing the triad of headache, vomiting and papilloedema may establish a diagnosis of tumour, but its position may remain uncertain. Of the general signs, it is to be noted that papilloedema and vomiting are often more pronounced in subtentorial than supratentorial tumours.

In the diagnosis of the nature of a tumour the patient's age takes a prominent part. Carcinoma, which is always secondary, is naturally found in older people. A primary focus should be sought (Figure 10.102). One of the commonest is carcinoma of the bronchus. Among primary tumours an important distinction is to be made between intracerebral and extracerebral growths. The former include various forms of glioma which replace brain tissue, while the extracerebral varieties, e.g. meningioma and pituitary tumours, cause special pressure effects and are more amenable to treatment (Figure 10.99). Whatever the nature of the tumour the signs of increased intracranial pressure depend largely on how it obstructs the free circulation of cerebrospinal fluid and how rapidly it grows.

MULTIPLE SCLEROSIS (DISSEMINATED SCLEROSIS)

This is one of the commonest organic nervous diseases. It affects both sexes, usually between the ages of 20 and 40 years, and is generally insidious in its onset. Its progress is marked by remissions in which the symptoms and signs may disappear partially or entirely.

Among early symptoms may be mentioned transient pareses, paraesthesiae (subjective sensory phenomena, see page 265), disturbances of micturition and ocular symptoms. The ocular manifestations, which include diplopia and blurring of vision, are perhaps most characteristic.

Blurring of vision may occur for a few days to a few weeks, indicating a retrobulbar neuritis, and may precede cord symptoms by months or years. It is often followed by a degree of optic atrophy, especially noticeable in the temporal halves of the optic discs. In a developed case, spastic paraplegia is the commonest clinical picture. But as the name of the disease indicates, the lesions are scattered, and before a diagnosis of multiple sclerosis is justifiable, the paraplegia must be accompanied by signs of damage to other parts of the nervous system. The triad of symptoms described by Charcot, nystagmus, staccato speech and 'intention' tremor, is by no means commonly found, but one of the triad with signs of a spastic paraplegia may suggest multiple sclerosis, indicating patches of sclerosis in the cerebellum and corticospinal systems. Both nystagmus and staccato speech are defects of postural fixation (tone) due to cerebellar involvement.

Evidence of sclerotic patches in the posterior columns or cerebellar pathways is to be found in ataxia, a common symptom (Figure 10.103). Loss of vibration sensation and of sense of position are more rarely found on objective examination. Damage to other sensory tracts may result in various anaesthesiae and paraesthesiae.

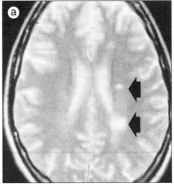

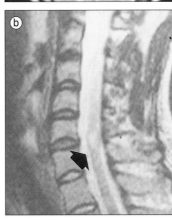

◀ **Figure 10.103 Multiple sclerosis.** MRI scans showing demyelinated plaques in white matter (a) and cervical cord (b)

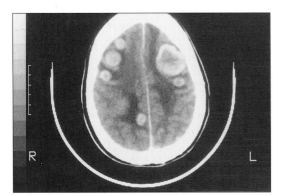

▲ **Figure 10.102 Multiple cerebral metastases from breast carcinoma**

SPECIAL INVESTIGATIONS

CEREBROSPINAL FLUID

This is secreted by the cells of the choroid plexus and absorbed via the arachnoid villi into the dural sinuses and spinal veins.

The information which it gives in diseases of the nervous system includes:

1 The pressure.
2 The presence of blood and turbidity from increased cellular content, observable by the naked eye.
3 The cell content, microscopically.
4 The chemical content.
5 The Wassermann reaction.

1 Pressure

The normal pressure, when measured at lumbar puncture in the lateral recumbent position, with the patient completely relaxed, varies between 100 and 180 mmH$_2$O. The fluid is contained in the ventricular system which has foramina communicating with the subarachnoid space. Any condition which causes a rise of intracranial pressure, e.g. tumour or abscess, may at first be compensated for by displacement of the fluid. As this runs into the sheath of the optic nerve it may cause papilloedema, and when it affects the posterior fossa of the skull there may be crowding of the cerebellum and medulla into the foramen magnum. This process is easily aggravated by lumbar puncture and may cause serious ischaemia of the medulla which can be fatal. By these pressure effects the escape of the cerebrospinal fluid into the spinal theca and its absorption from this part of the subarachnoid space are prevented. A failure of absorption in the ventricles also occurs if the foramina are blocked, and hydrocephalus may result. See also Queckenstedt's test (page 270).

2 Presence of blood

The presence of blood in considerable quantities may be noted in subarachnoid haemorrhage (page 10.63), or the fluid may be yellow due to altered blood from an earlier bleed ('xanthochromia'). The fluid may be turbid if there is a large number of cells, as in certain types of coccal meningitis.

3 Cell content

An increase of cells occurs as in the case of infections in other parts of the body. These cells are usually polymorphonuclear leucocytes in coccal infections and certain other acute infections, or lymphocytes when the infection is more chronic. When the cells are increased, a specific organism, e.g. the meningococcus or tubercle bacillus, may be identified immediately on microscopy or only after culture. Cellular changes may, however, occur in certain nervous diseases in which no organism is present.

4 Chemical content

The chemical constituents of the cerebrospinal fluid are not dissimilar from those in plasma, except for a much lower protein content. There is an increase in protein and a decrease in sugar and chlorides in many types of meningitis. Gross increase in the protein content is seen when the free flow of the cerebrospinal fluid is prevented by blockage of the theca in cases of spinal-cord tumour (Froin's syndrome). A very high protein level may also occur with certain forms of cerebral tumour and peripheral neuropathy.

The normal values of the main constituents of the cerebrospinal fluid and the changes commonly found in disease of the central nervous system are set out in Table 10.10.

RADIOLOGY

A plain radiograph of the *skull* may show evidence of fractures; raised intracranial pressure ('beaten silver' appearance of the vault and erosion of the clinoid processes); bone destruction by tumour or infection (e.g. of sinuses or mastoid cells); expansion of the pituitary fossa or of the various neural foramina (e.g. optic and auditory) due to tumours; calcification within tumours or vascular lesions such as aneurysm and angioma.

Directional Doppler ultrasonography is an accurate safe and atraumatic technique to identify narrowing in the common carotid artery and its branches including internal carotid and ophthalmic arteries.

Arteriograms are radiographs of the cervical and cerebral vessels taken after the intra-arterial injection of a radio-opaque contrast material. They may be used to locate and display cerebral aneurysms and obstruction or displacement of arteries.

Pneumoencephalography consists of injecting air into the spinal subarachnoid space (or directly into the ventricular system) to outline the cerebral ventricles. Radiographs may then help to demonstrate cerebral atrophy, distension or displacement of the ventricles and the site of obstruction to the flow of CSF.

Myelography is used to determine the level of a lesion compressing the spinal cord. A radio-opaque dye is injected into the lumbar subarachnoid space, and radiographs are taken with the patient tilted so that the dye can move up or down the spinal canal.

THE CEREBROSPINAL FLUID IN HEALTH AND DISEASE					
	Appearance	Pressure (mm CSF)	Cells (per mm^3)	Protein (mg/100 ml)	Other
Normal	Clear Colourless	100–180	0–5 Lymphocytes	15–45	glucose (3.3–4.4 mmol/l)
Traumatic	Bloody at first	100–180	Red blood cells	Elevated 4 mg per 5000 red blood cells	Supernatant clear
Subarachnoid haemorrhage	Bloody throughout	Raised	Red blood cells	As above	Supernatant xanthochromic
Purulent meningitis	Turbid	Raised	Polymorphs	100–400 100–5000	Glucose low, organisms on smear
Viral meningitis	Clear to opalescent	Normal	Lymphocytes 20–2000	150	Sterile PCR positive
Tuberculous meningitis	Clear to cloudy	Raised	Lymphocytes up to 500	80–400	Glucose low, organisms on smear or culture
Neurosyphilis	Clear	Normal	Lymphocytes up to 50	Up to 100	Positive antibody titres
Multiple sclerosis	Clear	Normal	Normal or up to 20 lymphocytes	Normal up to 120	Raised γ-globulins Oligoclonal bands
Spinal tumour with block	Yellow xanthochromia	Normal or low	Normal or up to 20 lymphocytes	200–600	May coagulate

▲ Table 10.10

COMPUTERIZED AXIAL TOMOGRAPHY (CT SCAN)

This technique has largely replaced the more invasive methods already mentioned for the location of intracranial lesions. X-rays penetrate the head from different angles, and by a process of triangulation the exact density of each point is obtained from the hindrance to the X-ray beams. A series of cross-sections of the brain is mapped out by a computer, and the various tissues, both normal and abnormal, are clearly distinguished by the difference in their densities.

MAGNETIC RESONANCE IMAGING

This is a useful non-invasive technique and preferable to CT in delineating lesions in the posterior fossa and the craniocervical spinal canal. As with CT, contrast medium may enhance lesions and demonstrate brain and spinal cord vascular abnormalities. It can reveal abnormalities in the brainstem such as syringomyelia and, by

distinguishing between white and grey matter, it is also helpful in the diagnosis of multiple sclerosis.

ISOTOPE BRAIN SCAN

Certain radioactive substances (e.g. technetium isotopes) are selectively localized in tumours and other lesions of the brain, especially those near the surface. This local concentration of the isotope can be detected by means of a scintillation scanner and displayed on suitable paper or film.

ELECTROENCEPHALOGRAPHY

The rhythmical activity of the cortical neurons is recorded by the electroencephalograph.

Departures from normal may be seen in many brain disorders, notably epilepsy, but also in some cerebral tumours and occasionally in certain metabolic and psychiatric diseases (Figure 10.104).

The electroencephalogram is a valuable aid in neurological diagnosis, even in localization of the lesion as in tumour, but needs special skill in its interpretation and close correlation with the clinical findings.

VISUAL EVOKED RESPONSES

These are performed by detecting the electrical potential arriving at the occipital cortex after stimulation of the retina by a flash of light or patterned stimuli. The response is measured through the intact skull and the presence, character and latency of the visually evoked response can be helpful in the differentiation of disorders of visual function.

ELECTROMYOGRAPHY, MUSCLE BIOPSY AND NERVE CONDUCTION STUDIES

The records of electrical variations made by insertion of a needle into muscle can give important information in various rare muscular diseases: myopathies, neuropathies and myasthenia. It may also indicate the presence or absence of muscular contraction where this is clinically abolished, as in traumatic lesions of nerves.

Muscle biopsy can be a similar aid to diagnosis.

Nerve conduction is determined by measuring the time taken for a stimulus to travel from one point on the nerve to another. This technique may be helpful in the assessment of peripheral nerve lesions (see Figure 10.105.)

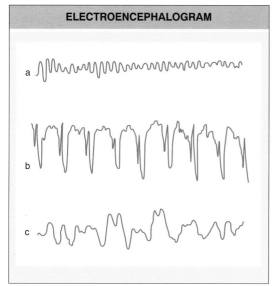

ELECTROENCEPHALOGRAM

▲ **Figure 10.104 Electroencephalogram**. (a) Normal record (alpha waves). (b) Petit mal epilepsy (spike and dome pattern). (c) Slow activity (delta waves): this can be generalized, as in epilepsy, or localized to one part of the brain, e.g. cerebral tumour

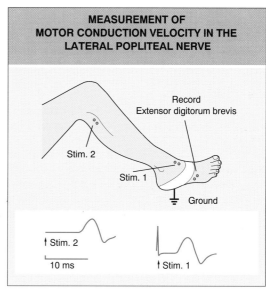

MEASUREMENT OF MOTOR CONDUCTION VELOCITY IN THE LATERAL POPLITEAL NERVE

▲ **Figure 10.105 Measurement of motor conduction velocity in the lateral popliteal nerve**. The anterior tibial branch is stimulated at the ankle (stim. 1) and the response recorded. The nerve is then stimulated at the head of the fibula (stim. 2) and the response is recorded. The time from the stimulus to the onset of the muscle potential is measured from each trace and the difference represents the time taken for the impulse to pass down the nerve between the two stimulus points

The diagnosis of
psychiatric disorders

ROBIN PHILPOTT

Psychiatric disorder is the second most common cause of patients seeking help from their general practitioner and affects about 15 per cent of the adult population at any given time. Acute psychiatric emergencies present at accident and emergency departments, particularly attempted suicide, drug intoxication or disturbed behaviour. More than half the elderly patients on general medical or geriatric wards have mental disorders. Obstetric departments need special links with drug dependency clinics for drug-dependent pregnant women. Sick children, including those with non-accidental injuries, may reflect hidden psychiatric morbidity in themselves, their parents or their families.

The reasons for the high co-existence of mental and physical disorder are complex. Partly they are causal; thus chronic painful conditions, such as arthritis or bowel disorders may result in depression, thyrotoxic patients are excessively anxious whereas myxoedematous patients may suffer almost any psychiatric symptom. Depressed or schizophrenic patients may neglect themselves so they become dehydrated, hypothermic or undernourished with secondary medical complications such as pneumonia or hypovolaemia and tertiary effects due to falls, cerebrovascular accident or myocardial infarct.

The treatment of medical conditions can induce psychiatric disorder. Admission to hospital may itself induce, or increase, confusion in the elderly and can precipitate acute delirium tremens in patients with undisclosed alcohol dependency. Drugs used in the treatment of medical conditions often have psychiatric side effects. Almost all treatments for Parkinson's disease can cause acute confusional or psychotic episodes. Steroids may induce mania or, more commonly, depression. Moreover, psychotropic drugs have physical side effects; anti-psychotic drugs induce Parkinsonian symptoms and some tricyclic anti-depressants are powerfully anticholinergic with effects on blood pressure, glaucoma and prostatism. Lithium may induce hypothyroidism or diabetes insipidus.

The presence of undiagnosed psychiatric morbidity may adversely affect and prolong medical treatment as an inpatient or outpatient. Depressed patients take longer to mobilize after trauma or hip replacement oper-

ation and anxious patients have higher morbidity and mortality rates after open-heart surgery.

A teenager diagnosed as diabetic will respond in ways that will reflect personality, intelligence and childhood influences. The response will be further affected by social deprivation, poverty and the presence of social, psychiatric or physical morbidity in close family members. A 16-year old diabetic woman from a deprived inner-city area with poor schooling, an unemployed father and drug-addicted brother will cope less well and will suffer more psychological disturbance, with poor treatment compliance and risk-taking behaviour such as unplanned pregnancy and attempted suicide. A similarly aged diabetic woman with professional parents, good school record and the prospect of university will suffer less psychological disturbance and thus better treatment compliance. Sadly, the deprived 16-year old may also receive worse care from her medical attendants as they may find it difficult to empathize with her psychological and social predicament.

For all these reasons medical students will need a firm grasp of the assessment of symptoms and signs of psychiatric disorder. It will be of benefit to their patients throughout their careers as doctors in hospital medicine or primary care.

THE PSYCHIATRIC INTERVIEW

This consists of four main points:
1 To form an understanding and empathic *relationship* with the patient.
2 To gather information about the patient's illness and personal and family background (*the history*).
3 To observe and systematically record the patient's psychiatric symptoms during the interview (*the mental state*).
4 Information from the history and mental state is synthesized into a diagnostic formulation (*the formulation*).

Initially, the student will probably find the need to form a warm and empathic relationship conflicting with the need for a structured interview. Most students will be aware of the need to approach all patients with tact and sensitivity, but this is of even greater importance when dealing with emotional and psychological disorder. The structure of the interview may need to be abandoned for brief, or longer, periods to enable patients to express their emotions in an unhurried and non-judgemental atmosphere.

Students will observe that experienced psychiatric interviewers slip easily from a role that appears empathic and supportive to one that is information gathering. They may assume that this is an inherent skill. It is not – it is one that results from practice and self-awareness.

THE DOCTOR/PATIENT RELATIONSHIP

The psychiatric interview, especially the first interview, plays a valuable role in establishing understanding with the patient and forms the basis of any subsequent work and relationships. Comments which make the patient realize he is being understood are likely to increase his confidence whilst too rigid an insistence on a formal interview structure, ill-timed interruptions or judgemental comments will have the reverse effect. Students should use open-ended questions and encourage the patient to discuss their feelings and emotions.

Before commencing the interview ensure from medical or nursing staff that the patient has been approached and has given his permission to be interviewed by a student. Find out if a room is available for a private interview. Psychiatric patients should, whenever possible, be interviewed privately in an office, not in an open ward. Some patients who are unduly anxious or frightened may wish to be accompanied by another member of staff, or a relative.

The physical setting of the interview is important; avoid sitting opposite the patient. If a desk is present sit on the same side of the desk as the patient, facing them, or without a desk in easy chairs at right angles to each other. The ability to write notes without the use of a desk is an important psychiatric skill. Think about your eye contact, facial expression and body language. You will not be expected to wear a white coat during your psychiatric student attachment, but a clean and reasonably smart appearance will inspire confidence in your professionalism. Do not let your appearance, speech or behaviour betray strong political, religious, moral or personal viewpoints.

You are now ready to commence the gathering of information that will enable you to make a diagnosis, and therefore treat the patient effectively. If you are distressed by information from the patient during the inter-

view try not to over-react. However, discuss your feelings immediately after the interview with qualified nursing or medical staff and with your educational supervisor when presenting the patient's history. You will find it useful during the first interviews to have an aide-mémoire of history taking readily available (the headings for history taking are included in Table 11.1). You will find it useful to copy this out onto a file card with History taking on one side and Mental state examination and formulation on the other. Do not be embarrassed to refer to this aid memoir during history taking. Almost all patients will be sympathetic to the fact you are a student and will be pleased that you are being conscientious.

Writing notes on your lap, referring to an unfamiliar *aide-mémoire* for history taking and remaining warm, empathic and non-judgemental with patients who may be distressed or disturbed will at first seem daunting. However, as each interview progresses you will become more competent, confident and more therapeutic in your relationship with your patients.

THE PSYCHIATRIC HISTORY

The format outlined here should be followed whenever possible for the sake of uniformity and accessibility. One interview may not be sufficient to obtain an adequate history. Facts and evidence should be stated in concise detail, including negative as well as positive factors. Jargon should be avoided and symptoms are often best recorded

AIDE-MÉMOIRE FOR PSYCHIATRIC EXAMINATION	
The psychiatric history	**Mental state examination**

Reason for referral
Complaints
History of present illness
Medication
Past medical history
Past psychiatric history
Family history
Personal history:
  Birth
  Infancy
  Schooling
  Occupations
  Sexual and marriage
  Habits
Premorbid personality
Social circumstances
	Appearance
	Motor activity
	Mood/affect
	Speech and language
	Thought content
	Perceptual disturbances
	Cognitive function
	Insight

	The formulation
	Summary Differential diagnosis Further investigations Treatment Prognosis

▲ **Table 11.1**

in the precise words of the patient. However, the record should not merely be a transcript of what the patient has said; the interviewer should abstract and organize the statements in a logical and sequential manner. Whenever possible a confirmatory history should be obtained from a close relative. Failing this, observations and information from nurses or social workers attached to the clinical team will be important confirmatory evidence.

REASONS FOR REFERRAL

Firstly, record the date and print your name and status at the top of all case entries. Then state the patient's name, sex, age, address, occupation, marital status and record when you have seen the patient, and in what circumstances; i.e. whether an inpatient or outpatient, whether a routine or emergency referral and, for inpatients, whether the patient is formally detained under the Mental Health Act. It is important to record the reason for referral by the referring agency.

COMPLAINTS

Ask the patient what it is they see as their problem, or what their current complaints are. Record verbatim their statements, even if seemingly irrelevant, such as 'I don't know why I'm here', or even, 'There's nothing wrong with me. I shouldn't be here'. Encourage the patient to enumerate as many complaints or problems as possible. What may appear to be completely irrelevant complaints, such as repetitive symptoms of backache, leg ache and headache may subsequently prove to be the somatic preoccupations of a depressed patient.

HISTORY OF PRESENT ILLNESS

Ideally, this should consist of a coherent and chronological account of the illness from its earliest onset, at which time change was first noticed, the subsequent development of symptoms, their duration, severity and effects on functions. However, the onset of psychiatric disorder is often notoriously difficult for patients to identify and questions such as 'When were you last completely well?' may be helpful, as may referring to fixed dates in the calendar, such as 'Were you well last Christmas or your last birthday?'.

The nature of the psychiatric disorder may also make it difficult for histories to be taken. A depressed patient may gloomily claim to have been unwell for many years whereas they have been remarkably well and symptom-free until 6 months previously. A psychotic patient may deny they are ill at all and a schizophrenic patient, perhaps acutely ill for only 3 weeks, may delusionally assume their symptoms are due to an event many years previously.

Organically confused patients of any age are unlikely to give any reliable history. In these circumstances information from relatives, nursing staff or social workers will be invaluable. The skills you have developed in taking histories of physical disorders will be useful here. Identify when each symptom occurred, its precipitant cause, severity and effect on functions such as work, leisure, personal relationships, appetite, weight and sleep. Thus:

An anorexic young female began to develop signs of excessive dietary preoccupation at the age of 14 with subsequent weight-loss. At the age of 16, when she failed exams, her parents noted she was vomiting after meals. Her weight loss was then accelerated and she developed amenorrhoea.

Or:

An 85-year old woman was noted by her relatives to have had memory loss for 3 years, which resulted in losing her keys and her pension book. Memory loss with self-neglect had become more apparent after her husband died 6 months' previously. A sudden worsening one week prior to referral was accompanied by visual hallucinations.

MEDICATION

List here all medication the patient is taking. Also, list here medication taken during the preceding 2–3 months and try to assess whether the patient has been compliant with medication. (A depressed or schizophrenic patient may well have been prescribed correct medication by a general practitioner, but non-compliance may be responsible for drug failure rather than the drug being inappropriate.)

PAST MEDICAL HISTORY

Note significant medical events, particularly during or immediately prior to the onset of the present illness, and any other significant medical conditions throughout the patient's life.

PAST PSYCHIATRIC HISTORY

Ask if any previous treatment has been received for psychiatric disease. It may be more tactful to ask if the patient has previously suffered from 'psychological problems', or 'nerves'. State if the patient has been treated by their general practitioner or required psychiatric services for each event. If there is a positive psychiatric history record this in terms of the year in which it occurred and also the age of the patient at the time. Check with the relatives or with nursing or social work staff because the patient may not admit to a previous psychiatric history.

FAMILY HISTORY

The family history should be recorded as described on page 2. In addition, the student should describe the home atmosphere during childhood, including emotional relationship with parents, siblings and other relatives and the patient's reaction to the death of a close relative. Note any long periods of separation from close relatives in childhood and reasons for this. Record any known family history of psychiatric disorder. A diagrammatic representation of the family history may be useful, particularly when there is a complex history of family disorder (Figure 11.1).

PERSONAL HISTORY

Birth

Record any complications associated with pregnancy or delivery.

Infancy

Record whether the patient was a delicate or healthy child, and whether they had normal developmental milestones: sitting up, walking, talking, etc. List any childhood neurotic traits such as nightmares, sleepwalking, tantrums, bed wetting, nail-biting, stammering or mannerisms. Most children have some neurotic traits but the presence of three or more may be significant for both childhood and adult psychiatric disorder.

Schooling

Age of beginning and finishing. Type of school attended. Educational standard attained, with evidence of abilities or backwardness (be sensitive here – if you suspect educational problems do not challenge the patient. Ask questions such as 'How are you at reading and writing?' and seek confirmatory evidence of educational problems with independent informants). Ask about relationships with schoolmates or teachers, whether they were punished or excluded from school for any reason. Also, whether they truanted or were frightened to go to school (school phobia).

Occupational history

Age of starting work, jobs held in chronological order, length of time held, reasons for changing occupation. Current ambitions, satisfaction in work and relationships with workmates. Include here past wartime or military history, including service rank and disciplinary record.

Sexual and marital history

Describe first sexual awareness, first sexual experiences and first sexual partner. Record details of significant sexual relationships, including children by these relationships and reasons for relationships ending. Record details of current partner, length of relationship and current quality of emotional and sexual relationship, frequency of sexual intercourse, particularly any recent change in frequency. Record chronological list of children, including miscarriages, ages, gender, personality and health. Are more children desired?

Habits

Ask about long-term use of alcohol, tobacco and drugs. Significant alcohol or drug misuse should be included in the history of presenting illness. Nevertheless, all patients should be asked about the possibility of substance misuse. The Cage questionnaire (see Table 11.2) is a useful and effective screen for alcohol misuse, and should be administered to all medical and psychiatric patients. Patients answering positively to two or more questions may well have alcohol problems.

Forensic history

Any contact with the law, past or present, including convictions should be recorded.

◀ **Figure 11.1 Schematic family history**

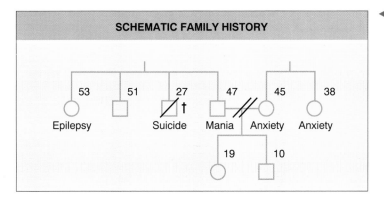

SCHEMATIC FAMILY HISTORY

Premorbid personality

The general form of the patient's family and personal history is probably the best guide to their premorbid personal adjustment. What is important here is the patient's general reaction to life and in particular their relationship with their family and workmates and their adjustment to domestic and leisure activities. Ask if the patient is normally cheerful and calm, or worrisome or anxious. Do they have a character that is timid, sensitive, suspicious, resentful, quarrelsome, irritable, impulsive, jealous, selfish, reserved, shy, self-conscious, strict, fussy or rigid? What are their moral, religious or social standards? What are their attitudes to themselves, others and to their health?

Social circumstances

Is the patient currently employed or retired, and what effect has this on their finances? Is the patient currently living with parents, a partner or alone? If the patient is living with someone else what is the nature of the relationship in terms of physical, financial or emotional dependence?

These headings constitute a comprehensive psychiatric history. At this stage ask if the patient has any further comments to make. Go back to your aide-mémoire to check if there are any major headings that you have forgotten to complete. Remember that the above guide will cover interviews in most circumstances with most patients but you will learn to use it flexibly as your experience increases.

In general terms, children and young adults will need a detailed history of family relationships, childhood and early adult development.

Elderly patients will require less detail in these areas, but nevertheless an autobiographical sketch of their background is needed with more emphasis on the history of present illness and current/past medical conditions.

A patient with alcohol misuse problems will require considerable emphasis on their past and recent history of alcohol intake, together with information regarding the physical effects of alcohol such as amnesia, blackouts, neurological and gastrointestinal complications. Patients with drug misuse problems will require a full history of medical complications of drug abuse and a forensic history.

Younger and middle-aged patients with mental impairment, patients with severe psychotic illnesses and older patients with organic dementing disorders require details of changes in their self-care skills, together with information regarding their current domestic living arrangements and the effect their disabilities have on their main carers.

You may need several interviews with the patient, or with other informants, to enable you to elucidate and record a psychiatric history. This part of the psychiatric examination equates to the history of present illness and systematic review of systems that you have undertaken for physical disorders. The personal and family history, and history of present illness, may be usefully summarized by use of a life chart (see Table 11.3). Record significant life, family and illness events sequentially down

THE CAGE QUESTIONNAIRE
Have you ever tried to *cut down* your drinking?
Have you felt *annoyed* when people have criticized your drinking?
Do you feel *guilty* about your drinking?
Do you need a drink on waking, an *eye opener*, to steady your nerves?
2 or more positive answers = alcohol problem

▲ Table 11.2

LIFE CHART	
Age	
2	Uncle commits suicide
2$\frac{1}{2}$	Father admitted to hospital with mania
6	Moves house and school
9	Brother born
11	Parents separate for 2 months
	Moves house and school
11–14	Bullied
	Truants
15	Father: manic episode
	Marital separation
15$\frac{1}{2}$	Raped on holiday
16	Leaves school
	Attacked by dogs in car park → Phobic symptoms
16	Seen by child psychiatric services → Advise anti-depressants – refused
17	Behaviour therapy for phobic symptoms → drops out of treatment
18	Attends day hospital for 9 months
18	First stable relationship with boyfriend for 6 months
19	This admission

▲ Table 11.3

the page with a new line for each event. Put the patient's age on the left-hand side of the page opposite each life event. You will now record your observations of the patient's mental state, which roughly equates to the physical examination for general medical problems. Seventy per cent of the information needed to make a diagnosis and formulation comes from the psychiatric interview, 25–30 per cent from the mental state examination and less than 10 per cent from subsequent investigations (mainly further interviews).

MENTAL STATE EXAMINATION

You are now ready to complete the mental state examination. Unlike a physical examination, which can only be completed when the history has been fully taken, you will be noting aspects of the patient's behaviour and mental pathology whilst taking the history. However, the history must be recorded separately from the mental examination. Describe accurately what you observe in the patient's behaviour and record any abnormal delusions or hallucinations. The mental state examination is usually recorded under eight headings:

1 Appearance.
2 Motor activity.
3 Mood/affect.
4 Speech and language.
5 Thought content.
6 Perceptual disturbances.
7 Cognitive function.
8 Insight.

APPEARANCE
Record the general appearance of the patient, including apparent age, obvious physical stigmata and general physical health, overt emotional display, manner relating to the interviewer and level of co-operation. The patient's general state of cleanliness should be recorded together with signs of self-neglect or incontinence. Manic patients may show exaggerated dress and make-up. Take into account the patient's social and cultural background.

ACTIVITY LEVELS
Motor activity may be increased or decreased or, in exceptional circumstances, show catatonic change. If increased, note whether purposeless e.g. foot-tapping, scalp-rubbing or purposeful, e.g. vigilantly looking out of the window. Record repetitive tics or mannerisms. Decreased motor activity is usually part of a psychomotor retardation which includes diminished move-

ments, speech and thinking. Patients may sit or stand relatively immobile with lack of facial expression or eye movement. Psychological and motor responses to questioning and examination are diminished. In very severe depressive or schizophrenic states patients may be stuporous, appear quite unresponsive to their environment and passively or actively resist food or fluids. A rare manifestation of catatonic schizophrenia is automatic obedience characterized by catalepsy when patients will sustain an awkward posture for lengthy periods, or waxy flexibility (flexibilitas cerea) when the examiner can move the patient's limbs rather like a wax rod.

MOOD AND AFFECT
Mood may be described as a sustained subjective feeling state of happiness, sadness, worry, anxiety, irritability, anger or lack of emotions such as detachment and indifference. Observe facial expression. Note whether the range of mood is constricted or expanded (i.e. excessive joyfulness or sadness). Note also the intensity, stability, persistence and lability of mood, its appropriateness to the patient's thoughts or predicament and whether affect remains static during the interview. Record the presence of biological symptoms, such as appetite and weight-loss, sleep disturbance – particularly early morning wakening (repeated or persistent wakening after 2.00 a.m.) – and diurnal mood variation (mood disturbance worse in the morning and improving as the day continues). Assess here suicidal ideas or active plans taken to commit suicide, such as hoarding and purchasing tablets, or exploring high buildings, railway tracks or rivers that may be suitable for a suicidal attempt.

SPEECH AND LANGUAGE
Speech and language provide the examiner with an indirect view of the patient's thinking. Formal speech or language abnormality can reflect psychiatric disorder or brain pathology, or both. Speech fluency should be noted. Excessive slowness of response or mutism, or paucity of speech, may be present in patients with motor retardation. Dysarthria, expressive speech deficits including nominal dysphasia, repeated grammatical errors and word finding errors should all be recorded. Manic patients may show excessive speech, pressure of speech (continual speech which is difficult to interrupt) or flight of ideas (moving rapidly from one topic to another, but with clear and meaningful links between topics).

Schizophrenic patients may show other forms of excessive or deranged speech in which the patient seems unable to arrive at the intended goal or point of the discussion; (circumstantial or tangential speech). They may suddenly stop (blocking), and when resumed the speech is on a different topic (derailment) or wanders aimlessly between topics (loosening of association). Differentiating the speech abnormalities of patients with mania, schizophrenia and organic mental disorder can be extremely difficult and in this context other aspects of the mental state, particularly affect, thought content and cognitive function will be of significance.

THOUGHT CONTENT

The student should initially record the patient's overriding thought content when allowed to speak freely. This will often be found in the initial complaints recorded verbatim at the beginning of history taking, though not necessarily so. Thought content may show preoccupation with somatic complaints, anxiety, worries, gloominess, pessimism, euphoria or persecution.

There may be specific abnormalities of thought content:

Patients with *phobic symptoms* will have an unrealistic fear of specific objects, locations or situations which are avoided if at all possible. The patient will recognize these fears as irrational, but out of their control.

Obsessive compulsive phenomena affect thinking and/or motor function. Obsessional behaviour is characterized by unwanted impulses that intrude into the patient's thoughts. These ideas concern contamination or dirtiness, illness or incompleteness which can only be relieved by the patient repetitively checking or cleaning. This will result in ritualistic behaviour, such as repetitive cleaning of lavatories or kitchen surfaces, or checking that lights have been turned off or locks locked. Checking often occurs in multiples which are counted by the patient, i.e. the patient may wash his hands four times after going to the toilet. Ruminations consist of repetitive intrusive thoughts without motor activity. Obsessive compulsive phenomena and phobias may represent a primary obsessive compulsive or phobic neurosis, but may complicate other disorders, particularly depression.

Delusional ideas are defined as unshakeable false beliefs that are not in keeping with the patient's social, cultural or religious background. They may be secondary when they arise from other pathological processes, such as hallucinations, abnormal mood or organic mental disorder, or primary when they cannot be understood as arising from any pre-existing disorder. Primary delusions usually signify the presence of schizophrenia. Patients with primary delusions may also have experienced passivity phenomena. These include experiences of influence where patients believe that their thoughts, speech or actions are being controlled by some outside agency or that thoughts have been inserted into their minds. Conversely, they may feel that their thoughts are broad-

cast or they hear an echo of their own thought or that voices continually comment upon their actions. These phenomena are known as first rank symptoms and are usually, but not always, associated with schizophrenia.

Less severe forms of abnormal thinking can occur. Patients who have not yet experienced delusional ideas may experience delusional mood in which they are convinced that something in their environment is unusual with a sense of an impending, usually adverse, occurrence. The term 'overvalued idea' describes a delusion-like idea that is not necessarily bizarre and about which the patient has insight.

The content of delusions is variable: delusions of persecution are likely to be related to schizophrenic disorders, grandiose delusions are usually found in manic states while somatic or hypochondriacal delusions and delusions of guilt, unworthiness or wickedness are associated with severe depressive disorder.

PERCEPTUAL DISTURBANCES

Any sensory modality may be affected by minor or severe perceptual aberrations.

Illusions are perceptions of stimuli which are misinterpreted, i.e. shadows are mistaken for figures or noises thought to be voices.

Hallucinations are sensory experiences which occur without any external stimulation. Hallucinations can affect any sensory modality. Auditory hallucinations and visual hallucinations are the most common. Auditory hallucinations which involve more than one voice, and talk about the patient are known as third person auditory hallucinations and usually signify schizophrenic disorder. Visual hallucinations in older patients usually signify organic mental disease.

Hallucinations may also affect smell, taste and bodily sensation. Hallucinations may give rise to secondary delusions. Thus, a primary hallucination of unusual odour may result in a secondary delusion of being poisoned by some external agency. Tactile hallucinations may be secondary to drug-induced psychotic states (cocaine addicts describe the sensation of insects crawling over their bodies as the 'cocaine bug').

Pseudo-hallucinations are similar to hallucinations in which there is no clear external stimulus, but the patient retains insight into the fact they are imaginary (pseudo-hallucinations are typical of grief reactions in which the recently bereaved will see, hear the voice or feel the touch of the recently deceased, but realize they are imaginary).

Perceptions of the self may be disturbed; thus, body image is distorted in patients with anorexia or bulimia. Patients (and normal individuals) may experience depersonalization or derealization in which they either feel themselves to have changed or their environment to have changed around them. In extreme cases this may result in out of body experiences in which the person observes themselves as an outside observer (these phenomena are commonly described in those involved in severe road or other trauma, or in combat situations).

COGNITIVE FUNCTION

Disturbances of cognitive function may result from psychiatric disorder, neurological disorder or overwhelming physical illness resulting in delirium.

Cognitive function is best considered as a hierarchy. The most basic cognitive function is level of consciousness followed by attention and concentration, language function, memory abstraction, calculation and other higher mental activities. If a lower level of function is disturbed then all higher levels will be affected; a delirious patient with a fluctuating conscious level will have difficulty in naming common objects, but is not truly dysphasic.

Assess the patient's level of consciousness by their awareness of their immediate environment, whether

◀ Table 11.4

MINI-MENTAL STATE EXAMINATION		
Patient	Examiner	
	Date	

Maximum score	Score	Orientation
5	( )	What is the (year) (season) (date) (day) (month)?
5	( )	Where are we: (country) (county) (town) (hospital) (ward)?
3	( )	Name three objects: 1 second to say each. Then ask the patient all three after you have said them. Give 1 point for each correct answer. Then repeat them until he learns all three. Count trials and score. **Trials:**
		Attention and calculation
5	( )	Serial 7's. 1 point for each correct. Stop after five answers. Alternatively spell 'world' backwards.
		Recall
3	( )	Ask for the three objects repeated above. Give 1 point for each correct.
		Language and copying
9	( )	Name a pencil, and watch (2 points)
	( )	Repeat the following: 'No ifs, ands or buts' (1 point) Follow a 3-stage command: 'Pick up a paper with your right hand, fold it in half and put it on the floor.' (3 points) Read and obey the following:
	( )	Close your eyes (1 point)
	( )	Write a sentence (1 point)
	( )	Copy design (1 point)
		Total score: Maximum 30.
		Assess level of consciousness: **Alert Drowsy Stupor**
A score of < 23 suggests organic disorder		

drowsy or fully alert and whether the level of consciousness fluctuates during the interview. Attention and concentration may be tested by asking the patient to name the days of the week or months of the year backwards and memory by ability to remember recent events and past events. Recent memory is tested by asking the patient the day of the week, and the full current date together with the patient's awareness of their whereabouts (recording the patient's answer verbatim). A judgement can be made as to past memory by the consistency of the patient's account of their life with that given by independent informants or by checking the internal consistency of the personal history given by the patient.

If there are doubts regarding the patient's memory or cognitive function the mini-mental states examination may be administered (Table 11.4). Patients scoring 23 or above on this examination probably have normal cognitive function. Patients scoring less than 23 are likely to have organic mental impairment.

INSIGHT

Make a judgement as to whether the patient has insight into their illness, i.e. whether they feel that they are ill and are aware of the significance of their symptoms and of life events in the production of their illness. Does the patient feel they are in need of treatment, and how do they see the future with or without treatment?

PHYSICAL EXAMINATION AND INVESTIGATIONS

A full physical examination (as described elsewhere in this book) should invariably be performed on all patients presenting for the first time with psychiatric symptoms.

Routine investigations at the first visit should also include the following:
- Hb WBC ESR
- Urea and electrolytes
- Liver function test
- Thyroid function test
- Random blood sugar
- Serology for syphilis
- Chest radiograph
- MSSU

When organic brain disease is suspected, a CT brain scan and EEG may also be needed (Figure 11.2).

Acutely psychotic patients should have their urine screened for substance misuse.

Check your *aide-mémoire* for the mental state examination to be sure you have covered all the important

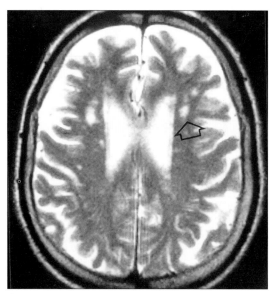

▲ **Figure 11.2 CT scan of multi-infarct dementia.** High signal infarcts (arrow) shown in periventricular white matter

points in mental state examination. You are now ready to proceed to the formulation of the patient's problems. The psychiatric interview is not finished until you have completed at least a basic formulation.

THE FORMULATION

Refer again to your *aide-mémoire* for the formulation. The formulation consists of a *summary* which will enable you to make a *differential diagnosis* that will lead to appropriate further *investigations*, *treatment* and *prognosis*. A specimen formulation is given in the following text. (It is a fairly detailed formulation of a relatively simple case.)

SUMMARY

The *summary* should include a brief résumé of important and relevant information from the psychiatric interview and the mental state examination.

Reason for referral
Mrs X is a 24-year-old housewife who presented at the A&E department following a panic attack, and was admitted to the ward informally as an inpatient.

Complaints and history
She complains of symptoms of anxiety and tearfulness for 6 months and has a 2-month history of anorexia

with weight loss of three-quarters of a stone. She has become increasingly fearful of leaving the house alone and in the last few weeks her marital and sexual relationships have deteriorated. She has been prescribed diazepam 5 mg bd by her GP, but has not taken this medication consistently.

Personal and family history
Previously a well-adjusted and outgoing person. She was born into a financially stable working-class family. Her mother died of carcinoma breast when the patient was 5 years old and her father subsequently remarried. She had a reasonable but distant relationship with her stepmother. Happily married since the age of 18, she has a healthy 4-year-old son and 2-year-old daughter. She has been worried by the financial and emotional effects of her husband's sudden and unexpected unemployment 9 months ago. There is no significant past medical or past psychiatric history.

Mental state examination
Initially calm and able to give a good account of herself she became increasingly anxious and distressed as the interview progressed, becoming tearful and expressing ideas that her life was futile and had fleeting ideas of ending her life. She had normal cognitive function with some insight into her predicament.

Physical examination and investigations
Physical examination and routine investigations are normal so far, but thyroid function test is still awaited.

DIFFERENTIAL DIAGNOSIS
The student should now enumerate the possible diagnoses that may be responsible for the patient's current condition. The most likely diagnosis is severe depression, but phobic neurosis, puerperal depression and thyroid dysfunction should be considered. (Use ICD 10 classification of psychiatric disorder – see Appendix 1.)

The most likely diagnosis in this patient is major depressive disorder. Phobic or other anxiety neurosis is unlikely as these symptoms have occurred in the clear setting of depressive illness and did not precede it. A puerperal depressive disorder is unlikely as the youngest child was over 1 year old when depressive symptoms first developed. Thyroid disorder has not yet been ruled out.

FURTHER INVESTIGATIONS
Further investigations include laboratory tests and other enquiries that are still required by medical staff and other members of the team, such as nursing staff, social workers or psychologists.

The nursing staff will observe the patient's self-care and social skills on the ward, her appetite, sleep and interaction with her husband and children. The team social worker will interview the patient's husband to check the factual details of the patient's history, examine the husband's attitude to the wife's illness and the quality of their marital relationship. A joint marital interview may be required.

TREATMENT
Treatment includes medication, as well as psychological and other treatment.

The patient described here requires inpatient care for a short period as she does pose a minor threat of suicide. She will benefit from general supportive nursing care, resocialization and attendance at an anxiety management group. She may prove to have unresolved grief for her mother, requiring therapy in its own right. Medical treatment for depression is strongly indicated here with a drug such as (give drug and dosage range).

PROGNOSIS
Prognosis includes not only short-term but also longer term prognosis together with factors which render the patient more vulnerable to further breakdown.

The prognosis here is extremely good in the short-term, but the husband's unemployment and presence of young children all increase the patient's vulnerability to relapse. The patient should remain under surveillance for two years after discharge with maintenance antidepressant medication during that time.

CONCLUSION

During your psychiatric student attachment you should aim to take a psychiatric history and perform an examination that will enable you to undertake a formulation as described above, using basic ICD 10 diagnostic categories (see Appendix 1). You will not be expected to have a full grasp of Freud or of neuropsychiatry.

During the first half of your attachment think about your doctor/patient relationship, take histories and perform mental state examinations referring, as required, to your *aide-mémoire*. Make yourself undertake a brief formulation of every patient however inadequate and embarrassing you feel your formulation to be.

During the second half of your attachment you will begin to feel more relaxed and to work more fluidly and flexibly with the schedules mentioned above. Your formulations will become briefer, more appropriate and accurate.

You will have acquired sufficient skills to pass your psychiatric clinical examination, but more importantly you will have acquired a set of skills that will set you in good stead whatever your future career path. You may even decide to become a psychiatrist.

APPENDIX 1:
ICD 10 CLASSIFICATION OF MENTAL AND BEHAVIOURAL DISORDERS

The International Classification of Disorders for Psychiatry (Mental and Behavioural Disorders) now has ten main categories. Seven of these refer primarily to disorders suffered by patients over the age of 16. One category refers to patients suffering from mental impairment and two categories refer specifically to mental and behavioural disorder in children. These categories are described below. (A full list of categories is included on pages 22–39 of the ICD 10 Classification of Mental and Behavioural Disorders World Health Organization.)

F00–F09: ORGANIC MENTAL DISORDERS
These include progressive organic disorders (the dementias) and acute confusional states (delirium). Delirium may be superimposed on an existing dementia. This category also includes the effects of static brain damage whether due to trauma or infection (encephalitis). Disorders of mood, schizophrenia and personality change due to organic brain disorder are also included here.

F10–F19: MENTAL AND BEHAVIOURAL DISORDERS DUE TO PSYCHOACTIVE SUBSTANCE USE
All disorders due to substance misuse or alcohol use are included here, including acute intoxication, dependency, withdrawal states and psychotic disorders or organic states induced by substance misuse.

F20–F29: SCHIZOPHRENIA AND DELUSIONAL DISORDERS
This includes all schizophrenic and delusional disorders which are not due to either organic disorder or substance misuse. Sub-types, such as paranoid, hebephrenic, catatonic and undifferentiated schizophrenia are included here as well as a description of the course of the illness; complete remission (acute), continuous, episodic or incomplete remission (chronic).

Patients with persistent delusions not reaching criteria for diagnosis of schizophrenia are included here, as well as patients with acute transient psychoses and schizo-affective disorder in which schizophrenic and mood disorders are both present.

F30–F39: MOOD (AFFECTIVE DISORDERS)
This includes manic disorder, bipolar affective disorder (in which manic and depressive episodes may be present either at the same time or, more commonly, alternate with each other). All depressive disorders are now included in this category. They include mild, moderate and severe depressive episodes and a category also for severe depressive episodes with psychotic symptoms. Mood disorders may also be described as recurrent or persistent.

F40–F48: NEUROTIC STRESS RELATED AND SOMATIFORM DISORDERS
This category includes phobic anxiety and other anxiety disorders, obsessive compulsive disorder, dissociative disorders (previously known as hysterical neurosis), somatiform disorders (previously known as hypochondriasis) and reactions to severe stress including post-traumatic stress disorder.

F50–F59: BEHAVIOURAL SYNDROME ASSOCIATED WITH PHYSIOLOGICAL DISTURBANCE AND PHYSICAL FACTORS
This includes eating disorders, such as anorexia and bulimia, sleep disorders, sexual dysfunction but not sexual deviation, and abuse of non-dependence producing substances such as laxatives, analgesics, steroids, etc.

F60–F69: DISORDERS OF ADULT PERSONALITY AND BEHAVIOUR
This includes personality disorders, including psychopathic disorder, habit disorders such as gambling, fire-setting and stealing, gender disorders such as transsexualism and transvestism (same sex preference, i.e. homosexuality/lesbianism is not a psychiatric disorder), sexual perversions and feigning of physical disorder (Munchausen syndrome and similar disorders).

F70–F79: MENTAL RETARDATION
Is classified in terms of severity of retardation and is dependent upon psychometric assessment.

F80–F89: DISORDERS OF PSYCHOLOGICAL DEVELOPMENT (IN CHILDREN)
This includes disorders of speech and language, disorders of development of scholastic skills and pervasive development disorders such as autism and hyperactivity with mental retardation.

F90–F99:
BEHAVIOURAL AND EMOTIONAL DISORDERS IN CHILDHOOD AND ADOLESCENCE

This includes hyperkinetic syndrome without subnormality, conduct disorder, emotional disorders, disorders of social functioning, tic disorder including De La Tourette's syndrome and other disorders including enuresis, feeding disorder and stuttering.

Patients may suffer from more than one category of mental or behavioural disorder; thus, a patient with a personality disorder may develop severe alcoholism and suffer a severe head injury resulting in organic impairment.

The endocrine system

INTRODUCTION

The endocrine system comprises various tissues secreting hormones which are conveyed by the circulation to distant organs. In general, the time scale over which hormones act is longer than that for the nervous system, the other major controller of body function. However, the ability to measure the minute concentrations of hormones using only small blood samples has caused a revision of certain older ideas, such as the relative constancy of hormone secretion. Indeed, many hormones are characterized by the notably pulsatile nature of their secretion. It is, nevertheless, true to say that hormones can have both rapid metabolic effects, as exemplified by adrenaline, and long-term effects on processes such as growth and sexual development. Many hormones exert multiple actions, spanning both rapid and prolonged activities, for example, insulin.

Although individual endocrine glands have certain specific functions, they also operate through their relationship with others. This applies particularly to the pituitary, which exercises control over other glands through its trophic hormones. The pituitary is, in turn, influenced by the secretions from these other members of the system, which provide 'feedback' regulatory signals that are of primary importance in maintaining homeostasis.

Whereas most hormones are secreted from condensed collections of cells termed endocrine glands, the large number of gut hormones are usually secreted from cells scattered over great lengths of the gastrointestinal tract; nevertheless, excess gut hormone hypersecretion is usually caused by localized, albeit sometimes multiple, endocrine tumours. In consequence of the small size of endocrine glands (and usually also their tumours) as well as the potency of their secretions, an endocrine disorder shows itself more often in the functional and morphological changes wrought by the abnormal state of hormone output rather than in local signs arising from the affected organ itself.

Hormonal dysfunction may also be secondary to disease in organs other than the endocrine glands. Examples include hyperaldosteronism secondary to cardiac failure, hyperparathyroidism in renal failure and the 'ectopic' production of hormones from several tumours, notably adrenocorticotrophic) hormone (ACTH) and vasopressin from small cell carcinomas of the lung.

The diagnostic approach to endocrine disorders can be considered in two stages. The first is an evaluation of hormonal status, which is essentially a physiological assessment, and the second is an effort to define precisely the nature of any underlying pathological process. Both approaches involve clinical skills of history and examination, backed up by an array of investigations involving hormone measurements in blood, urine (less frequently nowadays) and occasionally saliva, as well as various radiological, ultrasound and radio-isotopic imaging techniques. The complexity of these investigations lies outside the scope of this chapter but certain principles will be mentioned and it should be recognized that with their aid, documentation of endocrine status and pathology can often be made with a precision unrivalled in many other areas of modern medical practice.

LOCAL STRUCTURAL EFFECTS

It must again be stressed that an endocrine disorder can exist without any detectable clinical abnormality in the vicinity of the diseased gland.

The *thyroid* is the most accessible gland but is not usually visible or palpable. Any enlargement of the thyroid is termed a goitre without any implication of cause (Figure 12.1). To inspect the thyroid, it is best to give the patient water to sip as normally the thyroid is freely mobile but invested in fascia attached to the larynx which moves up on swallowing. Swallowing may disclose unsuspected enlargement of the thyroid, especially if a significant portion is retrosternal. Retrosternal goitre

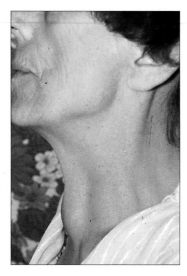

◀ **Figure 12.1**
Goitre

may impede venous return from the head which is more obvious when both arms are raised.

Palpation of the thyroid is performed by standing behind the patient, gently encircling the neck from each side with the hands and localizing the cricoid cartilage below the thyroid cartilage. The middle fingers are then largely used to palpate, starting medially below the cricoid cartilage where the isthmus generally crosses the trachea and up at the sides for the thyroid lobes. Texture and symmetry are noted and the patient is asked to swallow in order to assess size and mobility. The thyroid is usually asymmetrical with the right lobe slightly larger and this pattern often persists with diffuse enlargement of the gland. Localized lumps or nodules should be individually defined. When attempting this, it is helpful to place one hand on the top of the patient's head to 'steer' it downwards, forwards and rotated away from the side being palpated in order to relax the sternomastoid on that side. This provides visual access to localized lesions. Palpation continues with checking for tracheal deviation or local lymphadenopathy.

Thyroid cysts occasionally transilluminate. The vascularity of the thyroid is increased in thyrotoxicosis and may cause a palpable thrill or audible bruit. The latter is heard when the patient stops breathing (Figure 12.2). It is localized, sometimes loud and may be predominantly systolic or continue throughout the cardiac cycle. A thyroid bruit should not be confused with carotid bruits, conducted aortic murmurs or venous hums; these last are easily abolished by momentary light occlusion of jugular venous return. Goitres may compress the trachea to cause dyspnoea and stridor while invasive carcinomas may also result in dysphagia, change of voice and pain, which can radiate to the ear.

The *testes* are also readily amenable to clinical examination. It is often helpful to estimate the size of each testis. This is most accurately done using Prader's orchidometer, when each testis is matched most closely with one of a series of calibrated ellipsoids (Figure 12.3). These were originally devised for assessing testicular development through puberty, but it is also useful to quantitate testicular shrinkage, which commonly occurs with damage to seminiferous tubules, as these constitute 95 per cent of testicular volume. Any abnormality of testicular position, consistency and associated structures such as epididymis and vas deferens, or of venous drainage causing varicocele, should be recorded. *Ovaries* are far less accessible but cystic or generalized enlargement may be detectable per vaginam on bimanual examination.

The *pituitary gland* is normally seated within the aptly named sella turcica (Turkish saddle) or pituitary fossa, on the superior surface of the sphenoid. These close confines, together with effects on important neighbouring structures, are responsible for the local symptoms and signs of expanding pituitary lesions. These include headache, usually attributed to pressure on the diaphragma sellae, and the important consequences of impingement on the optic chiasma. Chiasmal compression from below will initially affect the lowermost decussating fibres causing upper, outer field defects. With increasing involvement, the field loss progresses to cause the classical bitemporal hemianopia. It is important to recognize that the optic chiasma occupies variable positions in different individuals and that tumour growth is more often than not asymmetrical, so that variation from the classical patterns of field loss is common. In keeping with the general principle of physical examination that subtle abnormalities are best elicited by using the minimal effective stimulus, it is often helpful to use a red hat pin (having established whether the patient has normal colour vision) to examine the peripheral visual fields. The pin should be slowly brought in from the periphery along each diagonal in a plane midway between the patient and the observer, while asking the patient to cover one eye and fix on the eye of the tester.

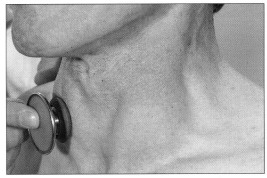

▲ **Figure 12.2 Auscultation of the thyroid**

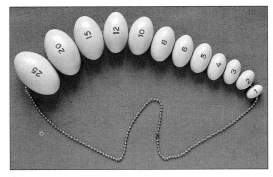

▲ **Figure 12.3 Prader's orchidometer**

The patient is asked to state immediately the pin is recognizably red. If there appears to be a hemianopia, its border can be mapped by bringing the pin horizontally across the visual field, starting out in the blind area and gradually working down the whole field. In this way, more reproducible information can be obtained than with crude finger wagging – since the retina is especially attuned to detecting movement that would still be recognized when colour vision is impaired.

Although pituitary tumours may raise intracranial pressure if they extend significantly above the sella turcica, it is exceptional for them to cause papilloedema. Instead, long-standing chiasmal compression causes optic atrophy, recognized by pallor of the discs on examining the fundi with an ophthalmoscope. Such changes may be associated with diminished visual acuity but, even in cases where surgery has successfully restored acuity and fields, the pallor tends to persist.

Despite lack of bony lateral walls to the pituitary fossa, invasion of the cavernous sinuses on either side is fortunately very rare but, when it occurs, may cause diplopia and ophthalmoplegia, especially through involvement of the oculomotor or third cranial nerve. Downward invasion is more frequent; the tumour may enter and fill the sphenoid air sinus and even very rarely erode into the nose, causing leakage of cerebrospinal fluid or rhinorrhoea.

GENERAL FUNCTIONAL EFFECTS

Because of the close integration between different parts of the system, the functional or metabolic features of endocrine disorder cannot always be attributed to disease of one particular gland. With experience, the major site of disturbance can readily be identified, however, and a detailed analysis of the contribution of different hormones to various metabolic processes is not warranted. This section will be confined to consideration of abnormalities of growth and development and those areas of metabolic disorder which can lead to critical illness and where the contribution of the endocrine system may not always be immediately obvious.

Abnormalities of Growth

Disorders of endocrine function can have profound effects on body form, size, proportion and development. These are most clearly seen in children and adolescents, but are by no means confined to the young. Assessment of growth can be made by height measurements and comparison with expected findings given by standard charts, with appropriate allowances for parental height

(see Chapter 14). Marked differences from the normal age-related distribution may be associated with discrepancies between the chronological age and skeletal development as assessed radiologically by the 'bone age', in which relevant areas, especially the hand and wrist, are examined for epiphyseal fusion, which tends to follow a characteristic age-related pattern. Various endocrine conditions can delay or even halt growth. These aspects of Turner's syndrome and hypothyroidism are dealt with in Chapter 14.

Growth hormone deficiency is often apparent within the first year of life but is frequently missed to the detriment of the child, as the potential for 'catch-up' growth diminishes with increasing delay in treatment. Affected children are very short and chubby due to excessive subcutaneous fat, and boys may have a micro-penis. Corticosteroid excess can also decelerate growth and induce obesity, in contrast to the simply obese child who normally has accelerated skeletal growth. Poorly controlled diabetes mellitus may retard growth.

Growth acceleration in childhood may result from hyperthyroidism or any cause of excessive sex steroid secretion, including the various causes of true precocious puberty. The latter group will have stunted ultimate height since premature epiphyseal fusion follows the early accelerated growth. On the other hand, the delay of puberty may prolong skeletal growth, especially of the long bones. This feature of hypogonadism leads to eunuchoid proportions in which the long limbs cause the span to exceed the total height by 5 cm or more – since the additional lengths of both arms are added (measurement in series) but not in the legs (measurement in parallel). Interestingly, this skeletal pattern is frequently seen during childhood in Klinefelter's syndrome – a condition of supernumerary X chromosomes, associated with gonadal failure (Figure 12.4). The early skeletal changes are probably genetic rather than endocrine in origin.

Water and Electrolyte Metabolism

It is essential to recognize the factors responsible for the separate regulation of body water and salts which in health are closely controlled. Disproportionate loss of water can occur in various ways, including impairment of vasopressin (antidiuretic hormone, ADH) secretion (cranial diabetes insipidus) or action (nephrogenic diabetes insipidus). It can also follow excessive osmotic load, as in uncontrolled diabetes mellitus. Excessive water retention is seen with inappropriate ADH secretion, which may result from a variety of intracranial or intrathoracic diseases and leads to stimulation of pathways activating hypothalamic release of ADH from the posterior pituitary gland. Some tumours, especially of

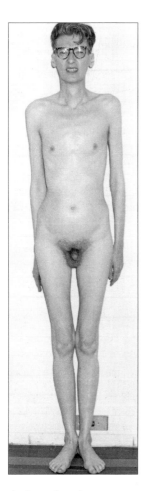

◀ **Figure 12.4 Klinefelter's syndrome in a man aged 50.** Note the youthful appearance, small genitalia, feminine hair escutcheon and pelvic contour and the long, thin limbs

the bronchus, have a propensity to secrete ADH: so-called ectopic hormone production.

Sodium retention is largely controlled by aldosterone. With increased aldosterone secretion there is normally concomitant potassium loss. It should also be recognized that hydrocortisone (cortisol) has some mineralocorticoid activity which may be significant in states of marked cortisol hypersecretion or Cushing's syndrome. Adrenal insufficiency can lead to excessive sodium loss with ensuing dehydration and postural hypotension manifesting as dizziness or syncope on standing. As mentioned above, salt and water metabolism and the hormones involved in their regulation may be disturbed by a variety of cardiac, renal, gut and hepatic disorders as well as drugs.

ENDOCRINE ASSESSMENT

Questions of endocrine dysfunction generally revolve about hyper- or hypo-function of specific glands with

the consequent clinical sequelae. In many more advanced cases spot diagnoses are possible owing to pathognomonic facies, but the attachment of a label is not enough. Thus in the conditions which readily fall into this situation, such as hypothyroidism, hyperthyroidism, acromegaly, Cushing's syndrome, to name but a few, it is essential to document in as quantitative fashion as possible the degree of local and systemic involvement, before embarking on the sometimes difficult further task of precise aetiological diagnosis.

ILLUSTRATIVE DISEASES

The illustrative diseases include those of the:
1 Thyroid.
2 Pituitary.
3 Adrenal cortex.
4 Adrenal medulla.
5 Gonads.
6 Parathyroids.
7 Pancreatic islets.

THYROID DISEASE

FUNCTIONAL DIAGNOSIS
The clinical assessment begins with assigning patients into one of these categories: hyper-, eu- and hypo-thyroid. It should be noted that most thyroid diseases are more common in women than men.

Hyperthyroidism
The clinical features of marked thyroid overactivity are termed thyrotoxicosis. Milder degrees of hyperthyroidism do not have all the 'toxic' aspects and may only be confirmed after biochemical investigation, instigated on the basis of one or two suspicious signs. Important features in the history include heat intolerance and excessive sweating; increased irritability and emotional lability; palpitations, dyspnoea, tremor and weakness; weight loss despite a good or enhanced appetite; increased frequency of bowel action; menstrual disturbance of any type, frequently with scanty periods; excessive thirst. The general appearance is often pathognomonic, with the patient frequently unable to sit still, pouring the history out and looking anxious or startled. Even on a cold day the patient may wear only light clothing. The hands may display a fine tremor which is best appreciated by placing a piece of paper on the outstretched hands (see Figure 10.43, page 240) and have a characteristically 'velvety' feel due to their hyperaemia

and perspiration. There is usually a tachycardia which persists during sleep, and a full volume to the pulse which is detectable through the palm while clasping the flexor aspect of the forearm. Atrial fibrillation is common especially in the older patient.

Hyperthyroidism due to any cause may cause two eye signs arising from the sympathetic component of the innervation of levator palpebris superioris: lid retraction and lid lag. In lid retraction, a rim of white sclera is seen above the iris when the patient is at rest and looks ahead. To elicit lid lag (von Graefe's sign), the observer moves his finger slowly downwards from above the seated patient, who is asked to watch the finger all the way without moving the head (which is best held steady by the observer's other hand); the upper eyelid is then seen to lag behind the eyeball (Figure 12.5). Weakness of proximal muscles is common in hyperthyroidism, often only mild, but detectable on asking the patient to rise from a squatting position, holding the back vertical and using only quadriceps to elevate the trunk.

Hyperthyroidism may be much more difficult to detect in the elderly in whom the disease may have a particular impact on the cardiovascular system. Osteoporosis may also occur with vertebral collapse. In some elderly patients, an apathetic form of the disease is seen with anorexia, marked weight loss, atrial fibrillation, cardiac failure, ptosis and deeply hollowed temporal fossae (Figure 12.6). On the other hand, some young thyrotoxics develop such ravenous appetites that, despite their increased metabolic rate, they actually gain weight. Rare complications include thyroid crisis, in which hyperpyrexia, psychosis and cardiac decompensation occur. Some oriental races are liable to develop hypokalaemic paralysis when thyrotoxic.

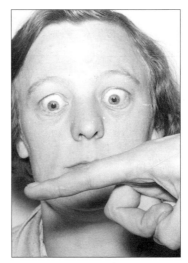

◀ **Figure 12.5 Von Graefe's sign, lid lag.** Although the lower margin of the iris is level with the lower eyelid, the upper eyelid has not moved downwards. The finger has been moved slowly from the level of the hair to its present position

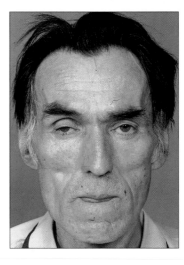

◀ **Figure 12.6 Ptosis with hollowed cheeks and temporal fossae: 'apathetic' hyperthyroidism**

Hypothyroidism

This characteristically creeps on insidiously. It is more commonly met with in the elderly (congenital hypothyroidism is dealt with in Chapter 14). In the older patient, the neurological system may be most profoundly affected with non-specific features of lethargy, loss of concentration and memory. Cold intolerance is a frequent complaint, as are paraesthesiae especially in the distribution of the median nerve in the hand due to carpal tunnel compression. Deafness and unsteadiness may occur, as well as aches and pains in muscles and joints. Cardiovascular symptoms are also common, including angina and intermittent claudication, both of which may improve strikingly on cautious replacement therapy, suggesting a biochemical as well as structural cause of tissue anoxia. Weight gain is frequently attributed to hypothyroidism but is rarely massive. Constipation is common.

Hypothyroidism is a good example of a disease in which 'the wood may be missed for the trees' as the overall first impression is often more telling than the individual items (Figure 12.7). There is a general slowness and sluggish response to questions. The voice may be husky with a changed timbre rather than deep, and this feature may have been commented on by people telephoning the patient. The skin is dry and cold and the face puffy with periorbital oedema – often with great bags under the eyes (Figure 12.8). By contrast, the loss of outer eyebrows is far less useful a sign than the myth retold in countless textbooks would suggest. Non-pitting myxoedema is only seen in advanced cases. The pulse is characteristically slow. Examination of the tendon jerks is especially useful, as they almost invariably have a slow relaxation phase or, as they have been

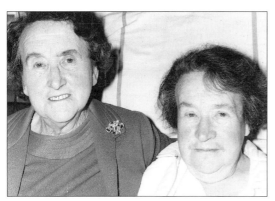

▲ **Figure 12.7 Hypothyroidism in identical twins, one (left) treated and the other (right) untreated**

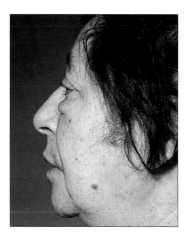

◀ **Figure 12.8 Hypothyroidism: infra-orbital myxoedema**

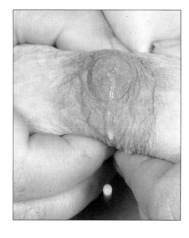

◀ **Figure 12.9 Galactorrhoea in hypothyroidism**

vividly described, are 'hung-up'. In the clinic, this sign is best elicited in the ankle reflex with the patient kneeling on a chair. Some grossly hypothyroid patients have cerebellar dysfunction especially affecting the trunk and causing difficulty with balance. Occasional patients have serous fluid accumulations, especially in the pericardium, but rarely ascites and hydrocele. Hypothyroidism can be difficult to diagnose in young women who may present with menorrhagia, infertility or recurrent abortion. Galactorrhoea occasionally also occurs as a presenting feature (Figure 12.9). The elderly are prone to hypothermia, intestinal obstruction from paralytic ileus and occasionally psychosis (myxoedema madness).

AETIOLOGICAL DIAGNOSIS

Most thyroid disease has an autoimmune basis and this should be suspected especially when another autoimmune disease such as pernicious anaemia is present. Vitiligo (see Figure 3.18) is also not uncommon in patients with autoimmune thyroid disease.

Hyperthyroidism

Autoimmunity causing thyrotoxicosis is called Graves's disease. In such patients extrathyroid manifestations are commonly found, especially in the eyes. The best known sign is exophthalmos (or proptosis) where the increase in orbital contents pushes the eyeball forwards. This can be observed by looking from above the patient while gently sweeping the brows and soft tissues backwards and observing whether the cornea can be seen (Nfziger's sign). This can be quantitated using Hertel's exophthalmometer but this requires skill for safe use and reproducible measurement.

Even more common is the complaint of grittiness in the eyes. It is important to see whether the eyelids fail to close completely at rest (lagophthalmos) as this puts the

cornea at risk of ulceration by abrasion during sleep. The eyes are often asymmetrically involved and indeed this may be the sole abnormality in some patients who are clinically euthyroid (dysthyroid eye disease). The ocular muscles may become infiltrated, thickened and weakened, leading to diplopia and ocular pareses, especially failure of upward gaze – which again may be obvious only unilaterally.

The ocular manifestations include conjunctival oedema (chemosis) and an oedematous angry inflammation – so-called malignant exophthalmos: a rather poorly defined term (Figure 12.10). Rarely, optic nerve compression leads to impairment of sight. It must be recognized that the state of the eyes in Graves' disease is independent of thyroid status and may suddenly worsen when the patient is euthyroid or even hypothyroid. Other extrathyroidal signs are less common but include pre-tibial myxoedema, where a plaque-like infiltration of the skin over the shin and sometimes encircling the calf or extending on to the foot, occurs. This has a characteristic sudden beginning or edge, easily felt on running the thumbnail along the skin. It is usually red, coarsely pitted and often bears black thick hairs and is cosmetically disfiguring. In some patients the fingers have an appearance very similar to clubbing – thyroid acropachy – in which a lace-like periosteal appearance may be seen on a radiograph. Splenomegaly and fat deposition over the angles of the jaws are occasionally found.

In Graves' disease the thyroid varies from the impalpable (especially in the elderly) to the diffusely large and vascular in which a bruit is of especial significance. Other forms of hyperthyroidism occur as toxic multinodular goitre in which the extrathyroid signs of Graves' disease are absent and the disease is usually milder; the goitre may be vast with great retrosternal extension and tracheal compression. A solitary nodule may become autonomously overactive and if this reaches hyperthyroid levels, will suppress the remaining normal gland (Plummer's disease).

Hypothyroidism

With most causes of primary thyroid failure the thyroid becomes a shrunken fibrous ghost, which is impalpable. In some cases, the thyroid enlarges due to autoimmune thyroiditis – Hashimoto's disease. This is partly a response to the rise in thyroid stimulating hormone secretion evoked as thyroid reserve fails; the gland is characteristically diffusely enlarged and very firm. Thyroid hormone replacement generally leads to shrinkage of the gland. Ablative therapy of thyrotoxicosis – whether by surgery or radio-iodine – is an increasingly common cause of hypothyroidism. Late treatment of cretinism will be detected by the neuro-logical sequelae, especially a low IQ and short stature. Secondary hypothyroidism due to deficiency of thyroid stimulating hormone usually has other features of pituitary failure.

PITUITARY DISEASE

Normal pituitary function is regulated by the overlying hypothalamus. Control of the anterior pituitary gland is mediated humorally by factors liberated from the median eminence into the hypothalamo–hypophyseal portal blood supply. The posterior pituitary gland is an evagination of the brain; its hormones are synthesized in the magnocellular neurons of the hypothalamus and travel down their axons to be liberated into the venous drainage of the posterior lobe of the pituitary.

FUNCTIONAL DIAGNOSIS
Hypopituitarism

Total loss of pituitary function is rare. Lesser degrees often develop along a characteristic path of anterior pituitary deficiency. Gonadotrophin deficiency develops early, manifesting in women as an ovulatory infertility, amenorrhoea, loss of libido, superficial dyspareunia due to vaginal dryness and, in the long term, osteoporosis: all due to secondary ovarian failure. Men become impotent, lose libido and fertility; the androgen loss is accompanied by poor muscular development. Hypogonadism in both sexes is associated with loss of secondary sexual hair. Men's beards may become softer and require less frequent shaving. These changes vary markedly in degree in patients with hypopituitarism (Figure 12.11).

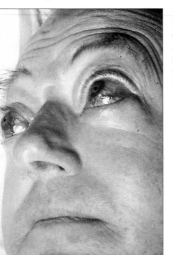

◀ **Figure 12.10 Exophthalmos with chemosis and congestion of conjunctival vessels.** A case of hyperthyroidism

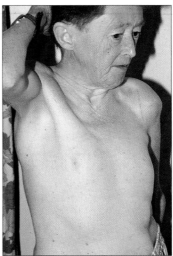

◀ **Figure 12.11 Man with hypopituitarism demonstrating loss of hair in axilla and beard**

Gonadotrophin deficiency in childhood is undetectable except for failure of phallic growth but later may appear as delayed puberty in either sex and eunuchoidal proportions due to delayed epiphyseal fusion (see above). Hypogonadism of any cause leads to finely wrinkled skin, especially on the face, with lines spreading up from the upper lip.

Deficiency of growth hormone makes for extra thinning of the skin, which also may be markedly pale (see below). Growth hormone loss tends to occur early but is unimportant clinically in adults, other than an increased liability to hypoglycaemia. This feature is more marked in growth hormone deficient children, where, however, the overwhelming impact is on growth (see above and Chapter 14).

ACTH and thyroid-stimulating hormone (TSH) secretion are generally preserved until much later. ACTH deficiency has two distinct effects. The first is due to loss of the skin pigmentation, which results from its extra-adrenal action (it is now known that separate melanocyte-stimulating hormones are not secreted in man); skin pallor is therefore disproportionate to mucous membrane pallor since the degree of anaemia that may accompany hypopituitarism is usually quite modest. The second effect of loss of ACTH is glucocorticoid deficiency, with general asthenia, hypotension and impaired response to stresses such as fever or trauma. Nausea and vomiting may occur but salt loss is mild, though water overload may be severe. TSH deficiency leads to all the changes of hypothyroidism but is frequently milder than that due to primary thyroid failure. Prolactin deficiency is very rare and its sole unequivocal effect is to render lactation impossible.

Of the two posterior pituitary hormones, only loss of vasopressin or antidiuretic hormone (ADH) is clinically important. This leads to diabetes insipidus with failure to concentrate the urine and liability to marked dehydration. It should be noted that the concomitant presence of adrenocortical insufficiency may mask the ADH deficiency, which only appears on glucocorticoid replacement therapy. The polyuria of absolute ADH deficiency is more marked than virtually any other polyuric state, but minor degrees are less easily recognized.

Hyperpituitarism

Prolactin is the pituitary hormone most frequently secreted in excessive amounts. It causes hypogonadism in both sexes. In women this may range from primary amenorrhoea to anovulatory infertility. In men it causes striking loss of sexual function due to diminished libido and sexual impotence – often to a much greater degree than the associated hypogonadism. Inappropriate lactation or galactorrhoea occurs in up to half hyperprolactinaemic women if sought for diligently (Figure 12.9). A small amount of galactorrhoea may be found in hyperprolactinaemic men, in whom there is frequently little or no palpable enlargement of breast tissue.

Growth hormone hypersecretion in adult life (following epiphyseal closure) causes acromegaly. Here there are changes in bones, viscera and soft tissues leading to pathognomonic features (Figure 12.12). The skull vault thickens with marked supraorbital and occipital bossing. The mandible enlarges, causing the lower teeth to jut in front of the upper, with an increase in interdental spacing (Figure 12.13). The bony changes affect also the hands, vertebrae and ribs. The hands and feet enlarge, due especially to soft tissue growth with consequent increase in ring and shoe sizes, often dating back several decades by the time the diagnosis is finally made – a testament to the slow and gradual changes that can sometimes be recognized by a series of dated photographs. The skin becomes increasingly sweaty and greasy, with occasional pigmentation, small skin tags or even papillomata. The enlarged nose, coarse features and thick lined skin gives a readily recognized facies (Figure 12.14). The thickened soft tissues in the upper airways may cause snoring and enlargement of the tongue and larynx with

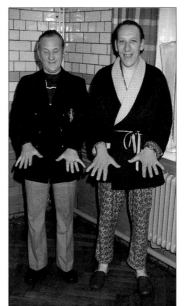

◀ **Figure 12.12**
Identical twins:
one with
acromegaly

deepening of the voice. About a quarter of acromegalics have nodular enlarged thyroid glands, and a similar proportion are hypertensive; a few are diabetic and many develop the carpal tunnel syndrome. Long-standing acromegaly causes severe osteoarthrosis. The rare occurrence of growth hormone secretion earlier in life leads to pituitary gigantism.

ACTH hypersecretion leads to Cushing's disease – the features of which are described below under 'Adrenals'. Primary overproduction of TSH and gonadotrophins, whilst being recognized more frequently nowadays, are still very unusual.

The overproduction of ADH is described above, and may cause severe or even lethal cerebral complications, including coma and fits, due to water retention.

Aetiological Diagnosis

Hypopituitarism most frequently results from a pituitary tumour. This may cause headaches or visual field defects and can be confirmed by appropriate radiological inves

tigation. Hypersecreting tumours, however, are often small and present a purely endocrine picture. They are characterized by their hormone products, and terms such as chromophobe, eosinophil and basophil adenoma are obsolete. Large hypersecreting tumours may have any of the space-occupying features of large non-functioning tumours, including the suppression of other pituitary functions.

Hyperprolactinaemia can result not only from prolactin secreting tumours but also from impairment of the hypothalamic influence, which in this case is inhibitory. Posterior pituitary failure – diabetes insipidus – is almost invariably the consequence of hypothalamic disease or at least high stalk section by tumour or trauma. The formerly common state of post partum pituitary necrosis, usually associated with a hypotensive episode caused by haemorrhage (Sheehan's syndrome), has been virtually abolished by improved obstetric practice. It is one of the few causes of hypoprolactinaemia.

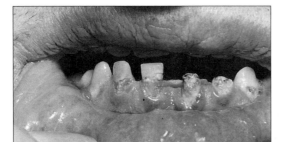

▲ Figure 12.13 Acromegaly: separation of the teeth

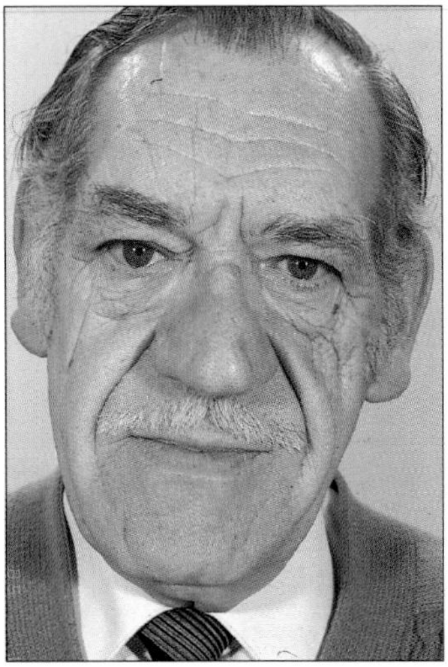

◀ Figure 12.14 Acromegaly: note enlarged nose and ears and prominent lower jaw

ADRENAL CORTICAL DISEASES

The groups of hormones produced by the adrenal cortex are the glucocorticoids, mineralocorticoids and androgens. Destructive processes of the glands may lead to diminished production of all hormones. Congenital enzyme deficiencies can lead to mixed pictures of hormone deficiency and excess, while hormone hypersecretion may involve one or more groups.

Functional Diagnosis
Hypoadrenalism
The majority of causes of primary adrenal insufficiency, or Addison's disease, act over a long time scale but often the diagnosis is not made until very late. The progress can be viewed in successive stages. The initial phase is one of progressive lethargy, anorexia and nausea, particularly in the morning, weight loss and symptoms of postural hypotension – dizziness on standing. Women may become amenorrhoeic and lose pubic hair. Later, there may be vomiting, diarrhoea or abdominal pain. The final stage is adrenal crisis which is often precipitated by an inadequate response to the stress of an intercurrent illness, especially gastroenteritis. The crisis is characterized by circulatory collapse, severe vomiting and pre-renal uraemia. Throughout the illness the falling cortisol levels lead to increasing levels of ACTH secretion which is responsible for the characteristic pigmentation especially on exposed areas, surfaces subject to friction,

recent scars, palmar creases and knuckles (Figure 12.15) and gingival and buccal mucosae (Figure 12.16). Very rarely septicaemia causes acute adrenal failure (Waterhouse–Friderichsen syndrome).

Hyperadrenalism
Cushing's syndrome
This is the result of excess of cortisol (hydrocortisone) or synthetic glucocorticoids. The commonly stressed features of truncal obesity with relatively thin legs, mooning and reddening of the face, hirsutes (most cases are women), 'buffalo hump', mild diabetes and hypertension are not always present. More useful are signs suggestive of protein wasting, clinically apparent in three main tissues: skin, muscle and bone. The skin becomes thin and fragile, bruises spontaneously (Figure 12.17) and the weakened collagen tears in stretched areas giving livid, thin, purple striae (Figure 12.18) which are readily distinguishable from those seen following childbearing, or in some adolescents who gain weight rapidly. Proximal muscle weakness is the rule and wasting commonplace (Figure 12.19). This is best shown by asking the patient to rise from squatting. Osteoporosis may cause vertebral collapse with the appearance of horizontal creases and loss of height as well as neurological sequelae. Cortisol excess may lead

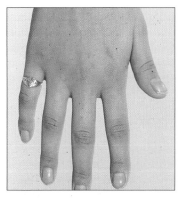

◀ **Figure 12.15 Addison's disease:** pigmentation of the knuckles

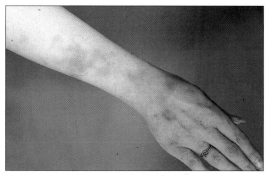

▲ **Figure 12.17 Cushing's syndrome:** spontaneous bruising

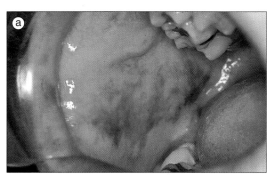

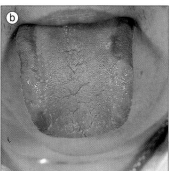

◀ **Figure 12.16 Addison's disease:** buccal pigmentation. (a) Cheek. (b) Tongue

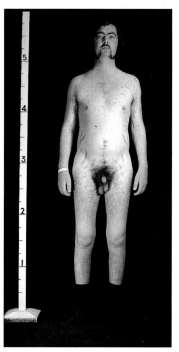

◀ **Figure 12.18 Cushing's syndrome:** purple striae

to aseptic necrosis of the femoral neck. When a patient with Cushing's syndrome has been treated surgically with bilateral adrenalectomy, wide spread pigmentation results from excessive production of pituitary ACTH (Nelson's syndrome) (Figure 12.20).

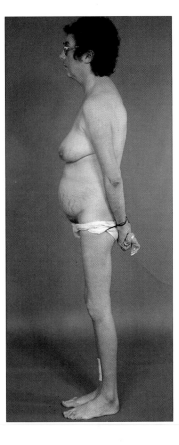

◀ **Figure 12.19 Cushing's syndrome:** wasting especially of thighs; note also the abdominal striae

Virilization

This may result from adrenal or ovarian androgen hypersecretion. The clinical features include hirsutes (hair growth on face and body of women in excess of racial norms), acne, greasiness of the skin, clitoral enlargement, enhanced muscularity, loss of the female pattern of fat deposition, temporal recession of head hair and deepening of the voice.

Conn's syndrome

Primary hyperaldosteronism may have no signs other than hypertension. Oedema does not occur. Muscle weakness and tetany may be present.

AETIOLOGICAL DIAGNOSIS

The commonest cause of Addison's disease is autoimmune adrenalitis and this may be associated with vitiligo and other autoimmune disorders. Tuberculosis is today a relatively less frequent cause.

Cushing's syndrome is most commonly due to pituitary ACTH excess (Cushing's disease). This may rarely cause sufficient ACTH to pigment the skin (Figure 12.21). Of the numerous tumours capable of ectopic ACTH secretion, bronchial small cell carcinomas are the commonest. The ACTH excess may be so high that a distinct syndrome arises of pigmentation, severe wasting, weakness and oedema due to hypokalaemic alkalosis from the massive hypercortisolaemia and diabetes but without the classical stigmata of long-standing Cushing's syndrome. Adrenal tumours hypersecreting cortisol autonomously may be benign adenomas, usually small, or carcinomas, often large and even palpable. The differential diagnosis of the underlying cause of Cushing's syndrome is a difficult and specialized matter relying heavily on biochemical and imaging techniques.

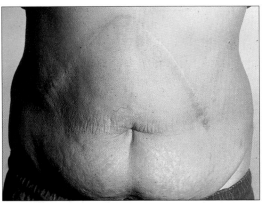

▲ **Figure 12.20 Pigmentation in Nelson's syndrome following bilateral adrenalectomy**

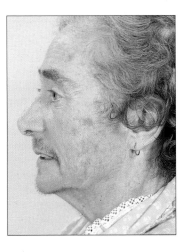

◀ **Figure 12.21 Cushing's syndrome:** hirsutes and pigmentation

ADRENAL MEDULLA

Loss of adrenal medullary tissue is without significant clinical consequences. Hypersecretion of adrenal catecholamines occurs from phaeochromocytomas, tumours which are most often intra-adrenal, single and benign. They cause symptoms of sweating, trembling and fear associated with pallor and episodic hypertension, sometimes followed by hypotension especially on standing and with intervening normal or raised blood pressure. Hypertensive crises are usually spontaneous but can follow local pressure, hence abdominal palpation should be especially gentle when phaeochromocytoma is suspected. This tumour may occur together with medullary cell carcinoma of the thyroid.

GONADAL DEFECTS

Hypogonadism has been described under the heading of hypopituitarism. There are many types of primary hypogonadism in men, ranging from Klinefelter's syndrome (see Figure 12.4) to myotonic dystrophy, but in most cases the cause remains unknown and simple testicular atrophy will be found. A history of cryptorchidism, testicular torsion or mumps in postpubertal life may be significant. Hypogonadism may be the consequence of diseases such as hepatic cirrhosis and haemachromatosis ('bronzed diabetes'). It may frequently be associated with features of feminization such as gynaecomastia (true, palpable, sometimes tender breast tissue – to be distinguished from excess fat) and a female fat pattern (Figure 12.22). This is common in Klinefelter's syndrome, cirrhosis and spironolactone therapy. In women there are less frequently diagnostic stigmata of ovarian failure. A notable exception is Turner's syndrome, with amenorrhoea, short stature, widely spaced nipples, puffy hands and feet, often present from birth, nail defects and webbing of the neck (Figure 12.23).

PARATHYROID DISEASE

FUNCTIONAL DIAGNOSIS
Hypoparathyroidism

In this condition, hypocalcaemia causes tetany, convulsions, psychiatric disorder and ectodermal changes such as cataract and nail dysplasias, often with moniliasis. Tetany may present as painful carpopedal spasms – fingers tightly apposed, thumb flexed and adducted across the palm: the *main d'accoucheur* (Figure 12.24). This

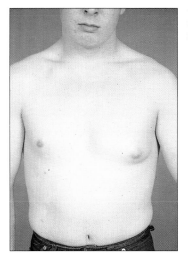

◄ Figure 12.22 Left gynaecomastia

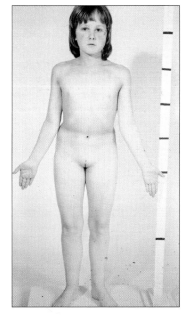

◄ Figure 12.23 A woman of 22 years with Turner's syndrome. Note the broad chest, short neck, lack of pubic hair and childlike appearance

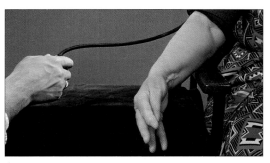

▲ Figure 12.24 Trousseau's sign: main d'accoucher

indicates increased neuromuscular excitability, which may also cause laryngeal spasm and stridor. It may be demonstrated by two signs:

1 *Chvostek's sign*: elicited by tapping over the facial nerve as it emerges from the front of the parotid gland. This causes twitching of the upper lip and drawing up of the angle of the mouth. It is relatively non-specific and may be elicited in many normal people.
2 *Trousseau's sign*: involves eliciting latent carpopedal spasm by pumping a sphygmomanometer cuff above systolic pressure for up to three minutes. This is invariably uncomfortable but if carpopedal spasm occurs the posture is unmistakable, and the spasm does not subside immediately on deflating the cuff, unlike the reaction seen with some hysterical subjects.

Hyperparathyroidism

The hypercalcaemia may initially cause non-specific aching in limbs, anorexia or depression, thirst and polyuria. Gastrointestinal symptoms include dyspepsia, vomiting, abdominal pain and constipation. Renal and ureteric stones may be the mode of presentation and late cases develop renal failure and severe skeletal problems including painful bone swellings.

AETIOLOGICAL DIAGNOSIS

Hypoparathyroidism may result from previous neck surgery for goitre. The occurrence of operative damage to the recurrent laryngeal nerves makes the possibility of tetany potentially lethal. Hypoparathyroidism may be of auto-immune origin and associated with Addison's disease or thyroid disorder. The secretion of abnormal parathyroid hormone, which is biologically inactive, causes pseudohypoparathyroidism. These patients often have short fourth and fifth metacarpals so that on making a fist they have dimples in the place of knuckles.

Hyperparathyroidism is usually due to parathyroid adenoma. These are for all practical purposes too small to palpate. The one sign that can be useful is corneal calcification, best seen with a slit lamp but often also visible when shining a slanting pencil of light across the cornea where a thin white band may be seen in the 3 o'clock and 9 o'clock positions (as opposed to arcus senilis which is most marked at the 12 and 6 o'clock positions). A convenient source of light is an auroscope bulb, when the instrument is used without an earpiece. The adjacent sclera frequently appears gritty and a little inflamed.

PANCREATIC ISLET DISEASE

FUNCTIONAL DIAGNOSIS
Hypoglycaemia

This presents classically with symptoms of cerebral dysfunction and sympathetic activation. The former depend on the speed and severity of the hypoglycaemia and may cause coma of rapid onset with neurological changes such as extensor plantar responses and convulsions; hemiplegia may occur, usually rapidly reversible. Lesser degrees may cause mental confusion and amnesia and chronic hypoglycaemia may cause personality changes which can be hard to identify. The sympathetic features include palpitations, sweating and hunger.

Hyperglycaemia

This causes thirst and polyuria because of the osmotic diuresis, weight loss often without anorexia and, especially in older women, pruritus vulvae. The underlying insulin lack can lead to diabetic ketoacidosis with vomiting, dehydration and hyperventilation due to air hunger, a ketotic odour on the breath, hypotension and drowsiness leading to coma. The complications of diabetes include retinopathy, cataracts, vascular insufficiency causing foot ulcers or gangrene (Figure 12.25), peripheral neuropathy and nephropathy.

AETIOLOGICAL DIAGNOSIS

Hypoglycaemia is most frequently the consequence of overtreatment of diabetes mellitus with insulin or sulphonylurea drugs. Hyperinsulism as a result of islet

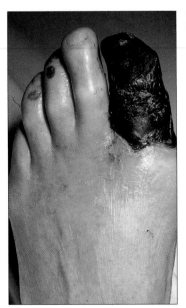

◀ **Figure 12.25 Diabetic gangrene**

cell tumour is rare and may present with hypoglycaemic symptoms in the fasting state or after exertion. The patient may learn to counteract symptoms with sugar-containing food and gain weight as a result.

Diabetes mellitus is generally of unknown origin but rarely may be due to excess insulin antagonists.

INVESTIGATION OF ENDOCRINE DISORDERS

THYROID
Thyroid hormone levels
Total serum thyroxine (T4) and triiodothyroxine (T3) measured by radioimmunoassay may be raised in hyperthyroidism and low in hypothyroidism. Thyroid stimulating hormone (TSH) is especially valuable in hypothyroidism when a high value indicates thyroid gland insufficiency and a low value suggests a pituitary cause. Radioactive iodine/technetium scans are useful for imaging lumps but are not used as a first-line evaluation of thyroid status. Thyroid auto-antibodies are helpful in establishing thyroid autoimmunity: they are *not* a function test.

PITUITARY
The insulin tolerance test (ITT) should only be performed in patients with no known cardiac disease or epilepsy and with normal basal morning cortisol levels. The induction of hypoglycaemia with insulin should stimulate ACTH and hence cortisol secretion.

Posterior pituitary function is screened by measuring both plasma and urine (preferably early morning) osmolalities.

Diabetes insipidus
Water deprivation test: collect urine in hourly aliquots, measure urine and plasma osmolality; this is reduced in diabetes insipidus but increases in response to exogenous vasopressin analogue (DDAVP).

Hyperprolactinaemia
The best test is a series of three basal prolactin measurements. Women usually have higher levels than men.

Acromegaly
During an oral glucose tolerance test the growth hormone level is abnormally maintained above 4 mU/l and may even rise paradoxically. Bromocriptine test: 80 per cent of acromegalics show a marked fall in growth hormone after a 2.5 mg oral dose of bromocriptine.

Radiology
Pituitary tumours may cause abnormalities of the pituitary fossa apparent on plain lateral or postero-anterior skull radiographs. Computerized tomography (CT) scanning of the pituitary is useful for detecting small pituitary microadenomas (<1 cm diameter) as well as for delineating larger tumours (Figure 12.26).

ADRENALS
In adrenal insufficiency the 0900 hours cortisol level is reduced. The plasma ACTH is high in adrenal disease and low in hypopituitarism. The plasma urea and potassium are high and the plasma sodium may be low when compensatory mechanics fail.

Synacthen test
Measure cortisol levels for 1 hour after a synacthen (ACTH) injection to assess adrenal reserve.

Cushing's syndrome
Screen by measuring 0900 hours cortisol after the patient has taken 2.0 mg dexamethasone at 2300 hours the previous night. If the cortisol level is greater than 180 nmol/l, Cushing's syndrome is suspected. Fuller investigation includes ACTH measurement; this is undetectable in adrenal adenomas and carcinoma and in these disorders the circadian profile of plasma cortisol is also lost. High dose dexamethasone suppression of plasma cortisol is found in pituitary dependent Cushing's syndrome and metyrapone tests may help in distinguishing these cases from those associated with carcinoma and ectopic ACTH production. Twenty-four hour urine estimations of free cortisol, 17-oxogenic and 17-

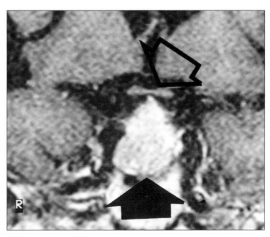

▲ **Figure 12.26 CT scan showing a pituitary prolactinoma (closed arrow).** Note normal optic chiasma (open arrow)

oxosteroid measurements complement the plasma estimation of cortisol and ACTH.

Conn's syndrome
The plasma potassium is abnormally low and the plasma aldosterone and renin levels are raised.

Congenital adrenal hyperplasia
In this condition, raised levels of plasma 17-hydroxy-progesterone, urinary preganetriol and (in women) plasma testosterone are found.

Assessment of adrenal size and morphology
This is best achieved by CT scanning. Radio-isotopic scanning may be useful, especially in adrenal tumours causing Cushing's syndrome and Conn's syndrome.

Phaeochromocytoma
Raised levels of vanillylmandelic acid (VMA) and meta-drenaline are found in 24-hour urine samples. Plasma noradrenaline is usually elevated but sampling and measurement requires specialized facilities. CT and radio-isotopic imaging may locate the tumour.

GONADS
Men: measure plasma testosterone, FSH/LH.
Women: premenopausal: record basal body temperature and measure plasma oestradiol, progesterone and FSH/LH levels.

In suspected *virilization*: plasma testosterone.

In suspected *Klinefelter's* and *Turner's syndrome*: check karyotype.

PARATHYROIDS
Measure total plasma calcium, albumen, inorganic phosphate and alkaline phosphatase, preferably fasting and in blood drawn without a tourniquet. In appropriate cases measure serum parathyroid hormone and vitamin D metabolites, also 24-hour urine calcium.

PANCREAS
Diabetes mellitus is usually diagnosed on the basis of a high random or fasting plasma glucose. If in doubt, perform an oral glucose tolerance test.

Diagnosis of insulinoma: low fasting blood sugar with high insulin. A suppression test may be necessary using exogenous insulin and measuring C-peptide to check the patient's own pancreatic response. Sampling for insulin via a catheter passed percutaneously trans-hepatically along the splenic vein may be needed to localize the source of insulin in the pancreas.

CT scanning may be helpful in localizing tumours, which are often very small.

Symptoms and signs in tropical disease

GEORGE WYATT

MEDICAL HISTORY

The principles of history taking have been fully described already. In the diagnosis of tropical disease the additional question 'Where have you been?' is vital. The geographical history may give the only clue to the diagnosis of a potentially lethal disease such as falciparum malaria. Residence in the tropics many years previously may be relevant since some tropical infections persist for decades. The families of former immigrants from the tropics are often at special risk when they return to visit relatives; business travellers, expatriate workers, sailors, the armed forces and children visiting their parents abroad during school holidays are other risk groups (Figure 13.1). The explosion of tourism to the tropics means that many who are not in traditional risk groups may also become infected. Find out exactly when and where the patient travelled and their living conditions abroad. Enquire about their immunizations and malaria prophylaxis including the regularity and duration of taking antimalarial drugs. Record any illness suffered, especially any accompanied by fever or rash.

In the tropics the pattern of disease can vary greatly from one country to another and even from one area to another within a country. A knowledge of the endemic diseases in the area from which the patient comes is often the most important guide to pertinent questions. In some instances religion is significant as with fasts or pilgrimages. Specific dietary habits such as eating raw fish or social customs such as pig feasts in New Guinea may be relevant. Clinics in many parts of the tropics operate

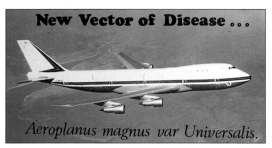

▲ Figure 13.1

under great pressure with long queues of patients. Many different languages are spoken necessitating use of interpreters and their understanding of the causes of disease may be quite different from the scientific model. A sound knowledge of the diseases in the area, a good brief medical history and a necessarily rapid, limited examination form the basis of a diagnosis. Simultaneous multiple infections are common so one should not be satisfied with having defined a single complaint.

FEVER

Fever is one of the most important signs of acute tropical infections. It is usually associated with a *rapid pulse* and sometimes with *rigors*.

The first attack of malignant *Plasmodium falciparum* malaria usually presents with an irregular fever without specific features. Classic malaria fever patterns such as tertian (fever every second day) and quartan (fever every third day) are usually due to relapses of benign tertian (*Plasmodium vivax* or *Plasmodium ovale*) or quartan (*Plasmodium malariae*) malaria and are unreliable in the initial attack. In *kala-azar* intermittent or remittent fever may peak twice in the day (double diurnal rise) and the patient often has fewer symptoms than expected from the height of the fever. *Relapsing fever* is characteristic of infection with *Borreliae* which may be transmitted by lice or ticks. Fever begins suddenly and lasts for several days, it subsides equally quickly and several days without fever are followed by one or more similar febrile episodes. In *dengue* there is often a saddleback fever curve. There are two phases of high fever separated by a remission. A generalized fine morbilliform rash often appears during the second febrile phase.

An unexpectedly slow pulse in relation to the height of the fever is sometimes present after the first few days in *yellow fever* (Faget's sign) and also in *typhoid*. On the other hand the pulse rate may be unexpectedly rapid in African trypanosomiasis and Chagas' disease. *Rigors* are common at the onset of many acute tropical diseases, particularly those associated with a rapid rise in temperature, such as *typhus*, *plague* and *relapsing fever.* In malaria rigors are particularly likely during relapses.

Prolonged fever in a patient from the tropics should lead to consideration of *tuberculosis, HIV* infection, *typhoid, brucellosis, amoebic liver abscess* and acute *schistosomiasis* as well as the ubiquitous causes of this syndrome.

SKIN MANIFESTATIONS

Rashes of various kinds are common in tropical infections, either as part of the disease process or resulting from treatment. Erythema and macular rashes are difficult to see in black skins. Many skin eruptions become complicated by scratching and secondary infection. *Scabies* is very common but mite burrows are often obscured by pyoderma.

Increased pigmentation of the skin sometimes occurs in *kala-azar* (the black sickness), while in *pellagra* the skin is heavily pigmented in parts exposed to the sunlight, e.g. the face, neck and the backs of hands and wrists. Diminished pigmentation occurs in the lesions of *pityriasis versicolor, leprosy, yaws, post kala-azar dermal leishmaniasis* and over the shins in *onchocerciasis*.

Localized areas of transient oedema occur in *loaiasis* (Calabar swellings), *trichiniasis, gnathostomiasis* and both American and African *trypanosomiasis*. In *leprosy* lesions vary from the numerous, symmetrical, hypopigmented or erythematous macules or nodules with normal sensation of lepromatous disease to the few, well-defined, roughened, anaesthetic and non-sweating lesions of the tuberculoid pole. Remember always to feel for enlarged superficial nerves.

Nodules are often felt over bony prominences in *onchocerciasis* (Figure 13.2) and may be present on the face or ears in lepromatous *leprosy*. Nodules on the extremities are sometimes due to *Kaposi's sarcoma*. Skin manifestations that may point to HIV infection include itching papular rash, severe seborrhoeic dermatitis or fungal infections, and especially the rash of, or scarring from, herpes zoster. An 'eschar' with blackened centre and surrounding erythema at the site of attachment of tick or mite is characteristic of both old world *tick typhus* or *scrub typhus*. Slowly growing ulcers of skin, ear pinna (Chiclero's ulcer) or nose are seen in *leishmaniasis* (Figure 13.3). Ecchymoses occur in South-East Asian haemorrhagic fever (Figure 13.4).

Creeping eruptions of the skin (*larva migrans*) are usually caused by hookworms of dogs or cats which penetrate human skin to form an itchy, slowly progressing, serpiginous track. Larvae of the human nematode

Strongyloides stercoralis can cause a similar but more rapidly progressing track up to forty or more years after the original infection, as seen in former Far-Eastern prisoners of war (Figure 13.5). Fly larvae may also develop in the skin. The African tumbu fly (*Cordylobia anthropophagia*) larva presents as a furuncle but with a central punctum through which it breathes. The classic skin lesions of dermal leishmaniasis in the Middle and

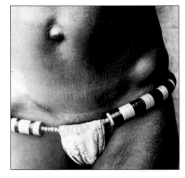

◀ **Figure 13.2 Subcutaneous nodules in onchocerciasis.** Taken from *A Colour Atlas of Tropical Medicine and Parasitology,* 2nd edition, 1981, W. Peters and H. M. Gilles (eds), London, Wolfe Medical Publications.

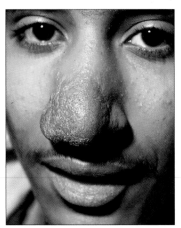

◀ **Figure 13.3 Cutaneous leishmaniasis involving the nose**

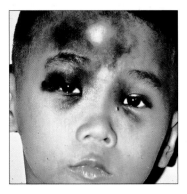

◀ **Figure 13.4 Facial ecchymoses in a boy with South-East Asian haemorrhagic fever.** Taken from *A Colour Atlas of Tropical Medicine and Parasitology,* 2nd edition, 1981, W. Peters and H. M. Gilles (eds), London, Wolfe Medical Publications.

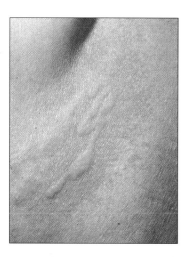

◄ Figure 13.5
A 'creeping'
elevation of the
skin by the larvae
of *Strongyloides*
stercoralis

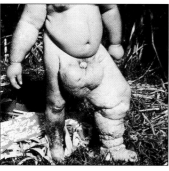

◄ Figure 13.6
Lymphoedema of
the leg and
scrotum due to
filariasis
('elephantiasis')

Near East are illustrated in Figure 13.3 and the gross lymphoedema associated with filariasis in Figure 13.6.

GASTRO-INTESTINAL MANIFESTATIONS

Symptoms
Diarrhoea

Diarrhoea is one of the most common symptoms in tropical medical practice. Only a few of the commonest causes can be mentioned here. Simple watery diarrhoea is often caused by enterotoxigenic strains of *Escherischia coli* or by viruses such as *rotavirus*. Simple diarrhoea with fever is also caused by falciparum malaria especially in children. Profuse watery diarrhoea and vomiting, 'rice-water' stools and rapid dehydration suggests *cholera* especially if others are affected. Prolonged diarrhoea with gaseous abdominal distension may be due to *Giardia intestinalis*. Prolonged diarrhoea with profound weight loss is common in HIV infection.

Frequent, severe diarrhoea with blood and mucus of sudden onset, combined with high fever and abdominal cramps often indicates bacillary dysentery due to *Shigellae*. *Amoebic dysentery* more often presents with slow onset, no fever, but a tendency to recur over weeks or months. Intestinal *schistosomiasis* may also cause dysentery.

Abdominal pain

Abdominal pain, simulating an acute abdomen in an anaemic child, should bring to mind the possibility of homozygous *sickle cell disease* (see Chapter 8). Laparotomy should not be undertaken until this possibility has been excluded. Pain over the liver or referred to the shoulder tip occurs in *amoebic liver abscess*, while pain in the left hypochondrium sometimes occurs in acute falciparum malaria and as a result of splenic infarction in sickle cell disease.

Haematemesis and melaena

Haematemesis and melaena arising from oesophageal varices is common in chronic intestinal *schistosomiasis* and cirrhosis caused by hepatitis B. Bleeding is also seen in the terminal phases of yellow fever and the viral haemorrhagic fevers.

Jaundice

Jaundice resulting from a combination of haemolysis and liver damage is an important symptom of severe falciparum malaria.

Signs
The mouth

During hot and windy spells in dry climates the lips are dry and may crack. Extreme dryness of the tongue and mouth with sunken eyes is seen in dehydration. Soreness of the lips with redness, crusting and fissuring at the angles of the mouth is seen with deficiency of the B group of vitamins. In riboflavin deficiency there is inflammation of the lips and a magenta coloured tongue (see Figure 3.7, page 30), while in pellagra (nicotinic acid deficiency) and sprue the tongue is smooth and red due to loss of papillae. Painless enlargement of the parotid glands is often seen in protein-energy malnutrition. Koplik's spots in an acutely ill, febrile infant often gives the clue to the diagnosis of measles – a very lethal disease in many parts of the tropics and one in which the rash is less obvious in dark-skinned people.

Hepatomegaly

An enlarged liver is a common finding in the tropics. Some frequent causes of hepatomegaly are given in Table 13.1.

With an amoebic liver abscess the liver is usually tender on pressure or by percussion. There may be signs

SOME 'TROPICAL' CAUSES OF LIVER ENLARGEMENT
Malaria
Cardiac failure*
Viral hepatitis*
Cirrhosis
Hepatocellular cancer
Amoebic liver abscess*
Schistosomiasis mansoni or japonicum
Protein-energy malnutrition
Hydatid disease
Visceral leishmaniasis
Haemoglobinopathies, sickle cell anaemia and thalassaemia
Liver flukes (*fasciola and opisthorchus*)
Toxocariasis
* Liver tenderness common, it also occurs with any condition which rapidly distends the capsule

▲ **Table 13.1**

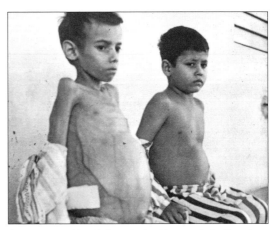

▲ **Figure 13.7 Chronic intestinal schistosomiasis.** Note the abdominal distension due to ascites and splenomegaly and, in the nearest child, engorged abdominal veins, eversion of the umbilicus and cachexia. Taken from *A Colour Atlas of Tropical Medicine and Parasitology*, 2nd edition, 1981, W. Peters and H. M. Gilles (eds), London, Wolfe Medical Publications.

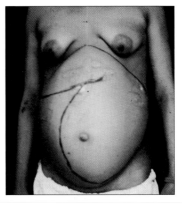

◀ **Figure 13.8 Class 5 splenomegaly**

at the right lung base but the diagnosis is best made by ultrasound examination of the liver. In chronic intestinal schistosomiasis all the classic features of portal obstruction are seen (Figure 13.7).

Splenomegaly

In many tropical areas splenomegaly is an extremely common finding. The physician has to decide whether the enlargement is related to the current illness of the patient or is the common manifestation of endemic malaria. In malarious areas the endemicity of malaria is measured by 'spleen and parasite rates'. Thus, in holoendemic areas of malaria the spleen is palpable in over 80 per cent of children between the ages of 2 and 9 years and in up to 20 per cent of adults as a 'normal' finding. Hackett has described a method of recording the spleen size which has been widely used in the tropics, particularly in relation to malaria surveys, but which is also useful as a routine clinical method. The classification is as follows:

Class of spleen	Findings on palpation
0	Spleen not palpable even on deep inspiration
1	Spleen palpable below the costal margin, usually on deep inspiration
2	Spleen palpable, but not beyond a horizontal line halfway between the costal margin and the umbilicus, measured in a line dropped vertically from the left nipple
3	Spleen palpable more than halfway to the umbilicus, but not below a line running horizontally through it
4	Spleen palpable below the umbilical level, but not below a horizontal line drawn halfway between the umbilicus and the symphysis pubis
5	Spleen palpable and extending lower than in class 4 (Figure 13.8)

Some common causes of splenomegaly in the tropics are given in Table 13.2.

SOME 'TROPICAL' CAUSES OF SPLENOMEGALY
Malaria*
Hyperreactive malarial splenomegaly †
Schistosomiasis mansoni and japonicum †
Portal hypertension from liver cirrhosis etc. †
Visceral leishmaniasis †
Brucellosis*
Typhoid*
Typhus*
Relapsing fever*
African trypanosomiasis*
Bartonellosis*
Haemoglobinopathies (sickle cell and thalassaemia)
* Indicates spleen often tender.   † Spleen sometimes grossly enlarged below umbilicus.

▲ **Table 13.2**

CARDIOVASCULAR SYSTEM
(see also Chapter 7)

Rheumatic heart disease causing mitral stenosis remains very common in the tropics. Hypertensive heart disease is also a major problem though ischaemic disease is still unusual in most rural areas. Dilated cardiomyopathies of uncertain cause are frequent in some countries. Severe anaemia from malaria or hookworm disease can cause heart failure. Beriberi is a rare but remediable cause of high output cardiac failure.

Chagas disease in South America is a cause of acute myocarditis in children and of dysrhythmias, embolic disease and heart failure in adults. *Trypanosoma rhodesiense* infection and trichinosis sometimes also cause myocarditis.

Pericarditis is seen in acute pyogenic infections and tuberculous pericarditis has become particularly common among those with HIV infection. Rupture of an amoebic abscess into the pericardium may cause cardiac tamponade.

A very high jugular venous pressure with gross ascites may be seen with constrictive pericarditis or with right ventricular endomyocardial fibrosis. Endomyocardial fibrosis of the left ventricle usually presents with signs of isolated mitral regurgitation and a third heart sound.

RESPIRATORY SYSTEM
(see also Chapter 6)

Cough, wheezing, transient lung shadows on X-ray and marked eosinophilia can be caused by allergic reactions to migrating larvae of the gut nematodes *ascaris*, *stongyloides*, hookworms and also of *toxocara*. Tropical pulmonary eosinophilia presents with nocturnal cough, wheeze and weight loss usually in people of Indian origin who have an intense response to filarial infections.

The Katayama syndrome of cough, fever, urticaria and eosinophilia occurs in the invasive stages of schistosomiasis. In the later stages of schistosomiasis eggs laid in pulmonary vessels may cause obliterative arteritis and cor pulmonale.

In paragonimiasis chronic cough productive of brownish blood-stained sputum occurs. Tuberculosis is so common in the tropics that it must always be excluded in those with chronic cough or haemoptysis. HIV infection is often complicated by pneumococcal pneumonia or tuberculosis. With an amoebic liver abscess there are commonly signs of consolidation or effusion at the right lung base. Embolic amoebic abscesses of the lung also occur.

Pulmonary oedema is a feared complication of severe falciparum malaria in adults; intravenous fluid overload must be avoided. In young children rapid, deep breathing with nasal flaring is associated with severe falciparum malaria.

Hydatid cysts of the lung are second in frequency only to liver cysts.

GENITO-URINARY SYSTEM
(see also Chapter 5)

Pain associated with obstruction due to stones in the kidneys, ureters and bladder is common in the tropics. In North-East Thailand, for example, children are particularly prone to bladder stones. Terminal *haematuria* is caused by *schistosoma haematobium* infection, especially during the acute phase of the disease. Blood may also be passed in the semen. In chronic infections there is dysuria with recurrent attacks of cystitis. Hydronephrosis may result from back pressure on the kidneys caused by obstruction of the ureters by granulomas or fibrosis.

Bancroftian filariasis may present with *hydrocele* or be complicated by *chyluria*. Falciparum malaria may cause acute renal failure with *oliguria* or *anuria*. Gross *proteinuria*, oedema and ascites (nephrotic syndrome) may be caused by infections with *Plasmodium malariae*, schistosomes or hepatitis B.

NEUROLOGICAL SYSTEM
(see also Chapter 10)

Delirium and *coma* are common in falciparum malaria, African trypanosomiasis and Japanese encephalitis. *Mental confusion* occurs with cerebral malaria, many acute infections including typhoid and typhus and with HIV encephalopathy. *Convulsions* are a feature of cerebral malaria, cerebral schistosomiasis (especially *schistosoma japonicum*), cysticercosis and cerebral toxoplasmosis.

Subjective sensory complaints may accompany vitamin deficiencies, e.g. the 'burning feet' syndrome of pellagra. Thiamine deficiency ('dry' beriberi) manifests itself with wrist drop, foot drop and marked wasting of the lower extremities.

In leprosy nerves are enlarged, hard and tender; the ulnar, posterior tibial and external popliteal nerves are most commonly affected (Figure 13.9). Of the superficial sensory nerves, the most frequently involved is the great auricular (see Figure 13.10). Neural damage is followed by paralysis and anaesthesia, sometimes with trophic damage to the skin and neuropathic injuries to bones and joints (Figure 13.11).

Psychosomatic disorders are common in the tropics: weakness, sexual incapacity, feelings of hotness and coldness, 'worms under the skin' and paraesthesiae of various kinds are frequent symptoms.

OCULAR SYSTEM

The eyes are affected in a large number of tropical diseases and some, e.g. onchocerciasis and trachoma, are among the world's leading causes of blindness.

In leprosy there may be a loss of eyebrows and eyelashes and bacilliferous granulomas may be found in any structure. Quite distinct are the hypersensitivity reactions occurring in the uveal tract during the acute exacerbations of lepromatous leprosy, and the paralytic lagophthalmos (inability to close the eye) that leads to exposure keratitis and corneal perforation.

In onchocerciasis a variety of eye lesions are seen ranging from 'snow flake' corneal opacities to sclerosing keratitis and optic atrophy. The appearance of small pale follicles in the palpebral conjunctiva of the everted upper eyelid is an early sign of trachoma. In vitamin A deficiency there is a loss of lustre and dryness of the conjunctiva (xerophthalmia), Bitot's spots (white foamy spots in the temporal conjunctiva), keratomalacia (softening), perforation of the cornea and finally blindness. Vascularization of the cornea with photophobia occurs in riboflavin deficiency. In loaiasis the movement of the

adult worm across the conjunctiva results in one of the most irritating and characteristic features of the condition. Subconjunctival haemorrhages are common in leptospirosis. Tumour-like nodules in the posterior segment of the eye may be due to toxocara larvae and must be differentiated from retinoblastoma. Retinal haemorrhages are a sign of severity in falciparum malaria.

Unilateral palpebral and facial oedema is characteristic of acute Chagas' disease; it also occurs in African trypanosomiasis.

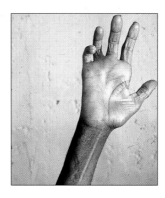

Figure 13.9 Ulnar nerve paralysis

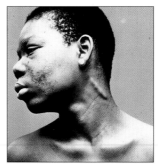

Figure 13.10 Great auricular nerve in leprosy thickening

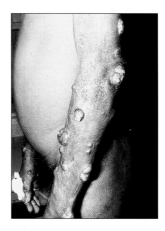

Figure 13.11 Multiple lepromatous lesions

HAEMATOLOGICAL MANIFESTATIONS

Many of the parasites that are responsible for tropical disease are found in the blood and frequently a diagnosis can only be made by blood examination.

PARASITAEMIA

The appropriate parasite is found in the blood in the following tropical infections:

1 Malaria (*Plasmodium falciparum, Plasmodium vivax, Plasmodium malariae, Plasmodium ovale*).
2 Filariasis (*Wuchereria bancrofti, Brugia malayi, Loa loa, Mansonella perstans, Mansonella ozzardi*).
3 Trypanosomiasis (*Trypanosoma brucei gambiense, Trypanosoma brucei rhodesiense, Trypanosoma cruzi*).
4 Relapsing fevers (*Borrelia recurrentis, Borrelia duttoni*, etc.).
5 Kala-azar (bone marrow, *Leishmania donovani, Leishmania infantum, Leishmania chagasi*).
6 Bartonellosis (*Bartonella bacilliformis*).

EOSINOPHILIA

Eosinophils are increased in number in many helminthic parasitic infections. This state is known as eosinophilia, and some of the conditions responsible are:

1 Filariasis.
2 Infections with non-human parasites e.g. Toxocara, animal hookworms.
3 Loaiasis.
4 Acute schistosomiasis.
5 Onchocerciasis.
6 Acute migratory phase of intestinal nematodes (e.g. *Ancylostoma duodenale, Necator americanus, Ascaris lumbricoides*).
7 Clonorchiasis.
8 Strongyloidiasis.
9 Trichinosis.
10 Dracontiasis.
11 Echinococciasis.
12 Gnathostomiasis.
13 Angiostrongyliasis.

LEUCOPENIA

Leucopenia is often associated with:

1 Kala-azar.
2 Dengue.
3 Yellow fever.
4 Brucellosis.
5 Typhoid.
6 HIV infection.

Because of the frequency of concomitant secondary infections this finding is not as consistent as might be expected.

THROMBOCYTOPENIA

Low platelet counts may accompany many infections but in a patient from the tropics malaria should always be sought first. It is sometimes a feature of HIV infection.

SIMPLE DIAGNOSTIC TECHNIQUES

Whereas sophisticated serological and other techniques have to be carried out in appropriate laboratories, the initial diagnosis of many tropical infections can be done in a clinic 'sideroom'.

For the morphological identification of the various parasites referred to in this section, the reader should consult *A Colour Atlas of Tropical Medicine and Parasitology*, 3rd edition, 1989, W. Peters and H. M. Gilles (eds), London, Wolfe Medical Publications.

BLOOD

Small quantities suitable for examination on glass microscope slides may be obtained by pricking the finger, the lobe of the ear or, in children, the heel or big toe. The blood can then be examined as a fresh wet preparation, a thin smear or a thick film (Figure 13.12).

Wet preparation

The wet preparation is particularly useful when there are present certain motile protozoa, e.g. trypanosomes or microfilarial larvae (*Wuchereria bancrofti, Loa loa, Mansonella perstans, Brugia malayi*).

The drop of blood is placed on the centre of a clean coverslip which is then lowered downwards onto the surface of a thoroughly clean glass slide. The film should be examined as soon as possible. The areas in which movement is observed are examined under the 4 mm objective and trypanosomes, if present, are easily identifiable. Microfilariae are much larger and can be easily distinguished under the 16 mm objective.

Thin films (Figure 13.12(b))

Prick the skin and put a small drop of blood near the end of the undersurface of a microscope slide and spread the film with the end of a second clean slide. The film should be allowed to dry thoroughly before staining with Leishman's or Giemsa's stain (for details see textbooks of parasitology).

Thick films (Figure 13.12(c))

Prick the skin and wait until a globule of blood has formed. Place the middle of the undersurface of clean slide against the blood and remove it, then spread the blood quickly and evenly. The film should be sufficiently thick to just allow recognition of the hands of a watch through it. After drying, the film can be stained with Giemsa's or Field's stain.

The blood should be examined on *several occasions* during a suspected attack of malaria, especially if *Plasmodium falciparum* is suspected, because the number of parasites present at any one time varies greatly during the day. Since more blood goes into the making of a thick film this acts as a concentration technique allowing more rapid recognition of small numbers of parasites under a 2-mm oil immersion objective.

Thin films are useful to distinguish the various species of malaria parasites. In general, if small rings are present in large numbers and no other forms of the asexual parasites are seen, the infecting parasite is *Plasmodium falciparum*. The presence of large trophozoites in small numbers and a polymorphic appearance – e.g. rings, trophozoites, schizonts, gametocytes – indicates infection with one of the benign malaria species (Figure 13.13).

Trypanosomes can be seen both in thick and thin-stained films as can amastigotes of *Leishmania*, although the latter are more easily found in aspirates of the spleen or bone marrow. Characteristic microfilariae are found in the peripheral blood provided blood is taken at the appropriate time, i.e. between 2200 and 0200 hours for the nocturnal microfilariae, and around midday for the diurnal ones.

FAECES

A portion of faeces is picked up on a bacteriological loop or matchstick and emulsified in a large drop of saline on a slide and covered with a coverslip. The specimen is examined systematically using the low-power objective (16 mm) with the light well cut down.

If adult worms or segments are present in the faeces they should be picked out and sent for detailed examination unless readily recognizable, e.g. ascaris worms.

During an attack of acute *amoebic dysentery* active vegetative amoebae are easily recognized provided that

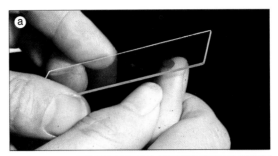
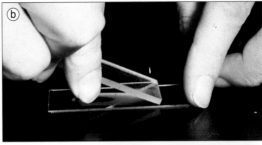
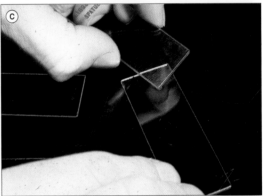

▲ **Figure 13.12 (a) collection of blood from finger-prick.** (b) Preparation of thin film (see text). (c) Preparation of thick film (see text)

the preparation is very fresh and is examined immediately; ingested red cells in the amoeba confirm the diagnosis. When the disease is quiescent the stools are formed and contain only cysts.

Helminth ova if present in moderate numbers will also be detected in saline preparations.

URINE

For the diagnosis of *Schistosoma haematobium* infection a 24-hour specimen should be used, but if random samples only are available, those collected around the middle of the day (1000–1400 hours) are likely to contain the most eggs. The urine specimens are allowed to stand for half an hour in a conical flask or are cen-

▶ **Figure 13.13 Malaria parasites**. Numbers 1 to 26 – thin films, Leishman's stain; Numbers 27 to 29 – thick films, Field's stain. Smears made from peripheral blood unless otherwise noted (x 660)

Plasmodium falciparum (malignant tertian malaria) – numbers 1 to 9:

1   Ring.
2   Ring with two chromatin dots.
3   Double infection of red cell. Marginal or accolé forms.
4   Ring in deeply stained cell showing coarse stippling (Stephen's and Christopher's dots).
5   Male sexual form. Gametocyte or crescent. Note purplish cytoplasm and scattered pigment.
6   Female sexual form. Gametocyte or crescent. Note slate-blue cytoplasm and compact pigment.
7   Half-grown asexual form from spleen smear of fatal case.
8   Fully grown asexual form (schizont) from spleen smear.
9   Macrophage containing ingested malarial pigment.

Plasmodium malariae (quartan) – numbers 10 to 15:

10   Ring.
11,12   Trophozoites. Note compactness of cytoplasm and heavy pigment. Number 12 shows an equatorial form.
13   Schizont. Typical rosette form consisting of a central mass of pigment surrounded by 8 merozoites
14   Male gametocyte. Shows diffusion of nucleus and scattered pigment
15   Female gametocyte. Shows compactness of nucleus and pigment
16   Blood-platelet superimposed on red cell. Often mistaken for a malarial parasite

Plasmodium vivax (simple or benign tertian) – numbers 17 to 21:

17   Ring
18   Trophozoite. Note amoeboid cytoplasm and paleness of red cell, which is enlarged and stippled with fine red dots (Schuffner's dots)
19   Schizont. Red cell enlarged, pale and stippled with Schuffner's dots
20   Male gametocyte
21   Female gametocyte. The gametocytes differ from those of quartan in being enclosed in enlarged, stippled cells, and in having finer pigment

Plasmodium ovale (tertian) – numbers 22 to 26:

22   Ring
23   Trophozoite. Differs from the trophozoite of Plasmodium vivax in being more solid, and is often found in an oval red cell with fimbriated edges. The stippling is heavier than in Plasmodium vivax
24   Schizont. The number of merozoites (12) is less than in Plasmodium vivax which has 16 to 24

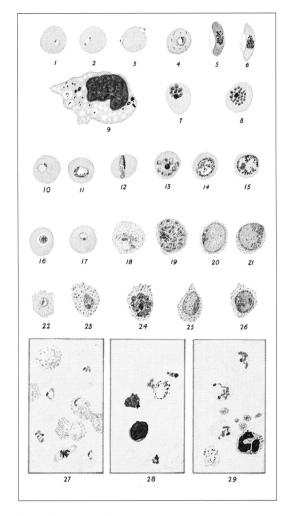

25   Male gametocyte
26   Female gametocyte
27   Plasmodium falciparum: thick film. Shows several rings lying at various angles, a gametocyte, and some blue-staining bodies, reticulocytes
28   Plasmodium malariae: thick film. Shows two trophozoites and a schizont. Included in the field are blood platelets, a punctate basophil, and a lymphocyte
29   Plasmodium vivax: thick film. Shows three trophozoites. Note apparent breaking up of cytoplasm, a typical feature. The outline of the infected red cells can be traced by the Schuffner's dots. Included are a neutrophil polymorphonuclear leucocyte, platelets and a reticulocyte

trifuged at 1500 rpm for 5 minutes. Samples of the wet sediment are transferred to microscope slides and examined under the 16 mm objective with the light cut down. The characteristic eggs of *Schistosoma haematobium* can be identified easily. Eggs of *Schistosoma mansoni* and more rarely *Schistosoma japonicum* may be found in the urine, although they are much more commonly excreted in the faeces.

SKIN

The best method for the parasitological diagnosis of onchocerciasis is the skin snip. A small piece of skin is raised on the end of a sterile needle and sliced off with a razor blade. Blood contamination should be avoided. The best site for taking the snip is the pelvic area in Africa but the scapular area should also be examined in Central America. The snip is transferred to a drop of normal saline in a microtitre plate well and examined for microfilariae after 30 minutes and again after 24 hours to give enough time for all to emerge.

ILLUSTRATIVE CASES

By way of summary two typical patients will be described, one with falciparum malaria and the other with amoebic dysentery.

FALCIPARUM MALARIA

A 40-year-old man went on holiday to the Kenya coast for two weeks but took no specific antimalarial precautions. He was well during his holiday and did not recall being bitten by mosquitoes. Four days after his return to the UK he began to notice generalized aches and pains and a low fever. Two days later he telephoned his doctor's surgery to say that he had 'flu' and was given advice.

His symptoms worsened markedly on the fifth day of illness when he had shivering attacks, began to drop things and could no longer tell the time. On admission to hospital he was slightly jaundiced, febrile and confused but liver and spleen were not felt. He was found to have falciparum parasites in 15 per cent of his red cells, a very low platelet count and evidence of liver and renal damage. He recovered fully after treatment with intravenous quinine but might well have died if there had been any further delay in beginning treatment.

The initial illness of falciparum malaria has few distinguishing features and the patient may not appear to be very ill for several days. Once complications begin the illness can lead to death within a few hours from involvement of many organs by schizogony occurring in the capillaries of the deep tissues. Cerebral, renal and pulmonary damage, hypotension and severe anaemia are some of the commonest complications. The diagnosis can only be made by asking about recent travel and arranging immediate blood film examination for those who have been at risk. Falciparum malaria usually presents within six months of leaving the malarious area (see Figure 13.14).

AMOEBIC LIVER ABSCESS

A 35-year-old Burmese seaman noted the rapid onset of severe upper abdominal pain with fever three days previously. The pain had been made worse by movement and kept him confined to his bunk. On examination he had a temperature of 39°C and there was marked tenderness with guarding in the right upper quadrant of his abdomen. His blood showed a polymorphonuclear leucocytosis and the alkaline phosphatase was raised. Ultrasound of his liver showed a 10 cm cavity in the right lobe and fluorescent antibody tests for amoebiasis which initially showed a low titre rose to a diagnostic level a week later. His fever and pain responded to treatment with oral metronidazole within 36 hours.

Amoebic abscess is another potentially fatal condition and may arise either during an attack of amoebic dysentery or as in this patient with no history of diarrhoea. Sometimes the onset is much less acute than in this patient and a picture of continued fever of uncertain origin may occur.

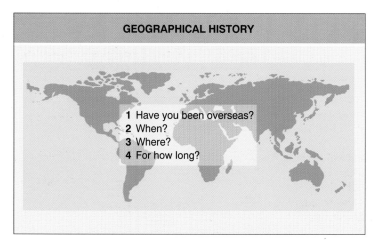

GEOGRAPHICAL HISTORY

1 Have you been overseas?
2 When?
3 Where?
4 For how long?

◄ **Figure 13.14 The geographical history is very important**

The examination of children

STEVEN RYAN

INTRODUCTION

There are three phases when considering physical examination of children. These are the newborn or neonatal period, infancy or toddlerhood, and childhood and adolescence. The priorities of examination are different for these three phases, depending on the child's growth, development and likely problems. In infancy, for instance, it is appropriate to make a careful assessment of gross motor development as part of a full examination, whereas this is rarely undertaken in teenagers.

Although three distinct phases are recognized, childhood is a continual process of growth and development. Physical growth is an important marker of child health, with abnormal growth resulting from a multitude of influences: both disease processes and environmental factors. Hence the accurate measurement of growth is an essential cornerstone of paediatrics and will be referred to frequently in this chapter.

In paediatrics there is usually a great deal of overlap between the history and the examination, as the child and family are observed during the interview. Valuable information about development, growth, behaviour and family interaction can be gleaned by careful observation. Such information is especially vital in the elucidation and management of conduct disorders. Frequently the diagnosis is made before the child is formally examined. Likewise there is an opportunity during the examination to chat to the parents and child in a more informal but none the less informative way, clarifying important points in the history.

THE EXAMINATION OF THE NEWBORN INFANT

The newborn infant or neonate is examined a number of times during the first month of life. The first examination is made, usually by a midwife, as soon as the baby is born. The purpose of this examination is to confirm that the baby has made a successful cardiorespiratory adaptation to extrauterine life, to detect gross abnormalities and also to detect any trauma suffered during the birth. At this time the weight is measured and an assessment made of the baby's gestational maturity. Head circumference and length should also be measured at birth.

CARDIORESPIRATORY STATUS

The normal term infant establishes respiration within the first minute after birth. Although usually accompanied by a loud cry it need not be, with many healthy postnatal lives starting relatively quietly. Over the next few minutes the baby becomes centrally pink – all babies are initially cyanosed. During this process babies maintain a heart rate above 100 beats per minute, they respond to gentle stimulation and have good muscle tone. Depression of some or all of the above features may indicate failure of extrauterine adaptation. This will have a cause which will need to be ascertained, e.g. intrapartum asphyxia, prematurity or depression by maternal drugs such as pethidine. The baby may also require cardiorespiratory resuscitation which is undertaken according to the same principles used in older children and adults.

One system used to standardize assessment of cardiorespiratory status at birth has gained almost universal acceptance – the Apgar score developed by Virginia Apgar in 1953. As can be seen in Table 14.1, it combines the clinical features mentioned above. Each feature is given a score of 0, 1 or 2, so that a score between 0 and 10 is recorded. The score is usually recorded at one and five minutes after birth and occasionally later in compromised babies.

THE APGAR SCORE			
	0	1	2
Colour	Blue or pale	Body pink Hands and feet blue	Completely pink
Heart rate	Absent	<100	>100
Respiration	Absent	Slow, irregular	Strong cry
Reflex irritability	No response	Grimace	Cry
Muscle tone	Limp	Some flexion of limbs	Active

▲ Table 14.1

Most healthy babies score 7 or over at one minute with a score of 9 or 10 at five minutes. The one minute score is a guide to the need for resuscitation. A baby with an Apgar score of 5 at one minute would be resuscitated initially with a bag, mask and oxygen. A baby with an Apgar score of 1 or 2 is likely to require endotracheal intubation and external cardiac massage. The score at five minutes is a guide to outcome, although large studies have called into question its validity in this respect.

TRAUMA

Severe birth trauma, resulting in long-term problems, is thankfully extremely uncommon. Minor degrees of trauma are more frequently seen. Bruising or haemorrhage is the most common and includes cephalo-haematoma which results from subperiosteal bleeding, usually over one or two parietal bones. This arises from a small underlying fracture which is usually not sought or detected – for this is a benign condition. The important feature of this swelling is that, being subperiosteal, it does not cross suture lines. This allows it to be differentiated from oedema overlying the presenting part of the scalp (caput succedaneum). This does cross suture lines and resolves within a few hours. Rarely a large haematoma may occur under the occipito-frontalis aponeurosis and lead to haemorrhagic shock. Another common site for bruising is the buttocks and genitalia in babies delivered by the breech.

Small petechiae may also be seen over the face following normal delivery and subconjunctival haemorrhages are not uncommon. The latter persist sometimes for many weeks, remaining red for longer than subcutaneous bruises. Parents may be reassured that they will eventually disappear.

Fractures occur occasionally commonly involving the clavicle or humerus. They usually present with paucity of movement on the affected side, either a spontaneous lack of movement or during the elucidation of a Moro response (see below). Incised wounds of the scalp are occasionally seen in babies delivered by caesarian section.

CLINICAL ASSESSMENT OF GESTATIONAL MATURITY

The gestational maturity of most infants is easily determined from maternal menstrual history and confirmed by antenatal ultrasound measurement of biparietal diameter around 16 weeks gestation. On most occasions no discrepancy is seen on physical examination of the infant. It is important to identify preterm infants who are at risk of feeding difficulty and jaundice (below 36 weeks gestation), hyaline membrane disease and apnoeic attacks (below 32 weeks gestation) and intraventricular

haemorrhages and retinopathy of prematurity (below 28 weeks gestation).

An accurate and widely used clinical assessment of gestation is that developed by Dubowitz in 1960. This assesses ten neurological features (Figure 14.1) and eleven physical features (Table 14.2). Each feature is scored and the total plotted on a graph (Figure 14.2). The gestational assessment calculated in this way is accurate to within ±2 weeks. For babies too sick to undergo the full Dubowitz assessment there are curtailed scores consisting of a subset of the original features. It is also possible to estimate gestational age by observing the retreating vascularization of the lens (using an ophthalmoscope set to +20 dioptres), which occurs in a centrifugal direction between 24 and 32 weeks gestation.

WEIGHT, LENGTH, HEAD CIRCUMFERENCE

All infants should be accurately weighed at birth. Taken together with an assessment of gestational maturity, weight will provide an estimate of fetal growth. Babies may be appropriately sized (between the 10th and 90th centile), small (below the 10th centile) or large (above the 90th centile) for gestational age (Figure 14.3). Babies who are large for gestational age include infants of diabetic mothers and infants with Beckwith syndrome (Figure 14.4), both groups suffering from hypoglycaemia post-natally. The latter infants may have malformations including exomphalos, macroglossia and horizontally creased earlobes resulting from fetal overgrowth.

Small for gestational age (SGA) babies can be divided into two categories. In the first group (proportionately small), all three commonly measured growth parameters (weight, length and head circumference) occupy equivalent centile positions. In this group one of two processes occurs relatively early in the second trimester: 'design fault', encompassing a large number of malformations and genetic conditions, or 'imposed intrauterine growth retardation (IUGR)' caused by placental nutritional inadequacy or intrauterine infection. In the case of IUGR, growth retardation is described as proportionate or symmetrical. Hepatosplenomegaly and a petechial rash often accompany intrauterine infection. If the growth retardation is severe a characteristic facial appearance of small sharp chin, small mid-face and bossed forehead is seen. This is the Russell–Silver syndrome, in which post-natal growth is extremely poor.

In the second group (disproportionately small), although weight occupies a position below the 10th centile, length and particularly head circumference occupy a more normal position. These babies look malnourished and often have a worried expression. They have

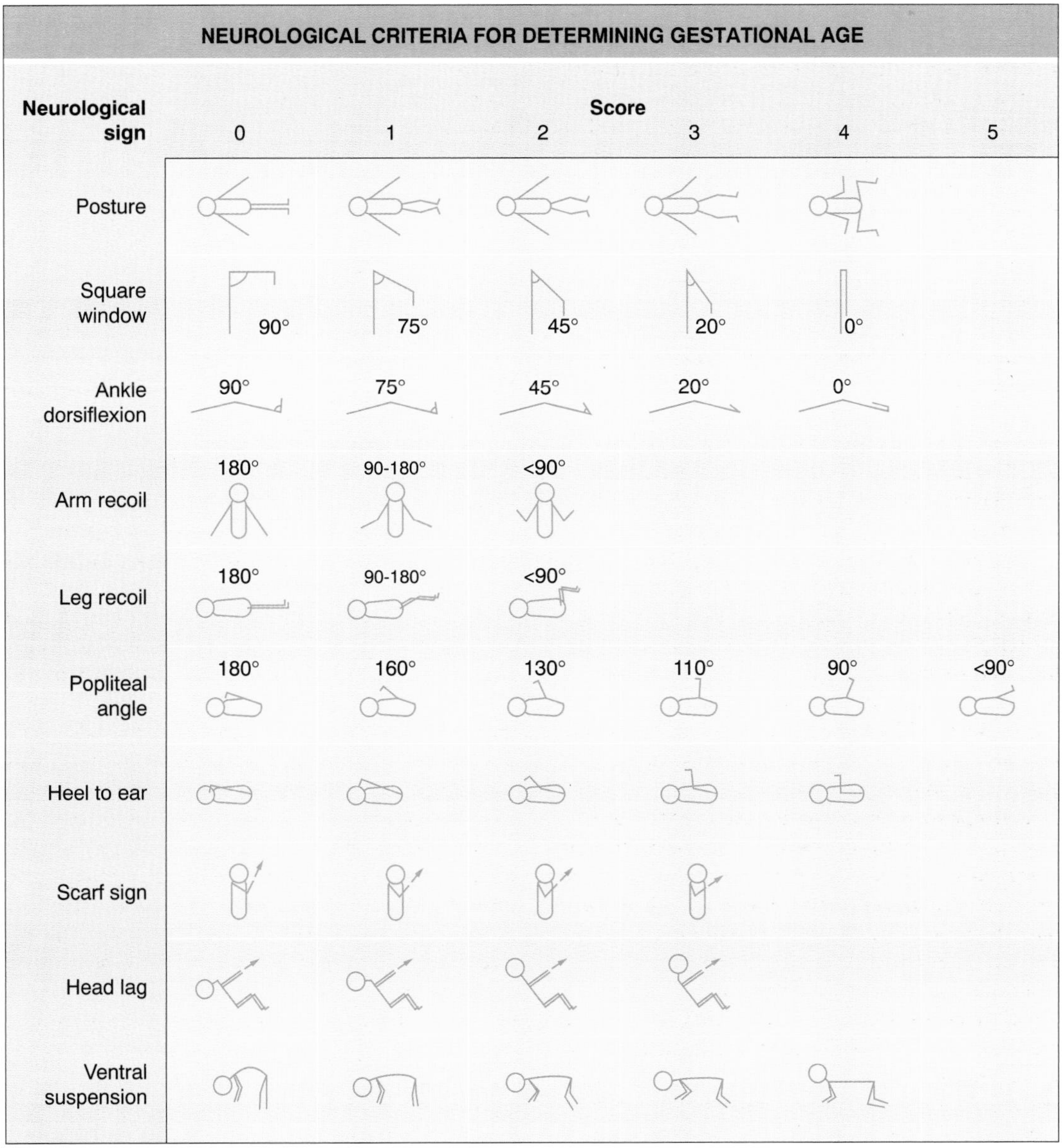

NEUROLOGICAL CRITERIA FOR DETERMINING GESTATIONAL AGE

Neurological sign	Score 0	1	2	3	4	5
Posture						
Square window	90°	75°	45°	20°	0°	
Ankle dorsiflexion	90°	75°	45°	20°	0°	
Arm recoil	180°	90-180°	<90°			
Leg recoil	180°	90-180°	<90°			
Popliteal angle	180°	160°	130°	110°	90°	<90°
Heel to ear						
Scarf sign						
Head lag						
Ventral suspension						

▲ Figure 14.1 Neurological criteria for determining gestational age

- **Posture.** Observe with infant quiet and in supine position
- **Square window.** Flex hand on the forearm
- **Ankle dorsiflexion.** Dorsiflex foot on to the anterior aspect of leg
- **Arm recoil.** Flex forearm for five seconds, then full extend and release
- **Leg recoil.** Flex hip and knees for five seconds, then fully extend and release
- **Popliteal angle.** Hold thigh in the knee-chest position, then extend leg
- **Heel-to-ear.** Draw the foot near to head. Observe degree of extension of knee and distance between foot and head
- **Scarf sign.** Draw hand towards opposite shoulder. Grade position of elbow according to illustration
- **Head lag.** Pull up slowly from supine position, grasping hands
- **Ventral suspension.** Suspend in prone position, holding under the chest

PHYSICAL CRITERIA FOR DETERMINING GESTATIONAL AGE				
	Score			
External sign	0	1	2	3	4
Oedema	Obvious oedema hands and feet; pitting over tibia	No obvious oedema hands and feet; pitting over tibia	No oedema		
Skin texture	Very thin gelatinous	Thin and smooth	Smooth; medium thickness. Rash or superficial peeling	Slight thickening Superficial cracking and peeling especially hands and feet	Thick and parchment-like: superficial or deep cracking
Skin colour (*infant not crying*)	Dark red	Uniformly pink	Pale pink: variable over body	Pale, only pink over ears, lips, palms or soles	
Skin opacity (*trunk*)	Numerous veins and venules clearly seen, especially over abdomen	Veins and tributaries seen	A few large vessels clearly seen over abdomen	A few large vessels seen indistinctly over abdomen	No blood vessels seen
Lanugo (over back)	No lanugo	Abundant; long and thick over whole back	Hair thinning especially over lower back	Small amount of lanugo and bald areas	At least half of back devoid of lanugo
Plantar creases	No skin creases	Faint red marks over anterior half of sole	Definite red marks over more than anterior half; indentations over less than anterior third	Indentations over more than anterior third	Definite deep indentation over more than anterior third
Nipple formation	Nipple barely visible, no areola	Nipple well defined; areola smooth and flat; diameter <0.75 cm	Areola stippled, edge not raised; diameter <0.75 cm	Areola stippled, edge raised; diameter >0.75 cm	
Breast size	No breast tissue palpable	Breast tissue on one or both sides <0.5 cm diameter	Breast tissue both sides; one or both 0.5–1.0 cm	Breast tissue both sides; one or both >1 cm	
Ear form	Pinna flat and shapeless, little or no curving of edge	Incurving of part of edge of pinna	Partial incurving whole of upper pinna	Well defined incurving whole of upper pinna	
Ear firmness	Pinna soft, easily folded, no recoil	Pinna soft, easily folded, slow recoil	Cartilage to edge of pinna, but soft in places, ready recoil	Pinna firm, cartilage to edge, instant recoil	
Genitalia (male)	Neither testis in scrotum	At least one testis high in scrotum	At least one testis right down		
Genitalia (female)	Labia majora widely separated labia minora protruding	Labia majora almost cover labia minora	Labia majora completely cover labia minora		

By kind permission of Dr Victor Dubowitz. Reproduced from the *Journal of Pediatrics*, 1970, 77, pages 1–10, by permission of C. V. Mosby, St Louis.

▲ Table 14.2

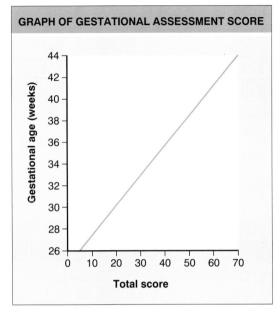

GRAPH OF GESTATIONAL ASSESSMENT SCORE

(Gestational age (weeks) vs Total score)

▲ Figure 14.2. Graph of gestational assessment score (see Table 14.2 and Figure 14.1)

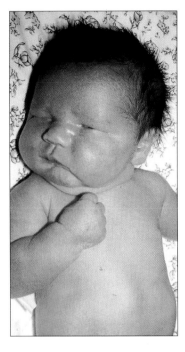

◀ Figure 14.3 Large-for-gestational age baby caused by maternal diabetes

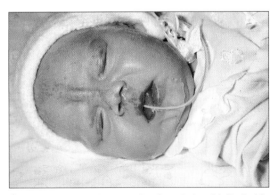

▲ Figure 14.4 Large-for-gestational age baby with Beckwith syndrome. Note protruding tongue and prominent naevus flammeus (stork mark), typical of the syndrome

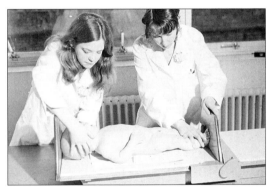

▲ Figure 14.5 Measurement of crown-heel length in an infant

all suffered disproportionate (asymmetrical) IUGR and are at the greatest risk of acute complications in the neonatal period: hypoglycaemia, asphyxia with meconium aspiration and necrotizing enterocolitis.

If length is measured, a supine infant stadiometer should be used (Figure 14.5). Tape measures give highly inaccurate results for body length. Head circumference is measured using a tape measure to find the largest circumference in the occipito-frontal diameter. Because of moulding and scalp oedema, considerable changes in head circumference may occur in the first few days.

ROUTINE NEONATAL SCREENING EXAMINATION

Within 24 hours of birth, all babies should be examined to detect any abnormalities that have not been found previously. It is important that the opportunity is taken during this examination to deal with any concerns of the parents, to give advice about immunization and sleeping position (especially in regard to preventing cot death) and to explain the procedures taking place. This will make what can be a repetitive task more rewarding.

OBSERVATION

The examination should begin with an inspection of the naked infant, although with practice palpation can be undertaken at the same time. Very important information can be gained by observation alone however.

The neurological status of the infant can be quite accurately assessed. Does the infant have the normal partially flexed posture? An infant with reduced tone will lose this posture, with the hips lying in the fully abducted position – the so-called 'frog's legs position'. Preterm neonates always adopt this position (Figure 14.6). Excessive tone may be difficult to discern, but may be revealed by an overactive grasp reflex (Figure 14.7) (see neurological examination) or difficulty in undressing the infant.

One is also able to judge the infant's degree of intrinsic activity and also that in response to handling. Most infants wake during the examination and respond with rather random but almost meaningful movements. Jitteriness or clonic movements may indicate an underlying brain or metabolic disorder. Lack of movement of an arm suggests a fractured clavicle or an Erb's palsy. The infant's cry may give useful information. Is it weak due to reduced tone or is it shrill because of cerebral irritation?

Peripheral cyanosis is common in the first 24 hours, especially if the baby is nursed in a cold room. Central cyanosis, best seen on the face and tongue, always has a pathological cause, which must be sought. Cyanotic conditions include a number which are life threatening:

1 Cyanotic congenital heart disease.
2 Diaphragmatic hernia.
3 Persistent fetal circulation.
4 Tracheo-oesophageal stricture.
5 Hypoventilation from a number of causes, e.g. hypoglycaemia.
6 Systemic infection.
7 Pneumonia.
8 Lung malformation.
9 Choanal atresia.
10 Surfactant deficiency.

If the infant is cyanosed, check for evidence of respiratory dysfunction. Tachypnoea alone (a sustained resting respiratory rate greater than 60 breaths per minute) can be the single subtle sign of early pneumonia, which is rapidly progressive and can be fatal. All tachypnoeic babies should always be fully assessed. Dyspnoea has characteristic features in the newborn. Grunting is accompanied by nasal flaring, sternal recession (Figure 14.8), lower costal retraction and abdominal breathing. Respiration may be irregular with apnoeic episodes.

Pallor may indicate poor peripheral perfusion, hypothermia or anaemia. Jaundice is common in newborn babies. It is usually easy to detect in good light

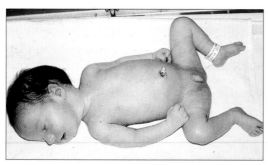

▲ Figure 14.6 Typical posture of preterm neonate showing reduced tone especially in the hips

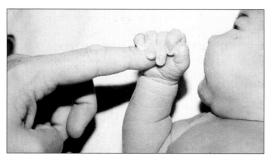

▲ Figure 14.7 Normal neonatal grasp reflex elicited by light pressure on the infant's palm

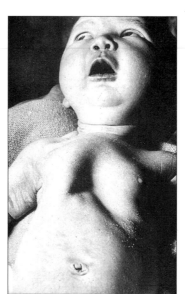

◀ Figure 14.8 Newborn baby with dyspnoea showing marked sternal retraction

conditions, but may be more difficult to spot in plethoric babies. Jaundice present at birth or appearing in the first 24 hours is usually caused by intravascular haemolysis. Later onset jaundice is commonly physiological, requiring no further investigations or treatment. Rapidly increasing jaundice, jaundice accompanied by other abnormalities or that requiring treatment (to prevent kernicterus), should be investigated. Clues to its cause include hepatosplenomegaly (haemolysis, intrauterine infection), cataract (intrauterine infection, galactosaemia) and periumbilical redness and induration (omphalitis – ascending infection of the umbilical tract).

Inspection of the nappy can help in the investigation of jaundice and provide other useful information. Infants with obstructive jaundice will have pale stools and dark urine. Such jaundice can arise from intrahepatic or extrahepatic biliary discontinuity and from infectious or metabolic hepatitis. Pink deposits in urine due to urate crystals may soak into nappies and be confused with blood. They are a benign finding, prompting reassurance. Any doubt can be dispelled by the use of a reagent stick test for blood. Failure of a baby boy to pass urine within 48 hours of birth should prompt a look for the enlarged bladder of posterior urethral valves. Failure to pass meconium within 24 hours of birth is seen in less than 5 per cent of infants. If accompanied by vomiting or abdominal distension, it suggests the low intestinal obstruction of either meconium ileus or Hirschsprung's disease.

SKIN

Any blemish on the skin can be referred to as a naevus and they come in a number of forms. The most common is naevus flammeus or 'stork mark', a pale pink capillary haemangioma found over the nasal bridge and upper eyelids (Figure 14.4) and the occiput. The anterior blemish always disappears, although the posterior can persist into adulthood. This should not be confused with the more intense red port-wine stain, usually found within the distribution of a branch of the trigeminal nerve. When associated with underlying brain haemangiomas, this represents Sturge–Weber syndrome. White pinhead lesions, milia, also seen on the bridge of the nose, are benign. Other vascular naevi include cavernous haemangiomas, which will enlarge before eventually disappearing in early childhood. Pigmented naevi are common, though thankfully large naevi including bathing trunk naevus and giant hairy naevus which have a high malignant potential are uncommon.

Pustular lesions surrounded by erythema are usually due to the benign condition erythema toxicum of unknown aetiology. Their general distribution and yellow centres differentiate them from staphylococcal skin infection. Any doubt can be dispelled by pricking a pustule and examining its contents microscopically. In erythema toxicum there are eosinophils, in staphylococcal infection there are neutrophils.

Petechiae present over the trunk may be due to thrombocytopenia which can result from intrauterine infection or isoimmune consumption by maternally derived antiplatelet antibodies. Larger purpuric lesions usually indicate a coagulopathy which can arise from septicaemia or inherited disorders of clotting. One benign condition which can be confused with bruising is that of Mongolian blue spot, a pigmented naevus more commonly seen in Asian Caucasians.

HEAD AND SCALP

Inspection will reveal any unusual shape to the skull. Most commonly this is due to the normal process of moulding, in which the various skull bones override to facilitate delivery. Such moulding disappears over the next few days. Most commonly the parietal bones override the occipital bone, with prominent ridges being palpable at this site. Occasionally the sagittal suture is closed by overlap between the parietal bones. The anterior fontanelle is normally patent, soft and pulsatile, whereas the posterior fontanelle is usually closed, or nearly so. The anterior fontanelle closes by the age of 2 years. Plagiocephaly is a common shape variation of the skull, in which the skull outline seen from above, normally contained within a rectangle, is contained within a trapezoid. This results in one side of the forehead being prominent and the other side being flattened. This is probably due to intrauterine compression and improves with time.

The midline of the scalp and nape of neck should be inspected for any small swelling or dimple which may be associated and sometimes communicate with an underlying abnormality of the central nervous system.

EARS AND FACE

The ears should be inspected to confirm normal formation and site of the pinna. Minor variations in pinna shape are extremely common. The absence of the normal helical pattern, the so-called primitive ear, has no audiological disadvantage – Mozart had two! Low set ears, lying below a line drawn between the outer canthus of the eye and occiput, may be associated with malformation syndromes but are compatible with normality. If ears are malformed and low set, other abnormalities such as Potter's or Down's syndrome are more likely.

The most common abnormality associated with ear development is the presence of skin tags anterior to the meatus, sometimes called accessory auricles. They may have a tenuous pedicle of skin or a thicker one containing cartilage or connective tissue.

Observation of the face may reveal minor individual malformations such as an external angular dermoid (a subcutaneous swelling at the upper lateral margin of the orbit) or a collection of features which may represent a malformation syndrome. Many such syndromes exist, but the most common is Down's syndrome (Trisomy 21) (Figure 14.9).

The eyes should not only be inspected, but the presence of a red reflex (best done with a funduscope) established. This will exclude the presence of a cataract.

MOUTH

A cleft lip is easily observed, as may be an associated cleft palate. Isolated cleft palates may be difficult to detect. The whole palate must be inspected using a tongue depressor and light and also palpated to exclude a submucous cleft.

A ranula, a benign glandular swelling below the tongue is rarely seen. Epstein's pearls represent accumulation of epithelial cells in white nodules in the midline of the palate. Natal teeth, usually incisors, should be left *in situ* if fixed but may be removed if loose. Thrush, infection of the mucous membranes with *Candida albicans*, presents with a spotty white rash on tongue and buccal mucosa.

NECK

The neck should be inspected and palpated. A midline swelling may be a goitre or a malformation of the thyroid gland. A hard swelling fixed to either sternomastoid muscle is referred to as a sternomastoid tumour. This represents a muscle tear and subsequent haematoma, not unlike a pulled hamstring. It resolves, but there may be a period of torticollis. Lateral swellings include branchial

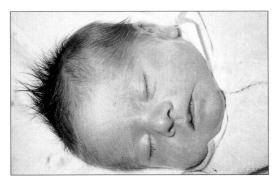

▲ **Figure 14.9 Down's syndrome.** Typical features include prominent epicanthic folds and upward slant of eyes

cysts and cystic hygromata. A branchial sinus can be found either on the face, anterior to the ear, or in between the lower heads of the sternomastoid muscle. Palpation should include the clavicles, checking for their presence and for crepitus due to a fracture.

THORAX

The signs which accompany cardiorespiratory failure are discussed above. The shape of the chest and its pattern of movement should be observed. Palpation reveals the position of the trachea and the heart apex and any cardiac thrills or heaves. In covert left diaphragmatic hernia, for instance, dextrocardia with tracheal deviation to the right is found.

Aortic coarctation is excluded by palpating good volume femoral pulses. If there is any doubt, the degree of right brachial-to-femoral pulse delay should be sought. In addition blood pressure in all four limbs can be measured using an automated cuff. Percussion may reveal a gross abnormality such as pneumothorax, but usually adds little useful information.

Auscultation should be undertaken with an appropriately sized stethoscope. Neonatal stethoscopes are available. The breath sounds of the newborn are harsher than those in older children and adults. Crackles may be heard, but the more erudite physical signs of the adult chest are not discernible in the newborn. Localization of abnormalities is usually impossible and, in any case, most lung disease in the newborn affects both lungs equally.

The heart should be auscultated in the classical four areas and also over the back. If a murmur is detected, its radiation should be established by auscultation of the lungs and neck. Occasionally a loud bruit over the skull indicates an arteriovenous malformation which may be large enough to cause heart failure.

Systolic murmurs are very common and are usually functional. If present, and in the absence of other physical signs, examination should be repeated in a few days. The nature of murmurs and their underlying causes are discussed in the section on infants and toddlers.

ABDOMEN

Start the examination of the abdomen by inspection of the umbilical stump, which should contain two arteries and a vein. A single umbilical artery, though usually a normal variant, may be associated with renal malformations. Potter's syndrome is a good example. The periumbilical area should be inspected for any redness or induration due to local infection which may spread along the umbilical tract. The most frequently seen abnormality is an umbilical granuloma, a pink fleshy swelling arising from the umbilicus in the first few weeks.

The rest of the abdomen can then be inspected for distension or asymmetry. The abdomen of a newborn baby often appears distended to a degree, but is soft. Palpation usually reveals the lower edge of a normal liver up to 2 cm below the costal margin. The spleen is also frequently palpable to 1 cm below the margin, but enlargement is usually towards the left and not the right iliac fossa as in adults. Liver enlargement may result from intrauterine viral infections, bacterial sepsis, inborn errors of metabolism or heart failure.

GENITALIA

In boys the descent of the testes is assessed. With warm hands an index finger is swept gently down from the inguinal area, stroking any retractile testis into the scrotum, where its presence can be confirmed between the index finger and thumb of the other hand in all but 2 per cent of infants. Apart from maldescent the other common abnormalities are indirect inguinal hernia and hydrocele. A very hard blue testis, discerned through the scrotal wall, is due to neonatal testicular torsion. Preterm infants are more likely to have either maldescent or inguinal herniae. Take note of any abnormal pigmentation of the scrotum which may be due to excess virilization in congenital adrenal hyperplasia. No attempt should be made to retract the prepuce which is normally firmly adherent to the glans. The site of the urethral meatus should be ascertained to exclude another common malformation – hypospadias. In this condition the urethral meatus may be found in any position in a line from the proximal ventral glans to the base of the penis.

In females the genitalia are inspected to rule out any degree of virilization. If a baby is found to have indeterminate sexual characteristics, no assignment of gender is undertaken until there has been detailed investigation by an endocrinologist and paediatric urological surgeon.

HIPS

The hips should be examined to exclude congenitally dysplastic or dislocatable hips. First the hips are inspected to determine any obvious apparent shortening of a femur. The posterior thighs are inspected for asymmetry in the number of creases – there is usually an extra crease on the abnormal side. The infant is then placed supine and both hips abducted to 90 degrees. This should be easily accomplished and reduced abduction indicates abnormality on that side. The Barlow and Ortolani manoeuvres are undertaken for each hip to test its stability. First, with the middle finger over the greater trochanter and the thumb over the lesser trochanter, the hip is flexed to 90 degrees and gentle pressure is applied along the line of the thigh as if to dislocate the hip posteriorly (Barlow

manoeuvre). A dislocatable hip may reveal itself by the sensation of giving way – telescoping. The hip is then abducted (Ortolani's test) and if it has been dislocated it will return to the acetabulum with a 'clunk' (Figure 14.10). A ligamentous click is a normal finding.

LIMBS AND DIGITS

Most abnormalities are obvious but check carefully for extra digits, accessory digits and syndactyly. Two types of talipes, abnormal position of the foot, are seen. Talipes calcaneovalgus is a benign condition in which heel position is normal. In talipes equinovarus (club foot, Figure 14.11), a malformation of the lower leg requiring surgical correction, the heel is fixed in an inverted position. There is also thinning of the calf and the forefoot is adducted.

SPINE AND ANUS

The infant is lifted and held in ventral suspension and the whole back examined for defects. A pit, hairy tuft or lipoma may overly a neural tube defect. A sinus above the second sacral vertebra is likely to communicate with the theca and requires surgical excision. A dimple or pit

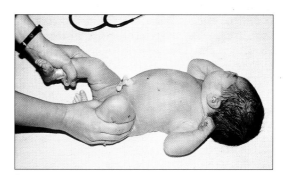

▲ **Figure 14.10 Examination for congenital dislocation of the hip.** Ortolani's test is being conducted on the left hip

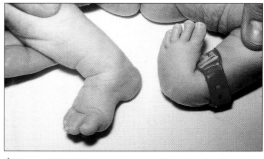

▲ **Figure 14.11 Talipes equinovarus.** There is a fixed inversion deformity of the heel and the forefoot is in a varus position

which overlies the coccyx is quite normal and requires no investigation or treatment. Other defects will be obvious. At this time the presence, position and patency of the anus can be determined.

NERVOUS SYSTEM

The examination of the newborn infant's nervous system requires a unique approach. Usually central neurological abnormalities do not present localizing features, so that one examines in an integrated fashion. The general inspection of neurological status has been dealt with above in terms of tone, posture and reactivity. Additional information is obtained when the baby is picked up to inspect the back. Is the baby easy to pick up, with good shoulder tone, or does he slip through your fingers like a rag doll? The baby's posture is checked in ventral suspension. The trunk should then be gently curved, the limbs flexed and the head briefly held in the neutral position before flexing. Similarly, when the arms are pulled, with the baby in the supine position, the head should initially be in line with the trunk before falling back (Figure 14.12).

A number of primitive reflexes are present in the newborn. Their absence at this time is abnormal, as is their presence beyond the age of 4 months.

The Moro reflex is elicited with the infant's trunk and head supported in the supine position. The neck is quickly but gently extended and the infant responds with a startle, throwing his arms out laterally with fingers extended. After this, arms and fingers are flexed. Bilateral failure of the response is a non-specific indication of central nervous system abnormality. Unilateral failure suggests either an Erb's palsy or a fractured clavicle or humerus.

The asymmetric tonic neck reflex occurs when the infant's head is rotated laterally, either actively or passively. The arm in the direction of gaze is extended, the other arm being flexed. The posture is reminiscent of that

taken up during the sport of fencing. This reflex typically persists in children (and adults) with cerebral palsy.

The rooting and sucking reflexes together allow the infant to assist with feeding. As the nipple touches the cheek, the baby turns his head to that side, opening his mouth and protruding his tongue. When the nipple reaches the baby's mouth, sucking commences by reflex. These reflexes can also be stimulated using a finger. The palmar grasp and plantar grasp reflex can be elicited by gentle contact with the appropriate surface (Figure 14.7). The former disappears by 4 months whereas the latter may take 12 months. Fisting is an exaggerated grasp reflex due to cerebral irritation.

THE INFANT AND TODDLER

Young babies should be examined lying down on an examination couch. Once infants reach the age of wariness, around 8 to 9 months, it is best at least to initiate the examination on their mother's knee.

The history in infants must, in addition to the presenting complaint, include a review of the child from conception, or even before in the case of potential genetic problems. The pregnancy and delivery history is sought together with social, family, feeding, immunization and neonatal history. Birthweight and gestation are also noted. The opportunity should also be taken for health education and to deal with any parental concerns.

The examiner will observe the child while taking the history and then engage them playfully before even undressing them. Undressing can occur in stages avoiding rapid movements which may be perceived as threatening. Useful social contact is obtained by talking quietly to both parents and child. With toddlers and older children, conversation about their likely interests will put them at greater ease. At the time of examination the child's face should be watched for signs of pain. Prolonged eye contact should however be avoided, since it may upset the infant.

The infant or younger child is usually less disturbed by continuous physical contact with the examiner's whole hand rather than by intermittent finger contact. For instance, after examining the hands, the examiner can gently move up to the patient's axillae and then to the neck. This regional approach to examination is preferred to a system based approach. The former is quicker and less likely to upset the child.

The period of infancy is characterized by very rapid growth and neurological development. The assessment of growth and development are the cornerstones of the examination.

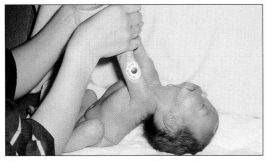

▲ **Figure 14.12 Floppy baby.** On pulling to sitting there is severe head lag and also hypotonia of the arms, which should show a degree of flexion

DEVELOPMENT

Four aspects of development are considered: gross-motor (e.g. sitting), fine motor/visual (e.g. pincer grasp of a small object), hearing and language, and personal/social development (e.g. toilet training). In each of these areas, achievements are known as milestones. Although there is wide variation between the achievement of individual milestones, these do allow the assessment of the broad front of development. Minor variations are unimportant, but two clear patterns must be recognized. Severe delay in all four areas (global developmental delay) can represent genetic conditions such as Down's syndrome or environmental factors such as neglect. A major delay in a single area represents a specific deficit, e.g. delayed language development in a deaf infant. An outline of the sequence of normal development is shown in Table 14.3.

◀ **Table 14.3**

CARDINAL MILESTONES IN DEVELOPMENT IN THE FIRST YEAR	
4–6 weeks	Smiles responsively at mother
6 weeks	Ventral suspension – head held up momentarily in the same plane as rest of body. Some extension of hips and flexion of knees and elbows Prone – pelvis largely flat, hips mostly extended
8 weeks	Gurgles responsively with smile, and eyes follow objects or person
3 months	Holds rattle placed in hand Turns head to sound in same plane as ear
5 months	Reaches for object and gets it
6 months	Supine – lifts head spontaneously Rolls prone to supine Pulled to sitting position with no head lag Sits supported by hands forward on floor Transfers cube from hand to hand Plays with toes Primitive reflexes have disappeared
7 months	Briefly sits on floor unsupported Rolls supine to prone Feeds self with biscuit
8 months	Sits unsupported Turns head to sound in plane above ear
9 months	Pulls self to stand or sit Crawls on abdomen
9–10 months	Index finger pointing to object Finger-thumb apposition
10 months	Waves bye-bye and plays pat-a-cake Helps to dress by holding out arm for coat or foot for shoe
11 months	Offers object to mother or adult Walks with support Says single word with meaning
1 year	Two or three words with meaning Walks with one hand held Casting objects begins Gives brick to mother or adult

By kind permission of Professor P. S. Illingworth. After his table in *Basic Developmental Screening*, 2nd edition, published by Blackwell Scientific Publications, Oxford, 1977.

Several caveats are necessary when drawing conclusions from a developmental examination:

1 Allowance must be made for prematurity.
2 Sick, hospitalized infants perform below expectations.
3 Children often 'fail to perform'. Listen to the parents and reassess where necessary. But beware the parents who, suspecting a problem in their child, overstate developmental milestones.
4 Children perform less well without security. This usually means with their parents, in their own house and in the absence of strangers.

When assessing development, first look for milestones within the framework suggested above. Then assess the child by play and examination, again within the framework of the four areas of development.

GROWTH

Prior to physical examination, the child should be weighed and measured. Measurement should include supine crown-heel length until the age of 2 years (Figure 14.5), standing height being measured thereafter (Figure 14.13). In order to ensure accurate supine length measurement, two people are required for the manoeuvre. The infant's head is held with the occiput touching the backplate and the crown of the head touching the base plate. Both legs are extended and the moveable footplate brought up to make contact with the full sole of the patient's foot, which is at right angles to the lower leg. Methods using a tape measure are inaccurate and should not be used.

Weight is measured using appropriate scales. Infants should be weighed naked. Head circumference should routinely be measured up to the age of 2 years. Most

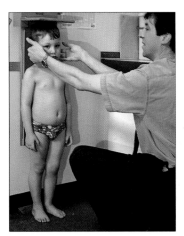

◀ **Figure 14.13** Measurement of standing height with the head held in the Frankfurt plane using a stadiometer

normal population height charts contain centiles for occipito-frontal circumference until the age of 2 years. Special charts are available for older children. All these measurements should be plotted on appropriate centile charts which are printed for both sexes. It is important to take into account previous values and the degree of prematurity. In infancy the plotted values may reveal failure to thrive: a weight below the third centile, or a weight line falling down the centiles with time. This condition is common and has many important causes both medical and social. Severe failure to thrive is associated with stunting but short stature alone is uncommon in infancy. Hydrocephalus or microcephaly may be revealed by measurement of occipito-frontal circumference.

GENERAL EXAMINATION OF THE INFANT AND TODDLER

With the infant naked or in a nappy, general observation is essential, paying attention to the following areas.

SKIN

The whole surface of the infant should be inspected. Important clues to the social well-being of the child can be found. Lack of care may be manifested in uncleanliness with dirt most usually found on the feet especially between the toes. The presence of a raw confluent red weeping rash in the napkin area which spares skin creases can indicate potentially serious neglect. This rash is a form of chemical burn caused when urea in stagnant urine is bacteriologically converted to ammonia. The presence of these two features should prompt detailed examination for other signs of neglect or even abuse. Thrush, the other common form of napkin rash, is due to superficial candida infection and presents as numerous small discrete lesions which particularly affect the skin creases.

Bruises in very small infants are of concern, since they may result from non-accidental injury. Bruises on the face, or fingertip sized bruises on the torso are extremely worrying. The latter may appear in a pattern which suggests that the child has been gripped very roughly and are associated with shaking injury (Figure 14.14). Common accidental bruises in toddlers are sustained on the forehead not the face and in more mobile children on the shins (Figure 14.15). An inconsistent or changing story, delayed presentation and a number of injuries of varying age are signs consistent with child abuse.

Most naevi in infancy and childhood will have been observed in the neonate. However some naevi may appear or become more prominent. Cavernous haemangiomas ('strawberry marks') may appear during the first few months but will disappear in time, first becoming pale in the centre. The appearance of café-au-lait

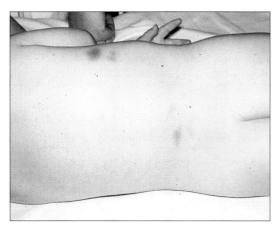

▲ **Figure 14.14 Non-accidental bruising**. The site is unusual for accidental bruising. Multiple bruises are present and no explanation could be given

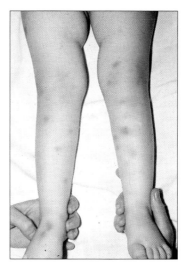

◀ **Figure 14.15 Non-accidental bruising (same patient as Figure 14.14)**. Although the shins are a common site for accidental bruises, there are a large number of fresh bruises and a suspicious bruise is present on the dorsum of the right foot

patches (neurofibromatosis) or pale ash leaf macules (tuberose sclerosis) can indicate a neurodermatosis. A Wood's light is useful for demonstrating ash leaf macules in a child or relatives.

GENERAL OBSERVATION

General inspection, as in the neonate, will reveal breathing difficulty, cyanosis or shock. In addition it is important to assess degree of hydration and nutritional status.

Dehydration may present as a dry mouth, sunken eyes, depressed fontanelle or decreased skin turgor (slow recoil after pinching), best assessed over the pectoral area. It is accompanied by tachycardia and a low volume pulse. In severe cases poor perfusion (shock) will be present. In malnutrition there is loss of fat and muscle bulk, best observed in the upper arms and buttocks. A measurement of the mid upper arm circumference (MUAC) can be made and centiles are available for comparison. Malnutrition with oedema and ascites (kwashiorkor), although rarely seen in developed countries, may occur in advanced cases of enteropathy (Figure 14.16).

Dysmorphic conditions frequently result in abnormal facies. The combination of abnormal facies and abnormalities of ears and hands is characteristic of malformation syndromes. The commonest of these is Down's syndrome which affects around 1 in 600 newborn babies in an unscreened population (Figure 14.9). There are several hundred other malformation syndromes including Turner's syndrome (Monosomy X) (see Figure 12.24). A single isolated abnormality may be familial, as a glance at one or other parent often reveals! Congenital hypothyroidism as a cause of abnormal facies is now rare because of a successful national screening programme.

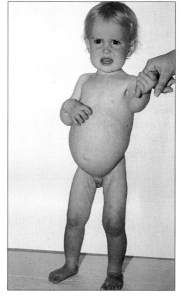

◀ **Figure 14.16 Coeliac disease**. Note protuberant abdomen, peripheral oedema and proximal wasting, mimicking kwashiorkor

SKELETON

It is not unusual to find some degree of skull deformity, particularly plagiocephaly in many infants but premature fusion of one or more sutures can lead to striking abnormalities of skull shape. Premature fusion of the sagittal suture leads to a long narrow skull (scaphocephaly). Early closure of the coronal suture leads to an elevated vertex and backward sloping frontal bone (oxycephaly). Bossing of the frontal bones is now most frequently caused by the extramedullary haematopoiesis seen in haemolytic anaemia such as thalassaemia.

The anterior fontanelle remains open until 18 months (range 9 to 27 months) and is pulsatile. Abnormalities include excessive bulging (tumours, hydrocephalus, subdural haemorrhages), depression (dehydration), premature closure (craniosynostosis, microcephaly) and delayed closure (hypothyroidism, rickets). In rickets, palpation may reveal the 'ping pong' sign as the parietal bone is pushed in and then springs back. It is occasionally found in normal infants up to age 3 months. Transillumination of the skull may reveal hydrocephalus or hydranencephaly.

Measurement of the occipito-frontal circumference at intervals will reveal whether an unusually small or large head is a normal variant or whether a pathological process exists.

The commonest deformity of the chest wall is related to air trapping in acute or chronic lung disease, such as asthma and cystic fibrosis. This is typified by an increased anterio-posterior diameter and lower costal recession which, if prolonged, results in the development of Harrison's sulci. Cardiomegaly due to congenital heart disease can result in a similar increase in diameter, often with deformity of the precordium.

Limb abnormality not seen at birth is uncommon in early childhood. The natural tendency of toddlers to bow-legs and preschool children to knock-knees is well recognized. Rickets is a disease of infancy characterized by enlarged epiphyses at the wrist and ankle, severe bow-legs and enlarged costo-chondral junctions ('rickety rosary') (Figure 14.17).

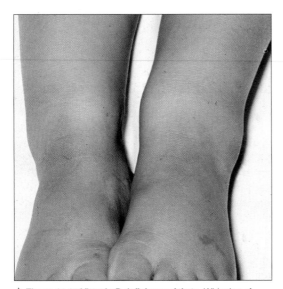

▲ **Figure 14.17 Vitamin D deficiency rickets**. Widening of epiphyses presenting as swelling of ankles

SPECIFIC EXAMINATION

HEART

Palpation will reveal any thrills or excessive precordial activity which are not so easily characterized as in an adult and localization of thrills is more difficult because of their wide conduction. The most readily demonstrable thrill arises in the central precordium from a ventricular septal defect. Palpation should be concluded by palpating the femoral pulses and checking for radio-femoral delay, a sign of aortic coarctation.

On auscultation, the heart sounds have a sharper quality than in later life and the resting heart rate is faster. The pulmonary second sound seems accentuated and is often split, although with a normal variation with respiration. Innocent or functional murmurs are many times more common than pathological murmurs. They are soft, systolic, ejection in type and vary with respiration and posture, increasing in intensity during inspiration. Other cardiovascular signs and symptoms are notably lacking. A venous hum is another though less common functional murmur which is continuous and heard over the base of the heart. It can be differentiated from the murmur of a patent ductus arteriosus because it is abolished by compression of the jugular veins.

Patent ductus arteriosus presents as a continuous machinery murmur under the left clavicle. Ventricular septal defect is characterized by a brash pansystolic murmur at the low left sternal edge. An atrial septal defect presents with a pulmonary murmur of increased flow and fixed splitting of the second heart sound.

Blood pressure measurement in toddlers is often neglected because of assumed technical difficulties. Given patience and the right cuff size it is quite feasible to obtain blood pressure measurements in most young subjects. The cuff should cover at least two-thirds of the upper arm. Inappropriately small cuffs give spuriously high readings.

EYES

Squints are commonly seen in infancy. Unlike squints acquired in adulthood which are usually paralytic, those in children are non-paralytic and usually concomitant; that is to say the angle between the ocular axes remains the same in all directions of gaze. Squints are more often convergent than divergent. To detect which eye is abnormal or to provoke a latent squint, a cover test is performed. The child is asked to look at an object with one eye covered. The cover is then removed laterally. If the abnormal eye has been covered, no change in fixation occurs. However, after a cover is removed from the normal eye, fixation changes and there is concomitant movement in both eyes.

Ears

The eardrums are inspected towards the end of a general examination and prior to inspection of the mouth and throat. Although frequently resented by toddlers, otoscopy can be facilitated by explaining the procedure and showing the child the otoscope and letting the child hold it. In this way few infants require restraint. In a struggling toddler, restraint is important to enable a good view to be obtained and to prevent pain or trauma. Secure but gentle restraint is obtained with the toddler seated on the mother's (or other adult's) lap with one arm placed around the trunk and arms, the other firmly holding the child's head against her chest (Figure 14.18). If necessary, the child's legs are held between her knees. It is important that the otoscope speculum is not too big for the size of the child's ear canal. It is better to choose one that is too small, since good views can still be obtained by moving it. The otoscope should be steadied against the child's face, so that it moves as the child's head moves.

The external canal is both shorter and straighter in infants. Hence it is usually unnecessary to pull on the auricle to straighten the canal. The normal eardrum is pale grey and shiny. A reflection of the examining light is seen as a triangular reflection on the drum, its apex at the handle of the malleus and its base inferiorly at the edge of the drum. Inflammation due to infection is revealed by loss of shine and redness. Bulging indicates excess fluid in the middle ear and retraction of the drum indicates eustachian tube dysfunction; the auditory ossi-

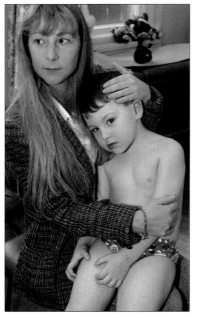

◀ **Figure 14.18 Method of holding a child for inspection of the ear canals with an otoscope**

cles are unusually prominent in the latter condition. A perforation is seen as a circular or oval deficit in the lower drum and is usually accompanied by purulent discharge into the ear canal.

Standard distraction hearing tests in infancy, even performed by well-trained health visitors, have fallen into disrepute. In many areas they have now been replaced by formal audiological assessment of children at increased risk of hearing loss. Family and personal medical history, together with the parents' comments, are taken into account when selecting children for such testing.

Mouth and Throat

The final procedure of the general examination is inspection of the mouth and throat. Frequently a full inspection without the use of a spatula can be undertaken if auroscopy has been straightforward. A spatula is reserved to the very end of procedure. A systematic approach is required, so that all physical signs are detected.

Vesicular lesions on the lips are usually due to herpes stomatitis. Such lesions may extend onto the buccal mucosa. The most characteristic abnormality seen on the buccal mucosa is the white plaque lesions of thrush. Koplik's spots, grey/white dots opposite the lower molars, are characteristic of early measles and oedema and redness surrounding the opening of Stensen's duct (opposite second upper molar) are characteristic of mumps. Petechiae on the soft palate are seen in a number of viral infections but particularly following Epstein Barr virus infection.

The gums are also affected in herpes stomatitis but most frequently gingivitis is caused by poor dental hygiene. Gingival hyperplasia with secondary gingivitis is a side effect of phenytoin treatment. A blue line on the gum is diagnostic of lead poisoning. The teeth should be inspected for number (delayed or abnormal dental development often accompanies similar processes in the skeleton), discolouration, the presence of caries and malformation.

Between the outer side of the upper and lower gums and the inside of the lips lie two frenula. It is important to observe their integrity. They can only be torn by trauma. Commonly this trauma is non-accidental, resulting from either the forcing of a hard object, usually a spoon, into the infant's mouth or a shearing force due to an external blow.

Accidental causes are seen, so that a clear explanation should be sought. Delayed reporting or the presence of other unexplained injuries should alert the clinician to possible non-accidental injury.

The tonsils are relatively large in childhood and especially during the first three years when the history reveals recurrent episodes of viral infection. Tonsillitis may present as follicles or an exudate on the surface (Figure 14.19). It may result from bacterial or viral infection. An exudative membrane on the tonsils is characteristic of either glandular fever or diphtheria, with the membrane in diphtheria being more adherent. Deviation of one tonsil towards or across the midline is due to peritonsillar abscess (quinsy) and is an indication for surgery.

An integral part of throat examination is palpation of the lymph nodes in the neck. The presence of a significant number of nodes is usual, in both anterior and posterior triangles. The jugulo-digastric nodes, lying behind the angle of the mandible, are easily felt.

No patient with stridor should have a spatula inserted into the mouth as it may precipitate complete airway obstruction. No attempt should be made to view the characteristic swollen red epiglottis of epiglottitis. Under such circumstances, the epiglottis is only examined in theatre with an anaesthetist and an ear, nose and throat surgeon present.

THE ABDOMEN

The abdomen is examined in the same way as in adults, but certain differences are found. The liver edge is ordinarily palpable up to 2 cm below the costal margin until 2 years of age and it is usually soft. Similarly the tip of the spleen may be palpable in early infancy. It should be noted that the direction of splenic enlargement is vertical into the left iliac fossa and not into the opposite iliac fossa as in adults. In young boys testes are usually retractile and it may be difficult to be certain of their position. If there is any doubt the boy can be examined while crouching on his haunches, which forces the testes into the scrotum. Umbilical herniae are frequently seen in the midline. They are always reducible, although they may have a wide base. They naturally resolve in most cases as the physiological divarication of the rectus muscle disappears with erect posture.

The abdominal examination should be completed by inspection of the genitalia in girls and the anus in both sexes. Examination for features of child sexual abuse is a difficult area requiring great expertise. Physical signs relating to this diagnosis are easily confused with other medical conditions. The diagnosis of abuse is not made with a single physical sign, but rather a jigsaw of physical features, a careful history and information from other agencies involved with the family. Reflex anal dilatation, the dilatation of the anus when the buttocks are gently parted in the lateral position, is one such sign.

CENTRAL NERVOUS SYSTEM

Toddlers and preschool children may be unwilling to co-operate with a systematic examination of the central nervous system. Fortunately it is possible by observation of spontaneous activity to determine the presence of gross deficits in the long tracts concerned with muscular power, co-ordination and posture.

The toddler or child should be encouraged to roam around the examination room, handle toys (including building bricks) and climb onto the couch. Once supine he should be allowed to sit up without assistance. If the young patient is able to clamber on to an examination couch, go from sitting to supine and vice versa, all without assistance, it is unlikely that significant weakness of limbs or trunk is present.

The manipulation of 2.5 x 2.5 cm blocks is not only an indication of visuo-spatial perception but also a test of fine movements. The child with a spastic upper limb will exhibit characteristic fanning of the fingers and external rotation of the wrist as he reaches towards an object.

The presence of a Babinski reflex may be masked by the persistence of a plantar grasp reflex. This can be avoided by testing for the Babinski reflex in two discrete movements using the thumb. Sharper objects should not be used on the soft sensitive feet of young children. Start by stroking the lateral border of the foot from the heel to the fifth toe. The second movement is a firm stroke

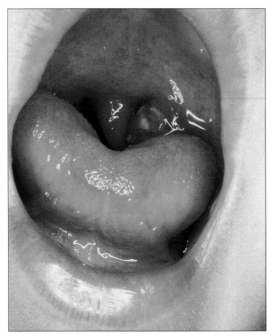

▲ **Figure 14.19 Tonsillitis.** Follicles are seen on the left tonsil

towards the medial border, across the sole at the base of the toes. A child with spastic diplegia may have an extensor plantar response with the first component but the presence of a grasp reflex elicited by the horizontal movement may then cause the toes to flex.

In the floppy infant, it is important to differentiate between central hypotonia and more peripheral weakness. The child with central hypotonia (Down's syndrome is a good example) will have a moderate amount of spontaneous movement and will withdraw from mildly noxious stimuli. Infants with peripheral weakness (e.g. spinal muscular atrophy) will have reduced reflexes with little spontaneous or responsive movement and fasciculation of the tongue may also be observed.

EXAMINATION OF THE OLDER CHILD AND ADOLESCENT

The examination can be conducted with a mixture of techniques based on formal adult techniques and the more informal approach detailed in this chapter. It is important, when the child is old enough, to ask for their consent to be examined as well as the assent of their parents. Teenagers are shy, particularly teenage girls, so it is important to respect their privacy. They should undress behind curtains and lie under a sheet or blanket. It should be remembered that many of the symptoms presenting in this age group have an emotional basis, so that a period of time with the parent absent may allow additional useful history to be obtained.

PUBERTAL STATUS

During puberty accurate height estimation is very important since growth is so rapid at this time. A standardized technique should be used to reduce intra- and inter-observer variability. Figure 14.13 shows the child standing in bare feet with the back against the measuring scale and the head held in the Frankfurt plane with gentle upwards pressure on both mastoids. Both height and weight values are then plotted on reference normal centile charts (Figure 14.20) which take into account the large variation in age of onset and duration of puberty.

The development of secondary sexual characteristics signals the beginning of the end of childhood. Within each characteristic there is an identifiable gradation of development rather like the milestones of infant development. These stages of puberty are well described and standardized according to the scheme of Tanner (Tables 14.4, 14.5 and 14.6).

STAGES OF PUBIC HAIR DEVELOPMENT IN BOYS AND GIRLS	
Stage 1	No pubic hair. Pre-adolescent
Stage 2	Sparse growth of long, slightly pigmented downy hair, straight or slightly curled, mostly at the base of the penis or along the labia
Stage 3	Considerably darker coarse and more curled hair spreads sparsely over the junction of the pubis
Stage 4	Adult type hair but less profuse
Stage 5	Adult in type and quantity

▲ Table 14.4

STAGES OF BREAST DEVELOPMENT IN GIRLS	
Stage 1	Pre-adolescent. Elevation of papilla only
Stage 2	Breast bud stage and projection of breast and papilla as a small mound. Areola enlarged
Stage 3	Breast and areola enlarged and elevated more than in Stage 2. No separation of contours
Stage 4	Areola and papilla project above the contour of the breast as a secondary mound
Stage 5	Mature stage. Papilla only projects

▲ Table 14.5

STAGES OF GENITAL DEVELOPMENT IN BOYS	
Stage 1	Pre-adolescent. Scrotum and penis same size as in early childhood
Stage 2	Slight enlargement of scrotum and testes (>4 ml) with some redness of scrotal skin. Penis shows little growth
Stage 3	Lengthening of penis and further enlargement of testes and scrotum
Stage 4	Further enlargement of penis in breadth, length and development of glans. Testes and scrotum enlarge further than Stage 3. Scrotal skin darker
Stage 5	Adult genital stage

▲ Table 14.6

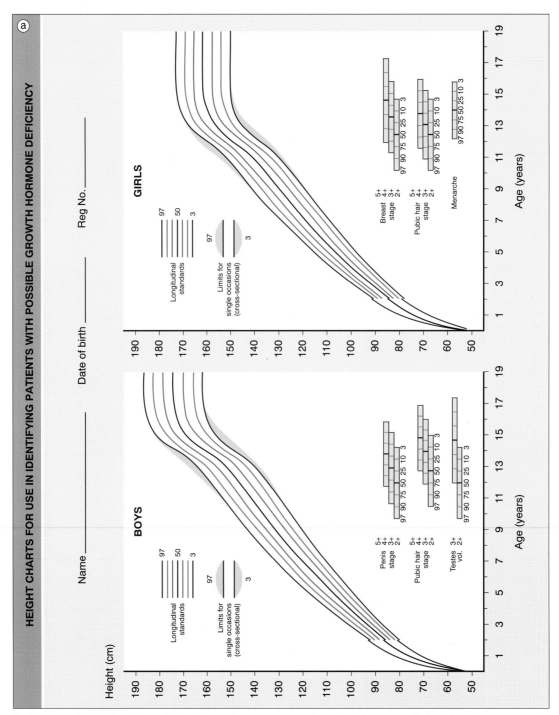

▲ **Figure 14.20 Height charts for use in identifying patients with possible growth hormone deficiency**. If height falls below the bottom of the lower shaded area, refer. If height falls within lower shaded area, re-measure a year later; if the plot progresses to nearer the lower border, refer. Velocity charts depict the individual rate of growth at different ages. (Redrawn from charts constructed by Professor J.M. Tanner and Mr R.H. Whitehouse, Department of Growth and Development, Institute of Child Health, London. Published with copyright by Castelmead Publications, Gascoyne Way, Hertford, Herts. Ref. LBH1A (boys) and LGH3A (girls)

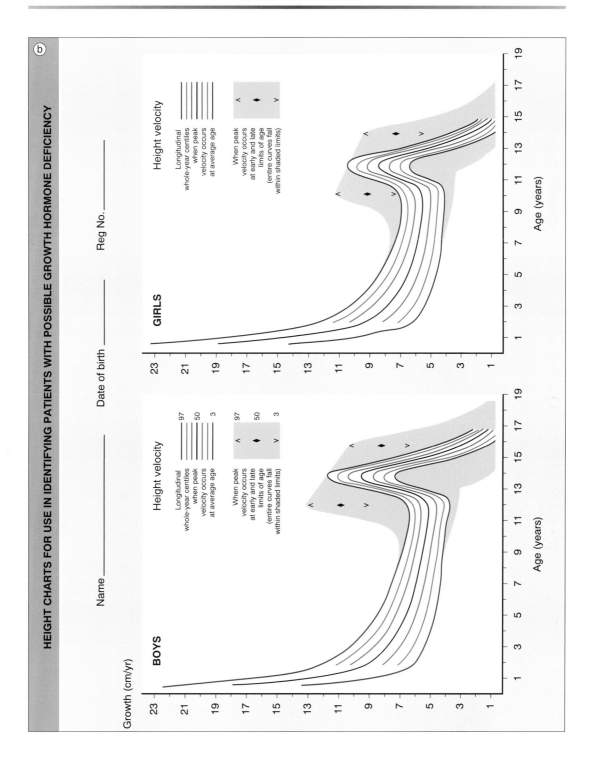

HEIGHT CHARTS FOR USE IN IDENTIFYING PATIENTS WITH POSSIBLE GROWTH HORMONE DEFICIENCY

Name

Date of birth

Reg No.

Growth (cm/yr)

b

BOYS

Height velocity

Longitudinal
whole-year centiles
when peak
velocity occurs
at average age

97
50
3

When peak
velocity occurs
at early and late
limits of age
(entire curves fall
within shaded limits)

97
50
3

Age (years)

GIRLS

Height velocity

Longitudinal
whole-year centiles
when peak
velocity occurs
at average age

When peak
velocity occurs
at early and late
limits of age
(entire curves fall
within shaded limits)

Age (years)

In both boys and girls the amount and quality of pubic hair is assessed. Girls have their breast development staged and in boys the development of the penis and scrotum is recorded. Additionally in boys an orchidometer is used to assess testicular volume (Figure 14.21). If testicular volume has reached 4 ml, further pubertal changes are imminent. In normal boys the increase in testicular volume starts between 9 and 14 years. The male growth spurt starts a year or so after initial testicular enlargement, reaching a peak an additional year later. By this stage (3 to 4), the penis is growing and pubic hair is becoming coarse and adult like.

In girls, pubertal changes begin with the development of the breast bud (stage 2) between 9 and 13 years. Onset of menstruation (11 to 15 years) occurs after peak height velocity has already been reached. At puberty most boys will have palpable breast tissue and even if unilateral, this is normal. A small number of adolescent males develop conspicuous gynaecomastia which only occasionally requires investigation and treatment.

While it is known that prepubertal children may be sexually active, it is very uncommon and consequently symptoms and signs of sexually transmitted disease are encountered rarely. On the other hand, sexual activity to a lesser or greater degree is a feature of the pubertal and post-pubertal teenage years. There should be no inhibition, but always sensitivity, to the examination of the genitalia in teenage patients when the symptoms are interpreted as those of a genitourinary infection. Signs of pregnancy should be sought when there is a history of sexual activity.

Along with sexual experimentation may come experimentation with drugs of all varieties. Few clinical signs exist in the early stages. Solvent abuse (glue sniffing) may give rise to perioral excoriation. Heroin sniffing can be associated with chronic changes in the nares whilst obvious evidence of multiple needle marks must be taken as pathognomonic of intravenous drug abuse. Smoking is also common and may be heavy enough to stain nails and teeth with nicotine.

SCOLIOSIS

Idiopathic scoliosis is a disorder of puberty of unknown aetiology which may result in progressive and serious deformity with significant long-term morbidity. It is more common in girls. Since it is frequently difficult to detect with the patient standing or lying, the young person should be asked to touch their toes, with the observer directly behind them. Scoliosis is seen as a curve in the trunk and asymmetry of the posterior ribs (see Figure 9.4, page 202).

GOITRE

Goitre is rare in childhood but enlargement of the thyroid may occur at puberty due either to autoimmune thyroiditis or a sporadic goitre of unknown aetiology (Figure 14.22). Children with the latter have normal thyroid function.

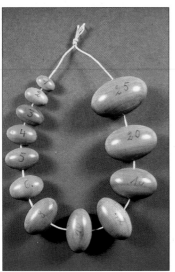

◀ **Figure 14.21**
Prader orchidometer for the assessment of testicular volume

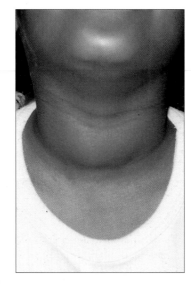

◀ **Figure 14.22**
Diffuse goitre

The history and examination of the older patient

MICHAEL LYE

INTRODUCTION

The core knowledge and the skills of clinical medicine are applicable to patients of all ages – differences between, for example, middle-aged and elderly patients are in the main swamped by their similarities. However the emphasis and focus of clinical examination, and the attitudes and approach of the clinician, have to be modified when there are 65 or more years between the ages of the student/doctor and the patient. Some conditions are either commoner or only occur in elderly patients. Also, diseases have to be considered more in the context of disability and handicap affecting the quality of the remaining years, rather than in the minutiae of pathology and the duration of life.

Elderly people are not homogeneous – they are at least as diversified as younger people and have much more life experience to draw upon. Even physiological ranges of 'normal results' over the 30-year span from 65 to 95 years of age is much wider than between 35 and 65 years. It may be helpful to consider the 'young old' as retirement age to 75 years, the 'old' 76–85 years and the 'old old' more than 85 years of age. As people continue to live longer, health services have to concentrate resources on the 'old old'. In the past there were so few 'old old' people that they could be ignored with impunity and often were.

Some students and doctors may have negative, 'ageist' attitudes towards older patients. These attitudes may stem from poor relationships within their own families, fear of dying or anxiety about their own ageing, but the acquisition of clinical experience combined with increasing age modifies our views. Elderly patients' attitudes are undoubtedly influenced by their previous experience. Clinicians must appreciate that a child's illness may bring back memories for grandparents of the deaths of one or more of their own siblings half a century previously. Equally a daughter's pregnancy may offer the prospect of a role as a babysitter to an unoccupied grandparent.

While a clinician needs to have insight into his patient's family relationships he must perforce stand apart from conflicts and not be judgemental. Many old-old individuals are remarkably tolerant and liberal in their attitudes despite their often strict upbringing. In particular, grandparents often accept with equanimity the immoderate foibles of teenage grandchildren whose own middle-aged parents have been driven to despair. Accumulated experience, the 'having seen it all before', generates tolerance of others and of life's vicissitudes including their own disability. The obverse of this is the common binding together which is seen when young grandchildren readily accept the carer role of an infirm grandparent.

HISTORY TAKING

The basic outline given in the first chapter of this book provides the framework for history taking and only requires 'fine-tuning' to cover specific problems presented by some older patients.

Old people seeking medical advice/assistance especially during admission to hospital are often fearful. They are of a generation when many illnesses were rapidly fatal and hospital admission for their contemporaries had proved a one-way process. These fears are invariably worse when admission occurs as an emergency. Even in the primary care setting anxiety and fear may not be absent. The student, by being open, friendly and sympathetic, and not condescending or patronizing in manner, is in a privileged position to reassure the patient.

Start by introducing yourself and who you are. There are so many people in hospital wearing white coats that they do not uniquely identify doctors any more! Address older patients formally as Mr or Mrs having, if possible, first made sure the lady is not a spinster. Do not rely on wedding rings for these may have been removed on the death of a husband (unusual) or even lost or stolen (alas, not unusual). You should find out the patient's age from the notes because asking directly may lead to being asked to guess and woe betide the young doctor who overestimates an elderly patient's age. If you underestimate by twenty years you have a friend for life.

Do not launch into formal history taking immediately. Ask about how they feel, sympathize and reassure in general terms if they are in pain or otherwise distressed.

Explain the necessity for taking a history and how it helps you to help them.

After an introduction and a general enquiry make sure the patient is comfortable. It is important that the patient does not become hypothermic in a draughty accident and emergency corridor or is unable to hear because of excessive background noise. It is best to gain eye contact by being at the same level as the patient – sitting on the bed may be necessary. An overbearing stance and an alien white coat do not ease communication.

Questions to ask yourself are:
1 Can the patient hear (hearing aid).
2 Can the patient see (spectacles/hemianopia).
3 Can the patient speak (teeth/dyspnoea/dysphasia).

Do not be afraid to reassure the patient during the interview by gently resting your hand on the back of their hand. This simple manoeuvre says so much to the patient – you are close, you care, you are interested in them, you are not too busy for their problem, you will help them and most of all you are their doctor and have time for them. This simple gesture, repeated as necessary, is better than any mission statement or patient's charter.

THE PRESENTING PROBLEM

It is unusual for the elderly patient to present with one crisp, cardinal symptom. More often than not their presenting complaint can be 'distilled' into one or more of the so-called *giants of geriatrics* (Isaacs, 1975). These 'final common pathways' may be due to many different causes, each of which may produce the same disability. It is then the task of the clinician to explore all the possible causes of the *giant* (Table 15.1).

In an emergency it may be necessary first to obtain an outline of the patient's problems by interviewing witnesses, relatives, carers or attendants. These people should be seen promptly as they have their own lives to lead and will not wait in accident and emergency for several hours – once they have gone it may be difficult to make contact later. It may be immediately apparent that the patient has communication problems (foreign language, dysphasia, stone-deaf, confusion) in which case a third party historian must suffice, at least initially. Don't let the opportunity slip by.

HISTORY OF PRESENT CONDITION

Elderly patients are often quite anxious and it is probably better to explore the immediate problem as perceived by the patient. The method of letting the patient tell his own story at his own pace, as described throughout this book, is followed but may need to be adapted for the verbose and rambling or for the reserved and terse. The art is not to be too directive – this may be difficult but the clinician, however hard pressed, who ends almost shouting for the patient to stick to the point, might as well give up any further attempts at communication. The temptation at times to give the patient a tranquillizer or to take one oneself should be resisted!

The history of the present complaint may have started 40 years or 4 hours ago. With elderly patients 40 years may be a common span and as has been stressed in this book it is vital to establish the start of a complaint and its precise evolution and progress over time. Unfortunately, temporal relationships are of little significance to the older patient. Twelve months to a 20-year-old student is 5 per cent of his expended life-span; to an 80-year old it is just over 1 per cent – almost an irrelevancy. Sometimes timing can be fixed more precisely in relation to Christmases, birthdays, weddings, etc., or even sadly to the highlights in the year of an old patient – such as visits to outpatient clinics.

The symptoms at the onset of many chronic serious disabling diseases seen in old age may be thought insignificant by the patient and dismissed until gently reminded by the clinician. Thus the start of chronic bronchitis may have been attributed to a smoker's cough, rheumatoid arthritis to work practices and shortness of breath with heart failure to lack of fitness with increasing age. It cannot be overemphasized that the duration and progression of a disease process are better signatures of diagnosis than any hi-tech investigation. A detailed account teaches the clinician much about the progress of disease and the impact of disease on individuals' lifestyles over the years.

Interaction between the 'normal' process of physiological ageing and the consequences of age-related diseases, i.e. those diseases that increase in frequency with increasing age, causes the presentation of disease in old age to alter (Table 15.2).

Multiple pathology

Throughout this book the emphasis on diagnosis has been the process of reducing symptoms and signs to fit

PRESENTATION OF DISEASE IN OLD AGE – THE GIANTS OF GERIATRICS	
Immobility	(dependency)
Incontinence	(social disintegration)
Incompetence	(intellectual impairment)
Instability	(recurrent falls)

▲ **Table 15.1**

one or, at the most, two diagnoses. Older patients invariably cheat by having more than one disease. Thus patients over the age of 75 years attending their family doctors have on average 2.8 diseases and those attending hospital as inpatients, 4.2 diseases.

Atypical symptoms

Many pathological conditions in old age may present as one of the *giants*. Thus conditions as diverse as epilepsy, osteoarthrosis of the knees, aortic stenosis, Parkinsonism, pneumonia, may all present as 'falls' or instability. Equally, perhaps because few elderly patients have read this book, they may present with acute myocardial infarction without pain, infection without fever and cerebrovascular accident without paralysis. Similarly the sudden onset of confusion in an elderly individual may herald a multitude of acute, non-neurological problems.

Polypharmacy

'For every ill, a pill.' The alternative aphorism – 'for every pill, an ill' is equally valid in geriatric medicine. Thus treatment of four or more diseases will lead to many interactions between drug and drug, and between drug and pathology. Remember that the most powerful therapeutic agents have equally powerful adverse effects and it is not unusual to see drugs added to counter the adverse effects of other drugs. This creates a downward spiral of increasing drugs and increasing iatrogenic symptoms. The student must always consider whether a prescribed or over-the-counter drug may be the cause of some or all of the patient's symptoms.

Iatrogenic dependency

Few diseases are confined to elderly patients but the state of *learned dependency* is a particular and perhaps a unique problem in old age. Following a fall or after a period of bed-rest, especially following surgery, an elderly patient may become entirely dependent on others for even the simplest activity. Well-meaning relatives, carers and indeed professionals unintentionally reinforce this state by being overprotective. Immobilization,

FEATURES OF DISEASE IN OLD AGE
Multiple pathology
Atypical symptoms
Polypharmacy
Iatrogenic dependency
Impaired homeostatic reserve

▲ Table 15.2

especially in bed, leads to loss of many functions and in particular postural reflexes. A reduction in cerebral perfusion on standing is a powerful drive to stay seated! Symptoms of postural hypotension in old age are so vague as not to alert the patient or the doctor to their aetiology. Because the final degree of dependency is so disproportionately more than the immediate pathology would suggest, it may lead the clinician to start searching for an underlying carcinoma or another cause for the gross debility.

Impaired homeostatic reserve

Finally, in elderly patients, even minor trauma or pathology greatly affects function and may cause a domino effect on other systems. Thus, pneumonia may lead to acute confusion, dehydration, uraemia and heart failure. Elderly patients must therefore have immediate access to the full facilities of the district general hospital because diagnosis and correct treatment are so urgent in this age group. The young could wait, the elderly must not.

SYMPTOMS REVIEW

After the history of the presenting condition has been recorded, a systematic enquiry for other problems and symptoms should be undertaken in the usual manner. However, the clinician needs to be circumspect because, after all, the 'strike rate' from questions – have you ever had headaches, indigestion, etc. – aimed at an 80-year-old, is going to reveal too many hits. Put the enquiry into a period of relevance to the presenting problem(s). Specific enquiry, beyond the usual ones, should however be made for:

1 Urinary problems including incontinence (both sexes) – does your water ever come so fast that you are unable to stop it?
2 Sleep – has there been a recent change from the usual pattern?
3 Mood – do symptoms get you down, do you ever go to sleep wishing you would never wake up?

PAST HEALTH

Again be prepared for a long list! Equally be prepared for incomplete details either because the event was a long time ago or the patient never had complete information at the time. It is only recently that doctors have fully informed patients. Many elderly people have scars from major surgery and were never told what operation had been performed. It is important to ask about the symptoms at the time and duration of any hospital stay remembering that the latter would have been much longer in the past than now.

Specific enquiry for previous 'nervous breakdowns' etc. should be pursued with the patient gently but firmly. Unfortunately many psychiatric conditions may return in old age after lying dormant for quarter of a century.

FAMILY HISTORY

A detailed family history is less useful than in younger patients and indeed may be counter-productive. When the 80-year-old patient has listed twelve members of the family who all died of different cancers around 80 years of age, a fearful penny may drop. If parents and grandparents all had very long lives you can be sure that your patient comes from good stock and is therefore also likely to be long-lived.

SOCIAL HISTORY

Some doctors and some students see all elderly patients as 'social problems'. *Primary* social problems occur in young adults – late teens to early thirties. It is this age group that is unable to cope with their romantic failures, with their sexuality, with pregnancy, with the responsibilities of homes and jobs. The elderly have been sufficiently robust in their social life to survive into old age; their social problems are almost invariably secondary to pathology.

Thus the elderly woman brought to an accident and emergency department in the evening after a fall who is found to have 'no bony injury' is not a social problem *because* it is now late at night and she lives alone. It is no use referring her to the social worker who cannot effect a cure. The question must be asked: 'Why is she falling,' and appropriate examinations and investigations performed – it is not due to old age alone. Unfortunately some elderly people have to earn the right to medical attention by fracturing the femur. Social crises are secondary to medical or surgical problems and therefore the domain of the clinician who may ultimately need to provide, with the help of the social worker, a social support package. This however should not supersede detailed diagnosis.

The usual questions about foreign travel, smoking, alcohol (especially elderly patients who fall), diet, pets, etc. should be asked. Particular attention should be paid to the housing circumstances – upstairs/outside toilet, stairs and steps between rooms, easy contact with neighbours, shops.

Social contacts

'Do you live on your own?' is better than 'Is your wife/husband still alive?' The patient may have divorced or separated or, if the spouse has died, the direct question may be upsetting. Look into the health of the spouse or partner – it may be worse than the patient's. Ask about children and grandchildren and always try to say 'You must be proud of them.' Do they visit regularly, or *vice versa*?

Social support

Enquire about home helps, meals on wheels, day centres, residential or nursing home accommodation. If positive, always find out the reason for the support and for how long the patient has been receiving it. Who does the shopping, collects the pension? Contrary to popular opinion financial problems do not seem to loom large in pensioners lives. Old people who will not spend money on food or accommodation are more likely to be depressed than impoverished though many may claim the latter.

FUNCTIONAL HISTORY

A precise diagnosis is of extreme interest to the clinician but of little import to the patient; he is more concerned about how the disease has or will affect his function (Table 15.3). Thus Parkinson's disease may range between an incidental, albeit important finding, on physical examination, to being the cause for admission to long-term nursing accommodation with all gradations between these extremes. Alternatively, a raised serum calcium may evoke more interest from the physician than the patient's immobilizing ingrowing toenail. Both require attention even if for the former the attention is but observation. However, the grateful patient is the one relieved of the latter.

If the hierarchy of impairment, disability and handicap is appreciated, a realistic management plan can be evolved. It is often impossible to reverse the disease process but it is always possible to alleviate to some extent the handicap.

Pre-morbid function

A clear and detailed recording of functional level before the onset of the presenting event defines the target of treatment. This is best described by 'a day in the life of.' An elderly patient who does the shopping, house cleaning, attends Church or bingo or both and goes on SAGA holidays contrasts with the patient who has home helps seven days a week, meals on wheels, lives downstairs and hasn't been out of the house for three years.

It is vitally important with the latter patient to find out how long they have been receiving social support and *why*. Some minimally handicapped patients may receive excessive social support – usually because their families are particularly articulate. The reason the patient has been receiving support allows the clinician to define the handicap, locate the disability and hope-

	PATHOLOGY IN CONTEXT			
Impairment	Pathological condition affecting:	Gene Cell Organ System		*Disease*
Disability	Consequence of impairment limiting:	Mobility Stability Cognition Continence		**Giants**
Handicap	Outcome of disability preventing:	Dressing Housework Cooking Shopping Independence		*Lifestyle*

◀ Table 15.3

fully arrive at a diagnosis or, more likely, diagnoses. The urgency of the presenting complaint may obscure other important diseases.

Sometimes elderly patients exaggerate their abilities and independence in the face of overwhelming evidence of severe and long-standing handicap. They may fear being kept in hospital or being institutionalized. If denial is a result of misplaced pride the clinician has not obtained the confidence of the patient. Finally, elderly patients may be unaware because of acute or chronic confusion. Corroboration of a patient's history is always useful but beware of taking the history from a relative when the patient is fully or even partially capable. Never put the patient in the position of being third-party to what is their history. It may be necessary to talk separately to a relative.

DRUG HISTORY

Polypharmacy can be a real problem for elderly patients (Table 15.2). Very commonly older patients are not taking the drugs their doctors think they are taking. This is not usually the patient's fault. Different doctors in a practice may be prescribing besides several hospital specialists. Sadly good communication is not always available to prevent this situation. For example, the locum GP may visit at home or the patient is seen in the clinic without their medical notes.

Patients should be seen with their drugs, asked to go through them one by one and to say when taken, for how long and for what? Be prepared for surprises. For example, digoxin may be taken on an 'as necessary' basis for pain relief and paracetamol taken 'once daily' for the heart. Ointments may be swallowed or inserted

in the most astonishing ways. Check for adverse effects in the usual way but do not forget 'social adverse effects'. Powerful diuretics may chain a patient to the toilet and prevent shopping, etc. They need not be taken in the morning and if the patient is travelling they could be omitted for a day or so without harm. The patient should be informed of this.

As a rule elderly patients do not consume as many over-the-counter (OTC) drugs as younger people but with an increasing market for OTCs this may be a larger problem in the future. Beware of elderly people 'sharing' drugs (not however in the dangerous way of some of their grandchildren using 'recreational' drugs!). Elderly subjects living in, for example, sheltered accommodation, discuss their medical conditions and the virtues of different prescribed drugs with all the enthusiasm of shoppers in the bazaar. This may lead to patients exchanging drugs.

MENTAL HISTORY

Most of us have clerked in the young overdose patient and recorded – *too drowsy to give history* – or the old patient – *too confused to give history* – when with a little more time and patience adequate histories could have been recorded. The crime however may be tolerable in the younger patient, where the sobriquet, drowsy, will rapidly disappear. Not so the older confused patient – confusion lives on in the notes and what started as a houseman's time saver grows into a diagnosis of dementia with all its negative connotations.

If the patient is confused then it is vital to measure it and decide whether it is acute or chronic, intermittent

ABBREVIATED MENTAL TEST
Time (to nearest hour)
Year
Address for recall
Age in years
What is this place?
Date of birth (day and month)
Recognition of two persons
Year of start of First World War
Count backwards 20–1

▲ **Table 15.4**

or progressive. Measurement using an abbreviated mental test (Table 15.4) establishes a baseline for monitoring change and additionally provides an appropriate measure for the degree of impairment. Always repeat and record the measurement 1–2 days later and before the patient is discharged. Remember the record of AMT 2/10 in the medical notes may mean that subsequently a patient's will may be overturned.

Always record an elderly patient's cognitive state in the medical notes even if perfectly normal. If in any doubt use the AMT. Beware patients with a good social facade who until formally tested seem to be mentally intact though a little peculiar. Many such patients may be shielded by their families who wish to avoid the stigma of mental illness. However, when introducing the AMT do not put the patient at risk of failing by saying 'just checking everything is all right' with the implication that one question wrong means to the patient at least, inadequacy.

PHYSICAL SIGNS IN THE OLDER PATIENT

The physical examination of the older patient follows the same principles already described throughout this book. These can best be summarized by an intelligent assessment, a sensitive approach and a comprehensive appraisal. It is important for the student to see history taking and physical examination as a continuing endeavour and not as two distinct and separate processes. Thus, abnormal signs discovered on examination will prompt further history taking while symptoms from the history will focus on physical examination. This is particularly the case with many elderly patients who have long histories and multiple signs!

ASSESSMENT OF INTELLIGENCE

Students should always be asking – what does this mean? What derangement of physiology is taking place? What is the significance of this complaint, this physical finding? Using our clinical skills means that we have an idea about likely physical signs from the previously obtained history. Thus, when examining the elderly patient with a recent history of exertional faints (effort syncope), special attention should be paid to the radial pulse and blood pressure which may reveal the plateau pulse and narrow pulse pressure of aortic stenosis. It is then easy to hear the characteristic murmur to confirm the presence of aortic stenosis. As every student doing short cases in finals knows, it is so much harder to recognize physical abnormalities in isolation.

In general, the specificity of physical signs is reduced in the older patient. For example, a few basal crackles heard in the chest of an elderly, relatively immobile patient, may not indicate pathology. Distal neurological signs do not have the same significance as in younger patients. It is vital to *interpret* physical signs in the light of the history and other findings.

SENSITIVE APPROACH

Always explain as far as one can why you are doing a particular manoeuvre and what you have planned. To be examined in silence by a white-coated automaton must be frightening for a patient of any age. It is especially so for an older patient who imagines everything in the worst possible light. Their anxiety may be compounded by reduced sensory input (poor vision or hearing). Nothing relaxes the older patient more than to be told that they have the blood pressure of a 21-year-old. Do not take this approach to extremes however or your patient will cease to trust you.

Remember most of your patients have not been expensively trained in the art of physical examination. Be quite clear and demonstrate in as much detail, using the patient's limbs if possible, exactly what you want them to do. Watching inexperienced clinicians almost screaming at the patient to relax while assaulting him with a patella hammer, says a lot about the doctor but nothing about the patient's neurological state!

Equally we should not strip patients naked and lay them on a couch surrounded by flimsy curtains with billowing gaps. It is not dignified, not comfortable, liable to lead to hypothermia and makes any physical examination almost useless. Allow patients the minimum of underclothing and a full length blanket, removing *and replacing* coverings as the examination proceeds. Elderly women may appreciate the presence of a female nurse if being examined by a male clinician.

Before moulding limbs into extreme contortions to elicit a reflex make sure, by asking, that joints are not painful. The older patient who has stoically adapted to arthritis over several decades may complain little but suffer considerably during physical examination. Old people truly wish to be helpful and may see complaining as a criticism of 'their doctor' and therefore not to be contemplated. Be gentle. Do not percuss so clumsily that the patient suffers a flail chest.

COMPREHENSIVENESS

Woe betide the clinician who concentrates his examination on the heart of the elderly patient with chest pain and misses the subtle neurological signs due to aortic dissection. Urgent thrombolysis is not the order of the day. Because of the high prevalence of multiple pathology, all systems of the elderly patient have to be examined in as much detail as possible. Time pressures or tiredness (the patient, the clinician or both) may require initial concentration on what seems to be the most immediate problem but do not neglect to return and complete the examination as soon as possible. It is dangerous to wait even until the next morning to finish the examination. Head (temporal arteritis) to toe (hallux valgus) examination will form the basis for a problem list and subsequent management plan involving investigation and treatment. An incomplete examination could render any strategy incomplete and therefore potentially dangerous.

SPECIAL ASPECTS

Confusion

Make sure the patient has heard you and can see you. Remember, elderly patients will invariably be trying very hard to help as much as they can. Unfortunately, in their enthusiasm, they may provide unrelated answers to your questions. If there is any doubt about a patient's cognitive function, measure it using the AMT (Table 15.4).

Vision

Approximately 50 per cent of elderly people admitted to hospital have significant visual impairment though very few complain. In three-quarters of these patients the visual impairments will be, in part at least, reversible. Therefore, *check* vision with a Snellen chart when the patient's clinical state will allow. This is especially important in patients with unexplained repeated falls.

Hearing

Old people have an expectation that hearing will decline, even more than eyesight, with increasing age.

It is one of the major unreported disabilities in old age and should therefore be assessed as part of the routine physical examination. Simple acuity testing with voice and the use of the auroscope is all that is usually required. Removal of impacted wax may earn the clinician the thanks not only of the patient but also the family who have tolerated loud television at home for many years.

Skin

Young looking skin suggests a good biological survivor. Thin skin may indicate thin bones – osteoporosis, steroid therapy. Tattoos may give insights to a colourful past – always worth exploring but be tactful and confidential. Always check for pressure sores on heels, buttocks and sacrum. When found, record with drawing and measurements in the patient's notes.

Feet

Elderly patients who have followed the dictates of fashion in their youth may now suffer crippling deformity leading to relative immobility. Chiropody and attention to footwear can easily effect a cure.

Aids and appliances

Many elderly patients have spectacles, dentures, hearing aids, walking sticks, etc., which seem as old as they are. Spectacles repaired by Elastoplast across the bridge combined with smeared lenses do not aid mobility. Loose fitting, clacking dentures do not aid speech or diet. A short walking stick, sans ferrule, not only doesn't aid mobility but makes any attempt a fearsome adventure. How many clinicians know the meaning of O, T and M on hearing aids?

Mobility

Asking an elderly patient to rise from a chair, to stand and to walk with or without an aid reveals much about the patient's present functional state. The immediate proffering of both outstretched arms characterizes the patient who has become dependent on overindulgent nurses or carers for even the simplest task. The patient who assumes the rigid oblique posture, with feet stuck out from the chair like a sparrow with rigor mortis, has lost all 'righting' reflexes due to prolonged bed rest. Beware the patient who stands, sways then falls because of postural hypotension. Check lying (sitting) and upright blood pressures with caution and with an assistant.

When walking, does the patient lean backwards – too much bed rest, frontal lobe problems; to the side – lower limb arthropathy, hemiparesis; forwards – kyphoscoliosis, festinant gait of Parkinsonism? The patient who has fallen, especially if they live alone, may show irrational fear by grabbing for any type of support including highly mobile and dangerous wheeled bed-tables or even the hapless doctor. Patients who take twice as long going from the chair as they do to return to the chair are also frightened of falling. These patients require expert rehabilitation by a team of physiotherapists and nurses.

This review has emphasized that elderly patients are not a race apart. Those skills of history taking and physical examination, learnt perhaps with younger patients, serve us well when we tackle difficult problems in older patients. While pathology in older people may present differently and make a greater impact on physical and mental function, this does not lessen the need for precise diagnosis; indeed, it makes it more necessary. Elderly patients are part of the continuum of humanity; no more, no less deserving of our skills and attention.

The diagnosis of death

Doctors often receive an urgent call to attend a patient who is thought to be dying or dead. In preparation for this emergency, the student must be aware of:

1 Legal definitions of death.
2 The differential diagnosis of death.
3 Forensic requirements in the examination of a dead body.

LEGAL DEFINITION OF DEATH

Irreversible loss of function of the brain, the organ most essential to meaningful life, is now generally accepted as the principal criterion of death. Since both respiration and circulation can be maintained by artificial means, the absence of spontaneous breathing and heart beat can only be accepted as proof of death if prolonged sufficiently to cause permanent loss of brain function.

Death is rarely an event in which there is immediate, simultaneous and irreversible loss of all organic activity. Except in the case of violent explosion or incineration, death is more often a process whereby certain cells and organs die before others, usually because of their greater vulnerability to hypoxia. The brain is not only the organ most susceptible to hypoxia but it can also be destroyed by such local causes as trauma or haemorrhage. It follows that, if respiration and circulation are maintained, death of the brain (i.e. legal death) is not necessarily accompanied by death of other organs such as heart, lungs, liver and kidneys. The law now permits removal of these organs for purposes of transplantation from an individual with a beating heart but a dead brain.

It is clearly of importance therefore to define what is meant by brain death. Disorders of the brain may affect the cortex, the brain stem or both together. Cortical death alone results in coma but spontaneous breathing may be maintained. This so-called 'persistent vegetative state' can continue for months or even years but the patient cannot legally be certified as dead. Death of the brain stem abolishes spontaneous breathing because of damage to the respiratory centre in the medulla but coma also occurs due to interruption of the ascending reticular activating system. The *current legal definition of death requires evidence of irreversible brain-stem death.*

DIFFERENTIAL DIAGNOSIS OF DEATH

The differential diagnosis of death includes all states in which loss of cardio-respiratory or brain function is reversible. There are two clinical situations in which this distinction may have to be made:

1 Where cardiac and respiratory arrest are of very recent onset.
2 Where cardiac and respiratory action are being artificially sustained by mechanical ventilation.

CARDIAC AND RESPIRATORY ARREST OF VERY RECENT ONSET

It is important to be aware of those potentially reversible conditions which can induce sudden and transient cardiac and respiratory arrest. The commonest of these is myocardial ischaemia but transient arrest may also result from traumatic shock, electrocution and hypoxia due to causes such as drowning, asphyxia, carbon monoxide poisoning and narcotic drugs.

When a patient stops breathing, the first step is to feel for the carotid pulse and, if this is impalpable, to auscultate the heart. If there are no heart sounds, observations need be continued for only a few minutes if the patient was known to be suffering from a terminal disease. When a possible death is sudden, unexpected or unwitnessed, observation must be maintained for a longer period while resuscitatory efforts are made to test cardio-respiratory responsiveness. If cardiac function cannot be restored within ten minutes, death may be assumed on the grounds of irreversible damage to the brain.

In cold conditions, however, brain tissue can survive more prolonged periods of hypoxia. Hypothermia should be suspected when the ambient temperature is low and the patient has been found inadequately clothed in unheated surroundings or after submersion in cold water; it is confirmed by recording a rectal temperature of less than 32°C. The state of 'suspended animation' which accompanies hypothermia is the commonest cause for an erroneous diagnosis of death.

After the cessation of cardiac action, early supportive evidence of death includes softening of the eyeballs due to loss of intraocular tension, clouding of the cornea, segmentation or 'trucking' of blood in the retinal vessels on ophthalmoscopy and loss of brain-stem reflexes (see below).

PATIENTS ON MECHANICAL VENTILATION

Since the advent of modern methods of cardio-respiratory resuscitation, the presence of a heart beat is no more proof of life than its absence is proof of death (Figure 16.1). After the brain is dead and spontaneous respiration ceases, the heart may continue to beat if mechanical ventilation maintains adequate oxygenation of the blood. Before such a patient is pronounced dead, careful enquiry and examination are needed to establish that there is total and irreversible loss of brain-stem function. A diagnosis of death requires that the patient is in deep coma of known cause with loss of all brain-stem reflexes and no reversible component to these changes. The commoner conditions leading to this situation are direct brain damage from gross trauma or intracerebral haemorrhage and indirect injury due to hypoxia following cardiac arrest.

There are therefore three steps in the diagnosis of brain-stem death:

1 The patient must be in a coma and unable to breathe spontaneously and is therefore on a ventilator.
2 The cause of the coma and cessation of respiration is structural and irreversible. Potentially reversible functional causes which must be specifically excluded are drug intoxication, hypothermia, hypoglycaemia, metabolic disorders (diabetic, renal or hepatic), shock and neuromuscular paralysis.
3 All brain-stem reflexes are absent. These include:
(a) Loss of pupillary and corneal reflexes (see page 222).
(b) Loss of vestibulo-ocular reflexes: injection of iced water into the ear fails to produce nystagmoid movements of the eyes (Figure 16.2).

(c) Lack of facial response to pain: no facial grimacing on firm pressure over the supraorbital ridge.
(d) Loss of the gag and cough reflexes: no response to catheter stimulation of the pharynx or larynx.
(e) Lack of spontaneous breathing on hypercarbic stimulation: after ventilation with 95 per cent oxygen and 5 per cent carbon dioxide for ten minutes, the ventilator is withdrawn and pure oxygen is delivered into the patient's airway. This technique ensures that the patient's organs remain adequately oxygenated while the arterial $P\text{CO}_2$ rises to above 50 mmHg (7 kPa). This should provide a sufficient hypercarbic stimulus to respiration and will induce spontaneous breathing if the brain-stem centres are intact.

These tests must be performed by two medical practitioners (one qualified for more than five years) on two occasions over a period of at least twelve hours, or longer if there is uncertainty about the degree of structural brain damage as may apply in cases of hypoxia injury.

EXAMINATION OF A DEAD BODY

When the doctor is satisfied that a patient is dead, a certain minimum examination of the corpse is required depending upon the circumstances of the case. The death in hospital of a patient suffering from a terminal disease is clearly in a different category from the unwitnessed and unexpected death of an individual previously unknown to the doctor. In the latter case, a postmortem examination may be ordered by the coroner but

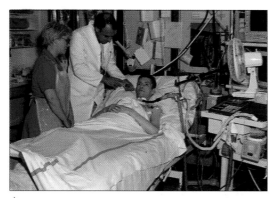

▲ **Figure 16.1 Intensive therapy unit**

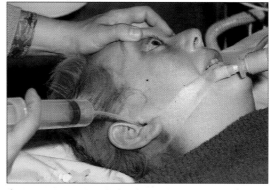

▲ **Figure 16.2 Testing vestibulo-ocular reflexes by injecting ice cold water into the external auditory canal.** Note the patient on the ventilator

the first doctor to see the corpse may find evidence relevant to the time of death which will not be available to the pathologist. On the other hand, a post-mortem would not normally be requested if the deceased had been seen by the doctor within the previous two weeks. When no further examination is likely to be required, a careful inspection of the corpse is essential before a certificate is issued.

The main objectives of examination after death are:

1 To determine the approximate time of death.
2 To seek the cause of death and especially to exclude 'unnatural' causes such as murder, suicide, accidental injuries, drug abuse and certain environmental hazards.

TIME OF DEATH

The accuracy achieved by fictional sleuths is not practical in the real world. It is possible only to make a crude estimate on the basis of body temperature, and the presence of rigor mortis or putrefaction. These vary considerably according to environment and climate but, in average temperate conditions, the following guidelines apply:

1 Dead less than 3 hours: body warm; no rigor.
2 Dead 3–8 hours: body warm; rigor present.
3 Dead 8–36 hours: body cold; rigor present.
4 Dead over 36 hours: body cold; no rigor.
5 Dead over 2–3 days: putrefaction.
6 Dead for weeks or more: insect and larva analysis may give date of death.

Temperature

Temperature can be roughly estimated by placing the back of the hand over central parts of the trunk. Accurate recording of body temperature (and simultaneous ambient temperature) may be of help to forensic experts in cases of unnatural death but, since this requires the insertion of a long thermometer deep into the rectum, it must not be undertaken in cases of suspected sexual assault.

Rigor mortis

Rigor mortis is detected by gently flexing the joints. It develops first in the small muscles of the fingers, face and jaws. Rigor occurs more quickly in a warm atmosphere and may be absent altogether in the cold. It must be distinguished from the rare cadaveric spasm which may accompany a violent death when a weapon or other object is clutched in the hand.

Putrefaction

Putrefaction is recognized by green or black discoloration of the skin, usually first evident in the abdomen over the caecum. This is followed by 'marbling' of surface veins, especially of the upper arms and thighs, due to proliferation of bacteria within the venous system. Later, there may be gaseous distension of the soft tissues, fluid exudation and protrusion of tongue and eyes.

CAUSE OF DEATH

The doctor must be satisfied that the condition in which he finds the body is compatible with other evidence available to him about the likely time and cause of death. When there is suspicion of unnatural death, the doctor's examination should be carried out with minimal disturbance of the corpse or its environment.

Surroundings and position

The surroundings and position of the body are recorded with special reference to its proximity to possible sources of harm, e.g. poisons and pills (Figure 16.3), gaseous fumes, electrical equipment, heights (e.g. foot of stairs) and water.

Skin colour

Skin colour is noted to exclude the bright pink of carbon monoxide or cyanide poisoning; less commonly, a brown or slate grey colour may be produced by methaemoglobin following ingestion of poisons such as sodium chlorate commonly used as a weed killer.

Scalp and head

The scalp and head are inspected and palpated for cuts, haematomata, depressed fracture or any other sign of injury.

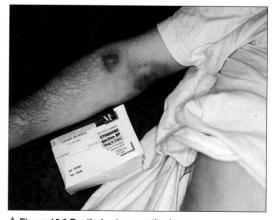

▲ **Figure 16.3 Death due to narcotic abuse**

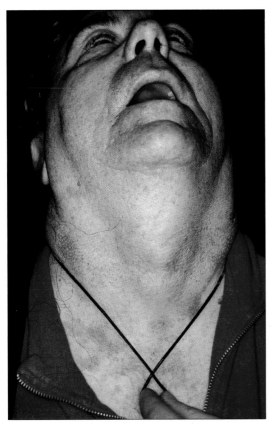

▲ **Figure 16.4 Lividity and rigor mortis in a man dying of natural causes due to myocardial infarction.** The cord round the neck carried an alarm device

Face and eyes

The face and eyes are examined especially for the petechiae of asphyxiation.

Neck

The neck is inspected for bruising, ligature marks or other evidence of strangulation.

Limbs

The limbs may show the puncture marks of injections (Figure 16.3). The hands are the commonest site for burns in cases of electrocution.

Trunk

The trunk is examined for any signs of injury and, if the body is found unclothed, the genital area is inspected for bruising, scratches, bleeding, seminal emission or other evidence of sexual assault. The body must be turned for examination of both sides of the trunk. Hypostatic lividity (Figure 16.4) may be observed in dependent areas; its presence elsewhere suggests that the body has been moved after death.

The circumstances of sudden death are such that the body is often found or placed in cramped and ill-lit surroundings. A common situation is where a doctor is asked to examine a presumed corpse in an ambulance. Death should not be pronounced nor a certificate issued until the body has been fully examined under conditions of adequate space and lighting. Auscultation of the heart must be performed with the chest fully exposed and over a sufficient period of time.

Index

Textual references, in addition to figures and tables, may be found on the pages marked *Fig.* or *Table*. Differential diagnosis or comparisons are denoted by '*vs*'.

A

Abbreviated mental test
  (AMT), 350 (*Table*
  15.4)
Abdomen
  acute, 77
  anatomy, 60–1
  auscultation, 61, 69
    peritonitis, 78
  contour and irregulari-
    ties, 63
  distension, 61, 63
    neonates, 333
    percussion, 68
  examination, 61–9
    infants/toddlers, 340
    newborn infants,
      332–3
    in renal/urinary tract
      disease, 88–9
  incisions, 61 (*Fig. 4.14*)
  inspection, 61–4
    peritonitis, 77, 78
  palpation, 61, 64–8
    newborn infants, 333
    peritonitis, 77, 78
    procedure, 64
  percussion, 61, 68–9
    peritonitis, 77–8
  physical signs, 61–9
    in cardiac disease,
      134
  regions, 60 (*Fig. 4.13*)
  skin, 61–2
    secondary nodules, 62
      (*Fig. 4.18*)
    surgical scars, 61 (*Fig.*
      4.14), 62 (*Fig. 4.15*)
    swellings, 63 (*Figs.*
      4.19, 4.20)
  questions/examina-
    tion, 18
  systolic murmurs, 69
  tenderness, 64
    rebound, 77
  tumours, 63, 67
    colorectal, 76
    percussion, 68
    position/site/consis-
      tency/mobility, 67
  viscera, enlargement,
    65–6
  X-ray, 76

Abdominal accidents, 77
Abdominal aorta
  aneurysms, 63, 86,
    134, 185
  pulsation, 63
Abdominal disease, 51–4
  symptoms, 51–4
    see also Abdominal
      pain; Vomiting
Abdominal pain, 51–2
  acute peritonitis, 77, 78
  analysis, 53 (*Table 4.2*)
  biliary tract disease, 57
  colic, 74
  description and history-
    taking, 52, 53 (*Table*
    4.2)
  epigastric, 71
  gastric/duodenal dis-
    ease, 54
  haemolytic anaemia,
    196
  pancreatic carcinoma,
    83
  pancreatitis, 83
  posture in, 35
  referred, 52
  right hypochondrial,
    57, 82
  tropical diseases, 317
  visceral, 51–2
Abdominal reflexes, 250,
  251 (*Fig. 10.62*)
Abdominal striae,
  Cushing's syndrome,
  309, 310 (*Fig. 12.19*)
Abdominal veins,
  enlarged, 341 (*Fig.*
  4.17)
Abdominal wall
  guarding, 7, 64–5
  inspection, 61–3
  laxity, 61–2
  movements, 63
  movements beneath,
    63–4
  oedema, 62–3
  rigidity, 64–5
  secondary nodules in
    malignant disease, 62
    (*Fig. 4.18*)
  tenderness, 64
Abducens nerve, *see*
  Cranial nerves, sixth

Abruption placentae,
  hypofibrinogenaemia,
  200
Abscess
  amoebic, *see* Amoebic
    abscess
  frontal lobe, 277 (*Fig.*
    10.96)
  intracranial, 32
  liver, 81
    see also Amoebic
      abscess
  lung, 49
  otitic, 262
  paraurethral, 91
  periodontal, 46
  peritonsillar, 340
  tuberculous, 188, 189
    (*Fig. 8.4*)
'Absence' attacks, 279
Accessory auricles, 332
Accommodation, visual,
  223
Acetone smell, of breath,
  49
Acetylcholine, pain cau-
  sation, 6
Achalasia, 51
  dysphagia, 50
Achondroplasia, 34
Acidosis
  dyspnoea, 105
  metabolic, in renal fail-
    ure, 87
  respiratory rate, 111
Acne vulgaris, 38
Acoustic nerve, tumour,
  283 (*Fig. 10.101*)
Acquired immunodefi-
  ciency syndrome, *see*
  AIDS
Acromegaly, 307 (*Fig.*
  12.12)
  facies, 28, 307–8, 308
    (*Fig. 12.14*)
  forehead and nose/ears,
    33 (*Fig. 3.15*)
  hands, 41 (*Fig. 3.36*)
  investigations, 313
  lips and nose, 31
  teeth, 308 (*Fig. 12.13*)
  tongue in, 47
ACTH
  deficiency, 307

ACTH (*cont.*)
  dexamethasone sup-
    pression test, 313
  ectopic secretion, 310
  hypersecretion/excess,
    308, 310
Actinomycosis, liver
  abscess, 81
Acute abdomen, 77
Acute tubular necrosis,
  98
Addison's disease,
  308–9, 309 (*Figs.*
  12.15, 12.16)
  aetiological diagnosis,
    310
  facial appearance, 28
  hair loss, 34
  hypoparathyroidism
    with, 312
  pigmentation, 28, 36,
    308–9, 309 (*Figs.*
    12.15, 12.16)
  of buccal membrane,
    48 (*Fig. 4.4*), 309
    (*Fig. 12.16*)
Adenoids, chest defor-
  mity association, 111
Adenoma
  gastrin-secreting, 83
  parathyroid, 312
  pituitary, 216 (*Fig.*
    10.2)
ADH, *see* Antidiuretic
  hormone (ADH)
Adie–Holmes syndrome,
  227
Adiposis dolorosa
  (Dercum's disease), 35
Adolescents
  behavioural and emo-
    tional disorders, 289
  examination, 341–4
Adrenal crisis, 308
Adrenal gland
  congenital hyperplasia,
    314
  cortical diseases,
    308–10
  aetiological diagnosis,
    310
  functional diagnosis,
    309–10
  investigations,